PLASTIC SURGERY SECRETS

PLASTIC SURGERY SECRETS

JEFFREY WEINZWEIG, MD

Formerly, Chief Resident
Division of Plastic Surgery
Brown University School of Medicine
Rhode Island Hospital
Providence, Rhode Island

Currently, Craniofacial Surgery Fellow
Division of Plastic Surgery
University of Pennsylvania School of Medicine
Children's Hospital of Philadelphia
Philadelphia, Pennsylvania

HANLEY & BELFUS, INC./ Philadelphia

Publisher: HANLEY & BELFUS, INC.
Medical Publishers
210 South 13th Street
Philadelphia, PA 19107
(215) 546-7293; 800-962-1892
FAX (215) 790-9330
Web site: http://www.hanleyandbelfus.com

Notice: A portion of all royalties received from the sale of this text will be donated by the editor to the National Endowment for Plastic Surgery and the Plastic Surgery Educational Foundation.

Library of Congress Cataloging-in-Publication Data

Plastic surgery secrets : questions you will be asked on rounds, in
    the OR, on oral exams / edited by Jeffrey Weinzweig.
         p.   cm. — (The Secrets Series®)
    Includes bibliographical references and index.
    ISBN 1-56053-219-X (alk. paper)
      1. Surgery, Plastic—Examinations, questions, etc. I. Weinzweig,
Jeffrey, 1963–   . II. Series.
    [DNLM: 1. Surgery, Plastic examination questions.
    2. Reconstructive Surgical Procedures examination questions.   WO
18.2P715 1999]
RD118.P5385   1999
617.9'5'076—dc21
DNLM/DLC
for Library of Congress   98-33916
                                       CIP

PLASTIC SURGERY SECRETS   ISBN 1-56053-219-X

Last digit is the print number: 9 8 7 6 5 4 3 2 1

DEDICATION

For my father,
Whose memory is my greatest inspiration.

For my mother,
In whose eyes I can do no wrong.

For my brother,
In whose vast footsteps I proudly tread.

For my sister,
Whose normal life remains a source of hope.

CONTENTS

CONTRIBUTORS

Ghada Youssef Afifi, MD
Instructor and Chief Resident, Division of Plastic and Reconstructive Surgery, Department of Surgery, Hospital of the University of Pennsylvania, Philadelphia, Pennsylvania

Edward Akelman, MD
Professor, Department of Orthopaedics, Brown University School of Medicine; and Chief, Division of Hand, Upper Extremity, and Microvascular Surgery, Rhode Island Hospital, Providence, Rhode Island

Eric Arnaud, MD
Consultant in Craniofacial Surgery, Craniofacial Unit, Department of Pediatric Neurosurgery, Hôpital Necker-Enfants Malades, Paris, France

Duffield Ashmead, IV, MD
Assistant Clinical Professor, Departments of Surgery (Plastic) and Orthopedics, University of Connecticut School of Medicine, Farmington; Director, Division of Hand Surgery, Connecticut Children's Medical Center; and Active Staff, Hartford Hospital, Hartford, Connecticut

Daniel J. Azurin, MD
Fellow, Institute for Aesthetic and Reconstructive Surgery, Baptist Hospital, Nashville, Tennessee

Nabil A. Barakat, MD
Hand and Microsurgery Fellow, Division of Plastic Surgery, Harvard Medical School and Massachusetts General Hospital, Boston, Massachusetts

David T. Barrall, MD
Clinical Assistant Professor, Department of Plastic Surgery, Brown University School of Medicine; and Chief, Department of Plastic Surgery, Miriam Hospital, Providence, Rhode Island

Scott P. Bartlett, MD
Associate Professor, Department of Plastic Surgery, University of Pennsylvania School of Medicine, University of Pennsylvania Medical Center, Hospital of the University of Pennsylvania, and Children's Hospital of Philadelphia, Philadelphia, Pennsylvania

Bruce S. Bauer, MD
Associate Professor of Surgery, Northwestern University Medical School; Head, Division of Plastic Surgery, Children's Memorial Hospital, Chicago, Illinois

Stephen P. Beals, MD, FACS
Assistant Professor, Department of Plastic Surgery, Mayo Medical School, Rochester, Minnesota; Adjunct Professor, Department of Speech and Hearing, Arizona State University School of Medicine, Tempe; Chief, Section of Plastic Surgery, Phoenix Children's Hospital and St. Joseph's Hospital; and Craniofacial Consultant, Barrow Neurological Institute, Phoenix, Arizona

Michael J. Belanger, MD
Clinical Instructor, Department of Orthopedics, Brown University School of Medicine, Providence, Rhode Island

Samuel J. Beran, MD
Assistant Professor, Department of Plastic Surgery, University of Texas Southwestern Medical School at Dallas, Parkland Memorial Hospital, Zale-Lipsky University Hospital, and Dallas Veterans Affairs Medical Center, Dallas, Texas

Richard A. Berger, MD, PhD
Associate Professor and Consultant, Departments of Orthopedic Surgery and Anatomy, Mayo Clinic/Mayo Foundation and Mayo Medical Center, Rochester, Minnesota

Jack R. Bevivino, MD
Assistant Clinical Professor, Department of Surgery, Brown University School of Medicine and Rhode Island Hospital, Providence, Rhode Island

Kirby I. Bland, MD, FACS
J. Murray Beardsley Professor and Chairman, Department of Surgery, Brown University School of Medicine; Executive Surgeon-in-Chief, Brown University Affiliated Hospitals, Providence, Rhode Island

Lynn Breglio, PT, CHT
Hand Therapist, Connecticut Combined Hand Therapy, Glastonbury, Connecticut

Stephen D. Bresnick, MD, DDS
Assistant Professor of Surgery, University of Southern California School of Medicine; Attending Plastic Surgeon, Children's Hospital of Los Angeles, Los Angeles, California

Michael Brucker, MD
Resident, Division of Plastic Surgery, Department of Surgery, Brown University School of Medicine and Rhode Island Hospital, Providence, Rhode Island

Harry J. Buncke, MD, Hon DHC (France)
Clinical Professor of Surgery, Division of Plastic Surgery, University of California, San Francisco, School of Medicine; Associate Clinical Professor of Surgery, Stanford University School of Medicine, Stanford; and Co-Director, Microsurgical Replantation/Transplantation Division, Davies Medical Center, San Francisco, California

Rudolf F. Buntic, MD
Attending Microsurgeon, Microsurgical Replantation/Transplantation Division, Davies Medical Center, San Francisco, California

James Ben Burke, MD
Plastic and Reconstructive Surgery, Jackson Hospital, Montgomery, Alabama

Richard I. Burton, MD
Marjorie Strong Wehle Professor and Chair, Department of Orthopaedics, University of Rochester School of Medicine and Dentistry, Rochester, New York

Anthony A. Caldamone, MD
Professor of Surgery, Department of Urology, Brown University School of Medicine, Rhode Island Hospital, Providence, Rhode Island

David L. Callender, MD, MBA
Associate Professor of Surgery, Vice President for Clinical Programs, Department of Head and Neck Surgery, University of Texas M. D. Anderson Cancer Center, Houston, Texas

Jeffrey E. Caplan, MD
Fellow, Microsurgical Research Center, Eastern Virginia Medical School, Norfolk, Virginia

Lois Carlson, OTR/L, CHT
Director, Connecticut Combined Hand Therapy, Glastonbury, Connecticut

Lloyd P. Champagne, MD
Resident, Division of Plastic Surgery, Department of Surgery, University of Pittsburgh School of Medicine, Pittsburgh, Pennsylvania

Benjamin J. Childers, MD
Assistant Professor, Division of Plastic and Reconstructive Surgery, Department of Surgery, Loma Linda University School of Medicine, Loma Linda, California

Gloria A. Chin, MS, MD
Chief Resident, Division of Plastic Surgery, University of Illinois College of Medicine, and University of Illinois Hospital and Cook County Hospital, Chicago, Illinois

William G. Cioffi, MD
Professor of Surgery, Brown University School of Medicine; and Chief, Trauma and Burns, Rhode Island Hospital, Providence, Rhode Island

Marilyn A. Cohen, BA
Speech Pathologist and Administrative Director, Regional Cleft–Craniofacial Program, Camden, New Jersey

Mimis Cohen, MD, FACS
Professor and Chief, Division of Plastic Surgery, University of Illinois College of Medicine and Cook County Hospital, Chicago, Illinois

Stephen P. Daane, MD
Plastic Surgery Fellow, New York University School of Medicine, and Manhattan Eye, Ear and Throat Hospital, New York, New York

Andrew L. Da Lio, MD
Assistant Professor, Division of Plastic and Reconstructive Surgery, Department of Surgery, UCLA School of Medicine, Los Angeles, California

Joseph L. Daw, Jr., MD, DDS
Division of Plastic and Reconstructive Surgery, Department of Surgery, University of Utah School of Medicine, Primary Children's Medical Center, Salt Lake City, Utah

A. Lee Dellon, MD
Professor, Departments of Plastic Surgery and Neurosurgery, Johns Hopkins University School of Medicine, Baltimore, Maryland

Rudolph F. Dolezal, MD
Clinical Associate Professor, Division of Plastic Surgery, University of Illinois College of Medicine, Chicago, Illinois

Scott A. Don, MD
Chief Resident, Department of Plastic Surgery, Scott and White Memorial Hospital and Clinic, Temple, Texas

Raymond G. Dufresne, Jr., MD
Associate Professor, Department of Dermatology, Brown University School of Medicine and Rhode Island Hospital, Providence, Rhode Island

Christian A. Dumontier, MD.
Consultant, Orthopedic Department, St. Antoine University and Institut de la Main, Paris, France

Raymond M. Dunn, MD, FACS
Associate Professor of Surgery and Anatomy, Division of Plastic Surgery, Department of Surgery, University of Massachusetts Medical Center, Worcester, Massachusetts

Lee E. Edstrom, MD
Chairman, Division of Plastic Surgery, Brown University School of Medicine; and Surgeon-in-Chief, Division of Plastic Surgery, Rhode Island Hospital, Providence, Rhode Island

W. G. Eshbaugh, Jr., MD
Fellow in Endoscopic and Anesthetic Plastic Surgery, Plastic and Anesthetic Surgical Center of Maryland, Baltimore, Maryland

Gregory R. D. Evans, MD, FACS
Associate Professor, Department of Plastic Surgery, University of Texas M. D. Anderson Cancer Center, Houston, Texas

Geoffrey C. Fenner, MD
Assistant Professor of Surgery, Northwestern University Medical School, Chicago; Attending Surgeon, Division of Plastic Surgery, Children's Memorial Hospital, Chicago, and Evanston Hospital, Evanston, Illinois

Jack Fisher, MD
Assistant Clinical Professor, Division of Plastic Surgery, Vanderbilt University School of Medicine; Attending Physician, Institute for Aesthetic and Reconstructive Surgery and Mid-State Baptist Hospital, Nashville, Tennessee

R. Jobe Fix, MD
Associate Professor, Division of Plastic Surgery, Department of Surgery, University of Alabama at Birmingham School of Medicine; Attending Physician, Children's Hospital of Alabama, and Chief of Plastic Surgery, Veterans Administration Medical Center, Birmingham, Alabama

Jeffery S. Flagg, MD, DDS
Chief Resident, Division of Plastic Surgery, University of Illinois College of Medicine, University of Illinois Hospital, Cook County Hospital, Chicago, Illinois

Earl J. Fleegler, MD
Hand Surgeon, Department of Surgery, Albert Einstein Medical Center, Philadelphia, Pennsylvania

James W. Fletcher, MD
Resident, Division of Plastic Surgery, Department of Surgery, Brown University School of Medicine, and Rhode Island Hospital, Providence, Rhode Island

Robert S. Flowers, MD
Director, Hawaii Postgraduate Fellowship in Aesthetic Plastic Surgery; Director, Plastic Surgery Center of the Pacific; and Assistant Clinical Professor, Division of Plastic Surgery, Department of Surgery, University of Hawaii John A. Burns School of Medicine, Honolulu, Hawaii

Paul Fortes, MD
Resident, Division of Plastic Surgery, Department of Surgery, Northwestern University Medical School, Chicago, Illinois

Jack A. Friedland, MD, FACS
Associate Professor of Plastic Surgery, Division of Plastic and Reconstructive Surgery, Department of Surgery, Mayo Medical School, Rochester, Minnesota

Karen E. Frye, MD, FACS
Assistant Professor of Surgery, Department of Surgery, and Director, Burn Center, University of South Alabama College of Medicine, and General Surgeon, University of South Alabama Hospitals, Mobile, Alabama

J. William Futrell, MD
Head, Division of Plastic Surgery, Department of Surgery, University of Pittsburgh School of Medicine, Pittsburgh, Pennsylvania

Giulio Gherardini, MD
Pediatric Plastic Surgery Fellow, Department of Plastic Surgery, Texas Children's Hospital, Houston, Texas

Louis A. Gilula, MD, DABR, FACR
Professor of Radiology, Orthopaedic Surgery, and Plastic and Reconstructive Surgery, and Director, Musculoskeletal Section, Mallinckrodt Institute of Radiology, Washington University School of Medicine, St. Louis, Missouri

Kerry A. Golden, MPT
Southwest Craniofacial Center, Phoenix, Arizona

Mark H. Gonzalez, MD
Professor of Orthopaedic Surgery, University of Illinois College of Medicine and Cook County Hospital, Chicago, Illinois

Mark S. Granick, MD
Professor and Chief of Plastic Surgery, Department of Surgery, Allegheny University of the Health Sciences, Philadelphia, Pennsylvania

Daniel P. Greenwald, MD, FACS
Clinical Associate Professor, Department of Surgery, University of South Florida College of Medicine, and Tampa General Hospital, Tampa, Florida

Kristine J. Guleserian, MD
Clinical Instructor in Surgery and Chief Resident, Department of Surgery, Brown University School of Medicine and Rhode Island Hospital, Providence, Rhode Island

Shalini Gupta, MD
Formerly, Resident, Division of Plastic Surgery, Department of Surgery, Brown University School of Medicine, Providence, Rhode Island; presently, Resident, Department of Dermatology, University of Washington School of Medicine, Seattle, Washington

Mark N. Halikis, MD
Assistant Clinical Professor, Department of Orthopaedic Surgery, University of California, Irvine, College of Medicine and UCI Medical Center, Orange, and Chief of Hand Surgery Service, Veterans Administration Medical Center, Long Beach, California

Geoffrey G. Hallock, MD
Consultant, Division of Plastic Surgery, Lehigh Valley Hospital, Allentown, Pennsylvania

Raymond J. Harshbarger, MD
Resident, Division of Plastic Surgery, Department of Surgery, Brown University School of Medicine and Rhode Island Hospital, Providence, Rhode Island

Christine Haugen, MD
Resident, Department of Surgery, Brown University School of Medicine and Rhode Island Hospital, Providence, Rhode Island

Tad R. Heinz, MD
Assistant Professor of Plastic Surgery, Division of Plastic Surgery, Department of Surgery, University of Alabama–Birmingham School of Medicine, Children's Hospital of Alabama, and Veterans Administration Medical Center, Birmingham, Alabama

Vincent R. Hentz, MD
Professor of Functional Reconstruction and Chief, Division of Hand and Upper Extremity Surgery, Stanford University School of Medicine, Stanford, California

Rosemary Hickey, MD
Professor of Anesthesiology, University of Texas Medical School at San Antonio, and University Hospital and South Texas Veterans Healthcare System, San Antonio, Texas

Roy W. Hong, MD
Department of Plastic and Reconstructive Surgery, Palo Alto Medical Foundation, Palo Alto; Stanford University Hospital, Stanford, California

M. Rusen Kapucu, MD
Craniofacial Fellow, Division of Plastic Surgery, Department of Surgery, University of Pittsburgh School of Medicine, Pittsburgh, Pennsylvania

Bobby Kapur, BA
Medical Student, Division of Plastic Surgery, Department of Surgery, Baylor College of Medicine, Houston, Texas

Henry K. Kawamoto, Jr., MD, DDS
Clinical Professor, Division of Plastic Surgery, University of California, Los Angeles, School of Medicine, Los Angeles, California

Carolyn L. Kerrigan, MD
Professor of Surgery, Section of Plastic Surgery, Dartmouth Medical School, Lebanon, New Hampshire

David C. Kim, MD
Attending Physician, Division of Plastic and Reconstructive Surgery, Temple University Hospital, Philadelphia, Pennsylvania

Daniel S. Kim, MD
Resident, Department of Surgery, Brown University School of Medicine and Rhode Island Hospital, Providence, Rhode Island

Kyoung C. Kim, MD
Resident, Division of Plastic Surgery, Department of Surgery, Brown University School of Medicine and Rhode Island Hospital, Providence, Rhode Island

Jane H. Kim, MD
Resident, Division of Plastic Surgery, Department of Surgery, Brown University School of Medicine and Rhode Island Hospital, Providence, Rhode Island

Thomas J. Krizek, MD
Professor and Vice-Chairman, Department of Surgery, and Chief, Division of Plastic Surgery, University of South Florida College of Medicine, and Tampa General Hospital, Tampa, Florida

Don La Rossa, MD
Professor of Surgery (Plastic), Division of Plastic Surgery, Department of Surgery, University of Pennsylvania School of Medicine; and Director, Cleft Palate Clinic, Children's Hospital of Philadelphia, Philadelphia, Pennsylvania

Donald R. Laub, Jr., MD
Assistant Professor, Division of Plastic Surgery, University of Vermont College of Medicine, Burlington, Vermont

Raphael C. Lee, MD, ScD, FACS
Professor of Surgery, Section of Plastic and Reconstructive Surgery, Professor of Organismal Biology and Anatomy, and Director, Surgical Research/Electrical Trauma Program, University of Chicago, Chicago, Illinois

W. P. Andrew Lee, MD
Assistant Professor of Surgery, Department of Surgery, and Chief of Hand Service, Harvard Medical School and Massachusetts General Hospital, Boston, Massachusetts

Dennis E. Lenhart, MD
Resident, Division of Plastic Surgery, University of Illinois College of Medicine, and University of Illinois Hospital, Chicago, Illinois

Salvatore C. Lettieri, MD
Assistant Professor, Division of Plastic, Reconstructive, Maxillofacial, and Oral Surgery, Duke University School of Medicine, Durham, North Carolina

David M. Lichtman, MD
Director, Fort Worth Affiliated Hospitals Orthopedic Residency Program, and Chairman of Orthopedics, John Peter Smith Hospital, Fort Worth; Adjunct Professor, Baylor College of Medicine, Houston, Texas

James Lilley, MD
Resident, Department of Orthopedic Surgery, University of California, Irvine, School of Medicine and UCI Medical Center, Orange, California

John William Little, MD, FACS
Clinical Professor of Surgery (Plastic), Department of Surgery, Georgetown University School of Medicine and Georgetown University Hospital, Washington, DC

Charles D. Long, MD
Assistant Professor, Division of Plastic Surgery, Department of Surgery, Allegheny University of the Health Sciences, Philadelphia, Pennsylvania

Michael T. Longaker, MD
John Marquis Converse Professor of Plastic Surgery Research, Institute of Plastic and Reconstructive Surgery, New York University School of Medicine, New York, New York

H. Wolfgang Losken, MD, FRCS(Edin)
Associate Professor of Plastic Surgery, Division of Plastic Surgery, Department of Surgery, University of Pittsburgh School of Medicine, Pittsburgh, Pennsylvania

Arnold Luterman, MD, FACS, FRCS(C)
Ripps-Meisler Professor and Chairman, Department of Surgery, University of South Alabama College of Medicine, and University of South Alabama Hospitals, Mobile, Alabama

Sheilah A. Lynch, MD
Chief Resident, Division of Plastic Surgery, Department of Surgery, Brown University School of Medicine, and Rhode Island Hospital, Providence, Rhode Island

Susan E. Mackinnon, MD
Shoenberg Professor and Chief, Division of Plastic Surgery, Department of Surgery, Washington University School of Medicine and Barnes-Jewish Hospital, St. Louis, Missouri

Ahmed S. Makki, MD, FRCS
Senior Specialist in Plastic Surgery, Plastic Surgery Department and Burn Unit, Hamad Medical Corporation and Hamad General Hospital, Doha, Qatar

Ernest K. Manders, MD
Professor of Surgery, Division of Plastic Surgery, Department of Surgery, University of Pittsburgh School of Medicine, Pittsburgh, Pennsylvania

Mahesh H. Mankani, MD
Craniofacial and Skeletal Diseases Branch, National Institute of Dental Research, National Institutes of Health, Bethesda, Maryland

Paul N. Manson, MD
Professor and Chairman, Division of Plastic Surgery, Department of Surgery, Johns Hopkins University School of Medicine, Baltimore, Maryland

Daniel Marchac, MD
Director, Craniofacial Unit, Department of Pediatric Neurosurgery, Hôpital Necker-Enfants Malades, Paris, France

Derlis Martino, MD
Resident, Department of Surgery, The New York Hospital of Queens, Flushing, New York

G. Patrick Maxwell, MD, FACS
Assistant Clinical Professor, Department of Plastic Surgery, Vanderbilt University School of Medicine, Nashville; Director, Institute for Aesthetic and Reconstructive Surgery, Baptist Hospital, Nashville, Tennessee

Robert M. McFarlane, MD, FRCS(C)
Professor Emeritus, Hand and Upper Limb Centre and Division of Plastic Surgery, University of Western Ontario Faculty of Medicine; Consultant, St. Joseph's Health Centre, London, Ontario, Canada

Mary H. McGrath, MD, MPH
Professor of Surgery and Chief, Division of Plastic and Reconstructive Surgery, Department of Surgery, George Washington University School of Medicine, and Children's National Medical Center, Washington, DC

Julie A. Melchior, MD
Attending Hand and Orthopaedic Surgeon, Southern California Permanente Medical Group; Consulting Hand Surgeon, Olive View-UCLA Medical Center, Los Angeles, California

Frederick J. Menick, MD
Private Practice, Tucson, Arizona

Viktor M. Metz, MD
Professor of Radiology, Clinic for Radiodiagnostics, University of Vienna, Vienna, Austria

D. Ralph Millard, Jr., MD, FACS, Hon FRCS(Edin), Hon FRCS, OD Ja
Light-Millard Professor and Chairman Emeritus, Division of Plastic Surgery, University of Miami School of Medicine, Jackson Memorial Hospital and Miami Children's Hospital, Miami, Florida

Daniel C. Mills, II, MD, FACS
Associate Clinical Professor of Plastic Surgery, Loma Linda University School of Medicine, Loma Linda, California

J. Gerald Minniti, MD
Resident, Division of Plastic Surgery, Department of Surgery, Brown University School of Medicine, and Rhode Island Hospital, Providence, Rhode Island

Louis Morales, Jr., MD
Clinical Associate Professor, Division of Plastic and Reconstructive Surgery, Department of Surgery, University of Utah School of Medicine, and Primary Children's Medical Center, Salt Lake City, Utah

John B. Mulliken, MD
Associate Professor of Surgery, Harvard Medical School; Director, Craniofacial Center, Division of Plastic Surgery, Children's Hospital, Boston, Massachusetts

Thomas A. Mustoe, MD, FACS
Professor and Chief, Division of Plastic Surgery, Department of Surgery, Northwestern University Medical School, Chicago, and Northwestern Memorial Hospital, Evanston, Illinois

Jeffrey N. Myers, MD, PhD
Assistant Professor, Department of Head and Neck Surgery, University of Texas M. D. Anderson Cancer Center, Houston, Texas

Chet L. Nastala, MD
Assistant Professor, Department of Plastic Surgery, University of Texas at San Antonio School of Medicine, San Antonio, Texas

Rahul K. Nath, MD
Assistant Professor, Division of Plastic Surgery, Department of Surgery, and Department of Neurosurgery, Baylor College of Medicine, Texas Children's Hospital and Methodist Hospital, Houston, Texas

Mary Lynn Newport, MD
Associate Professor, Department of Orthopedic Surgery, University of Connecticut School of Medicine, Farmington, Connecticut

Zahid Bin Masud Niazi, MD, FRCS(Ire)
Assistant Professor of Surgery, Associate Director of Microsurgery, and Chief of Craniofacial Surgery, Division of Plastic Surgery, Department of Surgery, New York Medical College, Valhalla, New York

Marcello Pantaloni, MD
Chief Resident, Division of Plastic Surgery, Department of Surgery, Brown University School of Medicine
and Rhode Island Hospital, Providence, Rhode Island

Gregory H. Pastrick, MD
Chief Resident, Division of Plastic Surgery, Department of Surgery, Brown University School of Medicine
and Rhode Island Hospital, Providence, Rhode Island

Jagruti C. Patel, MD
Resident, Division of Plastic Surgery, Department of Surgery, Brown University School of Medicine and
Rhode Island Hospital, Providence, Rhode Island

George C. Peck, MD
Department of Plastic and Reconstructive Surgery, St. Barnabas Medical Center, Livingston, New Jersey

George C. Peck, Jr., MD
Department of Plastic and Reconstructive Surgery, St. Barnabas Medical Center, Livingston, New Jersey

Wilfred C. G. Peh, MBBS, DMRD, MRCP, FRCR
Professor of Diagnostic Radiology, Department of Diagnostic Radiology, University of Hong Kong;
Honorary Consultant Radiologist, Queen Mary Hospital; and Clinical Head of Radiology, Duchess of
Kent Children's Orthopaedic Hospital, Hong Kong

Rexford A. Peterson, MD, FACS
Founder/Director, Phoenix Plastic Surgery Residency, 1963-1986; Emeritus Associate Professor of
Surgery, Mayo Medical School, Rochester, Minnesota

Tia Peterson
Clinical and Academic Assistant, Phoenix, Arizona

Jane A. Petro, MD, FACS
Professor of Surgery, Associate Director of Microsurgery, Associate Director, Burn Unit, Division of
Plastic Surgery, Department of Surgery, New York Medical College, Valhalla, New York

John W. Polley, MD
Director and Associate Professor, Craniofacial Center, Division of Plastic Surgery, University of Illinois
College of Medicine, and University of Illinois Hospital, Cook County Hospital, Michael Reese Hospital
and Medical Center, and West Side Veteran Administration Hospital, Chicago, Illinois

Julian J. Pribaz, MD
Director and Associate Professor, Harvard Plastic Surgery Training Program, Harvard Medical School;
Division of Plastic and Reconstructive Surgery, Brigham and Women's Hospital and Children's Hospital,
Boston, Massachusetts

Somayaji Ramamurthy, MD
Professor of Anesthesiology, University of Texas Medical School of San Antonio, San Antonio, Texas

Sai S. Ramasastry, MD, FRCS
Associate Professor of Surgery (Plastic), Division of Plastic, Reconstructive, and Cosmetic Surgery,
University of Illinois College of Medicine, and University of Illinois Medical Center and Cook County
Hospital, Chicago, Illinois

Oscar M. Ramirez, MD, FACS
Clinical Assistant Professor, Department of Surgery, Johns Hopkins University and University of
Maryland Schools of Medicine, and Greater Baltimore Medical Center, Baltimore, Maryland

Peter Randall, MD
Emeritus Professor of Plastic Surgery, Division of Plastic Surgery, Department of Surgery, University of Pennsylvania School of Medicine; and Senior Surgeon, Children's Hospital of Philadelphia, Philadelphia, Pennsylvania

John F. Reinisch, MD
Associate Clinical Professor of Surgery, University of Southern California School of Medicine; Head,
Division of Plastic Surgery, Children's Hospital of Los Angeles, Los Angeles, California

Ramon Angel S. Robles, MD
Chief Resident, Department of General Surgery, Maricopa Medical Center, Phoenix, Arizona

W. Bradford Rockwell, MD
Associate Professor, Division of Plastic and Reconstructive Surgery, Department of Surgery, University of
Utah School of Medicine, Salt Lake City, Utah

Alan Rosen, MD
Division of Hand and Microvascular Surgery, Hospital for Special Surgery, Cornell University Medical College, New York, New York

Cynthia L. Rosenberg, DDS, MSD
Clinical Assistant Professor of Surgery, Division of Plastic Surgery, Department of Surgery, Brown University School of Medicine; Orthodontist, Rhode Island Hospital, Providence, Rhode Island

Gary J. Rosenberg, MD, FACS
Clinical Instructor, Department of Plastic Surgery, University of Miami School of Medicine, Miami, Florida

Douglas C. Ross, MD, FRCS(C)
Assistant Professor, Hand and Upper Limb Centre and Division of Plastic Surgery, University of Western Ontario Faculty of Medicine; Consultant, St. Joseph's Health Centre, London, Ontario, Canada

Jhonny Salomon, MD
Craniofacial Fellow, Department of Plastic Surgery, University of Texas Southwestern Medical Center, Dallas, Texas

Homayoun N. Sasson, MD
Attending Plastic Surgeon, The New York Hospital of Queens, Flushing, New York

Paul L. Schnur, MD
Chairman, and Associate Professor of Plastic Surgery, Division of Plastic and Reconstructive Surgery, Department of Surgery, Mayo Medical School, and Mayo Clinic Hospital, Scottsdale, Arizona

Richard C. Schultz, MD, FACS
Clinical Professor of Surgery, Department of Surgery, University of Illinois College of Medicine and University of Illinois Hospital, Chicago, and Lutheran General Hospital, Park Ridge, Illinois

Brooke R. Seckel, MD, FACS
Chairman, Department of Plastic and Reconstructive Surgery, Lahey Clinic Medical Center, Burlington; Assistant Clinical Professor of Surgery, Harvard Medical School and Tufts University School of Medicine, Boston, Massachusetts

John T. Seki, MD
Resident, Division of Plastic Surgery, Department of Surgery, Brown University School of Medicine, and Rhode Island Hospital, Providence, Rhode Island

William W. Shaw, MD, FACS
Professor and Chief, Division of Plastic and Reconstructive Surgery, Department of Surgery, UCLA School of Medicine, Los Angeles, California

Saleh M. Shenaq, MD
Professor and Chief, Division of Plastic Surgery, Department of Surgery, Baylor College of Medicine, Methodist Hospital, Texas Children's Hospital, St. Luke's Episcopal Hospital, and Texas Institute for Rehabilitation and Research, Houston, Texas

Kenneth C. Shestak, MD, FACS
Associate Professor, Division of Plastic Surgery, Department of Surgery, University of Pittsburgh School of Medicine, and Chief of Plastic Surgery, Magee-Women's Hospital, Pittsburgh, Pennsylvania

Prasanna-Kumar Shivapuja, BDS, MDS(Ortho), DDS, MS(Ortho)
Staff Orthodontist, Craniofacial Anomaly and Cleft Palate Team, Children's Hospital of Michigan, Detroit, and Providence Hospital, Southfield, Michigan

Faizi A. Siddiqi, MD
Resident, Department of Surgery, The New York Hospital of Queens, Flushing, New York

Eugene M. Smith, Jr., MD
Fellow, Hawaii Postgraduate Fellowship in Aesthetic Plastic Surgery, University of Hawaii, Honolulu, Hawaii

John W. Smith, MD
Fellow in Microsurgery and Breast Reconstruction, Memorial Sloan-Kettering Cancer Center, New York, New York

Scott L. Spear, MD
Professor and Chief, Division of Plastic Surgery, Department of Surgery, Georgetown University School of Medicine, Washington, DC

Nicholas J. Speziale, MD
Department of Plastic Surgery, Palos Community Hospital, Palos Heights, Illinois

Melvin Spira, MD, DDS
Professor of Surgery, Division of Plastic Surgery, Department of Surgery, Baylor College of Medicine, and St. Luke's Episcopal Hospital, Houston, Texas

John L. Spolyar, DDS, MS
Assistant Clinical Professor, Department of Orthodontics, University of Detroit Mercy School of Dentistry, Cleft Palate Team, Children's Hospital of Michigan, Detroit, Michigan

Michael P. Staebler, MD
Clinical Instructor, Department of Orthopaedics, Brown University School of Medicine and Rhode Island Hospital, Providence, Rhode Island

Samuel Stal, MD, FACS
Associate Professor, Division of Plastic Surgery, Department of Surgery, Baylor College of Medicine; Chief of Plastic Surgery, Medical Director, Cleft Palate and Craniofacial Team, and Co-Chief, Birthmark Center, Texas Children's Hospital, Houston, Texas

Eric J. Stelnicki, MD
Clinical Instructor, Division of Plastic and Reconstructive Surgery, Department of Surgery, Washington University School of Medicine, and Barnes-Jewish Hospital, St. Louis, Missouri

Mitchell A. Stotland, MD
Assistant Professor of Surgery, Division of Plastic Surgery, Department of Surgery; and Instructor of Pediatrics, Department of Pediatrics, Dartmouth Medical School, Hanover, and Dartmouth Hitchcock Medical Center, Lebanon, New Hampshire

James W. Strickland, MD
Clinical Professor, Department of Orthopaedics, Indiana University School of Medicine, Indiana Hand Center, and St. Vincent's Hospital of Indianapolis, Indianapolis, Indiana

Brent V. Stromberg, MD, FACS
Plastic Surgery Images, St. Louis, Missouri

Patrick K. Sullivan, MD
Associate Professor of Plastic Surgery, Division of Plastic Surgery, Department of Surgery, Brown University School of Medicine and Rhode Island Hospital, Providence, Rhode Island

Jeffrey W. Szem, MD
Resident, Division of Plastic Surgery, Department of Surgery, University of Pittsburgh School of Medicine, Pittsburgh, Pennsylvania

Leslie D. Tackett, MD
Chief Resident, Department of Urology, Brown University School of Medicine, Providence, Rhode Island

Julio Taleisnik, MD
Clinical Professor, Department of Orthopaedic Surgery, University of California, Irvine, College of Medicine and UCI Medical Center, Orange, California

Julia K. Terzis, MD
Professor of Microsurgery, Microsurgical Research Center, Eastern Virginia Medical School, Norfolk, Virginia

Raoul Tubiana, MD
Professor of Orthopedic Surgery, Hôpital Cochin, Paris V University, Paris; Director and Orthopedic and Plastic Surgeon, Institut de la Main, Paris, France

John W. Tyrone, III, MD
Resident, Department of Surgery, University of California School of Medicine, Davis-East Bay, Oakland, California

Joseph Upton, MD
Associate Clinical Professor of Surgery, Division of Plastic Surgery, Department of Surgery, Harvard Medical School, Beth Israel Hospital, Children's Hospital, and Brigham and Women's Hospital, Boston, Massachusetts

Craig A. Vander Kolk, MD
Director, Johns Hopkins Cleft and Craniofacial Center; Associate Professor, Division of Plastic Surgery, Johns Hopkins University School of Medicine, Baltimore, Maryland

Armand D. Versaci, MD
Clinical Professor of Surgery (Plastic), Division of Plastic Surgery, Brown University School of Medicine, Rhode Island Hospital, Providence, Rhode Island

William F. Wagner, Jr., MD
Clinical Instructor, Department of Orthopaedics, University of Washington School of Medicine, and Staff Surgeon, Seattle Hand Surgery Group, Seattle, Washington

Richard J. Wassermann, MD, MPH
Assistant Professor, Division of Plastic Surgery, Department of Surgery, University of South Carolina School of Medicine, Attending Surgeon, Richland Memorial Hospital, Columbia, South Carolina

H. Kirk Watson, MD
Director, Connecticut Combined Hand Surgery Service, Chief, Hand Surgery, Connecticut Children's Medical Center, and Senior Staff, Department of Orthopedics, Hartford Hospital, Hartford; Clinical Professor, Department of Orthopedics, University of Connecticut School of Medicine, Farmington; and Assistant Clinical Professor of Orthopedics, Rehabilitation, and Surgery (Plastic), Yale University School of Medicine, New Haven, Connecticut

Andrew J. Weiland, MD
Professor of Orthopedic Surgery, Division of Orthopedic Surgery, Department of Surgery, Cornell University Medical College, and Hospital for Special Surgery, New York, New York

Adam B. Weinfeld, BA
Medical Student, Division of Plastic Surgery, Department of Surgery, Baylor College of Medicine, Houston, Texas

Jeffrey Weinzweig, MD
Formerly, Chief Resident, Division of Plastic Surgery, Department of Surgery, Brown University School of Medicine, Rhode Island Hospital, Providence, Rhode Island; currently, Craniofacial Surgery Fellow, Division of Plastic Surgery, Department of Surgery, University of Pennsylvania School of Medicine, Children's Hospital of Philadelphia, Philadelphia, Pennsylvania

Norman Weinzweig, MD, FACS
Associate Professor of Plastic Surgery and Orthopaedic Surgery; Head, Hand and Microsurgery, and Co-Director, Multidisciplinary Foot Clinic, University of Illinois College of Medicine, and Cook County Hospital, Chicago, Illinois

Arnold-Peter C. Weiss, MD
Associate Professor, Department of Orthopaedics, Brown University School of Medicine, and Hand Surgeon, Rhode Island Hospital, Providence, Rhode Island

Deborah J. White, MD
Private Practice, Scottsdale, Arizona

S. Anthony Wolfe, MD, FACS
Clinical Professor, Plastic and Reconstructive Surgery, University of Miami School of Medicine; Chief, Division of Plastic and Reconstructive Surgery, Miami Children's Hospital, Miami, Florida

R. Chris Wray, Jr., MD
Professor and Chairman, Division of Plastic Surgery, University of Rochester School of Medicine and Dentistry, and Strong Memorial Hospital, Rochester, New York

Soheil Younai, MD
Resident, Department of Plastic and Reconstructive Surgery, Lahey Clinic Medical Center, Burlington, Massachusetts

Eser Yuksel, MD
Research Fellow and Instructor, Division of Plastic Surgery, Department of Surgery, Baylor College of Medicine, Houston, Texas

David D. Zabel, MD
Chief Resident, Division of Plastic Surgery, Department of Surgery, University of Pittsburgh School of Medicine, Pittsburgh, Pennsylvania

Richard J. Zienowicz, MD
Assistant Professor of Surgery, Division of Plastic Surgery, Department of Surgery, Brown University School of Medicine and Rhode Island Hospital; Chief of Plastic Surgery, Veterans Administration Medical Center, Providence, Rhode Island

Acknowledgments

The character and integrity of a man are often judged based on those with whom he associates. His ability and potential based on those who have trained him. His instinct and insight based on those who have guided him.

As I enter the challenging world of plastic surgery, I do so with the comforting knowledge that I have been extremely fortunate, indeed blessed, to have been surrounded by an elite group of men, indeed giants, each of whom I am grateful and honored to call my mentor, my teacher, my friend:

Lee E. Edstrom, MD
Armand Versaci, MD
Richard J. Zienowicz, MD
H. Kirk Watson, MD
Paul L. Schnur, MD
Norman Weinzweig, MD

Tous Mes Remerciements

To Docteur Paul Tessier,

For reviewing the chapter on "Craniofacial Clefts" and providing insightful comments.

PREFACE

There is no such thing as a stupid question. Socrates knew this more than two thousand years ago when the interrogative (Socratic) method of teaching was born. The success of The Secrets Series® reaffirms the effectiveness of this approach to teaching. The purpose of **Plastic Surgery Secrets** is to serve as a comprehensive guide to a field in which the earliest procedures, including nasal and earlobe reconstruction, were described by Sushruta in 600 BC, while new frontiers pioneered within the last three decades, including craniofacial surgery, microsurgery, and fetal surgery, continue to evolve.

Nearly 200 authors have contributed the 120 chapters that comprise this volume, many of whom have literally defined the area of the specialty about which they have written. They have provided more than 3000 questions that broach virtually every aspect of plastic surgery and stimulate as many. I am indebted to each of them. The vastness of the field of plastic surgery by necessity presents countless opportunities for collaboration in patient management and medical education with colleagues in numerous other specialties. The scope of this volume is intended to cross over to students and practitioners in these allied fields. It is intended to provoke thought and stimulate further inquiry and represents a distillation of the important concepts and pearls that form the foundation of that alluring discipline of medicine known as plastic surgery.

Jeffrey Weinzweig, M.D.

FOREWORD

One of the proudest traditions of surgery has been the passing of knowledge from one generation to another—what we have come to define as surgical education. Yet, this tradition has taken many forms and has undergone continued evolution.

In ancient times, undoubtedly, it was based on the oral tradition of the teacher verbally conveying dogma to the student. The written word was also an important component, as witnessed by the writings of Sushruta in 600 B.C., the famous papyri of Egypt, the monastic manuscripts of the Middle Ages and the later dissemination of books, the latter resulting from the discovery of the printing press by Johann Gutenberg in 1440.

The modern age greatly facilitated the dissemination of surgical knowledge. Improvements in travel allowed surgeons to move from country to country, continent to continent in pursuit of new surgical techniques. Individual master surgeons could then draw surgeons from around the world to their operating clinics. The discovery of the photographic process permitted the accurate printing of images in books and eventually led to discovery of the projected slide—hence, Sir Harold Gillies' famous quip that the greatest advance in plastic surgery in his lifetime was "the discovery of the Kodachrome slide."

In this century, each advance in telecommunications was followed by another: radio allowed the first simultaneous national and international surgical conferences; motion picture film was capably exploited by the American College of Surgeons as a means of teaching technical surgery to large numbers of surgeons; television allowed closed circuit meetings, which could be viewed simultaneously around the world by satellite; and the computer provided multimedia capabilities.

As we approach the new millennium, we have come to realize that the problem is no longer the acquisition of surgical knowledge but the personal processing or integration of an overwhelming mass of surgical data that increases daily on an exponential scale.

Fundamental to this proud tradition of surgical education is what Dr. Jeffrey Weinzweig has so accurately defined as the Socratic method, a pedagogic technique attributed to the Athenian philosopher. His educational method, called DIALECTIC, is derived from the Greek word meaning to "converse."

In this text, **Plastic Surgery Secrets**, nearly 200 authors, under the able direction of Dr. Weinzweig, have superbly demonstrated the value of the question-and-answer technique in imparting plastic surgery knowledge. But one must not forget that it is not only the student who benefits from the well-posed question but also the teacher—it is truly an intellectual interchange. And one must also not forget that it is the questions *without* answers that push the discipline forward as the questioner becomes determined to find the answers. This is the true beauty of our plastic surgical heritage.

> "There is only one good, knowledge, and one evil, ignorance."
> Socrates c. 470–399 B.C.

JOSEPH G. McCARTHY, MD
Lawrence D. Bell Professor of Plastic Surgery
Director, Institute of Reconstructive Plastic Surgery
New York University Medical Center
New York, New York

I. Fundamental Principles of Plastic Surgery

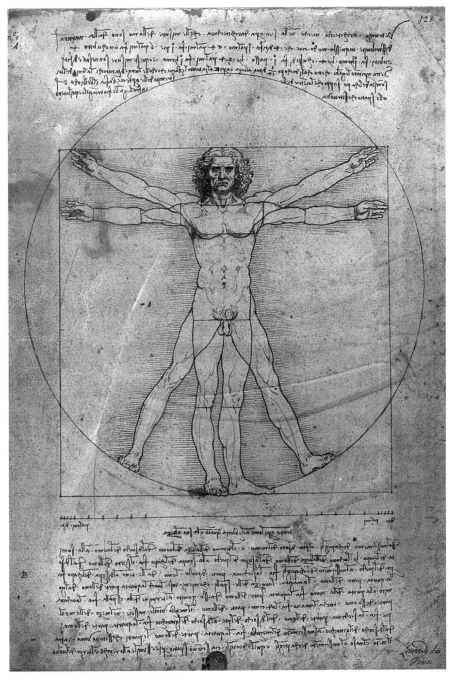

The Human Proportions According to Vitruvius
Leonardo da Vinci
ca. 1492
Pen, ink and light wash over silverpoint
Galleria dell'Accademia, Venice
© 1992 Alinari/Art Resource, New York

1. THE PRINCIPLES OF WOUND HEALING

John W. Tyrone, M.D., and Thomas A. Mustoe, M.D., F.A.C.S.

1. What events occur during each of the primary phases of wound healing?

Wound healing has three principal phases: inflammatory, proliferative, and remodeling. The **inflammatory phase** begins at the time of wounding and lasts for 24–48 hours. Platelets forming the initial thrombus release growth factors that are chemoattractant for macrophages and neutrophils. These cells cooperate to remove necrotic tissue, debris, and bacteria from the wound. By day 3, transforming growth factor beta (TGF-β) released from macrophages has attracted fibroblasts into the wound, signaling the start of the **proliferative phase**. Fibroblasts produce collagen and lay down extracellular matrix to strengthen the wound. Growth factors released from macrophages also stimulate angiogenesis and formation of new capillaries. The **remodeling phase**, which lasts up to 1 year, begins when remodeling of collagen reaches equilibrium, usually 2–3 weeks after wounding. All stages may vary in length because of infection, malnutrition, or other exogenous factors.

2. What role do macrophages play in wound healing?

During the inflammatory phase of wound healing, polymorphonuclear cells (PMNs) and macrophages infiltrate the wound. Macrophages play a critical role in removing debris and bacteria (along with PMNs) and, most importantly, orchestrate the events of wound healing. They are the primary source of growth factors (e.g., platelet-derived growth factor, TGF-β), which stimulate production of connective tissue proteins by fibroblasts. These growth factors also act in an autocrine fashion to amplify tremendously their expression.

3. During remodeling there is no net increase in collagen, but the wound breaking strength increases greatly. Why?

Initial wound healing is notable for large amounts of randomly laid down collagen. During remodeling, fibroblasts and macrophages cooperate to replace the random collagen with collagen that is cross-linked and oriented in a more orderly arrangement to the direction of mechanical stress. Like raw wool being woven into strong yarn, the remodeled collagen is compacted into fibers and is many times stronger than random collagen fibrils. The organization and strength of the new collagen never reach the strength of uninjured collagen.

4. What is the rationale for not allowing patients with hernias to do sit-ups for 6 weeks after a herniorrhaphy?

Wound tensile strength is relatively low in the first few weeks after wounding but increases linearly after 3–4 weeks. By 6 weeks, the wound has gained about 50% of its ultimate strength and is strong enough to tolerate moderate forces. However, in elderly patients it may be prudent to wait longer because gains in tensile strength are slower.

5. A well-healed wound eventually reaches what percentage of prewound strength?

Normally healed wounds reach 70–80% of prewound strength.

6. Is collagen makeup different in normal vs. newly healing wounds?

Type I collagen is the most abundant type of collagen in normal dermis (approximately 90%). Type II collagen is the collagen actively secreted by fibroblasts during the early stages of wound healing and may account for up to 30% of the collagen in a healing wound. By week 2 of the wound-healing process, type I collagen again becomes the principal collagen produced by fibroblasts. During remodeling, type III collagen is replaced by type I collagen to restore the normal dermal collagen profile.

7. What is the wound-healing defect in Ehlers-Danlos syndromes (EDS)?

Ehlers-Danlos syndromes are a heterogeneous group of connective tissue disorders characterized by hypermobile joints, hyperextensible skin, and generalized fragility of connective tissues. They are associated with defects in the synthesis, cross-linking, or structure of collagen. The collagen defect in

2

patients with EDS causes a decrease in wound strength and delay in wound healing. Patients are prone to wound dehiscence and formation of broad, thin, shiny scars resembling cigarette paper.

8. How long should a wound be kept dry after closing a surgical incision?
Well-approximated surgical incisions are usually epithelialized in 24–48 hours, forming a fluid barrier. Washing a wound once it is epithelialized to removed dried, crusted blood can reduce bacterial proliferation and prevent a potential delay in healing. For example, in a facial laceration, the benefits of washing and removing dried blood far outweigh any risks to the wound. However, in areas such as the lower extremity in elderly patients, epithelialization may not be complete for much longer. If a foreign material such as a prosthetic joint is beneath the incision, it may be desirable to keep it dry for much longer to prevent potential contamination of the prosthesis.

9. What effect does radiation have on wound healing?
Radiation causes endothelial cell, capillary, and arteriole damage, which results in progressive and cumulative loss of blood vessels in the affected area. Perfusion to the radiated tissues may be affected, leading to delayed healing. Radiated fibroblasts show decreased proliferation and collagen synthesis, leading to diminished deposition of extracellular matrix. Lymphatics likewise may be damaged, causing edema and poor clearance of infection in the healing tissues.

10. Are PMNs essential for strengthening wounds?
PMNs digest bacteria but play no role in strengthening the wound. Unlike macrophages, PMNs are not a source of growth factors in a healing wound.

11. What factors commonly impair wound healing?
Although many factors influence wound healing in surgical patients, the most important are nutritional deficiencies (albumin < 2.5 gm/dl), vitamin deficiencies (unusual), aging, subclinical wound infection, hypoxia, steroids, diabetes, and radiation.

12. After giving birth to her first baby, a patient asks if any treatments are available for stretch marks (striae distensae). What causes stretch marks? Are they amenable to treatment?
Stretch marks form when the dermis is stretched to the point of disruption of collagen fibers, but the epidermis remains intact. The dermis forms a scar that is visible through the translucent epidermis. Because stretch marks are scars in the dermis, any rational treatment entails removing the scar. Abdominoplasty with resection of the involved skin is the only consistent way to remove striae distensae.

13. Is a wound less likely to spread if closed with intradermal polyglactic acid suture (Dexon, Vicryl) vs. a nylon suture that is removed in 7 days?
Wounds can spread if closed under tension or if exposed to stretching forces. In the first 3 weeks of wound healing, the strength of a wound is only a small fraction of its eventual strength. Sutures removed or degraded before this time have little effect on wound spreading. Polyglactic acid suture retains strength for 3 weeks, at which time the wound is still relatively weak. The results are similar to removing a nylon suture from the wound in 1 week. Leaving a permanent intradermal suture in place for several months has been shown to decrease spreading, and it is possible that a synthetic suture that retains strength for 6–8 weeks may have the same effect.

14. You are about to remove an actinic/seborrheic keratosis from a patient's face when he asks if there will be any scarring. How do you respond?
Actinic and seborrheic keratoses extend only into the superficial (epidermal) layer of the skin. Scarring occurs following injury to the deeper layer of the skin, the dermis. Injuries to the superficial (reticular) dermis and epidermis can heal without scarring, but if wound closure is delayed or deeper layers are injured, scarring results. Therefore, superficial skin lesions such as actinic/seborrheic keratoses can be removed without scarring if care is taken not to injure the deeper dermis.

15. A patient has two burns on his chest, one of which epithelialized in 1 week, the other in 3 weeks. The second wound now has a hypertrophic scar. Why?
Partial-thickness burns or abrasions that remain open for more than 2 weeks have a high incidence of hypertrophic scarring. Scarring is believed to be secondary to prolonged inflammation and can be minimized by achieving a closed wound through skin grafting or other techniques.

16. Why does edema impair wound healing?

In normal tissue, each cell is only a few cell diameters away from the nearest capillary and receives oxygen and nutrients by diffusion. Edema impairs wound healing through several mechanisms. First, the additional extracellular water increases diffusion distances, resulting in lower tissue pO_2. Second, chronic edema may result in protein deposition in the extracellular matrix, which can act as a diffusion barrier for growth factors and nutrients, making them less available to cells. Finally, growth factors and nutrients are relatively diluted in the edematous fluid.

17. You perform a split-thickness skin graft (12/1000ths of an inch) for burns in a young and an elderly patient, using the same technique and equipment. Several weeks later the young patient is doing well, but the elderly patient has blisters forming on the graft. What may the cause be?

Basal epidermal cells are attached to the underlying dermis by hemidesmosomes. Cells of aged individuals have been shown to be ineffective at forming new hemidesmosomes. Without an adequate dermal base, coverage of the wound by epidermis is unstable and characterized by chronic and recurrent breakdown. The skin of elderly patients is therefore less tolerant to shearing forces. When shearing occurs, blisters are likely to form.

18. What is the mechanism of wound contraction?

Human wounds heal by wound contraction, reepithelialization, and scarring. As an integral part of wound healing, myofibroblasts orient themselves along lines of tension and pull collagen fibers together. They are responsible for contraction of the wound. Wound contraction is part of the normal healing process that closes the wound to the external environment. Scar contracture is an abnormal shortening and thickening of a scar that may cause functional (if across a joint) and/or cosmetic deformities.

19. Does any medical supplement, dressing, or drug accelerate wound healing?

The Food and Drug Administration (FDA) has approved several moist dressings for topical wound care, but no convincing evidence indicates that they improve wound healing compared with standard treatments. Vitamin A has been used to return healing time to normal in patients that use steroids. Dietary replacement in persons with a dietary deficiency normalizes wound healing. Recently, the FDA considered platelet-derived growth factor (PDGF) for use in diabetic ulcers because in clinical trials healing was reported in an increased percentage of wounds treated with PDGF.

20. Define wound infection.

It is the product of the entrance, growth, metabolic activities, and resultant pathophysiologic effects of microorganisms in the tissues. A wound with bacterial counts greater than 10^5 organisms per gram of tissue is considered infected and unlikely to heal without further treatment.

21. What effect does aging have on wound healing?

Aged patients have slower wound healing, less scarring, less contraction, decreased breaking strength, decreased epithelialization, delayed cell migration, and decreased collagen synthesis. Aging can be an advantage in performing cosmetic surgery because scarring can be minimized. It also can be a disadvantage because wound strength is lower, and a wound may easily be separated if placed under tension.

22. What factors are responsible for local wound ischemia?

Smoking, radiation, edema, diabetes, and peripheral occlusive disease can affect the perfusion and oxygenation of a wound and cause local wound ischemia.

23. What is a chronic wound?

Chronic wounds are those that fail to close in 3 months, and they fall into three broad categories: diabetic ulcers, pressure ulcers, and ulcers secondary to venous hypertension. With meticulous wound care, most chronic wounds will close without surgical intervention.

24. When does collagen production in a healing wound peak?

It peaks by 6 weeks, whereas the maximal amount of collagen accumulation occurs 2–3 weeks after wounding. Although no net increase in collagen occurs after this point secondary to remodeling, collagen synthesis and degradation continue at elevated rates for up to 1 year after wounding.

25. What are the benefits of occlusive dressings?

Occlusive dressings (e.g., polyurethane) maintain a moist environment that promotes rapid re-epithelialization and more effective wound healing than when the wound is allowed to dry out. "Epithelialization under a scab does not occur as quickly as it does under a moist dressing." Care should be taken to monitor for infection when occlusive dressings are used, because fluids also make an excellent medium for bacterial growth.

26. What causes hypertrophic/keloid scars? What treatment options are available?

Hypertrophic/keloid scars are believed to be due to an excessive inflammatory response during healing. Proven treatment options include intralesional injection of steroids, radiation therapy, or surgical resection combined with another treatment. More recently, interferon has shown some benefits in reducing scarring. Other therapies, including tamoxifen, calcium antagonists, pressure therapy, cryotherapy, and pulsed dye lasers, have yet to gain widespread acceptance.

27. What features distinguish between a keloid and hypertrophic scar?

Keloids usually extend beyond the original incision and become progressively larger. Hypertrophic scars are elevated but do not extend outside the original borders of the wound. Keloids are more common in people with dark complexions, whereas hypertrophic scarring occurs more often in fair-skinned people. Keloid scarring is transmitted in some patients in an autosomal dominant pattern. Both conditions are remarkable for overproduction of all components of the extracellular matrix, but absolute numbers of fibroblasts are not increased.

28. What roles do the growth factors PDGF and TGF-β play in wound healing?

PDGF is released by platelets during formation of the initial thrombus. It is chemoattractant for macrophages, which are responsible for orchestrating the events of healing. TGF-β is secreted by macrophages, is chemoattractant for fibroblasts, and stimulates formation of extracellular matrix by fibroblasts.

29. You are reluctant to debride a decubitus ulcer with necrotic tissue in a chronically ill patient who has multiple medical problems and a coagulopathy. What are the alternatives to surgical debridement?

Several options are available. Topical creams that break down necrotic tissue may be applied to the wound. Commonly used agents include autolytic and enzymatic debridement creams. Autolytic debridement agents work by activating endogenous collagenases within the open wound to separate the necrotic tissue. Enzymatic debridement agents, which are concentrated collagenases, act by directly digesting the nonviable tissues.

BIBLIOGRAPHY

1. Abbott RE, Mustoe TA: Enhancement of wound healing: Pharmacologic strategies. J Surg Pathol 2:183–192, 1997.
2. Clark AF: The Molecular and Cellular Biology of Wound Repair, 2nd ed. New York, Plenum, 1996.
3. Cohen IK, Diegelmann RF, Lindblad WJ: Wound Healing: Biochemical and Clinical Aspects. Philadelphia, W.B. Saunders, 1992.
4. Committee on Control of Surgical Infections of the Committee on Pre- and Postoperative Care of the American College of Surgeons: Manual on Control of Infection in Surgical Patients. Philadelphia, J.B. Lippincott, 1976.
5. Greenfield LJ: Surgery: Scientific Principles and Practice, 2nd ed. Philadelphia, Lippincott-Raven, 1997.
6. Khouri RK, Mustoe TA: Trends in the treatment of hypertrophic scars. Adv Plast Reconstr Surg 8:129–146, 1991.
7. LaVan FB, Hunt TK: Oxygen and wound healing. Clin Plast Surg 17:235, 1990.
8. Lawrence WT: In search of the optimal treatment of keloids: Report of a series and a review of the literature. Ann Plast Surg 27:164, 1991.
9. Leibovich SJ, Ross R: The role of the macrophage in wound repair: A study with hydrocortisone and anti-macrophage serum. Am J Pathol 78:71, 1975.
10. Madden JW, Peacock EE: Studies on the biology of collagen during wound healing. Rate of collagen synthesis and deposition in cutaneous wounds in the rat. Surgery 64:288, 1968.
11. Pierce GF, Mustoe TA: Pharmacologic enhancement of wound healing. Annu Rev Med 46:467–481, 1995.
12. Robson MC: Wound infection: A failure of wound healing caused by an imbalance of bacteria. Surg Clin North Am 77:637–650, 1997.
13. Winter GD, Scales JT: Effects of air drying and dressings on the surface of the wound. Nature 197:91, 1963.

2. TECHNIQUES AND GEOMETRY OF WOUND REPAIR

Jeffrey Weinzweig, M.D., and Norman Weinzweig, M.D.

1. What are important considerations in surgical wound closure?

Surgical wound closure is performed in conjunction with biologic events such as fibroplasia, epithelialization, wound contraction, bacterial balance, and host defense mechanisms. All suture materials, including both absorbable and nonabsorbable monofilaments, should be considered as foreign bodies that evoke a tissue inflammatory reaction. This reaction may result in delayed wound healing, infection, or dehiscence. Selection of suture material should be based on the healing properties and requirements of the involved tissue, the biologic and physical properties of the suture material, location of the wound on the body, and individualized patient considerations.

2. Why is the choice of suture material critical in the early stages of wound healing?

In the early stages of wound healing, the suture is primarily responsible for keeping the wound together. In the first 3–4 days after wound repair, the gain in tensile strength is related to fibrin clot, which fills the wound cavity. At 1 week, tensile strength is less than 5% of unwounded skin; it is 10% at 2 weeks, 25% at 4 weeks, 40% at 6 weeks, and 80% at 8–10 weeks.

3. What percentage of normal unwounded tensile strength do wounds ultimately achieve?

Classic studies by Levenson et al. in 1965, using a rat model, demonstrated that wounds never achieve more than 80% of normal unwounded tensile strength.

4. Which layer of a wound repair contributes the most to wound strength?

The dermal layer. Absorbable sutures placed in the dermis, such as poliglecaprone 25 (Monocryl), polyglactin 910 (Vicryl), polyglycolic acid (Dexon), or polyglyconate (Maxon), provide tensile strength over an extended period prior to suture resorption. Sutures placed in the epidermis, usually 5-0 or 6-0 Nylon (depending on location), permit fine alignment of the skin edges only and should be removed within 5 days.

5. What are the basic principles of suturing skin wounds?

Skin edges should be debrided when necessary and always everted and approximated without tension. If simple stitches are not sufficient, horizontal or vertical mattress stitches may be necessary. After tying a knot, the suture appears pear-shaped in cross-section with raised borders. The everted skin edges gradually flatten to produce a level surface. It is important to place the suture so that the wound edges just touch each other. Postoperative edema creates additional tension with potential strangulation of tissue and resultant ischemia that may lead to necrosis.

6. What are the different methods of suturing skin wounds?

Simple interrupted sutures are placed so that the needle enters and exits the tissue at 90°, grasping identical amounts of tissue on each side to permit exact approximation of the wound margins. Of course, this principle applies only when the skin edges line up at exactly the same level. Occasionally, one side of the wound is higher and the other lower. To approximate the edges at the same level, it is necessary to grasp the tissue "high in the high" (closer to the epidermis) and "low in the low" (farther from the epidermis).

Vertical and horizontal mattress sutures are especially useful for everting stubborn wound edges. However, horizontal mattress sutures cause more ischemia than either simple interrupted or vertical mattress sutures.

Subcuticular or intradermal continuous sutures obviate the need for external skin sutures; thus, they avoid suture marks on the skin and result in the most favorable scar. This suture should be left in place for 2–3 weeks. Prolene is often used because it produces little inflammatory reaction, maintains its tensile strength, and can easily be removed.

Half-buried mattress sutures (McGregor stitch or three-corner stitch) are especially useful for closing a V-shaped wound or approximating skin edges of different textures or thicknesses. This stitch usually prevents necrosis of the tip of the V, which is sometimes seen with simple interrupted sutures. By placing the buried portion of the suture within the dermis of the flap, ischemia and damage to the overlying skin are avoided.

The **continuous over-and-over or running suture** is most often used for closure of scalp wounds because it can be performed rapidly and is hemostatic. Locking this stitch provides additional hemostasis. A nonlocking running stitch, using fine Nylon, may be used in areas such as the face where the wound is uncomplicated and under no tension.

7. What is the role of immobilization in wound healing?

Immobilization of the wound is as important in soft tissue healing as it is in bone healing. By immobilizing the wound, tension across the skin edges is eliminated, yielding a more favorable scar. Immobilization can be achieved by using Steri-strips, tapes, collodion, or even plaster splinting.

8. How are suture materials classified?

Suture materials are classified as **natural or synthetic, absorbable or nonabsorbable**, and **braided or monofilament**. Further classification takes into consideration the time until absorption occurs, extent of tissue reaction, and tensile strength.

9. What are the differences among the various absorbable suture materials?

Catgut, derived from the submucosal layer of sheep intestine, evokes a moderate acute inflammatory reaction and is hydrolyzed by proteolytic enzymes within 60 days. Tensile strength is rapidly lost within 7–10 days. Chromization (chromic catgut suture) slightly prolongs these parameters compared with plain gut. The main indications for use of catgut suture include ligation of superficial vessels and closure of tissues that heal rapidly, such as oral mucosa. Catgut sutures also may be used in situations when one wishes to avoid suture removal, as in small children.

Vicryl and Dexon are synthetic materials that behave similarly. They produce minimal tissue reactivity and are completely absorbed within 90 days. Tensile strength is 60–75% at 2 weeks and lost at 1 month. Both are useful as intradermal sutures because of their low reactivity, but they should be used judiciously as buried sutures because of their tendency to "spit" with inflammation. Monocryl (a monofilament), on the other hand, may be used comparably as intradermal or buried sutures. Because the braided structure of Vicryl and Dexon may potentiate infection, neither should be used in wounds with potential bacterial contamination.

Polydioxanone (PDS), a synthetic absorbable monofilament, is minimally reactive. Absorption is essentially complete within 6 months, although little occurs before 90 days. Because of this slow absorption, "spitting" is a significant problem; as a monofilament suture, however, PDS is less prone to bacterial seeding. PDS sutures maintain their tensile strength considerably longer: 50% remain at 4 weeks and 25% at 6 weeks. Absorption is essentially complete at 6 months.

Maxon and Monocryl are absorbable monofilament sutures with similar qualities and advantages as PDS. However, they retain their tensile strength for only 3–4 weeks; absorption of Monocryl is essentially complete between 3 and 4 months.

10. What are the differences among the various nonabsorbable suture materials?

Nonabsorbable monofilament (Ethilon/Nylon and Prolene) sutures incite minimal inflammatory reaction, slide well, and can be easily removed, thus providing ideal running intradermal stitches. Prolene appears to maintain its tensile strength longer than Nylon, which loses approximately 15–20% per year. Nonabsorbable braided materials (Nurolon, Ethibond, and Silk) elicit an acute inflammatory reaction that is followed by gradual encapsulation of the suture by fibrous connective tissue.

Staples cause less inflammatory reaction than sutures, have similar strength up to 21 days, and result in a similar final appearance when removed within 1 week postoperatively. Large wounds can be closed faster and more expeditiously with staples, which are useful for procedures such as abdominoplasty, reduction mammaplasty, and skin grafting.

11. What influences the permanent appearance of suture marks?

The key factors influencing scarring due to suture placement are (1) length of time that the skin suture remains in place; (2) tension on the wound edges; (3) region of the body; (4) presence of infection; and (5) tendency for hypertrophic scarring or keloid formation. The most critical factors in avoiding suture marks in the skin are tension-free closure and early removal. Sutures left in place for excessive periods result in severe scarring. Epithelial cells crawl along the path of the suture within the skin, resulting in sinus tract formation; cross-hatching occurs from prolonged compression of the suture on the epidermal surface. Wounds in which sutures are removed within 7 days usually produce a fine linear scar. Wound closure with a running dermal pull-out suture provides the optimal scar without interfering with the development of tensile strength. The finest sutures for any given wound should be used. The timing of removal depends on the region of the body in which the sutures have been placed and ranges from 3–5 days in the face to 10–14 days in the back and extremities.

12. What are Langer's lines?

Elastic fibers within the dermis maintain the skin in a state of constant tension, as demonstrated by the gaping of wounds created by incising the dermis or by the immediate contraction of skin grafts as they are harvested. In 1861, Langer demonstrated that puncturing the skin of cadavers with a rounded sharp object resulted in elliptical holes produced by the tension of the skin. He stated that human skin was less distensible in the direction of the lines of tension than across them. Short-comings of Langer's lines are that (1) some tension lines were found to run across natural creases, wrinkles, and flexion lines; (2) they exist in excised skin; and (3) they do not correlate with the direction of dermal collagen fiber orientation. Nonetheless, Langer's lines serve as a useful guide in the planning and design of skin incisions and excisions.

13. What are RSTLs?

Relaxed skin tension lines (RSTLs), also known as wrinkle lines, natural skin lines, lines of facial expression, or lines of minimal tension, lie perpendicular to the long axis of the underlying facial muscles. They are accentuated by contraction of the facial muscles as with smiling, frowning, grimacing, puckering the lips, or closing the eyes tightly. An example is the frontalis muscle, which runs vertically straight up the forehead; RSTLs on the forehead run transversely or perpendicular to the underlying frontalis muscle.

14. What is the optimal scar?

The optimal scar is a fine, flat, concealed linear scar lying within or parallel to a skin wrinkle or natural skin line, contour junction, or RSTL. There should be no contour irregularity, distortion of adjacent anatomic or aesthetic units or landmarks, or pigmentation changes.

15. What causes "stretch" marks?

Significant stretch may result in disruption of the dermis with loss of continuity of the elastic fibers. Once this occurs, elastic recoil and skin tension in the involved area are lost—the result is a stretch mark.

16. Which excisional methods can be used for removal of skin lesions?

Skin lesions may be removed by elliptical, wedge, or circular excisions. Most skin lesions are removed by **simple elliptical excision** with the long axis of the ellipse on, or paralleling, a wrinkle, contour line, or RSTL. The ellipse may be lenticular in shape with angular edges or have rounded edges. Ideally, the long axis should be four times longer than the short axis. **Wedge excisions** are performed primarily for lesions on the free margins of the ears, lips, eyelids, or nostrils. Lip lesions can be excised as either triangular or pentagonal wedges. Pentagonal rather than triangular excision often leads to less contracture and shortening along the longitudinal axis of the incision with a more favorable scar. Closure of **circular defects** can be performed by either a skin graft or a local flap.

17. What is the purpose of serial excisions?

Large lesions, such as giant nevi, can be removed by serial excisions. This approach takes advantage of the viscoelastic properties of skin and the creep and stress-relaxation phenomenon. It has been especially useful for improvement of male-pattern baldness by excision of non–hair-bearing areas of the scalp. However, with the introduction of soft tissue expansion, the technique of serial excision has become less popular.

18. What are the differences among rotation, transposition, and interpolation flaps?

Each of these flaps has a specific pivot point and an arc through which the flap is rotated. The line of greatest tension of the flap is the radius of that arc. The **rotation flap** is a semicircular flap, whereas the **transposition flap** is a rectangular flap, consisting of skin and subcutaneous tissue that rotates about a pivot point into an immediately adjacent defect. The flap donor site can be closed by direct suturing or with a skin graft. A small backcut from the pivot point along the base of the flap can be made to release a flap that is under too much tension. Because a skin flap rotated about a pivot point becomes shorter in length the farther it is rotated, the transposition flap is usually designed to extend beyond the defect; a sufficient flap design is verified with a cloth template. An **interpolation flap**, although similar in design to the rotation and transposition flaps, is rotated into a nearby but *not* immediately adjacent defect. The pedicle of this flap, therefore, must pass over or under the intervening tissue.

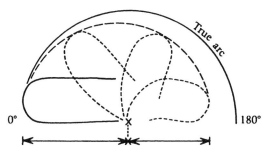

A skin flap rotated about a pivot point becomes shorter in effective length the farther it is rotated. Therefore, a flap should be designed to extend beyond the defect. (From Place MJ, Herber SC, Hardesty RA: Basic techniques and principles in plastic surgery. In Aston SJ, Beasley RW, Thorne CHM (eds): Grabb and Smith's Plastic Surgery, 5th ed. Philadelphia, Lippincott-Raven, 1997, p 22, with permission.)

19. What is a bilobed flap?

A bilobed flap is a transposition flap that consists of two flaps often designed at right angles to each other. The primary flap is transposed into the defect, whereas the secondary flap, usually half the diameter of the primary flap, is used to close the donor site.

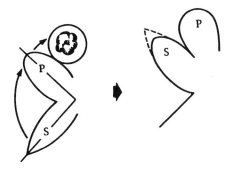

Bilobed flap. After excision of the lesion, the primary flap (P) is transposed into the resultant defect. The secondary flap (S) is then transposed to close the donor site defect. (From Place MJ, Herber SC, Hardesty RA: Basic techniques and principles in plastic surgery. In Aston SJ, Beasley RW, Thorne CHM (eds): Grabb and Smith's Plastic Surgery, 5th ed. Philadelphia, Lippincott-Raven, 1997, p 23, with permission.)

20. What is a "dog ear"? How can it be eliminated?

In excising a lesion in elliptical fashion, the long axis should be four times the length of the short axis. Dog ears form at the ends of a closed wound when either the ellipse is made too short or one side of the ellipse is longer than the other. Dog ears may flatten over time, but primary correction is best. If the elliptical excision is too short, one can lengthen the ellipse to include the excessive tissue or excise the redundant tissue as two small triangles. If one side of the incision is longer than the other, the dog ear can be corrected by making a short right-angle or 45° incision at the end of the ellipse with removal of the redundant tissue.

21. When should scar revision be performed? What are the goals?

Scar revision should be performed once the scar has matured—usually 9 months to 2 years after the original procedure. The goals of scar revision are to reorient the scar, divide it into smaller segments, and make it level with adjacent tissue.

22. What is a Z-plasty?

Referred to by Limberg as "converging triangular flaps," the Z-plasty is a technique by which two triangular flaps are interdigitated without tension, producing a gain in length along the direction of the common limb of the Z (useful in the management of scar contractures) as well as a change in the direction of the common limb of the Z (useful in the management of facial scars).

23. How is a Z-plasty designed?

A Z-plasty consists of a central limb, usually placed along the scar or line of contracture, and two limbs positioned to resemble a Z or reverse Z. The limbs must be equal in length to permit the skin flaps to fit together after transposition. The angles of the Z vary from 30–90°. The central limb, oriented along the line of contracture, is usually under considerable tension. After release or division of this contracture, the shape of the parallelogram immediately changes with spontaneous flap transposition and lengthening along the line of the central limb. Lengthening is related to the difference between the long and short axes of the parallelogram formed by the Z. The wider the angles of the triangular flaps, the greater the difference between the long and short diagonals and thus the greater the lengthening. In designing a Z-plasty, sufficient laxity must be available transversely to achieve the appropriate lengthening perpendicular to it. The limbs of the Z-plasty should follow the RSTLs.

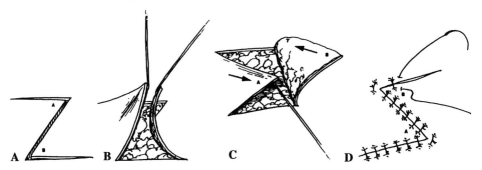

rClassic Z-plasty using 60° angles. *A* and *B*, Flap design and elevation. *C* and *D*, Flap transposition and suture without tension. (From Weinzweig N, Weinzweig J: Basic principles and techniques in plastic surgery. In Cohen M (ed): Mastery of Plastic and Reconstructive Surgery. Boston, Little, Brown, 1994, p 26, with permission.)

24. Why are angle size and limb length important in performing a Z-plasty?

The angle size determines the percentage increase in length. The original limb length controls the absolute increase in final limb length. As the angle size increases, the degree of lengthening increases. A 30° angle produces a 25% increase in length; a 45° angle, a 50% increase; a 60° angle, a 75% increase; a 75° angle, a 100% increase; and a 90° angle, a 120% increase. Although the length increase values are only theoretical, they provide a good approximation of the actual lengthening. In general, the actual increase in length is slightly less than the theoretical increase.

25. What is the optimal angle for Z-plasty design?

60°. Angles significantly less than 60° do not achieve sufficient lengthening, defeating the purpose of the Z-plasty and resulting in flap narrowing and vascular compromise. Angles much greater than 60° produce significant tension in the adjacent tissue, preventing transposition of the flaps.

26. What are the indications for multiple Z-plasties?
A similar degree of lengthening can be produced by a single Z-plasty and multiple Z-plasties, because the total length of the central limbs of multiple Z-plasties can equal the length of the single Z-plasty. Multiple Z-plasties, however, produce less transverse shortening. Lateral tension is reduced and more equally distributed over the entire length of the central limbs. Multiple Z-plasties are useful when insufficient tissue is available for a large single Z-plasty. In addition, multiple Z-plasties of facial scars often produce cosmetically superior results.

27. What is a four-flap Z-plasty?
A four-flap Z-plasty is an effective technique to correct thumb-index web space and axillary contractures. A 90°/90° angle or 120°/120° angle Z-plasty is designed. The two-flap Z-plasty is then converted to a four-flap Z-plasty by bisecting the angles, creating flaps that are 45° or 60°. This technique produces greater lengthening (124%) with less tension on the flaps.

28. What is a double-opposing Z-plasty?
Also known as the combination five-flap Y-V advancement and Z-plasty, the double-opposing Z-plasty is particularly useful for releasing contractures of concave regions of the body, such as the dorsum of the interdigital web spaces and the medial canthal region. The central flap is advanced in Y-V fashion while the flaps of the two Z-plasties on each side of the central flap are transposed.

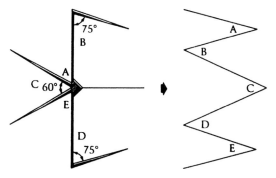

Five-flap Y-V advancement and Z-plasty. The central flap (C) is advanced in a Y-V fashion. The flaps of the two Z-plasties on each side of the central flap are transposed. (From Jankauskas S, Cohen IK, Grabb WC: Basic techniques in plastic surgery. In Smith JW, Aston SJ (eds): Grabb and Smith's Plastic Surgery, 4th ed. Boston, Little, Brown, 1991, p 76, with permission.)

29. What is a W-plasty?
A W-plasty is another technique for reorienting the direction of a linear scar. Triangles of equal size are outlined on either side of the scar with the tip of the triangle on one side placed at the midpoint of the base of the triangle on the opposite side. At the ends of the scar, the excised triangles should be smaller, with the limbs of the W tapered. The tips of the triangles should be sutured with three-corner stitches to prevent necrosis of the flap tips.

30. What is the main disadvantage of a W-plasty?
A W-plasty does not lengthen a contracted linear scar; a Z-plasty should be used for this purpose. A W-plasty increases rather than decreases tension in the area of the scar because of the necessary sacrifice of tissue and should be used only when there is an abundance of tissue adjacent to the scar.

31. What is the V-Y advancement technique?
The V-Y advancement technique allows forward advancement of a triangular flap (V) without rotation or lateral movement and closure of the resulting defect in a Y fashion. The skin that is actually advanced is on either side of the V.

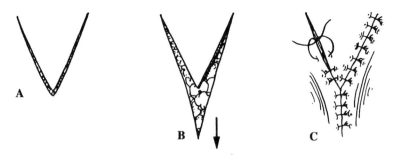

V-Y advancement technique. The central V is advanced forward and the defect is closed in a Y configuration. (From Weinzweig N, Weinzweig J: Basic principles and techniques in plastic surgery. In Cohen M (ed): Mastery of Plastic and Reconstructive Surgery. Boston, Little, Brown, 1994, p 26, with permission.)

32. When is a V-Y advancement flap used?

This technique is extremely useful for lengthening the nasal columella, correcting the whistle deformity of the lip, and closure of selected soft tissue defects. It also may be used in various other skin and mucosal flaps.

33. What is a rhombic flap?

The rhombic flap, originally described by Limberg and often referred to as the Limberg flap, is a combination of rotation and transposition flaps that borrows adjacent loose skin for coverage of a rhombic defect. A rhombus is an equilateral parallelogram with (1) acute angles of 60° and obtuse angles of 120°; (2) long and short diagonals perpendicular to each other; and (3) a short diagonal equal in length to each side of the rhombus. The flap is designed as an extension of the short diagonal opposite either of the two 120° angles of the rhombus. The short diagonal is extended by a distance equal to its length. From this point, a line of equal length is drawn at 60° parallel to either side of the rhombus. Four Limberg flaps are therefore possible for any given rhombic defect.

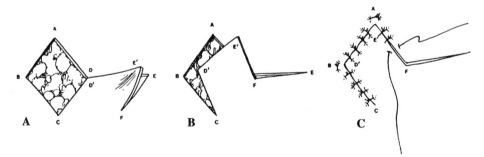

Rhombic flap. A, Flap design. B, Elevation of flap with wide undermining of the base to allow transposition. C, Suture of the flap without tension. (From Weinzweig N, Weinzweig J: Basic principles and techniques in plastic surgery. In Cohen M (ed): Mastery of Plastic and Reconstructive Surgery. Boston, Little, Brown, 1994, p 26, with permission.)

34. Should lesions be excised to create rhombic defects?

No. Lesions should be excised as circular defects or as necessary to permit adequate excision. A rhombus encompassing the defect and the four possible rhombic flaps can then be drawn. The selected flap is incised and elevated. Wide undermining beneath the base of the flap is necessary to allow the flap to fall into position in the rhombic defect without tension. The initial sutures are placed in the four corners of the defect.

35. What is the Dufourmental flap?

The Dufourmental flap is a variation of the rhombic flap in which the angles differ from the standard 60° and 120° angles in the Limberg flap. Although angles of 30° and 150° are usually used, angles up to 90° are also possible. This versatile flap is useful for coverage of a defect in the shape of a rhomboid rather than a rhombus. Although the two terms are often used interchangeably, a rhomboid differs from a rhombus in several important respects: (1) it has acute angles of various degrees; (2) only opposite sides are equal in length; (3) diagonals are not perpendicular; (4) diagonals are not equal in length; and (5) diagonals are not necessarily equal in length to the sides of the parallelogram. Planning is more complex than for the Limberg flap, and it is often easier simply to convert the defect into a rhombus with angles of 60° and 120°.

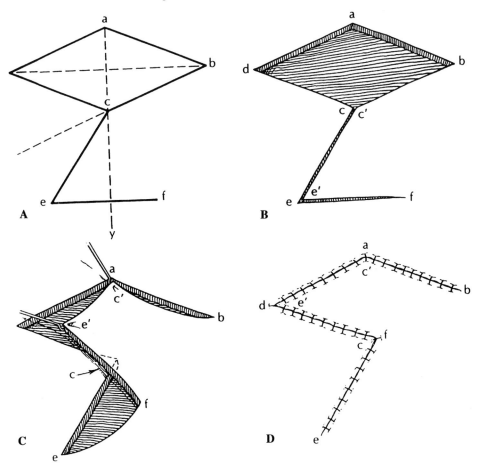

The Dufourmental flap. *A* and *B*, Flap design. *C*, Flap elevation and transposition. *D*, Resultant suture lines. (From Jackson IT: Local Flaps in Head and Neck Reconstruction. St. Louis, Mosby, 1985, p 20, with permission.)

BIBLIOGRAPHY

1. Borges AF: Elective Incisions and Scar Revision. Boston, Little, Brown, 1973.
2. Borges AF: Choosing the correct Limberg flap. Plast Reconstr Surg 62:542, 1978.
3. Borges AF: W-plasty. Ann Plast Surg 3:153, 1979.
4. Jackson IT: Local Flaps in Head and Neck Reconstruction. St. Louis, Mosby, 1995.
5. Limberg AA: The Planning of Local Plastic Surgical Operations. Lexington, MA, Collamore Press, 1984 [translated by SA Wolfe].
6. McGregor IA: The Z-plasty. Br J Plast Surg 19:82, 1966.
7. McGregor IA: Fundamental Techniques in Plastic Surgery and Their Surgical Applications, 7th ed. Edinburgh, Churchill Livingstone, 1980.
8. Jankauskas S, Cohen IK, Grabb WC: Basic technique of plastic surgery. In Smith JW, Aston SJ (eds): Grabb and Smith's Plastic Surgery, fourth edition, Boston, Little, Brown and Company, 1991, pp. 3-90.
9. Weinzweig N, Weinzweig J: Basic principles and techniques in plastic surgery. In Cohen M (ed): Mastery of Plastic and Reconstructive Surgery. Boston, Little, Brown, 1994.

3. ANESTHESIA

Brent V. Stromberg, M.D., F.A.C.S.

1. What is the maximal dose of lidocaine that can be safely used for local anesthesia?
Lidocaine is probably the most commonly used local anesthetic agent. The maximal safe dose is 4 mg/kg. The addition of epinephrine to the anesthetic solution (usually in a 1:100,000 concentration), which slows the absorption of lidocaine due to local vasoconstriction, allows a maximal dose of 7 mg/kg.

2. Which nerves exit the skull through foramina that lie in a sagittal plane?
The supraorbital, infraorbital, and mental nerves exit the skull along a straight line, approximately 2.5 cm from the midline of the face, that includes the pupil of the eye in a midgaze position. The ability to identify these nerves by surface anatomy is crucial to performing successful regional blocks of the face. Aspiration prior to instillation of an anesthetic agent is always advisable to avoid intraarterial injection.

3. How can the forehead and upper eyelid be blocked to permit excision of a large lipoma?
Regional blocks of the supraorbital and supratrochlear nerves provide effective anesthesia of the forehead area. The supraorbital nerve (V_1) emerges from the supraortibal foramen to supply sensation to the upper eyelid, conjunctiva, forehead, and scalp as far posteriorly as the lambdoid suture; the supratrochlear nerve emerges from the medial aspect of the supraorbital rim to supply the medial aspect of the forehead, upper eyelid, skin of the upper nose, and conjunctiva. A supraorbital nerve block is performed by inserting the needle just under the midportion of the eyebrow while palpating the foramen and injecting 2–3 ml of 1% lidocaine with epinephrine. A supratrochlear nerve block is performed similarly except that the needle is inserted in the medial portion of the orbital rim just lateral to the root of the nose. Both nerves can be blocked by infiltration along a horizontal line extending 2 cm above the eyebrow from the lateral orbital rim to the midline.

4. Which nerve provides sensation to the lower eyelid and upper lip? How can it be blocked?
The infraorbital nerve (V_2), after emerging from the infraorbital foramen, divides into four branches—the inferior palpebral, external nasal, internal nasal, and superior labial nerves. They supply the lower eyelid and upper lip as well as the lateral portion of the nose and ala, cheek, and mucous membranes lining the cheek and upper lip. Regional block of the infraorbital nerve is performed by first palpating the infraorbital foramen or notch along the infraorbital rim, which should lie below the midline of the pupil with the eye in a straight forward gaze. Instillation of 2–5 ml of 1% lidocaine with epinephrine at this site provides excellent regional anesthesia for 60–90 minutes.

5. How can the lower lip be anesthetized to permit excision of a basal cell carcinoma?
The mental nerve provides sensation to the lower lip and the submental cutaneous area. This nerve can be blocked transorally or transcutaneously as it exits the mental foramen. It can be palpated just posterior to the first premolar tooth 1 cm below the gum line. Intraorally the needle can be inserted into the mucous membrane between the bicuspids at a 45° angle, aimed toward the apex of the root of the second bicuspid, and advanced until bone is contacted. The needle is withdrawn 1–2 mm, and 2–3 ml of lidocaine are injected. An additional 0.5–1.0 ml of lidocaine can be injected if the foramen is located.

6. How can the masseter muscle be relaxed in cases of trismus?
A mandibular nerve (V_3) block can be performed as the nerve exits the foramen ovale by inserting the needle into the retromolar fossa at a point parallel to the mandibular teeth at a 45° angle. The needle is advanced to the posterior wall of the mandible, and the injection is instilled. This block anesthetizes the buccal, auriculotemporal, lingual, inferior alveolar, and mental nerves, providing adequate surgical anesthesia for the lower face, mandible, mandibular teeth to the midline, and anterior two-thirds of the tongue for 60–90 minutes.

7. **How can adequate regional anesthesia of the nose be obtained before performing a rhinoplasty?**

Regional anesthesia of the external nose can be obtained by blocking the infratrochlear, infraorbital, nasal palatine, and external nasal nerves. The block is performed by injecting 5–10 ml of 1% lidocaine with epinephrine along a line that begins at the nasolabial fold, continues just lateral to the ala and along the base of the nasal sidewall, and finally advances toward the radix on each side of the nose. Regional anesthesia of the internal nose can be obtained by blocking the inferior posterior nasal, nasopalatine, and superior posterior nasal nerves as well as branches of the ethmoidal nerve. The block is performed by placing small cotton applicators dipped in a solution of 4% cocaine directly on the areas or by packing the nose with plain gauze dipped in the cocaine solution.

8. **How can a regional block of the external ear be obtained before performing an otoplasty?**

The external ear is supplied by the auriculotemporal nerve anteriorly and by the great auricular and lesser occipital nerves posteriorly. A satisfactory block can be achieved by infiltrating the anesthetic solution (usually 1% lidocaine with epinephrine) around the ear in a ringlike fashion or by using a diamond-shaped pattern that encompasses the ear anteriorly and posteriorly.

9. **Just before an augmentation mammaplasty, bilateral intercostal nerve blocks are given with 30 ml of a 1% xylocaine solution. The patient soon appears agitated, and her pulse increases. What is the most likely cause?**

Sudden changes in the status of the patient are always a cause of concern. In this situation, the most worrisome possibility is a pneumothorax. Intercostal blocks are administered close to the pleura. Even a small increase in depth of penetration may result in injury to the lung. However, the most likely cause of the symptoms is lidocaine toxicity. Several areas of the body, including the intercostal area, have a high degree of vascularity and are known to have a much faster uptake of local anesthetics. The proximity of the intercostal vessels to the point of injection frequently results in a more rapid systemic uptake than expected. The dosage of xylocaine is at the upper limits of safety. A smaller volume and dosage are preferred. Fortunately, lidocaine toxicity usually passes quickly in a healthy patient because the compound is metabolized rapidly in the liver. Medication with a barbiturate, often already administered as a premedication, may be helpful. The usual treatment is monitoring and patience.

10. **How long should a patient fast before surgery?**

The tradition of nothing to eat or drink after midnight the night before seems to have few objective merits. For adults, several studies have shown that solid foods should not be given within 6 hours of surgery but that clear liquids may be given up to 3 hours before surgery. However, some believe that if a large meal has been eaten the night before, 6 hours may not be enough. For infants, reasonable amounts of fluids up to 3 hours before surgery seem safe. Several hours of fasting before surgery do not seem to decrease the amount of gastric contents or to increase the pH of the gastric fluid. It does significantly increase the discomfort of the patient. Prophylaxis against aspiration is of merit in high-risk patients, but it is not universally beneficial.

11. **Why does skeletal muscle contract if stimulated when D-tubocurarine is used as the paralyzing agent in anesthesia?**

D-tubocurarine blocks muscle contraction by acting as a nondepolarizing agent. As such, it blocks nerve transmission at the neuromuscular junction. It does not block direct muscle stimulation by an electrical stimulus such as electrocautery. If complete cessation of muscle contraction is needed, succinylcholine should be used because it depolarizes the muscle and keeps it depolarized.

12. **Twenty-four hours after suction-assisted lipectomy of the abdomen and upper thighs, a patient has become confused and somewhat disoriented. She has a petechial rash over the shoulders and anterior chest. Is she possibly allergic to the pain medication?**

This presentation is unusual for an allergic reaction to a medication. However, it is a relatively classic presentation for fat embolism. A fat embolism involves the blockage of small vessels by small globules of fat. Most commonly seen after long bone fractures, it also may be seen in other circumstances, such as after liposuction. Two theories address the mechanism. A physiochemical change in the circulating lipids (chylomicrons) may cause them to clump and form microemboli (fat droplets). The second theory states that the trauma from pressure or injury allows small veins to rupture and fat to enter directly through the area of injury. The emboli lodge in small caliber vascular structures, first the lungs and then the brain and kidneys. Although the cerebral manifestations are often the first noticed (confusion, lethargy, disorientation, delirium, and occasionally coma and stupor), the primary problem rests with the lungs. The diagnosis should be made quickly; it depends on prompt recognition of a pattern of pulmonary, cerebral, and cutaneous manifestations. Emboli may appear in retinal vessels. Other abnormalities may include a drop in hemoglobin and an EKG pattern of myocardial ischemia and right ventricular strain. Later lipuria may occur. Serum lipase elevation occurs in one-half of patients but may not be evident for several days and reaches its height on day 7 or 8.

Once the diagnosis is made, prompt treatment should include vigorous resuscitative measures, splinting of any fractures, intensive pulmonary care, oxygen, positive end-expiratory pressure (PEEP), intermittent positive pressure breathing, and consideration of digitalization. Corticosteroids are usually recommended (approximately 100 mg every 6 hours). Often low-dose heparin is given to increase the lipase activity (25 mg every 6 hours).

13. What are the appropriate preoperative preparations and intraoperative and postoperative considerations for a patient with possible sickle cell disease who is to undergo hand surgery?

Before surgery the patient should be well-hydrated. Preoperative transfusions are indicated only if blood loss has been massive or the hematocrit is below 20% (hemoglobin less than 7 gm/100 ml). Patients with sickle cell disease normally tolerate hemocrit levels of 25–30%.

During surgery the patient should be well-oxygenated. Inspired oxygen concentrations of 40–50% are adequate. Ideally the patient should be preoxygenated. In addition, the body temperature should be kept normal. Hypothermia may promote sickling. Many sources advise against the use of tourniquets. However, tourniquets have been safely used without evidence of sickling or precipitation of a crisis. If the patient is well-hydrated and well-oxygenated, tourniquets are safe. Postoperatively the same principles apply.

Sickle cell crisis is treated with bed rest, hydration, oxygenation, analgesics, sodium bicarbonate for acidosis, and possibly transfusions.

14. What are the anesthetic considerations for repair of a trochanteric decubitus ulcer in the lateral position?

During surgery, the position of the patient causes several changes that may be important to the surgeon. In the lateral decubitus position, blood pools in the lower or dependent portion. Pooling may be worsened if the patient is also paraplegic because autonomic regulation of the circulatory system is less effective. In addition, the lateral position limits expansion of the lungs by limiting chest movement. As the dependent lung is compressed, a ventilation/perfusion mismatch occurs, causing increases in physiologic dead space and carbon dioxide retention. Hypoxemia may result. The usual treatment is PEEP.

15. A patient vomits and aspirates during induction of anesthesia. What is the appropriate treatment?

Immediately upon consideration of aspiration the patient should be tilted to a head-down position, which allows residual gastric contents to drain. The mouth and pharyngeal regions should be suctioned, and endotracheal intubation should be performed immediately. Suctioning through the endotracheal tube should precede administration of positive pressure oxygen. After endotracheal suctioning 100% oxygen should be given. The insertion of a nasogastric tube should be prompt, and the pH of the aspirate should be determined. The significant pH level is 2.5. A pH above 2.5 yields a physiologic response that is not much different from aspiration of water. A pH below 2.5 significantly increases the risk of aspiration pneumonia. A pH below 1.5 involves significant risk of pulmonary damage.

Possibly the earliest sign of significant aspiration is hypoxia. If blood gas analysis shows any element of hypoxia, positive pressure ventilation should be instituted immediately. Adjunctive measures such as antibiotics and steroids have been proposed. Prophylactic antibiotics are not currently recommended. The use of corticosteroids remains controversial.

16. What preoperative instructions should be given for a 10-month-old child before cleft lip repair?

In the past, the policy was avoidance of oral ingestion for 8 hours. However, studies of younger children show that giving clear fluids to infants up to three hours before surgery is safe. This principle applies at least through adolescence. Preoperative sedation is also possible and sometimes helpful; a typical agent is pentobarbital, 5 mg/kg. For children less than 6 months old, pentobarbital is probably unnecessary.

Intraoperatively the use of lidocaine and epinephrine as a local injection is helpful. Large doses of epinephrine are not recommended in patients under halothane anesthesia. However, halothane is becoming less used as a general anesthetic agent. In addition, the maximal dose of epinephrine, 10 mg/kg, is rarely exceeded because of the small volumes required. Usually a 1-cc total of injection solution is adequate.

17. What is the critical anesthetic problem in a patient with cleft palate? How is it managed?

Establishment and protection of the airway are the key issues in repair of the cleft palate. During intubation and positioning, frequently with the neck hyperextended, maintenance of the airway is crucial, along with meticulous attention to positioning of the endotracheal tube. Postoperatively attention should be given to monitoring of airway obstruction, bleeding, and respiratory obstruction. Airway obstruction secondary to edema is possible. Significant blood loss may occur with repair of the palate, considering the size of the child. Requirement of blood transfusion is unusual, but loss of up to 200 cc of blood has been reported. Postoperatively careful attention to airway monitoring and careful suctioning of the pharynx are necessary. Some physicians recommend placement of a traction suture in the tongue in case posterior obstruction due to the tongue occurs. Use of an oral or a nasal airway is contraindicated because of the significant risk of disrupting the surgical repair. Either a lateral or prone position with the patient's head turned to one side and dependent is believed to be optimal. This position is easily achieved by placing a small towel or blanket under the child's hips.

18. A 10-year-old girl is scheduled to undergo a bilateral otoplasty for prominent ears. The parents are concerned because an uncle died during anesthesia several years ago. During the course of anesthesia the patient develops tachycardia, early cyanosis, and some increased rigidity in the muscles. What are the probable diagnosis and appropriate treatment?

Preoperative consideration of possible malignant hyperthermia is necessary. The family history of an anesthetic death is important. Approximately one-third of the cases of malignant hyperthermia occur in patients who have had previous uneventful anesthesia.

Malignant hyperthermia is a clinical syndrome characterized by accelerated metabolism, which usually manifests as tachycardia, cyanosis, sweating, rigidity, blood pressure abnormalities, and an increase in end-tidal CO_2. Only 30% of patients display an increase in temperature. However, when temperature is elevated, it commonly goes as high as 42° or 43° C. The family history is frequently positive for musculoskeletal abnormalities.

If possible, anesthesia should be performed using barbiturate sedation and local anesthetics. Both ester and amide local anesthetics are safe. All inhalation anesthetics, except nitrous oxide, are considered unsafe. Curare and phenothiazines are controversial. Most other drugs are considered safe, including antibiotics, propofol, barbiturates, opiates, antipyretics, and antihistamines.

If malignant hyperthermia is suspected during surgery, all anesthetics should be stopped and 100% oxygen should be administered. The patient should be hyperventilated, good access should be obtained for monitoring of central venous pressure, and an arterial line should be inserted. Dantrolene sodium should be administered at a dose of 2.5 mg/kg. This dose may be supplemented with 1-mg boluses to a total of 10 mg/kg. Rapid cooling should be initiated for core temperatures of about 40° C. Acidosis and hyperkalemia should be treated (sodium bicarbonate, 2 mEq/kg). Arrhythmias usually respond to procainamide (15 mg/kg). Cardiorespiratory support and monitoring should be available.

Postoperatively, coagulopathy, renal failure, hypothermia, pulmonary edema, hyperkalemia, and recurrence are possible. Dantrolene should be given for approximately 3 days after the attack. In addition, the family and patient should be counseled about the event and its significance.

19. Why is sodium bicarbonate sometimes added to local anesthetics?

Local anesthetics are in a balanced solution between ionized and nonionized forms. The nonionized form goes into the nerve tissue more rapidly. Alkalinization of the solution changes the concentration of the nonionized form and thereby increases the rapidity of onset and effectiveness. Appropriate doses of sodium bicarbonate are 1 mEq/10 ml of lidocaine and 0.1 mEq/20 ml of bupivacaine.

20. A patient with a 25% total body surface area burn is taken to the operating room for tangential excision and grafting of burn wounds 2 weeks after injury. During induction of anesthesia, succinylcholine is given as a muscle relaxant. The patient begins to show cardiac irregularities, and the procedure is terminated. What is the probable cause?

Although the exact mechanism of this response is somewhat unclear, a profound release of potassium from muscle has been well documented in burn patients after administration of succinylcholine. An increased number of muscle receptor sites for acetylcholine has been documented in burn victims. The agonist to acetylcholine, succinylcholine, may be responsible for the massive, and sometimes fatal, release of potassium. This response has been documented almost $1\frac{1}{2}$ years after the burn. For this reason, succinylcholine is not recommended as a muscle relaxer in burn patients for up to 2 years after injury. Nondepolarizing relaxants are recommended, such as D-tubocurarine, pancuronium, Atracurium, and Vecuronium. Even these agents show a variable response in burn patients. Although they are generally considered safe, patients may show variable degrees of resistance. Monitoring with a nerve stimulator is important.

21. During tangential excision of a 30% full-thickness burn, a patient begins to become hypotensive. What are the most likely causes?

Burn wound debridement, although relatively straightforward from a surgical point of view, involves complex anesthetic concerns. The patient is metabolically unstable because of the severe injury. Strict attention to fluid and electrolytes is required. A massive amount of fluids can be lost not only through the burn itself but also through exposure of injured skin and the heating effect of the dry air in the room. Underestimation of fluid loss is common. In addition, the possibility of sensitivity to medications should be considered. In burn patients, one of the most common sensitivities is transfusion reaction. Administration of blood intraoperatively is routine, but a hemolytic type reaction may occur when incompatible blood is administered. Although rare because of high blood bank standards, this problem still occurs. In awake patients signs include hypotension, fever, chills, shortness of breath, and pain. However, under general anesthesia the only sign is unexplained hypotension. Documentation by showing free hemoglobin in the urine is helpful, but response to the hypotension takes precedence. Treatment consists of cessation of surgery and all blood products, hydration, vasopressors, and inotropic agents, if necessary. Urine output should be maintained by rapid administration of fluids, and diuretics such as mannitol and loop agents should be considered. Historically, sodium bicarbonate has been proposed. The rationale is that alkalinized urine improves the solubility of the hemoglobin and its breakdown components. The actual value of this strategy has been poorly documented. Another possible cause of hypotension during anesthesia is the overadministration of narcotics and sedatives. The proper anesthetic protocol in a burn patient always consists of careful, slow titration of agents.

22. What is the maximal amount of bupivacaine (Marcaine) that can be added to 50 ml of 0.5% xylocaine in an intravenous regional anesthetic for the upper extermity to prolong duration of action?

None. The long action of bupivacaine on skeletal muscle results in a significant risk of cardiotoxicity if it is given intravenously. Although there are a few anecdotal reports of its use, intravenous injection is absolutely contraindicated.

23. A 65-year-old man is scheduled to undergo general anesthesia for extensive resection of an oral cancer 4 months after having a myocardial infarction. Should surgery be delayed?

This is a difficult problem. Multiple studies have consistently shown that perioperative morbidity, reinfarction, and mortality are significantly greater if general anesthesia is used within 6 months of a myocardial infarction. The general status of the patient as well as the status of his cardiac disease should be evaluated. If the patient can climb stairs and perform simple exercises without becoming short of breath, demonstrating cardiac arrythmia, developing chest pain, or having significant symptoms, he may be considered for surgery if medically necessary. On the other hand, presence of any of the above signs or symptoms is significant. Also important are the expertise of the anesthesiologist in dealing with cardiac patients and the severity and duration of the procedure.

24. When is it usually considered safe to discharge a patient after outpatient surgery under general anesthesia?

Although each facility needs to establish its own criteria, they usually include stable blood pressure and pulse, respirations within 20% of preoperative values, alert and oriented mental status, and steady gait with minimal or no assistance. Also important are absence of active bleeding, controllable pain, minimal nausea, and discharge with an appropriate, trustworthy adult.

BIBLIOGRAPHY

1. Apfelbaum JL: Current concepts in outpatient anesthesia. Anesthesia Research Society Review Course Lectures, 1989, p 104.
2. Barash PG, Cullen BF, Stoelting RK (eds): Clinical Anesthesia. Philadelphia, J.B. Lippincott, 1989.
3. Eckenoff JE, Vandam LD (eds): Introduction to Anesthesia: The Principles of Safe Practice, 7th ed. Philadelphia, W.B. Saunders, 1988.
4. Miller RD (ed): Anesthesia, 3rd ed. New York, Churchill Livingstone,
5. Schwarz SI (ed): Principles of Surgery, 5th ed. New York, McGraw-Hill, 1989.
6. Stromberg BV: Anesthesia. In McCarthy JH (ed): Plastic Surgery. Philadelphia, W.B. Saunders, 1990.
7. Vandam LD (ed): To Make the Patient Ready for Anesthesia: Medical Care of the Surgical Patient, 2nd ed. Menlo Park, CA, Addison-Wesley, 1984.
8. Weinzweig N, Weinzweig J: Basic principles and techniques in plastic surgery. In Cohen M (ed): Mastery of Plastic and Reconstructive Surgery. Boston, Little, Brown, 1994, pp 14–33.
9. White PF (ed): Outpatient Anesthesia. New York, Churchill Livingstone, 1990.

4. TISSUE EXPANSION

Ernest K. Manders, M.D.

1. Is controlled tissue expansion a phenomenon of the past 40 years or so?

No. It originated sometime in antiquity when our ancestors decided to expand earlobes or lips by inserting objects of ever larger diameter. In this century, Dr. Charles Neumann of New York was the first to carry out a controlled expansion of periauricular skin using a subcutaneous balloon filled with air. This work was reported in 1956, published in 1957, and forgotten. Soft tissue expansion entered the practice of plastic and reconstructive surgery through the efforts of the late Dr. Chedomir Radovan. Reviewers resisted his idea, and it took 3 years to get his discovery on a national program. His design of a silicone elastomer envelope with a remote self-sealing injection port became the first standard device. Periodic injections of saline were used to distend the overlying tissues to create flaps for reconstructive surgery.

2. What factors should one consider in selecting a patient for tissue expansion?

Not every patient is a suitable candidate for the use of soft tissue expansion as a reconstructive technique. The patient must understand that two operations are required, that the temporary deformity may be inconvenient and hard to disguise, and that it is impossible to say exactly when the expansion will be complete. Patients must understand that the process must be afforded the time required to generate the tissue necessary for reconstruction. Patients who specify that the expansion must be completed over the summer are imposing limitations on the technique and may be disappointed when the actual advancement falls short of the goal. All patients should be counseled that two expansions may be required.

3. Where should expanders be placed?

Expanders should be placed under tissue that best matches the lost tissue; similar tissue gives the best reconstruction. Normal landmarks must not be distorted. For example, the eyebrow should not be undermined and moved. It is of paramount importance that the surgeon ask, "Where do I want the final scars to lie?" The reconstruction should begin with the goal of imposing a minimum of scars. Vascular territories and patterns of innervation should be preserved whenever possible.

4. What expanders are available?

Expanders come in a wide variety of sizes and styles. They may be small, perhaps a few cubic centimeters in size, or designed to hold a liter or more. The devices may be fitted with remote injection ports or ports integrated into the envelopes themselves. The envelopes may be bonded to stiff backers or have no back. The expanders may be round, rectangular, oval, or crescent-shaped (the croissant expander). The envelope may be of uniform thickness and compliance or may be constructed to expand differentially or directionally. The envelope may be smooth or textured on its outer surface.

5. What are the advantages of the various designs?

Expanders with integrated valves are often used for breast reconstruction. They are especially useful in the head and neck because no dissection of a pocket for the remote port is required. Differential expansion is used in the design of breast reconstruction devices because more tissue is needed at the lower pole of the reconstruction site than in the upper infraclavicular area. The croissant expander is well suited for reconstruction of defects on flat or cylindrical surfaces. The defect is half surrounded by the expander, allowing better geometry of expansion with the largest expansion developed in the line of greatest advance. Remote ports can be placed atop the edge of an expander if desired; this technique effectively simulates the convenience of an integrated injection port.

6. Where do you place the incision for a tissue expander insertion?

Where to place the incision for expander insertion is somewhat controversial. Some authorities argue for a remote incision. Some assert that the incision should be oriented radially to the edge of the expander. The author believes that the best incision is usually placed at the edge of the defect. The scar in this position will be removed at the time of advancement of the expanded flap. If the defect to be replaced is a nevus, the incision should be placed entirely within the nevus so that the normal skin is not scarred and wasted. The reader is reminded of the question, "Where do I want the final scars to lie?" The incision must be made in stable tissue that is expected to heal.

7. What technical failures at the time of insertion will cause an expansion to fail?

The most common reason for the failure of an expansion is the construction of a pocket of inadequate size for the expander that is placed into it. Protrusion of the expander through the incision or projection of wrinkles of envelope through the overlying tissue often results from the surgeon's overestimation of the size of the pocket. The expander must lie flat, and the expander back, if one is present, must not be curled or flexed so that the edge pushes into the line of closure.

8. When do you begin filling an expander? How much saline do you add each time?

It is our practice to begin filling an expander 1 week after surgery if the wound is stable. The process of filling depends on the pressure in the expander. One cannot prescribe a given volume for injection at regular intervals. Often the expansion proceeds fairly rapidly and then becomes more difficult with higher ending pressures in the expander and discomfort noted by the patient. At this point the tissues need a rest. One can easily forego a weekly injection or simply inject less saline. On every occasion the safest strategy is to inject until the patient reports that the expansion is just starting to feel tight.

9. When is the patient ready to return to the operating room for advancement?

The patient is ready for advancement when the flap will produce the desired result. If the flap is to be advanced, it must have sufficient dimensions and suitable geometry to cover the defect. One measures the arc over the top of the expander and subtracts the width of the expander mass. The difference is an estimate of the advancement that can be made. The difference should equal or exceed the width of the defect.

For breast reconstruction, the expansion should proceed until the distance from the clavicle to the midmammary line at the inframammary fold on the expanded side equals or exceeds the same distance on the normal, unoperated side. Then fluid should be removed until the volume of the expander resembles that of the normal breast. The distance from the clavicle to the inframammary fold should be measured again. Most likely the distance will have shortened because the pressure on the skin and capsule are reduced by partial deflation of the expander. The fluid should be returned and expansion should continue until the partially deflated dimensions of the reconstructed skin envelope equal those of the normal breast.

10. How do you make the advancement?

The advancement should be simple. The skin in incised with a scalpel, and then an electro-cautery blade with a round, not sharp, tip is used to open the subcutaneous tissues and capsule. A needle point usually results in a punctured envelope; avoid using a needle tip. It should not be neces-sary in most cases—except nasal and ear reconstructions—to excise the capsule formed around the expander. Simply advance the expanded flap and determine that it will replace the defect *before* the defect itself is excised. If the trial advance shows that you will come up short, do a subtotal resection of the defect, leave an expander in place, and plan to finish the job on another day.

11. What aftercare is required?

Very little aftercare is required. Patients may shower on the first day after advancement. Drains are managed as usual. Do not rush to touch-up surgery, especially for dog-ears, which usually re-solve with time.

12. What touch-up surgery may be required?

The area of the body undergoing surgery determines the size of the final scar. The back usually produces a larger scar than the scalp. Infrequently dog-ears may need to be revised; be patient before attempting revision. Local areas of alopecia from hair follicles in telogen phase often reverse them-selves and hair density returns to normal. Concavities usually disappear, especially the concavities, or bathtub deformities, seen over the skull.

13. Where does the expanded skin come from?

Austad and Pasyk addressed this question. Both short-term, immediate factors and long-term changes yield an increase in dimension. In the short term, pressure forces interstitial fluid out of the tissues, allowing greater extension. Viscoelastic deformation, termed "creep," and recruitment of ad-jacent mobile soft tissue also contribute to the arc of skin over the acute expansion. Growth occurs with an increase in the collagen content and ground substance of the skin flap as dimensions increase.

14. What happens to the mitotic index of expanded skin?

In tissue culture 20–30 minutes of stretch is enough to initiate a round of DNA synthesis and cellular mitosis. The mitotic rate of skin has been demonstrated to increase with the application of tension. When the expander beneath expanded skin is deflated, the mitotic index falls to a subnormal level. This finding is thought to be consistent with clinical observations of skin contraction with weight loss and flattening of dog-ears after flap advancement.

15. Can the expander envelope rupture because of the internal expander pressure?

No. The expander envelope cannot rupture even when the patient lies on the expander. The ex-pander is contained and supported by a tough collagen capsule surrounding the expander. The cap-sule limits expansion and supports the elastomer envelope when external pressure is placed on the expander mound.

16. What limits the rate of expansion?

The rate of expansion is limited by the relaxation and growth of the tissues overlying the ex-pander. Pain is an important signal and must be avoided at all times. There should be absolutely no pain during the process of expansion. Prior irradiation and scar formation may slow expan-sion or even make it impossible. Tissues undergoing expansion must have the capacity for growth. Some tissues elongate more slowly than others and may limit the rate of expansion. Peripheral nerves do not tolerate pressures of more than 40 mmHg for sustained periods, and if a nerve is located in the expanding flap, or even immediately under an expander, paresthesias may slow the rate of inflation.

17. How many times can an expander be used?

Many times—but not in North America. The expander devices available in the North American market are extremely well engineered. The Food and Drug Administration has specified that the de-vices are meant for single use. It is our practice to save expanders after their removal. They are washed and wrapped, then sterilized and sent to surgeons and plastic surgery units in the developing world where they can be reused many times.

18. What is the effect of expansion on blood flow in the tissues over the expander?

Several independent studies have demonstrated that blood flow in expanded tissue is augmented. In our studies, the flow in a critical flap was doubled when measured with microsphere perfusion experiments. Expanded skin flaps survive to a length at least equal to that of a delayed flap. A new network of vessels just above the capsule has been demonstrated by histologic studies. These vessels involute with time after expander removal.

19. What histologic changes occur with expansion?

Other histologic changes of note are thinning of the dermis with eventual collagen realignment and deposition. The epidermis shows definite thickening. Fat may be compressed and, if subjected to high pressures, may atrophy. Thin muscles, such as the frontalis, also may suffer the same injury. Skin appendages are relatively unaffected. The hair follicles are moved apart by large scalp extensions. Bone may show resorption at the outer cortical surface. Typically this defect is repaired and a normal contour restored after removal of the expander.

20. What areas are especially suitable for soft tissue expansion reconstructions?

The scalp and breast are especially well suited to reconstruction using soft tissue expansion. Although some disagree, total nasal reconstruction is made straightforward when the forehead is expanded before raising it as a flap. An expanded forehead flap provides a complete nasal lining and allows immediate closure of the donor site. The capsule and frontalis in the area turned inward to form the alar rims must be removed to allow a thin, attractive reconstruction.

21. What will the future bring in the way of breast reconstruction? Will autogenous tissue reconstruction replace tissue expansion?

As reimbursement for breast reconstruction falls, pressures favoring outpatient reconstruction via soft tissue expansion will mount. It seems likely that the proportion of tissue expansion reconstructions will rise and the number of autogenous tissue reconstructions will fall. Although some have asserted that the costs were almost the same at their institutions, this has not been our experience. The cost of tissue expansion reconstruction has been about one-half the cost of a transverse rectus abdominis muscle (TRAM) flap. Some insurers give lower reimbursements for bigger procedures to drive doctors toward less cost-intensive alternatives in reconstructive surgery.

22. Where is it difficult or even inadvisable to use tissue expansion?

Defects of the central face seldom require expansion. The bathtub deformity in the facial fat is an unwanted outcome, even if temporary. The hands and feet are seldom rewarding sites for expansion. The neck remains one of the most frustrating sites for expansion. If soft tissue is needed for neck and/or face reconstruction, the best strategy is to expand the supraclavicular skin and turn it up as a large flap. The amount of tissue created by expansion on the neck is almost always overestimated because of the natural concavity under the jawline. Upward advancements over the jawline are frequently disappointing in outcome.

23. What are contraindications and relative contraindications to soft tissue expansion?

Contraindications include expansion near a malignancy, under a skin graft, under very tight tissue, near an open leg wound, or in an irradiated field. Relative contraindications include expansion near an open wound (not in the leg), near a hemangioma, under an incision, or in a psychologically incompetent patient.

24. Should families and patients be trusted to do their own expansions at home?

Most certainly. Injection of saline into a tissue expander is certainly less risky than administering insulin. Families can learn to perform home expansion safely and effectively for family members.

25. How can you—or a child's family—measure the intraluminal pressure of an expander during a home inflation?

If using a scalp vein needle with a short length of tubing between the needle and the hub connecting to the syringe, one has a built-in manometer. If the syringe is removed from the hub and the tubing is held extended straight up into the air, the standing height of saline is equivalent to about 20 mmHg.

If the meniscus falls in the tube, the intraluminal expander pressure is less. If fluid overflows from the hub, the pressure is greater then 20 mmHg. No tissue is injured if a 20 mmHg limit is observed.

26. Does a textured surface on an expander make a difference?
Although some enthusiasts claim that using an expander with a textured surface is beneficial, in at least one double-blind perspective study, no benefit was demonstrated. We have not found a textured surface to be of benefit. No differences were observed when one side of a symmetric expander was textured and the other side was smooth.

27. What are some of the inherent advantages of tissue expansion?
Tissue expansion provides tissue for reconstruction that is most like the lost tissue. It is matched in color, texture, and hair-bearing characteristics. The tissue may be sensate. The donor defect is minimal. Usually the contour is superior to that achieved with another technique. Tissue expansion often can be performed entirely on an outpatient basis under local anesthesia. Seldom is tissue lost; if an exposure or infection occurs, the expander is removed and replaced in 2–3 months in most cases. Large flaps with increased vascularity may be created for the reconstruction of defects that were formerly approached with no alternatives but skin grafts.

BIBLIOGRAPHY

1. Argenta LC: Controlled tissue expansion in facial reconstruction. In Baker SR, Swanson NA (eds): Local Flaps in Facial Reconstruction. St. Louis, Mosby, 1995, pp 517–544.
2. Argenta LC, Austad ED: Principles and techniques of tissue expansion. In McCarthy JG (ed): Plastic Surgery. Philadelphia, 1990, pp 475–507.
3. Austad ED, Thomas SB, Pasyk KA: Tissue expansion: Dividend or loan? Plast Reconstr Surg 78:63, 1986.
4. Jankauskas J, Cohen IK, Grabb WC: Basic technique of plastic surgery. In Smith JW, Aston SJ (eds): Grabb and Smith's Plastic Surgery, 4th ed. Boston, Little Brown, 1991, pp 67–68.
5. Manders EK, Schenden MJ, Hetzler PT, et al: Soft tissue expansion: Concepts and complications. Plast Reconstr Surg 74:493–507, 1984.
6. Manders EK, da Paula P: Repeated tissue expansion. In Grotting JC (ed): Reoperative Aesthetic and Reconstructive Plastic Surgery. St. Louis, Quality Medical Publishing, 1995, pp 137–153.
7. Maxwell GP: Breast reconstruction following mastectomy and surgical management of the patient with high-risk breast disease. In Smith JW, Aston SJ (eds): Grabb and Smith's Plastic Surgery, 4th ed. Boston, Little Brown, 1991, pp 1203–1247.
8. Sasaki GH, Tissue Expansion. In Jurkiewicz MJ, Krizek TJ, Mathes SJ, Aryian S (eds): Plastic Surgery: Principles and Practice. St. Louis, Mosby, 1990, pp 1609–1634.

5. ALLOPLASTIC IMPLANTATION

Stephen P. Daane, M.D.

1. What are the advantages of alloplastic materials?
1. No donor site morbidity from a second surgical site.
2. Reduced operative time compared with harvesting a graft.
3. Unlimited supply of alloplastic materials.
4. Prefabricated implants may be tailored to the individual patient.
5. Unlike autogenous materials (bone, cartilage, dermis, fat, fascia), there is no scar formation or reabsorption of the implant over time.

2. How are biomedical alloplants classified?
Biomedical alloplants are classified as either liquids (injectable silicone, collagen) or solids (metals, polymers, ceramics). The physical form of the implants (solid or mesh, smooth or rough) determines whether the implant is encapsulated as a whole or whether fibrous tissue will penetrate the interstices of the implant. Selection of specific alloplastic implant materials can be advantageous in different clinical situations: vigorous tissue ingrowth into Marlex polypropylene mesh provides a

strong, long-lasting repair, whereas fibrous encapsulation of a Hunter rod silicone tendon prosthesis ensures free gliding of a subsequent tendon graft.

3. What are the properties of the ideal implant?

The ideal implant should fulfill certain conditions: (1) biologically compatible; (2) nontoxic; (3) nonallergenic; (4) productive of no foreign-body inflammatory response; (5) mechanically reliable; (6) resistant to resorption and deformation; (7) nonsupportive of the growth of microorganisms; (8) easy to shape, remove, and sterilize; and (9) radiolucent (not interefere with CT or MR).

4. What is the goal of alloplastic implantation?

The goal of implantation materials is to simulate a missing part while evoking minimal reaction from the host. Polymers are most commonly used as bulk space fillers for soft tissue contour restoration, as with nasal, chin, auricle, or breast implants. The biologic response to the polymer group of materials generally consists of a normal inflammatory response, deposition of collagen fibers, and maturation of fibrous connective tissue that completely encapsulates the implant in 4–6 weeks. In some instances a restrictive capsular fibrosis occurs, a biologic response that may be related to myofibroblast activity and may require surgical correction.

The quality of the tissue envelope holding the implant must also be considered. If the blood supply is marginal (as with irradiated tissues), the chance of extrusion is high, or the implant is placed in a tight pocket, the chance of bony resorption beneath the implant is high. Principles of placing hard implants include (1) shaping the edges to avoid hard corners, (2) burying the implant as deeply as possible under the skin and subcutaneous tissue, (3) avoiding tension in adjacent tissues or tension against the overlying skin, (4) placing the incision as far from the implant as possible, (5) handling the implant gently, and (6) using the proper stiffness of material (hard implants should not be used for tissue replacement).

5. What is the Oppenheimer effect?

In 1948, Oppenheimer reported that metal implants placed in experimental animals could induce tumors. Further experiments showed that the composition of the material was unimportant; maximal tumorigenesis occurred when the material had a smooth, continuous surface. Other characteristics of this phenomenon were minimal size requirement (0.5×0.5 cm in rats) and minimal time requirement for the implant to remain in situ (6 months in rats). Tumors appeared after a latent period of approximately 300 days.

Rare clinical reports of tumor occurrence adjacent to alloplastic implants in humans are consistent with the Oppenheimer effect, although extensive human clinical experience has not demonstrated a strong association between carcinogenicity and medical alloplants. However, to rule out the oncogenic potential of implants, a follow-up period of 20–50 years would be necessary to match the short latent period of animal tumors.

6. What are bioabsorbable plates and screws?

Experimentation with absorbable polymers led to the development of poly-L-lactic acid (PLA) and polyglycolic acid (PGA) as resorbable implantable devices. When used alone, PLA forms a strong crystalline lattice that takes months or years to undergo hydrolysis, whereas PGA used alone produces an implant that loses its tensile strength quickly and is resorbed within weeks to months. Pure PGA was first marketed as Dexon suture; Vicryl suture is a mix of 8% PLA and 92% PGA. A chondrocyte-seeded PLA/PGA polymer similar to Vicryl has recently been used in the tissue engineering of cartilage scaffolding. A copolymer of PLA (82%) and PGA (18%) consistently demonstrated adequate initial strength and complete resorption after 9–15 months. This combination had been used in resorbable surgical clips and microvascular couplers and was introduced as the LactoSorb craniofacial plate fixation system in 1996.

The theoretical advantage of absorbable PLA/PGA over titanium hardware in pediatric craniofacial surgery is that the plates are resorbed and do not put the patient at risk for intracranial migration of hardware or growth restriction. Metallic fixation also interferes with postoperative radiographic imaging, oncologic follow-up, and evaluation of fracture healing. The characteristics of initial strength followed by complete resorption at 1 year may make LactoSorb a valuable tool for rigid bony fixation in craniofacial surgery.

7. Which metals are suitable for implantation in plastic surgery?

(1) Stainless steel, (2) Vitallium, and (3) titanium. Their uses include plate-and-screw fixation sets for craniofacial surgery and hand surgery and as hemoclips, cranial plates, artificial joints, and dental implants.

The term **stainless steel** refers to a large group of iron-chromium-nickel alloys that were first used as biomedical implants in the 1920s. Orthopedic devices of stainless steel were adapted to craniofacial surgery for rigid fixation; however, they were found to undergo a high degree of corrosion with a potential for implant failure after several years. Compared with stainless steel, Vitallium and titanium have superior corrosion resistance, partially due to a protective oxide layer that forms on their surface.

Vitallium is a cobalt-chromium-molybdenum alloy introduced in the 1930s. It has a higher tensile resistance to fatigue or fracture than stainless steel or titanium. Because of its high tensile strength, lower-profile plates that have narrow interconnecting bars between the holes can be implanted.

Titanium was introduced as an implant material in Europe in the 1940s. Unalloyed titanium is much more malleable than stainless steel or Vitallium. Malleability facilitates bending to fit the complex topography of the facial skeleton (e.g., titanium mesh is useful for orbital floor reconstruction in blowout fractures). Titanium alloy (titanium-aluminum-vanadium) has a tensile strength similar to Vitallium. Titanium is the least corrosive for implantation and has the least artifact on CT and MR imaging studies.

8. How are injectable collagens used?

Collagen is a large protein made up of repeating peptide triple helices, representing 25% of the body's protein. The use of injectable collagen for the correction of small wrinkles and contour deformities was first reported in 1977, and in 1981 a highly purified form of injectable bovine collagen was developed. Zyderm I and the follow-up products, Zyderm II and Zyplast, are administered by injection during outpatient visits. The injectable collagens shrink as they extrude water and ultimately biodegrade within the host. Zyderm I and II are sterilized fibrillar bovine collagen, 95% type I and 5% type III. The peptide end regions, thought to be the most antigenic sites on the molecule, are enzymatically removed. Zyplast, introduced in 1985, results from cross-linking the collagen with glutaraldehyde to give it a longer lifespan. These products differ primarily in rates of resorption.

Zyderm I has a collagen concentration of 35 mg/cc. It is useful for superficial dermal defects in thin skin, such as fine periorbital and perioral wrinkles. Zyderm II has a collegen concentration of 65 mg/cc, which may leave transient bumps at injection sites. This material is usually used for defects in thicker skin, such as glabellar lines, nasolabial lines, transverse forehead lines, or acne scarring. Zyplast is a more rigid material and should be injected into the deep dermis to prevent a superficial bump. Zyplast is recommended for glabellar folds, nasolabial folds, and postrhinoplasty defects in the deep dermis. Lip augmentation is not an approved use for bovine collagen. Using Zyderm I or II, overcorrection to 1.5 or 2 times the initial depth of the deficiency is recommended, because absorption of the saline carrier leaves 30% of the injected voume. Zyplast retains the injected volume and overcorrection is not advocated.

Another commonly used collagen implant is catgut suture, harvested from the fibrous tissue of beef or sheep intestinal wall.

9. What are the major concerns with the use of injectable collagens?

The main concerns about injectable collagens are the need for repeated injections and the presence of circulating antibodies to bovine collagen, although they are not known to cross-react with human collagen. Skin testing is performed preoperatively, and localized hypersensitivity reactions develop in 1–4% of patients. Reinjection for maintenance is required every 6 months to 2 years. In areas where mechanical stresses may be higher (e.g., facial wrinkles), ongoing correction is required more frequently. Contraindications to injectable collagen include autoimmune disease, viral pock marks, "ice-pick" acne scars or indurated scars, and hypersensitivity reactions to skin testing.

10. What is hydroxyapatite?

$Ca_{10}(PO_4)_6(OH)_2$, or hydroxyapatite (HA), is the major inorganic constituent of bone. Corals of the genus *Porites* create a calcium carbonate exoskeleton resembling human bone with an average pore size of 200 μ. Surgical vendors convert the calcium carbonate skeleton into HA through an exchange reaction of the carbonate for phosphate. The resultant material has the porous anatomy of bone with identical chemical composition. HA is capable of strongly bonding to adjacent bone.

Compared with onlay bone grafts, HA demonstrates excellent maintenance of contour and volume. HA implants elicit no foreign-body or inflammatory response.

11. How is HA used in plastic surgery?

HA is available in block form (porous or solid) and as granules. It is used most commonly to augment the contour of the facial skeleton or as a bone graft substitute in orthognathic surgery. Contouring of HA blocks is performed with dental burrs. Lag screw fixation is suggested when HA blocks are placed in an onlay manner, because osteointegration will not occur if the blocks are mobile.

Porous HA blocks and HA granules are rapidly invaded by fibrovascular tissue; within 2–3 months there is histologic evidence of direct osseous union between implant and bone. HA is osteoconductive in that it provides a matrix for deposition of new bone from adjacent living bone. HA is not osteogenic because it will not induce new bone formation when placed in ectopic sites such as muscle or fat. Long-term radiographic follow-up shows a lack of resorption of HA implants. The typical composition of HA granules or porous HA implants on follow-up biopsy specimens is approximately one-third HA, one-third new bone, and one-third soft tissue.

HA blocks are brittle but gain rapidly in strength as the implant pores are invaded by fibrovascular tissue and bone; the ultimate compressive strength exceeds masticatory forces of the jaws. Complication rates for porous HA implants in large clinical series have been in the 4–10% range. The low infection rate is thought to be due to an abundant blood supply. Infection is likely to occur with a deficiency of soft tissue coverage.

HA granules may be mixed with Avitene or blood and microfibrillar collagen, then placed into a carefully dissected subperiosteal pocket to produce a desired contour. Granular HA is somewhat more difficult to handle. Although solid HA has a high extrusion rate when used for alveolar ridge augmentation, HA granules have been used quite successfully for this application; they become strongly anchored by fibrous tissue.

12. How is synthetic HA used in plastic surgery?

BoneSource is a synthetic HA cement that was first used clinically in 1991. When mixed with water and a drying agent (sodium phosphate), BoneSource powder forms a paste that hardens to form a microporous implant within 15 minutes. It is completely biocompatible with no inflammatory tissue response. In addition to its ease of application, the infection rate is extremely low.

Although experiments in feline cranial defects and initial anecdotal clinical reports indicated resorption of BoneSource, longer follow-up in humans has shown that HA cement maintains its shape and volume over time. The wound bed must be dry at closure. HA cement stimulates bony ingrowth when placed in contact with bone, whether in an inlay or onlay position in the facial skeleton. Currently, the approved indication for HA cement is for calvarial defects of up to 25 cm^2, although it is also commonly used for facial skeletal augmentation. Experiements mixing HA cement with protein growth factors to enhance bony ingrowth are under way.

13. Which polymer is most often used for facial augmentation? Why?

High-density porous polyethylene (Medpor) is replacing silicone as the most commonly used material for facial augmentation procedures. Medpor has a void volume of up to 50%. Pore sizes ranging from 100–250 μ allow stabilization of the implant through bony and soft tissue ingrowth. The foreign body reaction to Medpor is minimal, with only a thin fibrous capsule and few giant cells. It has low infection and extrusion rates, with no loss of the implant on long-term follow-up.

Medpor is available in sheets and blocks that can be sculpted at the time of surgery and as preformed implants for chin augmentation, malar augmentation, and microtia reconstruction. It is also useful for orbital floor blowout fractures and as a columellar strut for cleft rhinoplasty.

14. What are the physical properties of silicone?

Polydimethylsiloxane (PDMS), or silicone, is a repeating chain of –Si–O– units, with methyl groups attached to the silicon atoms. Silicone can simulate different soft tissues as a liquid, gel, or rubber by varying the length and cross-linking of the PDMS chains. Silicone fluids are short, straight chains of PDMS, gels are lightly cross-linked chains of PDMS, and elastomers are longer chains of PDMS that are cross-linked to a greater degree. Amorphous silica particles (30 μ) may be added to increase the tensile strength of silicone rubber.

Silicone is highly biocompatible, nontoxic, nonallergenic, and resistant to biodegradation. The tissue response is limited to a mild foreign body reaction followed by encapsulation. Silicone cannot be rendered porous to improve its incorporation into tissues; instead, a fibrous capsule forms around the implant. Capuslar contracture is the most common complication after breast augmentation and may occur unilaterally in patients with bilateral implants.

15. What are the disadvantages of using silicone?

1. Propensity of silicone rubbers to tear easily or fail in heavy stress applications (e.g., Swanson finger joint implants).

2. Difficulty removing gel foam from soft tissues in case of implant failure.

3. Bone resorption beneath silicone implants placed subperiosteally for augmentation (e.g., chin).

4. The smoothness of silicone implants makes them prone to extrusion when placed superficially (e.g., Silastic placed in the nose or ear).

5. Silicone rubbers are permeable, allowing proteins or lipids to become adsorbed onto the surface of an implant, which may alter its physical properties and lead to failure.

16. How is silicone currently used?

Currently silicone is used in ventriculoperitoneal shunts, pacemakers, heart valves, myringotomy tubes, and intraocular lenses. In plastic surgery silicone is used for aesthetic contour restoration in breast and facial reconstruction; orbital floor implants in facial fractures; tissue expanders and prosthetic penile devices; and finger joint replacements. As an injectable liquid, silicone was once used for augmentation of facial soft tissues and breast enlargement. However, silicone injections were ultimately affected by gravity with loss of the augmentation effect after a period of years. Infection and chronic inflammation, migration of the material, and inappropriate usage led to its withdrawal from the market. However, an injectable form of gel-coated silicone microbeads (Bioplastique) has recently been approved for clinical trials.

17. How is methylmethacrylate used in plastic surgery?

Methylmethacrylate, a self-curing acrylic resin, is used for securing joint components to bone and as a craniofacial bone substitute. Advantages of this inexpensive material include ease of surgical manipulation, density similar to bone, radiolucency, and good long-term tissue tolerance. Methylmethacrylate is available in two forms: as a heat-cured, preformed implant or as a cold-cured implant that can be molded in the operating room and contoured with burrs after hardening. The body's response to methylmethacrylate is minimal, consisting of a typical foreign body reaction that subsides as the implant becomes enveloped by fibrous tissue.

Methylmethacrylate forms an exothermic reaction while curing. This reaction may damage tissues; cardiac arrest also has been reported during the curing process due to absorption. The major late problems are infection, extrusion, or mechanical failure due to deterioration of the bone–polymer interface. Risks of infection are decreased by keeping the edge of the implant at least 1 cm away from a skin incision and avoiding the use of methylmethacrylate under skin grafts or scarred tissues.

Methylmethacrylate is used in orthopedics as a bone cement for joint replacements, in neurosurgery for reconstruction of cranial defects, and in dentistry for denture plates. In plastic surgery, gentamicin-impregnated methylmethacrylate beads are used in conjunction with muscle flaps to treat infected long bone fractures. Methylmethacrylate is also used for forehead augmentation and chest wall reconstruction. For difficult reconstructions, implants can be created before an operation based on a moulage or from CT scan data and computer-assisted milling. HTR, a recently available composite of methylmethacrylate, is porous and negatively charged to stimulate bony growth.

18. What is cyanoacrylate? How is it used?

Cyanoacrylate ("superglue") is a strong, biodegradable tissue adhesive that polymerizes in contact with tissues. It may be used as a hemostatic agent or to "glue" tissues together in a surgical wound. Its binding is not affected by moisture or blood. Cyanoacrylate is widely used in orthopedics for hardware fixation and has been used for aortic and liver trauma, but it has found limited use in plastic surgery for blood vessel anastomoses, wound closure, flexor tendon repair, application of skin grafts, or hemostasis. In strength comparison studies, cyanoacrylate is comparable to plate and screw fixation in the facial skeleton and comparable to suture for wound closures. Cyanoacrylate is easy to handle in the operating room. There is a mild toxicity from the degradation products, formaldehyde and cyanoacetate, which can be detected in the urine.

Recently, the FDA approved Dermabond, a cyanoacrylate "topical skin cohesive." In a multicenter trial of more than 800 patients, Dermabond compared favorably with sutures in the emergency repair of lacerations and punctures, general surgical incisions, and facial plastic procedures. Dermabond polymerizes within one minute and begins to peel off in 7–10 days.

19. Which fluorocarbon polymers are used in plastic surgery?

Fluorocarbon polymers as a group are resistant to chemical degradation and minimally reactive when placed in the body. Of the fluorocarbon polymers used in plastic surgery, Teflon is limited to vocal cord reconstruction and Proplast was withdrawn from the market in 1990. Only PTFE (GoreTex) is in common use today.

Proplast I is a black-colored composite of Teflon and carbon that was developed in 1970. With a void volume of 75% and pores ranging from 80–400 μ in size, its tissue ingrowth property led to its use as an augmentation material for the chin, zygoma, and orbital rim area. **Proplast II** is a white-colored composite of Teflon and aluminum oxide that is more suitable for superficial implantation. In addition to rapid tissue ingrowth, Proplast can be sculpted and impregnated with antibiotics. However, frequent biomechanical failure of Proplast temporomandibular joint implants led to the withdrawal of Proplast by the FDA in 1990.

Polytetrafluoroethylene (PTFE) consists of non–cross-linked linear polymers of fluorinated carbon units with molecular weights of 6–10 million. The carbon-fluorine bonds are highly resistant to degradation. PTFE is inert, nonadhesive, and nonfrictional; it elicits virtually no inflammatory response within the body. It is nonallergenic and noncarcinogenic and has no immune reactivity.

GoreTex is a polymer sheet of expanded PTFE interconnected by Teflon fibrils, yielding tremendous strength. Pores of up to 30 μ result from the expansion, allowing a small amount of tissue ingrowth. GoreTex is useful for vascular reconstruction and soft tissue augmentation. GoreTex has been used in the face for the correction of wrinkles and for lip, chin, nasal, and forehead augmentation. It also is used for ligament repair, chest wall or abdominal wall reconstruction, static suspension of the paralyzed face, and guided tissue regeneration (GTR). Problems with extrusion or migration of GoreTex implants are reduced when the implants are properly fixed to the tissues. Infection rates with GoreTex implants are very low.

20. What are osseointegrated implants?

Osseointegration is the harmonious coexistence of implant, bone, and soft tissue. Osseointegrated percutaneous implants allow the attachment of a prosthesis to an implant that is anchored to bone but penetrates the skin or mucosa. In the first stage, a titanium implant is placed into bone and buried beneath the periosteum or soft tissues for 3 months to provide osseointegration. At a second stage, the implant is uncovered and a permanent prosthesis is made for fixation to the implant. The implant must be absolutely stable during the first 3–6 months of healing; otherwise, connective tissue rather than bone may form at the implant surface. Threaded implants with small pores are more likely than smooth implants to establish initial stability, and titanium is used because the oxide layer that readily forms on the implant's surface is important to tissue interaction. More recently, HA-coated titanium implants have been used. Success rates greater than 95% have been reported using osseointegrated implants for dental restoration and prosthetic facial parts on long-term follow-up.

21. Should patients with implants undergo antibiotic prophylaxis?

The potential of an implant material to promote infection is an important consideration. For example, experiments have shown that the requirement of 10^6 organisms to produce a pus-forming infection is lowered to 100 orgainisms in the presence of a braided silk suture. Although studies have shown a beneficial effect for perioperative antibiotic prophylaxis in patients undergoing implantation with alloplastic materials, usually only patients with prosthetic heart valves or hips receive antibiotics when undergoing dental procedures that cause a transient bacteremia. It seems possible that breast implants or other materials may serve as a nidus for bacterial colonization, although formal recommendations for antibiotic prophylaxis in such patients have never been made.

BILBIOGRAPHY

1. Albrektsson T, et al: Present clinical applications of osseointegrated percutaneous implants. Plast Reconstr Surg 79:721, 1987.
2. American Academy of Orthopedic Surgeons: Metals used in orthopedic surgery. In Orthopedic Knowledge Update I. Chicago, American Academy of Orthopedic Surgeons, 1984.
3. Constantino PD, Friedman CD: Synthetic bone graft substitutes. In Otolaryngol Clin North Am 27:1037, 1994.
4. Holmes RE: Alloplastic implants. In McCarthy JG (ed): Plastic Surgery. Philadelphia, W.B. Saunders 1990, pp 698–731.
5. Mole B: The use of Gore-Tex implants in aesthetic surgery of the face. Plast Reconstr Surg 90:200, 1992.
6. Montag ME, Morales L, Daane S: Bioabsorbables: Their use in pediatric craniofacial surgery. J Craniofac Surg 8:100, 1997.
7. Oppenheimer BS, Oppenheimer ET, Danishefski I, Stout AP: Carcinogenic effect of metals in rodents. Cancer Res 16:439, 1956.
8. Ousterhout DK: Prosthetic forehead augmentation. In Ousterhout DK (ed): Aesthetic Contouring of the Craniofacial Skeleton. Boston, Little, Brown, 1991, pp 199–219.
9. Scales JT: Discussion on metals and synthetic materials in relation to soft tissues: Tissue's reaction to synthetic materials. Proc R Soc Med 46:647, 1953.
10. Wellisz T: Clinical experience with the Medpor porous polyethylene implant. Aesthet Plast Srug 17:339, 1993.

6. THE PROBLEMATIC WOUND

Thomas J. Krizek, M.D.

1. What is a problematic wound? What causes it?

The goal of wound healing is to obtain successful closure of the wound with an intact epithelial layer. A wound becomes problematic when it presents unusual difficulty in obtaining such closure. The difficulty may relate to the configuration of the wound in which the technique or mechanics of closure is the main issue. The difficulty also may relate to problems intrinsic to the wound itself. Systemic (e.g., sickle cell anemia, administration of steroids) or local factors (e.g., bacterial contamination) may affect wound healing.

2. What are primary, secondary, and tertiary wound closure?

Closure of wounds in which the edges can be directly approximated is referred to as **first intention or primary closure**. The typical example is a surgical wound. Closure with sutures, staples, tape, or other means brings the edges together and maintains approximation while the wound experiences the healing stages of inflammation and early fibroplasia. In certain wounds, such as a burn wound, primary closure cannot be achieved; the surgeon awaits and promotes spontaneous reepithelialization of the wound from viable epithelial elements in the wound itself or from the epithelium at the margin. This approach, called **second intention or secondary closure**, is associated with the potential problems created by a wound that remains open: intense and prolonged inflammation, which, in turn, promotes excessive contraction and excessive fibroplasia. Secondary closure may result in an unsightly scar and, when across a joint, may limit motion due to contracture. One approach to the wound that otherwise would be closed only by secondary means is to close the wound surgically by bringing tissue from elsewhere in the form of a flap or graft. This technique is **third intention or tertiary closure**.

3. What systemic problems may make a wound problematic?

Systemic problems may affect the wound directly or indirectly. In patients with Ehlers-Danlos syndrome, for example, a defect in collagen deposition results in less tensile strength and more elasticity. A deficiency in vitamin C (scurvy) makes the hydroxylation of proline to hydroxyproline impossible and causes a collagen cross-linking deficiency. Sickle cell anemia has profound local effects on healing. Chronic administration of steroids interferes with fibroplasia. It is important to recognize how few systemic conditions result in wound closure difficulty. Such factors as malnutrition, anemia, age, and other systemic factors are clinically relevant only at their extremes and only marginally so; the body recognizes wound closure as a biologic priority.

4. What local factors may make a wound problematic?

Far more frequent are local wound problems that render the wound biologically rather than technically problematic. The most common examples include ischemia, pressure, radiation, foreign material/traumatic wounds, and bacterial contamination.

5. What are the guidelines for handling ischemic wounds?

Ischemic wounds must be evaluated for reversible vascular problems (for example, bypass surgery). Venous wounds are also ischemic, perhaps from functional shunting of blood from the arterial to the venous side of circulation, bypassing the ulcerated area. Some evidence suggests that microvascular free tissue transfer from the arm or scapular area provides venous drainage. Closure with tissue containing valves makes recurrence less severe than closure merely with grafts. Lymphatic disease is particularly difficult because, as in venous wounds, edema is an ongoing problem. Edematous tissue is particularly prone to streptococcal infection, which, when it heals, results in more lymphatic scarring and thus more edema. Unna boots (containing calamine, zinc oxide, and gelatin), elastic support, and prophylaxis against streptococci are of long-term value. Growth factors may soon be commercially available for use in diabetic arterial disease and other wounds. Sickle cell ulcers, when skin-grafted, usually recur promptly if the patient is allowed to have a crisis during the healing phase. If the hematocrit is maintained above 35% or so, crisis will not occur and the grafted skin has a chance to mature and become less easily traumatized.

6. What are the guidelines for handling pressure wounds?

Wounds resulting from unrelieved pressure, usually in patients without sensation (quadriplegics, paraplegics, neuropathics, and patients with chronic debilitating central neurologic problems) are extremely difficult and cannot be successfully managed unless the underlying cause is corrected. Successful wound closure in unselected patients, even with sophisticated muscle flaps, is probably less than 10%. With careful education and limitation of surgery to the most compliant patients, muscle closure of pressure sores is successful in about 75% of cases. Many problematic pressure wounds are best managed by creating a controlled wound—namely, a wound without excessive contamination that can be maintained indefinitely by local wound care. The wound, if not excessively large, is of no danger to the patient; this approach is useful in patients in whom the success of surgery is small. The use of growth factors in compliant patients may result in successful closure of pressure wounds by second intention to a degree formerly thought impossible.

7. How are radiated wounds managed?

Radiation injuries may be acute or chronic. Acute injury, which is seen only in industrial accidents, is rare because the dangers are so well known. Chronic injury may occur from industrial exposure or formerly from therapeutic treatment of acne or other benign conditions. Fortunately the generation of patients so injured has largely passed, and no new patients are being added. Most problematic wounds that we encounter are due to therapeutic radiation for malignancy and fall into the category of subacute injury. The ultimate effect of radiation on the tissue is not necessarily to produce ischemia; in fact, radiated wounds are usually quite well vascularized and bleed easily. Instead, the radiation destroys stem cells necessary for both revascularization and fibroplasia. In many radiation wounds a split-thickness skin graft will close the wound nicely. In others, vascularized tissue, in the form of muscular or musculocutaneous flaps or free microvascular flaps, gives the wound a new start with tissue that brings its own blood supply and stem cells.

8. What about traumatic wounds?

Sir James Learmonth, surgeon to the Queen of England, provided guidelines on which it is hard to improve. The key to managing such wounds is adequate debridement:

Of the edge of the skin,   And muscle much more,
take a piece very thin.   until you see fresh gore,
The tighter the fascia,   And the bundles contract,
the more you should slash'er.   at the least impact.
                                  Leave intact the bone,
                                  except bits quite alone.

Learmonth emphasized the value of accurate debridement as the single most important factor in preparing the traumatic/contaminated wound for closure. The skin is highly vascular, and excessive removal is unnecessary. Intravenous fluorescein and examination of skin with a Wood's lamp offer accurate delineation of vascular compared with devitalized skin. Foreign bodies must be removed before closure. Wounds should be explored for metallic foreign bodies such as needles, only with radiographic control available. The needle in the haystack is easier to find than the needle in the sole of the foot. In addition to accurate debridement and removal of foreign bodies, irrigation is essential.

The figure below shows a grossly contaminated, neglected wound of the leg with an exposed tibial fracture. We need to debride, irrigate, and bring it into bacterial balance. When these goals are accomplished, our technical virtuosity will be used to close it. But first, **debride** the wound.

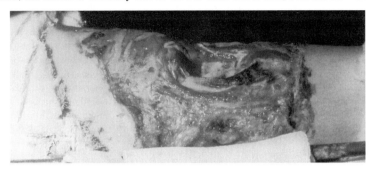

Open tibial fracture with contaminated wound. The wound needs to be debrided and irrigated under pressure, and bacterial flora in soft tissue and bone should be determined by quantitative microbiologic techniques. Only when bacterial control can be documented is the technical virtuosity of the reconstructive surgeon employed to close the wound.

9. Which irrigation fluid should be used? How much?

Most irrigation is designed to remove particulate matter, which is often difficult to see, and bacteria, which cannot be seen. If one measures particulate matter and bacterial flora in an open wound quantitatively, before and after irrigation, one has an excellent model to study the effect of irrigation. Surface irrigation—for example, with a bulb syringe—is only marginally effective and then only for surface bacteria. Bacteria lodged in the tissue are not reduced by this technique whether one uses 1 liter or 20 liters. "Dilution is the solution to pollution" only when irrigation is performed with pressure; pressure irrigation with the jet lavage or Systec-like systems at about 70 PSI (pounds per square inch) reduces bacteria counts and the amount of particulate matter. Although saline is readily available, Ringer's lactate is probably a better choice. The amount depends on the nature of the wound. Small wounds irrigated in the emergency department with a syringe and fine needle require only a few ounces, whereas large wounds require proportionately more.

10. What about bacterial contamination?

Humans are not germ-free. Our skin is contaminated by bacterial flora that are both transient and resident. Transient flora, which reflect contact with the environment, may be extremely high after contact with heavily contaminated material or relatively low if they are exposed to the air, dry up, and die from lack of nourishment. We remove transient bacteria when we wash our hands before patient contact or before entering the operating room. Resident flora, which reside in the hair follicles and skin glands, are "normal." A biopsy culture of normal skin identifies about 10^3 microorganism per gram of skin. Similarly the mucous membrane of the oral cavity and the mucosa of the bowel are colonized. The mere presence of bacteria does not constitute infection. Rather than being free of bacteria, we live in delicate balance with them—a balance that can be identified and measured with great precision.

11. What is quantitative microbiology?

All microbiology laboratories routinely culture urine to determine whether a level of 100,000 (10^5) microorganisms is present. A level less than 10^5 microorganisms indicates contamination, whereas a level more than 10^5 microorganisms indicates invasive infection. For the past 40 years surgical biologists have used the same technology to measure bacterial contamination in the tissue of open wounds. A specimen is obtained, weighed, and converted to liquid on a weight/volume basis and then cultured in the same fashion as urine cultures. The number of microorganisms per gram of tissue is determined. The surface bacteria in a wound are insignificant because they are so easily eliminated. Surface swabs for culture fail to recognize the bacteria in the depths of the wound—which make the difference.

The rapid slide test provides information about whether the wound has more than 10^5 microorganisms per gram of tissue in less than 30 minutes. It does not identify the exact organisms or their sensitivities, but it is useful in screening contaminated wounds.

12. Does quantitative microbiology make a difference?

Gertrude Stein has been quoted as saying, "A difference, to be a difference, must make a difference." All differences are not necessarily important, but quantitative microbiology *makes* a difference. When fewer than 10^5 microorganisms are present in the tissue, invasive infection will not occur, wounds will close spontaneously, and skin grafts will take with uniform success. When the counts are greater than 10^5 microorganisms per gram of tissue, skin grafts will not take and invasive infection will occur. Streptococci, which are dangerous in *any* quantity, are the exception that proves the rule.

Of interest, 10^8–10^9 microorganism per gram of tissue are necessary to produce clinical evidence of pus; the difference, therefore, between what can be seen with the naked eye and the critical level of bacteria is a difference of almost 1,000-fold. In a clinical study of random wounds in the emergency department, the number of wounds with more than 10^5 microorganisms per gram was 20%. This is the average infection rate in wounds managed in emergency departments nationally. When wounds with fewer than 10^5 microorganisms were closed, the infection rate dropped to less than 1%.

The importance of quantitative microbiology in bone also has been demonstrated. When sternal wounds are debrided and closed only when bone cultures show fewer than 10^5 microorganisms per gram, the infection rate for wounds is all but eliminated. Quantitative microbiology adds scientific precision to the measurement of soft tissue contamination and makes wound closure, by any modality, a matter of clinical accuracy rather than guesswork.

13. Should quantitative microbiology be used before closing all wounds?

No. The use of any test in every case, no matter how inexpensive or readily available, is as inappropriate as never using it. Neither approach is biologically sound. Clean surgical wounds and traumatic wounds under clean conditions (e.g., cuts around the home) are most likely free of unusual contamination. Our studies have shown that almost 80% of unselected wounds presenting to the emergency department fall into the clean category. It is the other 20% that cause the infections. Quantitative microbiology is indicated in wounds that are known, by history, to be contaminated. Human bites involve major bacterial contamination. Most dog bites are "clean," because the dog's mouth has fewer than 10^3 bacteria/gm *unless* the dog has eaten meat in the previous 8 hours. In this case, the counts go as high as 10^7 bacteria/gm. The imaginative surgeon will ask about the dog's eating pattern, recognizing the effect of meat (biscuits and dry food do not raise counts), and discern which wounds will benefit from quantitative counts.

Clean wound	**Contaminated wound**	
Example: elective surgical incision, traumatic wound from clean knife	Example: surgical wound in contaminated field	
↓	↓	
Debride, irrigate, close wound	Quantitative microbiologic bacterial count	
	↓	↓
	< 10^5/gm	> 10^5/gm
	↓	↓
	Debride, irrigate, close wound	Debride, irrigate, leave open, use topical antibacterials
		↓
		Repeat quantitative microbiologic count
	↓	↓
	< 10^5/gm	> 10^5/gm
	↓	↓
	Close wound	Repeat debridement, irrigate under pressure, apply topicals until count is < 10^5/gm

Algorithm for managing clean and contaminated wounds.

14. What is the value of antibacterial agents in problematic wounds?

Antibacterial agents must be appropriate for the organism most likely to cause the infection and must be given at the proper time, in the proper dose, and by the proper route to be effective.

Time. The proper time to give an antibacterial is *before* the contamination occurs so that an effective level is present in the tissue when bacterial contamination occurs. Most persons do not walk around on antibacterial therapy. In patients with lymphedema or edema of a healing burn, however, long-term prophylaxis against streptococcal infection is appropriate, and a narrow-spectrum agent (penicillin) is indicated. In many elective operations the intravenous administration of an antibacterial as surgery begins is appropriate and should be repeated at intervals if the operation is prolonged. Contaminated, traumatic wounds also are appropriately treated with systemic antibacterials if the danger of contamination is high and if the antibacterial can be delivered within the golden period of about 3 hours. Most clean lacerations have minimal contamination, and in large series of patients systemic antibacterials show no advantage. It cannot be emphasized enough that the widespread emerging resistance of microorganisms to most, in some cases even all, antibacterials can largely be traced to the indiscriminate, broad-spectrum use of antibacterials when they are not indicated.

Route. The bloodstream is the finest delivery system yet invented and is to be preferred for all antibacterials unless scientific evidence indicates otherwise. After about 3–4 hours, antibacterials in the bloodstream no longer reach the wound. An open wound may be measured by quantitative bacterial culture before and during administration of systemic antibacterials. When systemic administration of the antibacterial at many times the normal dosage has no effect on the bacterial level in the wound, one may conclude only that it is not the appropriate route. This, of course, is the scientific and biologic basis for the use of topical antibacterials, which reach the wound and, in fact, reduce the bacterial count. It is logical, therefore, when managing a contaminated wound to use the following steps:

1. Culture the wound by quantitative microbiologic techniques and determine the microorganism that is present, at what level, and which antibacterial is appropriate. If the count is more than 10^5 microorganisms per gram of tissue, it is not safe to close the wound; if fewer than 10^5 microorganisms per gram of tissue are present, close the wound.

2. Use the antibacterial by the proper route until you can demonstrate that the bacterial count has been reduced to a safe level of fewer than 10^5 microorganisms per gram of tissue. Then close the wound. The documented success rate for closure of wounds managed in this fashion is greater than 98%.

15. My laboratory does not perform quantitative microbiology. Please comment.

Hogwash. Every microbiologic laboratory in the United States performs quantitative bacterial cultures on urine on a daily basis. With simple equipment (less than $100.00) lab workers can weigh, crush, and dilute soft tissue and perform the test in about 30 minutes (rapid slide). They can also give you accurate cultures and sensitivities in 24 hours, as they do with urine samples. They do not perform quantitative analysis because you did not ask them to do so. Hospitals that spend millions of dollars on expensive equipment such as MRI will gladly perform the test free of charge if you show them that you can prevent even one wound infection or save even one patient a single day in the hospital. There are more resistant surgeons than there are resistant microorganisms.

BIBLIOGRAPHY

1. Krizek TJ, Gottlieb LJ: Acute suppurative mediastinitis. In Sabiston DC Jr (ed): Textbook of Surgery: The Biologic Basis of Modern Surgical Practice. Philadelphia, W.B. Saunders, 1997, pp 1929–1933.
2. Learmonth J, as quoted by Bowen TE: To the soldier medic [editorial]. Mil Med 156:638–639, 1991.
3. Robson MC, Krizek TJ, Heggers JP: Biology of surgical infection. In Ravitch MM, Austen WG, Scott HW, et al (eds): Current Problems in Surgery. Chicago, Year Book, 1973, pp 1–62.

7. THE FETAL WOUND

Eric J. Stelnicki, M.D., Michael T. Longaker, M .D., and Jeffrey Weinzweig, M.D.

1. What is the major phenotypic difference that distinguishes fetal from adult wound healing?

Unlike the adult cutaneous skin wound, which heals with scar, fetal cutaneous wound healing is scarless, appearing more like tissue regeneration than wound repair.

2. How was scarless fetal wound healing discovered?

The observation that the human fetus heals without scar was originally described by Rowlatt in 1979 but went unappreciated by the medical community until the early 1980s when surgeons at the University of California San Francisco made the observation that patients who underwent fetal surgery healed without scar. Only after this second observation did intense study into the process of fetal wound healing begin.

3. Does the process of fetal wound healing follow the same patterns as adult wound healing?

No. Adult wound repair is characterized by five stages: hemostasis, inflammation, proliferation, early remodeling, and late remodeling. The first three stages take several weeks to be completed, and the final remodeling stages may last for months to years. In contrast, the scarless fetal wound repair process occurs at an accelerated rate, with restoration of normal tissue architecture within 5–7 days after injury; the acute inflammatory stage of healing is absent.

4. Is the ability of the fetus to heal without scar purely a function of being in the womb, bathed by amnionic fluid?

No. Two experiments prove that such is not the case. First, fetal marsupials, which move outside the womb and develop in a maternal pouch, also heal without scar. Second, human fetal skin transplanted onto the backs of adult mice with severe combined immunodeficiency also regenerate. Neither of these cutaneous tissues is in contact with amnionic fluid during or after the time of wounding, indicating that the process is intrinsic to the fetal cells.

5. Are the same cells involved in the processes of fetal and adult wound healing?

No. The presence of the inflammatory cell, particularly the macrophage, is essential to normal adult wound healing. Without these cells normal epithelialization and fibroblast proliferation do not occur. The fetal wound, in contrast, contains few inflammatory cells and appears to be controlled purely by the activities of the fetal fibroblast and epidermis. In addition, the function of the macrophage in the fetal wound has yet to be determined.

6. What effect does inflammation have on the fetal wound?

The induction of inflammation in fetal cutaneous wounds induces adultlike scar formation. The same effect is seen on fetal wounds regardless of the type of inflammatory stimulus, indicating that inflammatory cells somehow alter the function of the fetal fibroblast and make it respond in a more adultlike manner.

7. What types of collagens are laid down within the fetal wound?

The fetal wound is repaired primarily by the rapid and highly organized deposition of type III collagen. The ratio of type III to type I collagen is 3:1. In the adult wound type III collagen is laid down early in the healing process but is quickly replaced predominantly by type I collagen. At the end of adult wound remodeling the ratio of type III to type I collagen is 1:3, the opposite of the fetal wound.

8. What is the role of the extracellular matrix (ECM) in fetal wound healing?

Several features of the extracellular matrix (ECM) other than changes in collagen deposition characterize the fetal wound-healing process. First, hyaluronic acid (HA) is abundant in the fetal wound; it is produced 2 weeks longer than in adults. The abundance of HA is thought to aid in fibroblast movement, to promote cellular proliferation, and to inhibit cellular differentiation. Second, fibronectin is deposited faster in fetal wounds (4 hours vs. 12 hours in adult wounds), rapidly providing a good scaffolding for epithelial cell migration. Finally, sulfated glycosaminoglycans (GAGs), such as decorin and heparin sulfate, are expressed at low levels in fetal wounds but increase with gestational age. This increase correlates with the development of scar formation after cutaneous wounding. It is thought that GAGs may play a role in the induction of cytodifferentiation.

9. How may HA provide the matrix signal that coordinates healing by regeneration rather than by scarring?

HA is a key structural and functional component of the ECM in instances of rapid tissue proliferation, regeneration, and repair. HA is laid down early in the matrix of both fetal and adult wounds; however, sustained deposition of HA is unique to fetal wound healing. Although the mechanism for prolonged HA deposition in fetal wounds remains unclear, the presence of HA-protein complexes in the fetal matrix may provide the signal responsible for promoting healing by regeneration rather than by scarring.

10. Do all fetal tissues heal scarlessly?

No. To date, fetal bone, skin, and palatal mucoperiosteum are the only elements of the mammalian fetus that appear to be able to regenerate after wounding. Studies of tendon, diaphragm, nerve, and GI tract have shown scar formation in response to wounding in both fetuses and adults.

11. Do fetal wounds heal differently in congenital models and surgically created models?

No. Models of dilantin-induced cleft lip in mice and anabasine-induced cleft palate in goats heal in the same manner as analagous surgically created models in both species—scarlessly.

12. Is there a time limit to the process of fetal cutaneous wound healing?

Yes. The fetus is able to heal its wounds without scar only up to the early third trimester of gestation. After this point, cutaneous wounds develop an increasing amount of scar.

13. Do all fetal cutaneous wounds heal without scar?

No. Excisional wounds greater than 9 mm contract and heal with scar at any gestational age. Most second trimester excisional wounds of smaller size heal scarlessly. After the early second trimester, as the fetus advances in age, the size of the excisional wound that can be repaired scarlessly decreases proportionately until the third trimester is reached and all wounds heal with scar.

14. Does amniotic fluid play a role in wound contraction?

Yes. Both fetal and adult fibroblast contraction are inhibited by human amniotic fluid. This effect progressively decreases with increasing wound size and advancing fetal age.

15. Is the lack of wound contracture in the fetus due to lack of myofibroblasts in the skin?

No. Multiple studies using immunohistochemistry and transmission electron microscopy have demonstrated the presence of myofibroblasts in the fetal wound. The mere presence of these cells does not correlate with the ability to form a scar contracture.

16. Can adult skin placed into a fetal environment heal without scar?

No. Adult skin wounds always heal with scar regardless of their location. Experimental work in a fetal lamb model, in which adult maternal skin was placed as a graft within a fetal cutaneous defect, demonstrated healing by scar formation consistent with typical adult wound healing.

CONTROVERSIES

17. What regulates the process of fetal wound healing?

Current theories range from growth factor regulation to the coordinated expression of DNA-binding proteins such as homeobox genes. Whatever the mechanism, it probably involves the process of decreased inflammation and regulation of increased fibroblast and epidermal proliferation.

18. How do growth factor profiles differ between fetal and adult wounds?

The fetal wound is characterized by a decrease in the activity of various growth factors such as transforming growth factor beta (TGF-β), platelet-derived growth factor (PDGF), and basic fibroblast growth factor (bFGF) compared with adult wounds. When activated in the fetus, these growth factors are expressed rapidly and for a short time. The addition of some exogenous growth factors to the fetal wound induces scar formation. This may explain why inflammatory cells that secrete these growth factors force the fetal fibroblast to produce scar. The level of growth factor expression in the fetal wound is controversial because of several conflicting reports in the literature. A review of these reports indicates that the variable changes in fetal growth factor expression are both species- and model-dependent.

19. What is the potential advantage of scarless fetal wound healing in the treatment of congenital craniofacial anomalies?

Scarless healing in utero may minimize or prevent facial dysmorphology associated with anomalies such as cleft lip and palate. Maxillary hypoplasia, with resultant midface retrusion and relative prognathism, is often the result of surgically induced scar formation after repair of cleft lip and/or palate. Increased lip pressure after postnatal repair of cleft lip in animals is also associated with progressive midface hypoplasia. Thus, the major advantage of scarless fetal wound healing is unimpaired facial growth without the adverse effect of the lip and/or palate scar.

20. Can scarless healing after in utero repair of cleft lip and palate completely eliminate the facial growth abnormality associated with postnatal, surgically induced scar formation?

Not likely. An intrinsic factor contributes to facial growth impairment in the repaired as well as unrepaired congenital cleft. The incidence of this factor is unpredictable and variably expressed. This intrinsic component of facial dysmorphology is unrelated to scar formation and, thus, is largely unaffected by the nature of the healing process. However, the presence of scar may adversely affect the expression of this intrinsic factor, resulting in a greater degree of facial growth impairment.

BIBLIOGRAPHY

1. Adzick NS, Lorenz HP: Cells, matrix, growth factors, and the surgeon. The biology of scarless fetal wound repair. Ann Surg 1994. 220:10-18, 1994.
2. Cass D, Bullard KM, Sylvester KG, et al: Wound size and gestastional age modulate scar formation in fetal wound repair. J Pediatr Surg 32:411–415, 1997.
3. Hallock GG: In utero cleft lip repair in A/J mice. Plast Reconstr Surg 75:785, 1985.
4. Howarth G, Ferguson MWJ: Marsupial models of scarless fetal wound healing. In Adzick NS, Longaker MT (eds): Fetal Wound Healing. New York, Elsevier Science, 1992, pp 95–124.
5. Leibovich SJ, Ross R: The role of the macrophage in wound repair: A study with hydrocortisone and anti-macrophage serum. Am J Pathol 78:71–100, 1975.
6. Longaker MT, Adzick NS: The biology of fetal wound healing: A review. Plast Reconstr Surg 87:788–798, 1991.
7. Longaker MT, Burd DA, Gown AM, et al: Midgestational excisional fetal lamb wounds contract in utero. J Pediatr Surg 26:942–947; discussion, 947–948, 1991.
8. Longaker MT, Whitby DJ, Ferguson MW, et al: Adult skin wounds in the fetal environment heal with scar formation. Ann Surg 219:65–72, 1994.
9. Longaker MT, Whitby DJ, Jennings RW, et al: Fetal diaphragmatic wounds heal with scar formation. J Surg Res 50:375–385, 1991.
10. Lorenz HP, Lin RY, Longaker MT, et al: The fetal fibroblast: The effector cell of scarless fetal skin repair. Plast Reconstr Surg 96:1251–1259; discussion, 1260–1261, 1995.
11. Lorenz HP, Longaker MT, Perkocha LA, et al: Scarless wound repair: A human fetal skin model. Development 114:253–259, 1994.
12. Martin P, Nobes C, McCluskey J, Lewis J: Repair of excisional wounds in the embryo. Eye 8:155–160, 1994.
13. Mast BA, Krummel TM: Acute inflammation in fetal wound healing. In Adzick NS, Longaker MT (eds): Fetal Wound Healing. New York, Elsevier Science, 1992, pp 227–240.
14. Meuli M, Lorenz HP, Hedrick MH, et al: Scar formation in the fetal alimentary tract. J Pediatr Surg 30:392–395, 1995.
15. Nath RK, LaRegina M, Markham H, et al: The expression of transforming growth factor type beta in fetal and adult rabbit skin wounds. J Pediatr Surg 29:416–421, 1994.
16. Rowlatt V: Intrauterine wound healing in a 20 week human fetus. Virchow's Arch 381:353, 1979.
17. Siebert J, Burd A, McCarthy JG, et al: Fetal wound healing: A biochemical study of scarless healing. Plast Reconstr Surg 85:495–502; discussion, 503–504, 1990.
18. Sullivan WG: In utero cleft lip repair in the mouse with an incision. Plast Reconstr Surg 84:723, 1989.
19. Weinzweig J, Sullivan P, Panter K, et al: The fetal cleft palate: Characterization and in utero repair of a congenital model. Plast Surg Forum 20:25–27, 1997.
20. Weinzweig J, Panter K, Pantaloni M, et al: The fetal cleft palate: A histomorphologic study of palatal development and function following in utero repair of a congenital model. Plast Surg Forum 21:86–88, 1998.

II. Integument

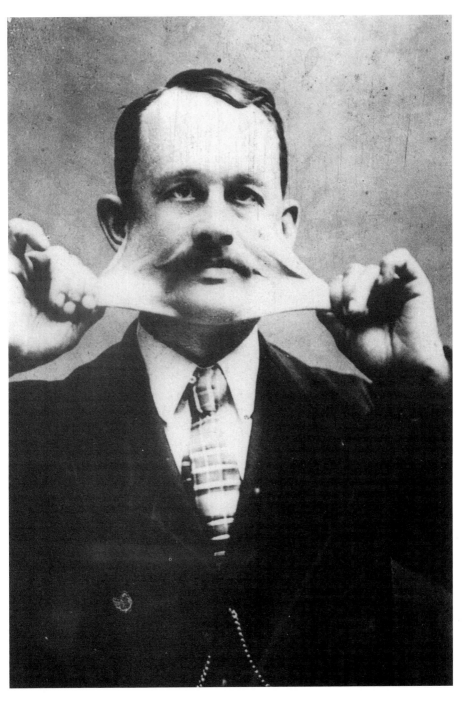

Elastic Skin Man
James Morris
ca. 1890
Albumen print
© 1998 The Wellcome Institute Library, London

8. MALIGNANT MELANOMA

Faizi A. Siddiqi, M.D., Derlis Martino, M.D., and Homayoun N. Sasson, M.D.

1. What causes cutaneous melanoma?

Overall, **genetic determinants** play a major role in the pathogenesis of melanoma and normal and dysplastic nevi. Melanoma has long been known to have a higher incidence in families. Between 5% and 10% of patients with melanoma have a family history of the disease independent of other factors such as sun exposure. Presently, several melanoma susceptibility genes are under study. One of the most significant is the tumor suppressor gene for protein p16, CDKN2, alterations of which have been found in about one-half of all melanoma-prone families. This protein is a negative regulator of the cell cycle. Mutations in the N-*ras* oncogene were detected in 36% of all patients with melanomas in one series. In addition to the above, certain risk factors have been identified for the development of the tumor:

1. **Sun exposure.** After extensive study, sun exposure was found to be the most important risk factor for melanoma. There is a closer association with ultraviolet (UV) B radiation (wavelength of 290 nm) than UVA (wavelength of 375 nm) and visible light (wavelength of 600 nm). On the other hand, studies of sunscreen use have suggested that exposure to UVA also increases the risk of melanoma. Commonly used sunscreens block UVB but are transparent to UVA, which makes up 90–95% of the UV energy in the solar spectrum. Thus, sunscreens may permit excessive exposure of the skin to portions of the solar radiation other than UVB and may increase the risk of melanoma. Studies relating sunburns to melanoma risk have shown a consistent association. Results showed an increased risk with an increase in the number of blistering sunburns. The evidence also suggests that sunburns are more dangerous in childhood than later in life. Of interest, intermittent sun exposure (e.g., during summer holidays at the beach) rather than chronic sun exposure (e.g., outdoor occupations like farming or construction) appears to be the main risk factor.

2. **Pigment traits.** Persons with blue eyes, fair or red hair, and pale complexion are at higher risk for melanoma. Hair color is a stronger factor than eye color.

3. **Skin reaction to sunlight.** People who get sunburned easily and tan poorly are at an increased risk for melanoma. However, pigment traits and skin reaction to sunlight are correlated with each other and may represent a common underlying sun-sensitivity trait.

4. **Freckling.** Freckling is a characteristic pigmentation pattern related to poor sun tolerance and an increased risk of melanoma.

5. **Benign melanocytic nevi.** The number of nevi rather than their size has been related to a higher melanoma risk in many studies. The presence of dysplastic nevi with irregular edges and irregular pigmentation or inflammation is associated with increased risk of melanoma, and the number of dysplastic nevi more strongly predicts the risk than the total number of nevi of all types.

6. **Anthropometric indices.** A prospective study showed an increased risk of melanoma with increasing height in both sexes.

7. **Immunosuppressive states.** Renal transplant recipients and patients who have had cancers such as lymphoma have an increased risk of developing melanoma.

2. What are the different types of melanoma?

There are four types of melanoma: lentigo maligna, acral lentiginous, superficial spreading, and nodular. All four types have two biologic phases: a horizontal (radial) growth phase (with epidermal involvement only) and a vertical growth phase (dermal invasion). Metastatic invasion does not pose a threat in the horizontal growth phase because blood vessels do not occur in the epidermis. In the vertical growth phase, however, the deeper the melanoma invades the skin, the greater the possibility of hematogenous and lymphatic spread.

Lentigo maligna melanoma accounts for 4–10% of cutaneous melanoma and is typically located in the head, neck, and arms of elderly individuals. The precursor in situ lesion, lentigo maligna, is usually present for more than 10–15 years and attains large size (3–6-cm diameter) before progressing to malignancy. The lesion appears as a tan-to-brown macule or patch with variation in pigment or areas of regression that appear hypopigmented clinically. Malignant degeneration is characterized by nodular development within the precursor lesion.

Acral lentiginous melanoma is the least common subtype, representing 2–8% of melanoma in Caucasians, although it accounts for 35–90% of melanoma in African Americans, Asians, and Hispanics. It typically occurs on the palms or soles or beneath the nail plate (subungual variant). Irregular pigmentation, large size (>3 cm diameter), and plantar location are characteristic features of acral lentiginous melanoma.

Superficial spreading melanoma is the most common subtype, accounting for about 70% of all cases. It occurs most frequently on the upper back of men and women as well as the lower extremities of women. The clinical lesion typically shows irregular, asymmetric borders with color variegation and size typically greater than 6–8 mm.

Nodular melanoma is the second most common subtype of melanoma, occurring in 15–30% of patients. As with superficial spreading melanoma, legs and trunk are the most frequent sites of occurrence. Rapid growth, which corresponds to the lack of an identifiable radial growth phase, is a hallmark of nodular melanoma. Clinically the lesion presents as a raised, dark brown-to-black papule or nodule; ulceration and bleeding are not uncommon.

3. Why is the incidence of melanoma rising?

The incidence of melanoma has been rising for the past several decades. In fact, it is estimated that 1 in 57 Americans will be diagnosed with melanoma by the year 2000. Melanoma mortality rates also have been on the rise, but survival rates are improving. One of the more plausible explanations for the increased incidence is the progressive depletion of the ozone layer. The stratospheric ozone layer is more effective in blocking UVA than UVB radiation. Thus, more UVB radiation reaches the earth's surface. As discussed above, UVB is the wavelength most associated with the development of melanoma. Since 1969, there has been a decrease of 3–7% in the ozone layer. It has been estimated that for each percentage decrease in the amount of ozone, melanoma incidence increases about 1%.

4. What are the indications to biopsy a lesion? What type of biopsy should be performed?

The cornerstone of management of malignant melanoma is early diagnosis, which leads to treatment at a curable stage. Inspection alone is about 60–80% effective in identifying malignant melanoma. Other techniques, such as baseline full-body photography of patients with atypical moles, may be helpful. Appropriate biopsy of a suspicious pigmented lesion is essential to establish the diagnosis and to optimize histologic exam and staging. Any lesion that produces patient concern or that demonstrates changing morphology, pruritus, or bleeding and all new lesions or scalp lesions should be biopsied. Melanoma is not always suspected clinically, particularly with unusual variants such as desmoplastic or amelanotic lesions.

An **excisional biopsy** is recommended. This approach allows adequate distinction of the neoplasm from surrounding normal tissue and, if the lesion proves to be melanoma, adequate measurement of the thickness of invasion. However, incisional biopsies or punch biopsies may be satisfactory for diagnosing melanoma, especially in large pigmented lesions in areas of cosmetic importance or where primary closure would be difficult. The shave biopsy technique should *not* be used if melanoma is suspected. Transection of the lesion during shave biopsy may compromise histopathologic interpretation and prevent accurate measurement of thickness.

5. What are the recommended prevention strategies?

Patient education about the warning signs of melanoma has been successfully achieved with the **ABCDE** criteria for a changing mole:

Asymmetry
Border-notching
Color variegation with black, brown, red, blue or white hues
Diameter greater than 6 mm (larger than a pencil eraser)
Elevation

In addition, increased public awareness of the dangers of excessive sun exposure should be an important target, especially avoidance of exposure in young children, in whom the melanocytic population is more unstable. Self-examination for melanoma is advocated and should be done by everyone, especially people with large numbers of melanocytic nevi (50 or more) before age 20 or after age 50 and people who have more than 100 benign pigmented nevi or more than 20 pigmented nevi on the trunk or an extremity.

6. How is prognosis determined?

Tumor thickness and **depth of invasion** are the most important prognostic factors and help to guide treatment and management plans. In perhaps no other cancer can we derive as much prognostic information from the primary tumor alone. This factor was first defined by Clark, who determined five levels of microinvasion. Clark et al. showed that survival rates worsened with the increasing levels of invasion of melanoma cells. In 1970, Breslow took Clark's work a step further with quantitative measurement of the maximal vertical height of the tumor using an ocular micrometer. Breslow's method avoids the confounding effect of the variable thickness of the reticular dermis. This measurement is easier and more accurate than the Clark level and appears to predict the risk of metastatic disease more precisely. Over the years, numerous thickness subsets, using large series of patients, have been measured for prognostic value. Breakpoints have been defined with respect to tumor thickness and statistical survival. The current breakpoints for staging are 0.75, 1.5, and 4.0 mm. In fact, there may not be natural breakpoints but rather a continuous linear correlation of survival and tumor thickness.

Other prognostic factors include:

1. **Ulceration**, which is a statistically significant independent factor, even after thickness of the tumor is taken into account;

2. **Lymphocyte infiltration**, which has been reported as a favorable prognostic factor;

3. **Mitotic rate**, which correlates inversely with survival.

In addition, anatomic site (extremity lesions indicate improved survival rates compared with truncal lesions) and gender (women survive melanoma better than men) are important prognostic factors.

Once the tumor has become metastatic, the prognosis is dramatically altered for the worse. The most common first site of metastasis is the regional lymph nodes. Presence of tumor in the lymph nodes makes the disease stage III in the American Joint Committee on Cancer Classification. As with certain other malignancies, the number of nodal metastases has been identified as the most important prognostic factor for patients with lymph node involvement.

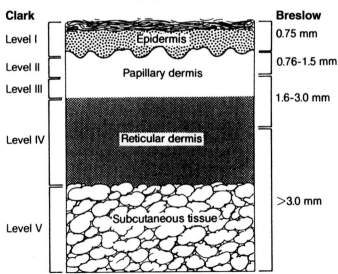

Classification of primary melanoma according to depth of invasion. (Adapted from Schwartz S: Principles of Surgery, 6th ed. New York, McGraw-Hill, 1996, p 526.)

Tumor-Node-Metastasis Classification of Melanoma of the Skin

Primary tumor (T)

TX	No evidence of primary tumor (unknown primary or primary tumor removed and not examined histologically)
T0	Atypical melanocytic hyperplasia (Clark level I), not a malignant lesion
T1	Invasion of papillary dermis (level II) or 0.75 mm in thickness or less
T2	Invasion of the papillary/reticular–dermal interface (level III) or 0.76–1.5 mm in thickness
T3	Invasion of reticular dermis (level IV) or 1.51–4 mm in thickness
T4	Invasion of subcutaneous tissue (level V) or 4.1 mm or more in thickness or satellite(s) within 2 cm of any primary melanoma

Nodal involvement (N)

NX	Minimal requirements to assess the regional nodes cannot be met
N0	No regional lymph node involvement
N1	Involvement of only one regional lymph node station; negative regional lymph nodes and < 5 in-transit metastases beyond 2 cm from primary site
N2	Any one of the following: (1) involvement of > 1 regional node station; (2) regional node(s) over 5 cm in diameter or fixed; (3) 5 or more in-transit metastases or any in-transit metastasis beyond 2 cm from primary site with regional lymph node involvement

Distant metastasis (M)

MX	Minimal requirements to assess the presence of distant metastasis cannot be met
M0	No known distal metastasis
M1	Involvement of skin or subcutaneous tissue beyond the site of primary lymph node drainage
M2	Visceral metastasis (spread to any distant site other than skin or subcutaneous tissues)

Adapted from Schwartz S: Principles of Surgery, 6th ed. New York, McGraw-Hill, 1996, p 525.

Staging System for Melanoma Adopted by the American Joint Committee on Cancer

STAGE	THICKNESS/LEVEL	TNM CATEGORY	5-YEAR SURVIVAL (%)
IA	≤ 0.75 mm or level II	T1, N0, M0	> 90
IB	0.76–1.5 mm or level III	T2, N0, M0	
IIA	1.51–4 mm or level IV	T3, N0, M0	70
IIB	> 4 mm or level V	T4, N0, M0	
III	Limited nodal metastasis	Any T, N1, M0	35
IV	Advanced local metastasis	Any T, N2, M0	< 2
	Distant metastasis	Any T, any N, M1 or M2	

Adapted from Rogers G, et al: New approaches to treating advanced melanoma: Adjuvant treatment of high-risk primary melanoma and boron capture therapy. Semin Cutan Med Surg 16:166, 1997.

7. What treatment strategies currently complement surgery?

No therapy is effective as a consistent cure for melanoma that has spread beyond the regional nodes. Combinations of chemotherapy, radiotherapy, and immunotherapy have been tried in patients with advanced melanoma, and the best response rates have been less than 25%. Of these approaches, **immunotherapy** seems the most promising, mostly because melanoma is one of the most immunogenic of all solid tumors. However, at this point no therapy appears to be better than dacarbazine alone. The ultimate goal is to develop a melanoma vaccine to block the initial pathogenesis of the tumor in high-risk patients. For this purpose, approximately 70 different antigens expressed in melanoma cells have been defined by monoclonal antibodies. None of these has proved to be truly melano-specific. Vaccines prepared with these antigens in various mixtures are currently under study. Currently, two innovative immunotherapeutic modalities are used to treat advanced disease: high-dose interleukin-2 (IL-2) therapy and high-dose interferon alpha-2b. Both treatments are highly toxic, and their exact indications are currently being defined.

8. How do melanomas metastasize?

Metastatic disease usually follows a sequential order: first to the regional lymph nodes and then to distant sites, including subcutaneous tissue, lung, liver, brain, bone, and visceral organs. Distant metastasis portends a poor prognosis with a 5-year survival rate of less than 10%. Peculiar types of metastatic disease in such patients are the so-called "satellites" and "in-transit" metastases, which develop in 2–20% of patients with melanoma. These cohesive aggregates of tumor cells are found within the dermal subcutaneous tissue or blood vessels (or both). They are separated from the main mass of the tumor by normal tissue and represent microscopic metastatic lesions. Satellites occur within an area of 5 cm from the primary tumor, whereas in-transit lesions are farther away than 5 cm. The incidence of nodal metastatic involvement correlates with the presence of these lesions. The presence of microscopic satellites and in-transit metastasis correlates with a poor rate of patient survival and is associated with an increased frequency of local and nodal disease compared with other tumors matched in thickness but without satellites.

9. What kinds of moles have malignant potential?

Malignant melanoma may arise de novo or from a precursor melanocytic nevus. Precursor lesions include congenital melanocytic nevi, common acquired melanocytic nevi, dysplastic nevi, and melanoma in situ. Remnants of a benign melanocytic nevus can be found in up to 35% of melanoma biopsy specimens. Patients with large congenital melanocytic nevi are at increased risk for the development of melanoma. These nevi have, or are predicted to have, a largest diameter of 20 cm in adulthood. It is recommended that they be evaluated for excision early in life.

10. What is a dysplastic nevus?

Dysplastic nevi represent a clinically heterogeneous group of melanocytic nevi that tend to be larger (usually >5mm) than ordinary nevi and have more ill-defined borders. The lesions are typically seen on the trunk and extremities but may be found anywhere on the body. Many have the overall morphology of a fried egg. They usually are acquired in adolescence but may appear in childhood. Dysplastic nevi may occur in two clinical settings:

1. Patients with a personal or family history of malignant melanoma or familial dysplastic nevus syndrome
2. Patients without such a history, the so-called sporadic dysplastic nevus syndrome.

The familial syndrome is a distinctive clinicopathologic entity, and patients in this group are at an increased risk for the development of melanoma. However, the sporadic syndrome is less well-defined, and the incidence of melanoma is relatively small. In terms of management, dysplastic nevi are not precancerous lesions in themselves but rather clinical markers for increased risk of melanoma. Such patients should be examined frequently with the aid of total body photography on either a semiannual or annual basis; excision is recommended with a change in clinical appearance.

11. What is the surgical approach to the primary melanoma lesion?

The fundamental principle in the surgical treatment of malignant melanoma, as with other malignant tumors, is excision of the melanoma with pathologically negative margins. In the past, excision margins of 4–5 cm were deemed necessary to obtain local control; they resulted in large defects requiring split-thickness skin grafting with accompanying morbidity, increased hospital stay, and increased cost. Once it was revealed that tumor thickness influenced prognosis, prospective randomized studies were initiated to determine the margins necessary to obtain local control. Based on these trials, it is clear that most primary cutaneous melanomas can be managed with excision and primary closure with acceptable local control. Advantages of this approach include less wound morbidity, reduced need for skin grafting, and reduced costs. Based on the findings of the studies, 1-cm margins are adequate for very thin lesions. For lesions deeper than 2 mm, a margin of 2 cm is adequate. If the lesion is 1–2 mm in thickness, a 2-cm margin is adequate; a 1-cm margin is associated with only a 3% local recurrence rate, which may have no impact on survival.

Recommended Margins of Resection for Primary Melanoma

THICKNESS (mm)	MARGIN (cm)
Melanoma in situ	0.5
< 1.0	1
1.0–2.0	1–2
2.0–4.0	2
> 4.0	2–4

12. What is the significance of the regional nodal basin?

The most common site of metastatic disease in patients with malignant melanoma is the regional nodal basin; risk of nodal metastases is related to depth of the primary lesion. The risk of identifiable synchronous nodal metastases is 2–10% in patients with primary lesions < 1 mm in thickness. In patients with intermediate lesions (1–4 mm in thickness), the risk of identifiable synchronous nodal metastases is 20–25%. For patients with thick primary melanomas (> 4 mm), the risk is 50–60%. Identification of nodal metastases is the most powerful factor for predicting survival. Survival is associated not only with the presence of nodal metastases but also with the number of positive lymph nodes. The 5-year survival rate for patients with pathologically negative lymph nodes is approximately 90%. For patients whose lymph nodes are clinically negative but pathologically positive, the 5-year survival rate is about 50–60%. In patients with clinically and pathologically positive lymph nodes upon presentation, the 5-year survival rate is about 15–20%. The 5-year survival rate in patients with 1 positive lymph node is about 50%. In patients with 2–4 positive lymph nodes, the 5-year survival rate is 20–40%. Finally, for patients with 5 or more positive lymph nodes, the 5-year survival rate is less than 20%.

13. How should patients with clinically positive lymph nodes be managed?

Patients who have palpable, clinically positive lymph nodes in the primary lymphatic draining area should undergo complete nodal dissection. The extent of inguinal dissection, however, remains controversial. Should patients undergo superficial dissection alone, or should it be combined with an en bloc deep inguinal lymph node dissection of the external iliac and obturator groups? Two major studies from Roswell Park Cancer Institute and Memorial Sloan-Kettering Cancer Center reported conflicting results. Although the basis for the differences between the two studies is unclear, it may be that the only curative option for patients with positive deep nodes is complete, en bloc dissection of superficial and deep inguinal as well as obturator nodes, which accounts for the improved survival noted in the Roswell data. A more conservative strategy is en bloc deep and superficial groin dissection for patients who undergo therapeutic superficial inguinal lymph node dissection and have histologically positive lymph nodes at the junction between superficial and deep chains.

14. What is elective lymph node dissection?

Elective lymph node dissection (ELND) refers to the anatomic lymphadenectomy of the primary draining nodal basin when it is clinically negative. The theoretic advantage of this procedure is obvious: if cutaneous melanoma spreads initially to the lymphatic groups and from there systemically, prophylactic dissection of the nodal basin will interrupt this progression in a proportion of patients at an early stage, thereby potentially improving survival. The disadvantage is that approximately 80% of the patients with melanomas of intermediate thickness (1–4 mm) have negative lymph nodes at presentation and therefore would not benefit from this procedure. Only patients with clinically negative nodal metastases and no distant metastases would potentially benefit from ELND.

15. What is the morbidity of ELND?

Patients undergoing ELND incur the expense and inconvenience of surgery along with a hospital stay of 1–2 days. Postsurgical complications of wound infection, dehiscence, and poor wound healing occur in 20–25% of patients. Symptomatic lymphedema occurs in 20–25% of patients even with appropriate prophylactic measures. Moreover, opponents of ELND claim that because melanomas metastasize via the hematogenous route as well as via the lymphatics, ELND would have no effect. They are also concerned that the removal of regional lymph nodes may decrease the immunologic response to tumor antigens. Furthermore, lymph node metastasis may be a manifestation rather than a predecessor of distant tumor spread.

16. Which patients benefit from ELND?

Both proponents and opponents of ELND generally agree that with melanomas less than 1 mm in thickness, ELND is not indicated because such lesions have a low rate of nodal metastases and a generally good prognosis. ELND in patients with melanomas greater than 4mm in depth is also not indicated because such lesions have a high incidence of systemic metastases and ELND is not thought to improve survival. The intermediate-thickness melanomas are the most controversial. However, prospective randomized trials of ELND vs. observation failed to show an overall survival advantage. The two most frequently quoted studies—the World Health Organization Study and the

Mayo Clinic Study—were criticized for the number of patients, a high percentage of female patients (known to have a good prognosis), and lack of tumor thickness verification.

There appears to be no clear benefit to the general population for ELND because of the inherent problems with retrospective analyses and the difficulty of explaining why patients older than 60 years of age do worse with lymph node dissection than patients younger than 60 years of age. It may be that patients with thin intermediate-thickness melanomas (1–2 mm) do better than patients with thicker intermediate-thickness melanomas (2–4 mm) because they have less propensity to spread hematogenously and benefit from nodal dissection.

17. How can lymphatic mapping with sentinel lymph node biopsy circumvent the problem of diagnosis of lymph node metastases by lymphadenectomy with its attendant morbidity?

The technique of intraoperative lymphatic mapping, first described in 1991 by Wong et al., allows the surgeon to identify the sentinel lymph node—i.e. the single lymph node or group of lymph nodes that first receives lymphatic flow from the area of skin involved with the melanoma. The sentinel node is the first node in the lymphatic chain to receive tumor cells from the primary site. If this node is free of tumor, the remaining lymph nodes in the regional lymph node chain also will be free of tumor. This technique allows the surgeon to determine the status of the regional lymph nodes after lymph node biopsy rather than lymphadenectomy, thereby sparing lymph node-negative patients the morbidity of extensive lymph node dissection. Moreover, because the pathologist receives the lymph node that is most likely to harbor metastatic disease, a more extensive evaluation of the lymph node with multiple sectioning and immunostaining will improve the accuracy of diagnosis.

18. How is lymphatic mapping performed?

At the time of lymph node surgery, the surgeon injects a vital blue dye into the skin at the site of the melanoma. The dye is quickly taken into the lymphatics and results in blue staining of the sentinel lymph node in the regional lymphatic basin. The nodes are then removed and examined for the presence of metastatic disease. By adding immunohistochemistry analysis and polymerase chain reaction to hematoxylin and eosin studies of the sentinel lymph node, the degree of identifying positive micrometastases for melanoma has increased by an additional 40%. The optimal technique for identifying sentinel lymph nodes is a combination of a blue dye that stains the nodes in the operating room and subdermal injection of a radioactive tracer that marks the nodes either preoperatively or intraoperatively with a hand-held gamma counter. In experienced hands, sentinel lymph nodes can be identified in more than 95% of patients with a false-negative rate less than 1%.

19. What are the advantages of intraoperative lymphatic mapping?

1. The technique can be done under local anesthesia.

2. Only patients with histologic proof of nodal metastases undergo formal lymphadenectomy; thus, lymphadenectomy is therapeutic and performed at an earlier stage of disease.

3. Patients without nodal metastases are spared the morbidity of unnecessary lymphadenectomy.

4. It is more feasible to perform a meticulous pathologic exam of just one or two sentinel nodes.

5. Because many of the ongoing systemic adjuvant trials require lymph node involvement as an entrance criterion, the use of sentinel lymph node biopsy followed by selective lymphadenectomy allows patients to enter trials earlier in the course of the disease.

20. What is the treatment of metastatic disease?

Systemic therapy for cutaneous malignant melanoma is relatively limited; even the best combination of chemotherapeutic agents has limited response rates and virtually no sustained complete response rates. One exception is high-dose interleukin-2 therapy, which results in a complete response rate of 7% that is sustained in 75% of patients who achieve it. As a result, a selective approach to resection of limited distant visceral metastases includes patients with in-transit and nonregional nodal metastases, pulmonary metastases, gastrointestinal metastases, adrenal metastases, and isolated brain metastases.

21. What is the only approved adjuvant therapy for resected melanoma?

Alpha interferon has been approved by the Food and Drug Administration as an effective adjuvant therapy for resected melanoma patients at high risk for systemic relapse. The Eastern Cooperative Oncology Group Trial EST 1684 randomized patients at high risk for systemic relapse (positive resected lymph node or primary lesions > 4 mm in thickness) to 1 year of high-dose interferon alpha-2b therapy vs. observation. At a median follow-up of 6.9 years, the group that received interferon had a significant improvement in disease-free survival and overall survival rates. Interferon alpha-2b is the first adjuvant demonstrated to show a significant benefit for patients with melanoma at high risk for systemic relapse.

BIBLIOGRAPHY

1. Ahmed I: Malignant melanoma: Prognostic indicators. Mayo Clin Proc 72:356–361, 1997.
2. Balch CM, Milton GW, Cascinell N, et al: Elective lymph node dissection: Pros and cons. In Balch CM, Houghton A, Milton GW, et al (eds): Cutaneous Melanoma, 2nd ed. Philadelphia, J.B. Lippincott, 1992, pp 345–366.
3. Balch CM, Soong S-J, Bartolucci AA ,et al: Efficacy of an elective regional lymph node dissection of 1 to 4 mm thickness melanomas for patients 60 years of age and younger. Ann Surg 224:225–266, 1996.
4. Balch CM, Soong S-J, Murad TM, et al: A multifactorial analysis of melanoma. III: Prognostic factors in melanoma patients with lymph node metastasis (stage II). Ann Surg 193:377–388, 1981.
5. Breslow A: Thickness, cross-sectional areas and depth of invasion in the prognosis of cutaneous melanoma. Ann Surg 172:902, 1970.
6. Brown M: Staging and prognosis for melanoma. Semin Cutan Med Surg 16: 113–121, 1997.
7. Clark WH, et al: The histogenesis and biological behavior of primary human malignant melanoma of the skin. Cancer Res 29:705, 1969.
8. Cockerell C: Biopsy technique for pigmented lesions. Semin Cutan Med Surg 16:108–112, 1997.
9. Coit DG, Brennan MF: Extent of lymph node dissection in melanoma of the trunk or lower extremity. Arch Surg 124:162–166, 1989.
10. Fraker DL: Surgical issues in the management of melanoma. Curr Opin Oncol 9:183–188, 1997.
11. Heasley D, et al: Pathology of malignant melanoma. Surg Clin North Am 76: 1223–1256, 1996.
12. Karakousis CP, Emrich LJ, Driscoll DL, et al: Survival after groin dissection for malignant melanoma. Surgery 109:119–126, 1991.
13. Kirkwood JM, Strawderman MH, Ernstaff MS, et al: Interferon alpha-2b adjuvant therapy of high-risk resected cutaneous melanoma: The Eastern Cooperative Oncology Group Trial EST 1684. J Clin Oncol 14:7–17, 1996.
14. Krag DN, Meijer SJ, Weaver DL, et al: Minimal access surgery for staging of malignant melanoma. Arch Surg 130:654–660, 1995.
15. Liu T, Soong S: Epidemiology of malignant melanoma. Surg Clin North Am 76:1205–1222, 1996.
16. NIH Consensus Development Conference Statement on Diagnosis and Treatment of Early Melanoma. Am J Dermatopathol 15:34–43, 1993.
17. Nelson M, et al: Clinical implications of cytogenetic abnormalities in melanoma. Surg Clin North Am 76:1257–1272, 1996.
18. Rigel DS: Malignant melanoma: Incidence issues and their effect on diagnosis and treatment in the 1990's. Mayo Clin Proc 72:367–371, 1997.
19. Sim FH, Taylor WF, Pritchard DJ, et al: Lymphadenectomy in the management of stage I malignant melanoma: A prospective randomized trial. Mayo Clin Proc 61:697–702, 1986.
20. Sondak V, Wolfe J: Adjuvant therapy for melanoma. Mayo Clin Proc 9:189–204, 1997.
21. Verones U, Adamus J, Bardieru DC, et al: Inefficacy of immediate node dissection in stage I melanoma of the limbs. N Engl J Med 297:627–632, 1977.
22. Wong JH, Cagel LA, Morton DL, et al: Lymphatic drainage of skin to sentinel lymph node in a feline model. Ann Surg 214:637–641, 1991.
23. Wornow IL, Soong S-J, Urist MM, et al: Surgery as palliative treatment for distant metastases of melanoma. Ann Surg 204:181–185, 1986.

9. BASAL CELL AND SQUAMOUS CELL CARCINOMA

Bobby Kapur, B.A., Samuel Stal, M.D., F.A.C.S., Melvin Spira, M.D., D.D.S., and Giulio Gherardini, M.D.

1. Name the major skin carcinogens that can initiate precancerous and cancerous growth.

Exposure to **ultraviolet radiation** (UV) correlates directly with the development of skin cancer. The incidence of skin cancer is highest in sunny climates, in people with light complexions, in people who work outdoors, and on areas of the body not covered by clothing. The typical patient has fair skin, fair hair, and blue eyes. The photochemical effects of UV irradiation are due to electron excitation in the absorbing atoms and molecules, which induces damaging chemical reactions. Radiation-induced chemical damage in DNA may be responsible for cell death and neoplastic transformation. Normal DNA synthesis and cell mitosis are inhibited early in UV-exposed epidermis. The effect of a UV dose on the skin is reduced somewhat by the presence of hair, a thick stratum corneum, and melanin. A patient's susceptibility to UV-induced cutaneous malignancies is inversely related to skin melanocyte content. Solar radiation consists of UVA (315–400 nm), UVB (290–315 nm), and UVC (200–290 nm) wavelengths. Atmospheric ozone absorbs the UVC waveband, and 95% of the radiation that reaches human skin is in the UVA waveband. However, the minimal UVB wavelength causes acute sunburns and most of the chronic sun damage and malignant skin changes. In addition, excessive UVB radiation interferes with the normal functioning of the immune system and increases the incidence and severity of skin cancer.

Ionizing radiation also has been recognized as causing skin cancer. Ionizing radiation includes electromagnetic radiations (x-rays and gamma rays) and particulate radiation (electrons, protons, neutrons, α-particles, and heavy nuclei). Both types of radiation elicit changes by ionizing important cell constituents. An important feature of radiation-induced tumor is that a single radiation exposure may produce a tumor after a long latent period.

Chemical carcinogenesis occurs through a biochemical interaction—the covalent bonding of carcinogen residues with cellular macromolecules, RNA, DNA, and protein. Arsenic, atmospheric pollutants, psoralens, and nitrogen mustard have been implicated in cutaneous malignancies.

2. What inherited conditions predispose to cutaneous malignancies?

Xeroderma pigmentosum is an autosomal recessive disorder with an acute sensitivity to sunlight secondary to a defective DNA repair mechanism and results in multiple epitheliomas with subsequent malignant degeneration.

Basal cell nevus syndrome, also known as Gorlin syndrome, is an autosomal dominant disorder with three characteristic findings: multiple basal cell nevi on the skin with malignant changes by puberty, jaw cysts (adontogenic keratocysts), and pitting of the palms and soles. Other associated anomalies include pseudohypertelorism, frontal bossing, syndactyly, and spina bifida.

Albinism manifests as hypopigmentation of the skin, hair, and eyes and increases the risk of squamous cell (SCC) and basal cell carcinoma (BCC).

Epidermodysplasia verruciformis consists of an autosomal recessive cell-mediated immunity disorder characterized by several subtypes of human papillomavirus that induce numerous polymorphic verrucous lesions with a high propensity for transformation into SCC.

Muir-Torre syndrome is a disorder of multiple internal malignancies, cutaneous sebaceous proliferation, keratoacanthomas, BCC, and SCC.

Porokeratosis is an autosomal dominant disorder of abnormal keratinization with malignant degeneration.

Baze-Dupre-Christol syndrome is an X-linked disorder characterized by follicular atrophoderma, congenital hypotrichiosis, basal cell nevi, and BCC.

3. What is a solar keratosis?

Actinic keratosis, often referred to as solar keratosis, represents the cumulative effect of UV light exposure. Therefore, lesions appear primarily on sun-damaged or exposed skin and are frequently multiple. Grossly, the lesions are discrete, well circumscribed, erythematous, and maculopapular. They vary in color from reddish to light brown and are dry and scaly due to adherent parakeratotic scales. Microscopically, hyperkeratosis and parakeratosis, together with dyskeratosis and acanthosis, are prominent features in the epidermal layer. Within primarily the upper dermis distinct alterations include an actinic elastosis with an associated inflammatory infiltrate consisting of lymphocytes. Almost all cases of actinic keratosis progress to SCC, and the percentage of lesions that become invasive SCC varies from 20–25%. These carcinomas rarely metastasize, and there is little place for wide margins in surgical treatment.

4. How is actinic keratosis treated?

Curettage and electrodesiccation form the foundation for treatment of most lesions. Liquid nitrogen is also an effective modality, and more recently 5-fluorouracil (5-FU) in a 1–5% concentration (Efudex) has proved effective. Chemical peel and dermabrasion of the skin also have been effective but have been replaced largely by 5-FU.

5. What is Bowen's disease?

Bowen's disease is seen in older patients in both sun-exposed and non–sun-exposed areas. It represents an intraepithelial SCC (carcinoma in situ) and may involve the skin or mucous membranes, including mouth, anus, and genitalia. Most of the lesions are solitary, and men are afflicted more often than women. Lesions have a long clinical course, generally years. Clinically the lesion appears as a solitary, rather sharply defined, erythematous, reddish, dull, scaly plaque. Pruritus, superficial crusting, and oozing may be noted.

Microscopic examination reveals the stigmata of an intraepidermal SCC with hyperkeratosis, parakeratosis, dyskeratosis, and acanthosis within the epithelial layers. Within the epithelium there is disorder. Cells are keratinized within the prickle cell layer, and hyperchromatic bizarre nuclei and increased cell mitosis are observed. There is no dermal invasion, but a heavy inflammatory infiltrate is frequently noted in the papillary dermis with multinucleated giant cells.

Surgical therapy includes either excision or a combination of curettage and electrodesiccation. The prognosis is excellent with appropriate treatment. However, the prognosis is poor if SCC develops; these lesions are much more aggressive than the SCCs that develop from actinic keratoses.

6. What is Bowen's disease of mucous membranes?

Erythroplasia of Queyrat is often referred to as Bowen's disease of the mucous membranes. It most often affects the glans penis and is seen during the fifth and sixth decades of life, primarily in uncircumcised men. Grossly, erythroplasia consists of solitary or multiple erythematous lesions that are well circumscribed, moist, glistening, and velvety. Microscopically, the lesion resembles Bowen's disease. Erythroplasia is much more likely than Bowen's disease to become invasive and has an increased tendency to metastatic disease.

7. Where is leukoplakia usually found? What is its appearance?

Leukoplakia, literally meaning *white patch*, is seen primarily on oral, vulvar, or vaginal mucosa. Leukoplakia in the mouth is seen mostly in older men with a history of smoking. Ill-fitting dentures and teeth in poor repair often are associated with this condition. Grossly, the lesions are elevated, sharply defined patchy areas of keratinization, generally lighter in color (white to gray) than the surrounding tissue and of variable thickness. Long-standing or chronic lesions may exhibit a verrucoid appearance. Microscopically, we see the classic quartet of hyperkeratosis, parakeratosis, keratosis, and acanthosis. Within the epidermal layer, cellular atypia abounds, and within the dermis is seen an inflammatory infiltrate. Of untreated lesions, 15–20% undergo malignant transformation. Evidence of ulceration or underlying induration increases the possibility of cancer. The SCCs that develop from premalignant lesions on the mucous membranes are much more malignant than those associated with actinic keratoses.

8. Pseudoepitheliomatous hyperplasia is found in what underlying condition?

Pseudoepitheliomatous hyperplasia is seen in long-standing chronic ulcers, typically decubitus ulcers; it is evidenced as an epidermal thickening that may be mistaken for neoplastic change or degeneration. Microscopic examination shows downward proliferation of epidermal cells associated with mild cellular atypia and an inflammatory infiltrate with microabscesses. The condition resembles SCC at times and may be difficult to differentiate from malignancy. Generally, cell and nuclear changes are not as prominent in blood vessels, and nerve invasion is not seen. The condition responds to conservative treatment. In more long-standing cases, excision of the ulcer and grafting may be required.

9. Describe a nevus sebaceous.

This superficial skin lesion is present at birth in the head and neck region. It is typically a well-circumscribed, irregularly raised plaque. It has a yellowish color, and hair is distinctly absent. The incidence of transformation to BCC is 10%.

10. BCC arises from which cells?

BCC arises from the pluripotential cells of the basal layer of the epithelium or from the external root sheath of the hair follicle and is the most common malignancy of Caucasians. Its onset is directly related to the UV radiation of sun exposure. BCCs occur most often at sites with the greatest concentration of pilosebaceous follicles. BCC differs from SCC in that it does not arise from malignant changes in preexisting mature epithelial structures; it requires stromal participation for survival. It does not possess the cellular anaplasia associated with true carcinoma, and it almost never metastasizes.

11. Where anatomically do most primary BCCs occur?

Approximately 93% occur in the head and neck region; the remaining 7% are found on the trunk and extremities. In the head and neck, BCC is distributed as follows: nose, 25.5%; cheek, 16%; periorbital, 14%; scalp and temple, 11%; ear and periauricular, 11%; forehead, 7.5%; neck, 7%; upper lip, 5%; chin, 2%; and lower lip, 1%.

12. List the different types of BCC.

1. **Nodular ulcerative carcinoma.** Lesions are usually single, occur mostly on the face, and begin as small translucent papules that remain firm and exhibit telangiectasia. They grow slowly and tend to ulcerate, which may result in tissue destruction. They are the most common of the BCCs.

2. **Superficial basal cell carcinoma.** Lesions often occur multiply, usually on the trunk. They are lightly pigmented, erythematous, scaly, and patchlike. They may resemble eczema or psoriasis.

3. **Sclerosing basal cell carcinoma.** Lesions are yellow-white, morpheaform epitheliomas with ill-defined borders and resemble small patches of scleroderma. They are most frequently associated with recurrent disease. Peripheral growth with central sclerosis and scarring is characteristic.

4. **Pigmented basal cell carcinoma.** Lesions combine the features of the nodular ulcerative type with a deep brownish-black pigmentation.

5. **Trabecular (Merkel cell) carcinoma.** This relatively new entity resembles BCC histologically and may occur as a single tumor in older people. The tumor may be epidermal, dermal, or even subcutaneous in origin, with a microscopic picture of irregularly anastomosing trabeculae and a rosette arrangement of deeply basophilic, uniform tumor cells. The name Merkel cell is derived from the fact that the tumor cells contain small granules identical to the neurosecretory granules of the epidermal Merkel cell. Tumors are aggressive and metastasize not only to local nodes but also to viscera and bone. Treatment for cure is difficult but consists of surgery and radiation therapy.

6. **Adnexal carcinoma.** These skin malignancies arise from sebaceous sweat glands. They are relatively uncommon and appear as solitary tumors in older patients. The tumors have no particular distinctive features, grow slowly, tend to recur locally after surgery, and metastasize regionally.

13. What are the microscopic and clinical distinctions among the types of BCC?

The microscopic characteristics of the different clinical types of BCC vary considerably. All cases show proliferation of similar cells, oval in shape with deeply staining nuclei and scant cytoplasm. The tumors are composed of irregular masses of basaloid cells in the dermis, with the outermost cells forming a palisading layer on the periphery. The surrounding stroma frequently exhibits a fibrous reaction. Microscopically, the nodular ulcerative type of basal cell tumor may show differentiation toward adnexal structures; there may be a solid, cystic, adenoid, or keratotic variety. The superficial BCC shows bands of basal cells in the dermis but maintains continuity with the overlying epidermis. This lesion contrasts with sclerosing BCC, which shows clusters and clumps of basal cells in the densely fibrotic stroma without continuity with the overlying epidermis (which in fact may be perfectly normal). A blue nevus generally can be differentiated from a deeply pigmented BCC by the character of the overlying epithelium (normal) and duration of the tumor without growth.

14. Which biopsy techniques allow a histologic diagnosis?

Curettage is done under local anesthesia by scraping the tumor with a dermal curet. Tumor cell groups are soft and often can be curetted. Normal underlying dermis or scar tissue is hard and almost impossible to curet. When BCC occurs in a scar or is morpheaform, it is too difficult to curet. The difference in ability to curet aids in differentiating normal tissue from some BCCs.

Shave biopsy of the upper half of the dermis is an excellent way to reveal a recurrent tumor, because a wide area can be sampled with minimal deformity. On rare occasions, a tumor is present so deeply that a shave biopsy does not reveal its presence. Rare BCCs present as a subcutaneous recurrence that would be missed by a shave biopsy. In such cases, however, there is a deep-seated nodule, and recurrence is easily recognized by tightly pulling normal or scarred overlying skin.

Punch biopsy, 3 or 4 mm in diameter, visualizes only a small area of the suspicious tissue but usually provides a specimen of sufficient size for diagnostic histologic evaluation.

Excisional biopsy is the treatment of choice in dealing with a primary BCC or a pigmented lesion. However, in the context of large tumors (as recurrences often are) and when location of the actual borders of the tumor are unknown, excisional biopsy is impractical.

Deep-wedge biopsy often gives valuable information about the depth below the dermis and extent of infiltration of a recurrent BCC.

15. How is BCC treated?

Most BCCs are treated by curettage and desiccation or by simple excision as a fusiform ellipse and primary closure.

Curettage and desiccation are best suited for lesions less than 1 cm in diameter and lesions that are nodular, ulcerative, and exophytic. The technique is not suited for morpheatype BCCs or recurrent disease. When a functional or anatomic deformity may result or when cartilage or bone is involved, other modalities are more effective.

Surgical excision provides an immediate pathologic inventory and an index of the adequacy of excision. The lesion can be removed as a fusiform ellipse positioned along the lines of least skin tension with a small perimeter (0.2–0.5 cm) of normal tissue. If margins are clear, the defect is undermined and the line of closure is delineated. Excessive tissue (dog ear) is excised, and closure is carried out with the surgeon's preferred technique.

Cryotherapy is used for small nodular or ulcerated lesions located over bone or cartilage, on the eyelid, or on the tip of the nose. Liquid nitrogen applied with a cotton-tipped applicator or a spray that freezes the tumor and a 5-mm area of normal tissue for approximately 30 seconds has proved effective. One sees immediate edema, exudation, subsequent necrosis, eschar formation, and healing. In recent years, cryotherapy has been increasingly used in the management of skin tumors, but it is associated with local tissue destruction and requires an incisional biopsy for tissue diagnosis before treatment.

Radiation therapy with low penetration x-irradiation to a tumor site in doses of 5000 rads may be useful, particularly around orifices (eyelids, nares, and mouth) or at sites where a scar due to surgical excision may be a difficult problem, as in the deltoid or sternal region. Scars from surgery generally improve with time, whereas scars from radiation therapy worsen. The late changes associated with any type of radiation treatment detract from its use in young and middle-aged patients; however, it can be effective for treating an older person with a large tumor in whom extensive resection is unacceptable or the goal is palliation.

Mohs' fresh frozen section technique employs serial tangential excisions and is particularly useful for the treatment of sclerosing BCC, especially in dealing with a recurrent lesion, and for large primary tumors with poorly delineated borders or perineural invasion.

16. Describe the indications for skin flaps, distant skin and musculocutaneous flaps, and split-thickness skin grafts.

Skin flaps and, in some instances, skin-muscle flap closures provide versatility in treating large defects and defects over cartilage or bone, where skin grafts may result in cosmetic deformity. The Limberg flap has replaced the simple sliding skin flap as the method of choice, particularly for large defects of the head and neck area. The sliding subcutaneous flap is effective, particularly for the forehead, cheek area, lips, and lower nose. Musculocutaneous flaps, including the Abbé flap, Estlander flap, and Karapendiz flap, are also effective.

Distant skin and musculocutaneous flaps are rarely required, except for more extensive lesions after resection for recurrent disease, accompanied by extensive loss of tissue during the extirpative process. Although the use of medial trapezius and deltopectoral flaps is well known, free flaps provide a more effective source of skin, soft tissue, and, when indicated, bone with less donor site morbidity.

Split-thickness skin grafting is a mainstay of treatment, particularly for large defects not involving bone or cartilage. Although a split-thickness skin graft can be placed directly over cartilage and bone, even bone in the mid-face without periosteum, the aesthetic result is compromised. However, application of a skin graft to a defect is preferable to any delay. A skin graft over a large area may be amenable to a tissue expansion technique several months later, allowing primary or staged excision of the graft and resurfacing with local tissue. In most instances, the best donor sites for skin grafts are the supraclavicular and postauricular regions.

17. What are high-risk anatomic areas for BCC recurrence?

High-risk areas for tumor recurrence include the center of the face (periorbital region, eyelids, nasolabial fold, nose-cheek angle), postauricular region, pinna, and forehead. Recurring lesions are most common in young women.

18. What are the clinical signs of recurrence?
1. Scarring with intermittent or nonhealing ulceration
2. Scar that becomes red, scaled, or crusted
3. Enlarging scar with increased telangiectasia in the adjacent area
4. Development of papule or nodule formation within the scar itself
5. Frank tissue destruction

When recurrence of a previously excised BCC is suspected, a biopsy is performed. The clinical types of BCC most likely to recur after excision are infiltrative nodular BCC with a poorly defined border and sclerosing, morpheaform BCC. The outer borders of such tumors often cannot be accurately defined by clinical examination. Mohs' micrographic surgery is the mainstay of treatment.

19. SCC arises from which cells?
SCC originates from the keratinizing or malpighian (spindle) cell layer of the epithelium; it is seen primarily in older patients, mostly men. As with BCC, the prime etiologic factor is solar radiation. In addition to radiation, however, chemicals, chronic ulcers (including osetomyelitis), cytotoxic drugs, immunosuppressant drugs, chronic lesions, a wide variety of dermatoses, discoid lupus erythematosus, and hydradenitis suppurativa play a significant role in the development of the relatively small number of SCC skin cancers. Initially the lesion appears smooth, verrucous, papillomatous, or ulcerative and later exhibits induration, inflammation, and ulceration.

20. Describe the two general types of SCC.
The first is a slow-growing variety that is verrucous and exophytic; although this type may be deeply locally invasive, it is less likely to metastasize. The second general type is more nodular and indurated, with rapid growth and early ulceration combined with local invasiveness and increased metastatic tendency.

21. Where are SCCs anatomically distributed?
Compared with BCC, SCC has a slightly increased incidence on the trunk and extremities. The lesions are distributed as follows: cheeks, 45%; nose, 13%; ear and periauricular areas, 12%; hand, 11%; neck, 10%; arms, 5%; trunk, 2%; and scalp and legs, 1% each.

22. What is the mainstay of treatment for SCC?
Treatment depends on the age of the patient and the size of the lesion. Surgical excision and Mohs' micrographic surgery are the mainstays of treatment. Older patients are treated conservatively. The location of the lesion is a factor in choosing the technique. Wound appearance may not matter so much to an older patient.

23. Name factors associated with SCC recurrence.
Degree of cellular differentiation is a significant prognostic indicator, ranging from 7% recurrence for well-differentiated tumors to 28% recurrence for poorly differentiated lesions. Depth of tumor invasion also raises the incidence of recurrence. Perineural invasion usually indicates increased tumor involvement and greater probability of recurrence. The tendency for recurrence of SCC treated by any technique is approximately twice that for the best results of treating BCC.

24. What is the best way to treat recurrent lesions?
A recurrent lesion is probably best treated by excision and skin grafting. Microscopically controlled excision (modified Mohs' technique) is a good way to handle difficult and recurrent lesions, specifically in medial canthal and alar areas. Radiation therapy can be used effectively in patients over 55 years of age, particularly around the eyelids, nose, and lip.

25. Where does Marjolin's ulcer arise?
Marjolin's ulcer is a term used to describe SCC in previously traumatized locations such as burn scars, healed fistula tracts, and draining osteomyelitis sites.

26. Describe the metastatic potential of SCC.
About 5–10% of lesions metastasize. SCCs resulting from Marjolin's ulcer or xeroderma pigmentosum have a much greater tendency to metastasize than SCCs resulting from sun-induced skin changes. In addition, SCCs of the ears, nostrils, scalp, and extremities are particularly prone to metastasis.

27. What is the significance of perineural and mucoperiosteal invasion?

Perineural, lymphatic, and mucoperiosteal invasion usually indicate advanced disease and worsen the prognosis for local cure and, in cases of SCC metastasis. The probability of cure when SCC has spread to the mucoperiosteum of the piriform aperture is remote. When such invasion is found, surgical treatment must be aggressive; wide extirpation represents the only hope for cure.

28. When should a patient treated for BCC or SCC be clinically reexamined?

The patient should be clinically examined every 6 months for 5 years because about 36% of patients who develop BCC develop a second primary BCC within the next 5 years. Diagnosis and treatment of recurring BCC in its early stages result in less morbidity. SCCs have definite metastatic potential, and patients should be reexamined every 3 months for the first several years and followed indefinitely at 6-month intervals.

29. What is an effective technique for periodic self-examination to catch lesions at an early stage?

To perform self-examination, the patient needs a full-length mirror, a hand mirror, and a brightly lit room. The following technique is appropriate:

1. Examine the body, front and back, in the mirror, then the right and left sides with arms raised.
2. Bend the elbows and look carefully at forearms, back of upper arms, and palms.
3. Look at the back of the legs and feet, spaces between the toes and soles.
4. Examine the back, neck, and scalp with a hand mirror.
5. Check the back and buttocks with a hand mirror.

BIBLIOGRAPHY

1. Barrett TL, Greenway HT, Massullo V: Treatment of basal cell carcinoma and squamous cell carcinoma with perineural invasion. Adv Dermatol 8:277–304, 1993.
2. Chao CK, Gerber RM, Perez CA: Reirradiation of recurrent skin cancer of the face. A successful salvage modality. Cancer 75:2351–2355, 1995.
3. Derrick EK, Smith R, Melcher DH, et al: The use of cytology in the diagnosis of basal cell carcinoma. Br J Dermatol 130:561–563, 1994.
4. Drake LA, Dinehart SM, Goltz RW, Graham GF: Guidelines of care for Mohs micrographic surgery. J Am Acad Dermatol 33:271–278, 1995.
5. Fleming ID, Amonette R, Monaghan T, Fleming MD: Principles of management of basal and squamous cell carcinoma of the skin. Cancer 75:699–704, 1995.
6. Fijan SD, Honigsmann S: Photodynamic therapy of epithelial skin tumours using delta-aminolaevulinic acid and desferrioxamine. Br J Dermatol 133:282–288, 1995.
7. Gherardini G, Bhatia N, Stal S: Congenital syndromes associated with non-melanoma skin cancer. Clin Plast Surg 24:649–661, 1997.
8. Ikic D, Padovan I, Pipic N, et al: Interferon reduces recurrences of basal cell and squamous cell cancers. Int J Dermatol 34:58–60, 1995.
9. Kempf RA: Systemic therapy of skin carcinoma. Cancer Treat Res 78:137–162, 1995.
10. Kopf AW, Salopek TG, Slade J, et al: Techniques of cutaneous examination for the detection of skin cancer. Cancer 75:684–690, 1995.
11. Marks R: An overview of skin cancers. Incidence and causation. Cancer 75:607–612, 1995.
12. Marks R: The epidemiology of non-melanoma skin cancer: Who, why and what can we do about it. J Dermatol 22:853–857, 1995.
13. Marks R, Motley RJ: Skin cancer. Recognition and treatment. Drugs 50:48–61, 1995.
14. Multicentre South European Study Helios. I: Skin characteristics and sunburns in basal cell and squamous cell carcinomas of the skin. Br J Cancer 73:1440–1446, 1996.
15. Multicentre South European Study Helios. II: Different sun exposure patterns in the aetiology of basal cell and squamous cell. Br J Cancer 73:1447–1454, 1996.
16. Nelson BR, Fader DJ, Gillard F: The role of dermabrasion and chemical peels in the treatment of patients with xeroderma pigmentosum. J Am Acad Dermatol 32:623–626, 1995.
17. Roberts DJ, Cairnduff F: Photodynamic therapy of primary skin cancer: A review. Br J Plast Surg 48: 360–370, 1995.
18. Stal S, Spira M: Basal and squamous cell carcinoma of the skin. In Aston SJ, Beasley RW, Thorne CHM (eds): Grabb and Smith's Plastic Surgery, 5th ed. Philadelphia, Lippincott-Raven, 1997, pp 107–120.
19. Wilson BD, Mang T: Photodynamic therapy for cutaneous malignancies. Clin Dermatol 13:91–96, 1995.

10. HEMANGIOMAS AND VASCULAR MALFORMATIONS

John B. Mulliken, M.D.

1. Is presence at birth helpful in distinguishing hemangioma from vascular malformation?

Hemangioma typically appears after birth; the median age is 2 weeks. However, about one-third of hemangiomas are nascent in the newborn nursery, manifesting as either a red patch or macule, pale spot, ecchymosis, or telangiectasia. At a cellular level, all vascular malformations are present at birth, but some do not appear until years later.

2. A newborn has a large vascular mass. Which is it more likely to be—a vascular malformation or a hemangioma?

The correct answer to this slippery question is probably vascular malformation. Lymphatic (LM) and venous malformations (VM) are often large at birth, whereas a neonatal arteriovenous malformation (AVM) usually manifests as only a blush. Less well appreciated is the fact that, in rare instances, hemangioma can present at birth as a large, fully grown tumor—a *congenital hemangioma*. Such a tumor must have proliferated in utero; it can be detected by prenatal ultrasonography. Other neonatal masses mimic hemangioma and vascular malformation, such as teratoma, nasal glioma, and sarcoma (e.g., infantile fibrosarcoma, rhabdoid sarcoma). MRI evaluation is indicated if the diagnosis is uncertain; never hesitate to biopsy a perplexing vascular mass.

3. Which is more accurate for diagnosis—ultrasonography or MRI?

Ultrasonography (US) is notoriously operator-dependent. MRI images are the unequivocal gold standard. However, precise characterization by US and MRI requires a radiologist with special knowledge of vascular anomalies. For example, both hemangioma (in the proliferative phase) and AVM are fast-flow lesions; they are frequently confused. Intralesional bleeding within a lymphatic anomaly muddles the radiologic images of a pure LM or VM or a lymphaticovenous malformation (LVM). MRI examination must be complete, including gradient sequences for visualization of fast-flow vessels and contrast enhancement for detection of lymphatic vs. blood-filled channels.

4. Is histopathologic study ever necessary to differentiate vascular tumor (hemangioma) from vascular malformation?

Over 90% of vascular birthmarks can be diagnosed accurately by physical examination and history, but in some patients radiologic and/or histopathologic studies are necessary. Biopsy is indicated when the history, physical examination, or radiologic imaging is confounding. Unfortunately, pathologists continue to use the old Virchowian terminology (e.g., cavernous or capillary hemangioma and lymphangioma). The pathologist must be familiar with a biologic nomenclature for vascular anomalies. The histologic patterns usually discriminate between tumor and malformation. For rare lesions, however, even an experienced pathologist can have difficulty in differentiating a vascular tumor from a benign vascular proliferation within a preexisting vascular malformation.

Classification of Vascular Anomalies of Infancy and Childhood

TUMORS	MALFORMATIONS	COMBINED MALFORMATIONS
Common	**Slow-flow**	Klippel-Trénaunay syndrome
Hemangioma	Capillary (CM): telangiectases	(CVM) (CLVM)
Uncommon	Lymphatic (LM)	Parkes Weber syndrome
Kaposiform hemangioendothelioma	Venous (VM)	(CLAVM) (CLAVF)
Tufted angioma	**Fast-flow**	
Congenital hemangiopericytoma	Arterial (AM): aneurysm, coarc-	
Epithelioid hemangioma/	tation, ectasia, stenosis	
hemangioendothelioma	Arteriovenous fistula (AVF)	
Angiosarcoma	Arteriovenous (AVM)	

5. What is Kasabach-Merritt syndrome?

Contrary to what is stated in the literature, severe thrombocytopenia never occurs with common hemangioma. This coagulopathy accompanies kaposiform hemangioendothelioma, a more aggressive infantile vascular tumor. There are also rare cases of thrombocytopenia with congenital tufted angioma and congenital hemangiopericytoma. Unfortunately, the double eponym Kasabach-Merritt has also been misapplied to a low-grade bleeding disorder that may complicate a large venous anomaly. This disorder is more properly termed a localized rather than disseminated intravascular coagulopathy.

6. Is hemangioma ever associated with syndromes characterized by dysmorphic features?

Unfortunately, many geneticists and syndromologists incorrectly apply the word *hemangioma* to the common macular vascular birthmark, also known as angel's kiss, salmon patch, or naevus flammeus neonatorum. These macular patches usually fade by the first year of life. Like true hemangioma, they are so common as to occur fortuitously in the presence of congenital anomalies—this does not mean that they are "associated" in the syndromic sense.

In rare instances, a large cervicofacial hemangioma may be associated with various structural anomalies (e.g., sternal cleft, supraumbilical raphe, persistent embryonic arteries, right-sided aortic arch, ocular anomalies, cystic anomaly of the posterior cranial fossa). There is a marked female predilection in many of these associations.

7. Can hemangioma in the midline axis be associated with underlying malformative anomalies?

A lumbar hemangioma can be a red flag signalling spina bifida occulta, i.e., lipomeningocele, diastematomyelia, and tethered cord. Sometimes there is a tail-like skin appendage (acrochordon). The diagnosis can be ruled out by US during the first 6 months of life; usually MRI is necessary. This condition should not be confused with Cobb syndrome, which involves capillary stain of the trunk with underlying spinal AVM.

8. Does hemangioma ever cause skeletal overgrowth?

Minor bony hypertrophy may occur beneath a large cutaneous hemangioma. It is most frequently seen with facial hemangioma producing minor maxillary overgrowth or enlargement of an involved ear. A large craniofacial hemangioma also may cause a mass effect, such as deviation of the nasal pyramid or deformation of the neonatal calvaria. Hemangioma does not cause skeletal hypertrophy or axial elongation of a limb. In contrast, bony overgrowth, distortion, and deformation are common problems with slow-flow vascular malformations. Bony erosion and osteolysis may occur with fast-flow vascular malformations.

9. Does a cavernous hemangioma regress more slowly than a capillary hemangioma?

This is a trick question, because there is no such vascular lesion as cavernous hemangioma. Hemangioma is hemangioma! There is no difference in rapidity of regression for a deep cutaneous or subcutaneous hemangioma, with almost normal overlying skin (formerly known as "cavernous") compared with a superficial cutaneous tumor (formerly known as "capillary"). Unfortunately, the 19th-century term *cavernous hemangioma* is entrenched in medical parlance. Often it is used incorrectly to describe venous malformation, whether in skin, hollow or solid viscera (particularly liver), or brain.

10. None of the following characteristics influences speed of regression or residuum of a cutaneous hemangioma *except* (a) gender, (b) race, (c) site, (d) size, (e) presence at birth, (f) appearance, (g) occurrence of ulceration, or (h) duration of proliferating phase.

The answer is (e), presence at birth (see question 2).

11. Are phleboliths seen on plain radiography of hemangioma?

No. Phleboliths (calcified thrombi) are characteristic of VM or LVM. Rarely, dystrophic calcification occurs in congenital hemangioma or hemangioma of the liver.

12. A pediatrician consults you to evaluate a neonate with over 20 tiny, red, dome-shaped cutaneous vascular lesions. What are your recommendations?

The child probably has multiple hemangiomas (hemangiomatosis). Palpate for **hepatomegaly**, investigate for early signs of **congestive heart failure**, and check the hematocrit for **anemia**. This clinical triad occurs with hemangiomas of the liver, lungs, and other viscera. Suggest hepatic US or MRI. This is a life-threatening diagnosis. Heart failure may result from increased blood flow through hepatic hemangiomas. Mortality is 20–30%, even with therapy.

13. Why is hemangioma of the upper eyelid an endangering lesion? What are the treatment options?

An upper eyelid tumor can obstruct the visual axis, causing deprivation amblyopia and failure to develop binocular vision. Less well appreciated is the fact that adnexal hemangioma can deform the infantile cornea, producing astigmatism and secondary myopia. These visual distortions give rise to anisometropia and amblyopia over a period of weeks or months. Even a small hemangioma of the upper eyelid or supraorbital area can cause these refractive disturbances. However, it is rare for a large hemangioma in the lower eyelid or cheek to distort the cornea. Prompt treatment is mandatory. Options include corticosteroids (intralesional or systemic), interferon, and surgical excision. The normal eye is patched for several hours per day to encourage use of the affected eye.

14. At what age does spontaneous involution of a hemangioma usually cease?

The bright red color usually fades by 5 years; however, hemangiomas continue to shrink thereafter. Regression is complete in 50% of children by age 5 years and in 70% by age 7 years. Improvement continues in the remaining children until age 10–12 years.

15. Can laser therapy of hemangioma during the early proliferative phase prevent a small tumor from growing larger?

Flashlamp pulsed-dye laser penetrates skin to a depth of 0.75 mm. Hemangioma often begins as a field transformation—the tumor is deeper than 0.75 mm and more extensive (radially) than initially appreciated. Thus, a cutaneous hemangioma, programmed to remain superficial and small, can be successfully treated by prompt laser application. Laser does not influence the proliferation or regression of the deep portion of the tumor. Possible complications of flashlamp pulsed-dye laser are superficial ulceration, scarring, and hypopigmentation.

16. If an endangering facial hemangioma fails to respond to 2 weeks of oral corticosteroids, given at 2 mg/kg/day, should the dosage be increased or administered intravenously?

No rigorous published evidence indicates that an unresponsive hemangioma will respond to a higher dosage or intravenous administration. In general, 30% of hemangiomas respond quickly, 40% show an equivocal response, and 30% are unresponsive to systemic corticosteroids.

17. What are the considerations in deciding whether to remove a facial hemangioma before a child's entry into school?

The preschool period is a logical time to consider excision, but only in certain instances is removal indicated. For example, a pedunculated lesion that surely will leave expanded skin or fibrofatty residuum or a lesion with central scarring due to infantile ulceration should be removed. It is reasonable to excise a hemangioma during the involuting phase before the child attends school if (1) the scar will be well-hidden or (2) the scar will be the same length and quality if the resection were to be done at a later age. Involuting hemangioma of the nasal tip or lip frequently is trimmed in the preschool period. Staged excision is often the best strategy, notwithstanding the age of the child.

18. Which of the following characterize Sturge-Weber syndrome: (a) port-wine stain in V_2 distribution; (b) choroidal angiomatosis; (c) leptomeningeal vascular anomalies; or (d) skeletal and fibrovascular hypertrophy?

The correct answers are (c) and (d). Capillary malformation (port-wine stain) of V_2 neurotome alone is not associated with Sturge-Weber syndrome. The at-risk distributions are V_1, V_1 and V_2, or V_1, V_2, and V_3. Vascular changes of the choroid (so-called tomato catsup fundus) consist of tortuosity and dilatation of choroidal vasculature, a malformation rather than angioma (i.e., there is no endothelial proliferation).

19. Can capillary malformation in the midaxial dorsal line be associated with an underlying structural deformity?

Midline capillary stain is a cutaneous signpost that requires investigation. For example, a congenital stain of the occiput, often with a central tuft of dark hair (hair collar sign) may be associated with underlying craniodural defect (encephalocoele). A stain in the lumbar area requires radiographic assessment for spinal dysraphism (see question 7).

20. What is the mechanism by which flashlamp pulsed-dye laser therapy causes blanching of a capillary malformation (port-wine stain)?

The process is called selective photothermolysis. Pulsed-dye laser uses a wavelength of 585 nm, which is close to the third (577 nm) absorption spectral peak of oxyhemoglobin. The pulse duration is set at 400 μsec to cause coagulation of the vessels without extensive thermal diffusion to the surrounding tissues. The laser beam penetrates skin to 0.75 mm and is absorbed by the red blood cells in the ectatic vessels. The absorbed light is released as heat, damaging the red cells, perivascular wall, and perivascular collagen. Histologic studies show that pulsed-dye laser produces selective intravascular and perivascular coagulative necrosis, seen clinically as purpura. One month later, microscopic study shows a diminished number of dermal ectatic vessels, resulting in a more normal cutaneous hue. With dark skin types, laser treatment can cause damage to melanocytes in the basal epidermis, resulting in hypopigmentation.

21. What is the significance of a prenatal ultrasonographic finding of a dorsal midline cervicocephalic lymphatic anomaly?

So-called lethal midline cystic lymphatic malformation is easily diagnosed by US as early as 12–14 weeks of gestation. A thin-walled, multiseptated cystic mass is seen in the posterior aspect of the fetal head and nuchal region, usually associated with fetal hydrops. Amniocentesis for karyotyping is essential for parental counseling. Over one-half of these fetuses have Turner syndrome (XO); other common aneuploidies are trisomy 13, 18, and 21. Terathanasia (spontaneous elimination of a defective embryo) is common.

22. Does either lymphangioma or cystic hygroma spontaneously regress by adolescence?

No. Lymphangioma and cystic hygroma are quaint 19th-century terms for microcystic and macrocystic LM, respectively. Reported cases of spontaneous diminution in the size of lymphatic anomalies are extremely rare and probably result from rapid deflation, perhaps via persistent lymphaticovenous shunts. Like other vascular malformations, lymphatic anomalies grow proportionately with the patient; they can suddenly expand as a result of either intralesional bleeding or infection.

23. Is injection of OK-432 currently the best therapy for LM?

OK-432, an agent made from killed streptococcal protein, is believed to be an immunologic stimulant. It is currently in limited clinical trial and has not been approved by the FDA. Like the sclerosants (e.g., ethyl alcohol, tetracycline, Ethibloc), OK-432 can be effective in shrinking macrocystic LMs but is relatively ineffective for microcystic LM.

24. Is surgical resection the best treatment for VM?

With the exception of small, well-localized venous anomalies, surgeons should stand behind the interventional radiologists in the therapy of VMs. The first-line strategy is direct injection of sotrachol (1% or 3%) for small lesions or ethyl alcohol (100%) for large anomalies. After sclerotherapy, surgical resection is easier and more likely to be successful. Flashlamp pulsed-dye laser can destroy a small, superficial VM. Neodynium-YAG laser can be used for larger VMs, but scarring is common.

25. Should preoperative evaluation of a patient with a large VM include clotting studies for disseminated intravascular coagulopathy?

VM does not cause disseminated intravascular coagulopathy (DIC). The coagulopathic pattern is similar to DIC (i.e., low fibrinogen, elevated prothrombin time, activated partial thromboplastin time, and D-dimer), but the mechanism is different. A large VM causes localized intravascular coagulopathy (LIC) by formation of thrombus and consumption of clotting factors, probably due to stasis.

26. Which of the following eponymous vascular syndromes are considered fast-flow anomalies: (a) Bonnet-Dechaume-Blanc (Wyburn-Mason), (b) Sturge-Weber, (c) Klippel-Trénaunay, (d) Parkes Weber, or (d) Rendu-Osler-Weber (hereditary hemorrhagic telangiectasia)?

Bonnett-Dechaume-Blanc syndrome is a telangiectatic facial birthmark with intracranial AVM involving the mesencephalon. Patients with Sturge-Weber syndrome typically have capillary and venous leptomeningeal anomalies. Patients with Rendu-Osler-Weber disease may have microscopic and macroscopic AVMs and arteriovenous fistulas (AVFs) in the skin, mucous membranes, lungs, and abdominal viscera. Although microscopic AVFs are sometimes documented in the lateral thigh of patients with Klippel-Trénaunay syndrome, this disorder is primarily a slow-flow, combined malformation. Parkes Weber syndrome is characterized by multiple AVFs, usually involving a limb.

27. What is Maffucci syndrome?

Unfortunately, physicians continue to use the term *hemangioma* in a generic sense by referring to Maffucci syndrome as hemangiomas in association with enchondromas. The vascular anomalies in this rare disorder are venous in type. Patients may develop spindle cell hemangioendotheliomas, painful, benign vascular proliferations in preexisting malformed vascular tissue, typically in the limbs. Patients with Maffucci syndrome have a predilection to develop various malignancies.

28. Which cutaneous vascular anomalies have a genetic cause?

Rendu-Osler-Weber disease (hereditary hemorrhagic telangiectasia [HHT]) is an autosomal dominant disorder characterized by gradual formation of mucosal, cutaneous, and visceral AVMs. HHT is caused by mutations in two genes that code for endoglin (9q) and activin receptor-like kinase (12q). A point mutation in TIE 2, an endothelial receptor tyrosine kinase on chromosome 9p, has been found to segregate in two unrelated families with autosomal dominant mucocutaneous venous malformations. Glomangiomas are familial, but the causative gene has not been located. In rare instances, capillary malformation (CM) can be inherited as an autosomal dominant trait.

29. Which are more frequent, intracranial or extracranial AVMs?

Intracerebral AVMs are 20-fold more common than extracerebral AVMs.

30. Should an AVM be treated by embolizing the feeding arteries?

No. Embolization should be through the feeding arteries and into the nidus (epicenter) of the AVM. Proximal embolization of a feeding vessel is just as injurious as proximal ligation, causing collaterals to form with expansion of the AVM. The majority of experienced interventional radiologists agree that "cure" by embolization is unlikely unless the AVM can be subsequently and completely resected.

BIBLIOGRAPHY

1. Boon LM, Enjolras O, Mulliken JB: Congenital hemangioma: Evidence for accelerated involution. J Pediatr 128:329–335, 1996.
2. Boon LM, Burrows PE, Paltiel J, et al: Hepatic vascular anomalies in infancy: A twenty-seven-year experience. J Pediatr 129:346–354, 1996.
3. Enjolras O, Mulliken JB: The current management of vascular birthmarks. Pediatr Dermatol 10:311–333, 1993.
4. Gorlin RJ, Kantaputra P, Aughton DJ, Mulliken JB: Marked female predilection in some syndromes associated with facial hemangiomas. Am J Med Genet 52:130–135, 1994.
5. Meyer JS, Hoffer FA, Barnes PD, Mulliken JB: MRI-correlation of the biological classification of soft tissue vascular anomalies. Am J Roentgen 157:559–564, 1991.
6. Mulliken JB, Glowacki J: Hemangiomas and vascular malformations in infants and children: A classification based on endothelial characteristics. Plast Reconstr Surg 69:412–420, 1982.
7. Mulliken JB, Young AE: Vascular Birthmarks: Hemangiomas and Malformations. Philadelphia, W.B. Saunders, 1988.
8. Mulliken JB: Vascular anomalies. In Aston SJ, Beasley RW, Thorne CHM (eds): Grabb and Smith's Plastic Surgery, 5th ed. Philadelphia, Lippincott-Raven, 1997, pp 191–203.
9. Scheepers JH, Quaba AA: Does the pulsed tunable dye laser have a role in the management of infantile hemangiomas? Observations based on 3 years' experience. Plast Reconstr Surg 95:305–312, 1995.
10. Sarkar M, Mulliken JB, Kozakewich HPW, et al: Thrombocytopenic coagulopathy (Kasabach-Merritt phenomenon) is associated with kaposiform hemangioendothelioma and not with common hemangioma. Plast Reconstr Surg 100:1377–1386, 1997.

III. *Craniofacial Surgery I—Congenital*

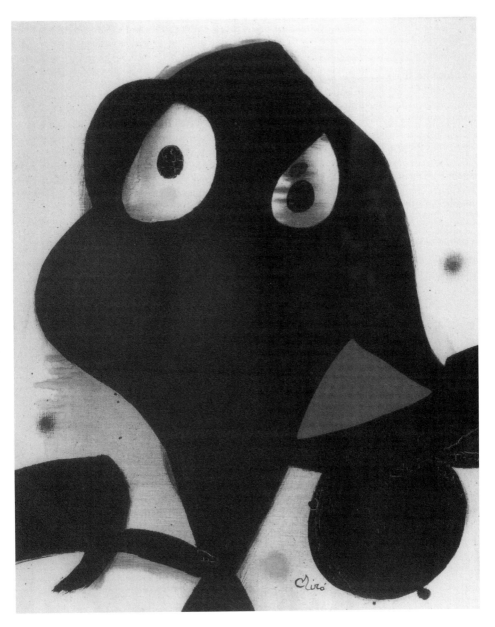

Head I
Joan Miró
1974
Acrylic and oil on canvas
Fundació Joan Miró, Barcelona
© 1998 Artists' Rights Society (ARS), New York/ADAGP, Paris

11. PRINCIPLES OF CRANIOFACIAL SURGERY

Daniel Marchac, M.D., and Eric Arnaud, M.D.

1. What is the specialty of craniofacial surgery?

Craniofacial surgery is plastic surgery of the cephalic extremity, including the skull, the face, and, in particular, the orbit. Paul Tessier, the pioneer of craniofacial surgery, defined the field as *orbitocentric*. It involves the cephalic skeleton as well as surrounding soft tissues.

2. What three types of pathology can be treated by the craniofacial surgeon?

Congenital anomalies, defects after tumor ablation, and posttraumatic deformities. Congenital conditions should be treated early in infancy to optimize final results. Reconstruction of resultant defects after tumor ablation and trauma often requires the input of the craniofacial surgeon for both pediatric and adult patients.

Types of Craniofacial Pathology

CONGENITAL ANOMALIES	POSTTRAUMATIC DEFORMITIES	DEFECTS AFTER TUMOR ABLATION
Craniosynostosis and faciocraniosynostosis	Frontoorbitonasoethmoidal fractures	All tumors of the anterior base of the skull
Facial clefts and related hypertelorism	Le Fort fractures (especially Le Fort III fractures)	Fibrous dysplasia
Hemifacial microsomia		
Craniofacial syndromes		

3. What are the goals of craniofacial surgery in patients with craniosynostosis or faciocraniosynostosis?

The goals of surgery include correction of the dysmorphogenesis and prevention of functional impairment, such as mental retardation and visual disturbances.

4. What is the incidence of craniosynostosis?

Based on European statistics, the incidence of common craniosynostosis averages 1 of 2200 live births. Conversely, a rare faciocraniosynostosis, such as Apert's syndrome, is likely to appear in 1 of 150,000 live births. Although some cases of craniosynostosis are clearly familial, most are sporadic.

5. What is the pathogenesis of craniosynostosis?

Premature fusion of the sutural system of a growing skull is the common mechanism of craniosynostosis. As a result, there is a cessation of calvarial growth perpendicular to the affected suture. The classic law of Virchow predicts compensatory calvarial growth in a direction *parallel* to the affected suture.

6. How is craniosynostosis classified?

Classification is based on the affected suture and its associated morphologic deformity:

Morphologic deformity	Affected suture
Trigonocephaly	Metopic suture
Scaphocephaly	Sagittal suture
Plagiocephaly	Unilateral coronal suture
Brachycephaly	Bilateral coronal sutures
Oxycephaly	Sagittal and both coronal sutures

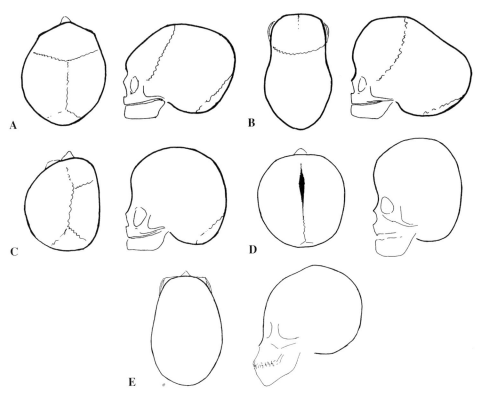

Types of craniosynostosis. *A*, Trigonocephaly. *B*, Scaphocephaly. *C*, Plagiocephaly. *D*, Brachycephaly. *E*, Oxycephaly. (From Marchac D, Renier D: Craniofacial Surgery for Craniosynostosis. Boston, Little, Brown, 1982, with permission.)

7. What is the main feature of faciocraniosynostosis compared with craniosynostosis?

In addition to the skull deformities, the facial involvement in pure craniosynostosis is limited to the forehead and orbital regions (hypo- or hypertelorism). In addition, faciocraniosynostosis is associated with midface hypoplasia characterized by centrofacial retrusion with a class III intermaxillary relation (malocclusion).

8. Are all craniosynostoses or faciocraniosynostoses present at birth?

No. Although most craniosynostoses are congenital and present at birth as a result of a fetal sutural problem, genuine oxycephaly and Crouzon's disease are delayed conditions, often appearing after 3 or 4 years of age. Because the synostoses appear later, the shape of the skull is different and the functional consequences, such as increased intracranial pressure (ICP) or visual impairment, more insidious. Increased ICP is present in at least 60% of cases of oxycephaly or Crouzon's disease.

9. What is the main functional risk of craniosynostosis?

The main functional risk is increased ICP, the consequences of which are visual loss and brain impairment.

10. In acrocephalosyndactyly (such as Apert's syndrome), which factors may be associated with a better mental outcome?

Frontal advancement before 1 year of age and a good psychosocial environment are associated with a more favorable mental outcome.

11. Describe the preoperative evaluation of the craniofacial patient.

1. Analysis of the morphologic abnormality
2. Evaluation of functional risks
3. Detection of associated malformations (e.g., cerebral, cardiac)

   4. Classification of any existing syndrome
   5. Preparation for surgery

12. Which imaging studies are necessary before surgery?

Standard radiographs of the cephalic skeleton and a CT scan are essential before surgery. An MRI is indicated in cases of trigonocephaly because of the higher risk of brain abnormalities and in all syndromic patients.

13. What are the principles of frontoorbital remodeling in craniosynostosis?

The forehead has two components: the supraorbital bar (or bandeau) and the forehead convexity. After being mobilized separately, these components are joined by resorbable or nonresorbable fixation. Reconstructive goals are tailored to the particular type of synostosis:
   1. Symmetric advancement in brachycephaly
   2. Asymmetric advancement in plagiocephaly
   3. Anterior rotation and Z-plasty in oxycephaly
   4. Widening in trigonocephaly

14. Compare the growth of the brain and skull in the first 2 years of life.

The size of the brain doubles in the first year of life. The anterior base of the skull has reached 70% of its adult size by 2 years of age, whereas the cranial capacity has expanded fourfold since birth.

15. What is the main factor responsible for frontal sinus growth after frontocranial remodeling?

The degree of frontoorbital advancement has a significant effect on postoperative sinus growth. The degree of frontal sinus pneumatization correlates inversely with the amount of supraorbital bar advancement.

16. What complications are associated with craniofacial surgery? How can they be prevented?

Craniofacial surgery combines the disciplines of plastic surgery and neurosurgery. The complications of craniofacial procedures are mainly neurosurgical and necessitate postoperative management in specialized intensive care units. The perioperative mortality rate remains approximately 1%, depending on the types of procedures performed. The main complications include bleeding, coma, blindness, meningitis, intracranial hematoma, and hydrocephalus. Additional morbidity may result from rhinorrhea, osteitis, and resorption of bone flaps. The incidence of these complications can be reduced by appropriate preoperative planning and an experienced surgical team.

BIBLIOGRAPHY

1. Marchac D (ed): Proceedings of the Sixth International Congress of the International Society of Craniofacial Surgery. Bologna, Monduzzi Editore, 1996.
2. Marchac D: Radical forehead remodeling for craniostenosis. Plast Reconstr Surg 61:823, 1978.
3. Marchac D, Renier D: Craniofacial Surgery for Craniosynostosis. Boston, Little, Brown, 1982.
4. Marchac D, Renier D, Arnaud E: Evaluation of the effect of early mobilisation of the supraorbital bar on the frontal sinus and frontal growth. Plast Reconstr Surg 95:802, 1995.
5. Marchac D, Renier D, Broumand S: Timing of treatment for craniosynostosis and fasciosynostosis: A 20-year experience. Br J Plast Surg 47:211–222, 1994.
6. Tessier P: Relationship of craniostenoses to craniofacial dysostoses, and to faciostenoses: A study with therapeutic implications. Plast Reconstr Surg 48:224, 1971.

12. CLEFT LIP

D. Ralph Millard, Jr., M.D., F.A.C.S., Hon. F.R.C.S.(Edin), Hon. F.R.C.S., O.D. Ja.

1. What is the cause of a cleft of the lip and palate?

Before the first trimester of pregnancy, the five facial elements—the frontonasal, two lateral maxillary, and two mandibular segments—fuse by mesenchymal migration to create the face and jaws. When, for whatever reason, these fusions are interrupted, a cleft (or clefts) results.

2. What is the cause of clefting in a specific case?

The cause in specific cases is not known, but genetics, viral infection, lack of certain vitamins, and other factors during the first trimester of pregnancy may be involved.

3. What is the anatomy of a cleft?

A cleft is not just a division through the lip and palate; it is distortion of the anatomy that may involve the lip, nose, septum, vomer, alveolar segments, levator palati muscles, and other structures.

UNILATERAL CLEFTS

4. What is the key factor involved in the treatment of a unilateral cleft?

Correction of asymmetry.

5. Summarize the evolution of unilateral cleft surgery.

For patients with a unilateral cleft lip, early surgeons merely freshened the edges of the lip cleft and approximated them with sutures. Later attempts were made to lengthen the lip on the cleft side with local flaps.

6. What is the Mirault-Blair-Brown method of lip repair?

The lip length on the cleft side is increased by a triangular flap taken from the cleft side. The Cupid's bow is destroyed.

7. What is the Hagedorn-Le Mesurier method?

A rectangular flap from the cleft side is inset into a releasing incision on the noncleft side to create an artificial Cupid's bow.

8. What is the Tennison-Randall method?

A Z-plasty of the cleft lip edges that positions the Cupid's bow but at the expense of an unnatural lip scar across the philtrum column and partial flattening of the philtrum dimple.

9. What is the rotation-advancement method?

The distorted anatomy of the unilateral cleft of the lip is corrected by a rotation incision that releases lip tissue, including the Cupid's bow, downward into normal symmetrical position with the opposite side and advances the lateral lip element into the rotation gap to maintain rotation and complete the lip reconstruction. The advancement action assists the correction of the flaring ala, and the C-flap aids in unilateral columella lengthening. The scar of lip union is in the line of a natural philtrum column position and what philtrum dimple is present is preserved as such (See figures, next page.)

10. What are the most common mistakes made in the rotation-advancement method?

1. Inadequate rotation due to failure to cut back on the rotation incision.

2. Inadequate use of the lateral advancement flap by failure to pare the cleft edge sufficiently.

3. Failure to use the C-flap to reduce the cutback gap in the upper lip and to lengthen the columella on the cleft side.

4. Vertical lengthening of the entire lip by extending the cutback across the normal philtrum column.

5. Too much reduction of nostril size in incomplete clefts.

11. What are the recent advances in unilateral cleft lip surgery?

Presurgical orthodontics using the Latham appliance to align the alveolar segments carefully so that the cleft of the alveolus and anterior hard palate can be closed with a gingivoperiosteoplasty. Bone grows into this area, negating the need for secondary bone grafting. This alveolar construction presents a symmetrical platform on which definitive lip and nose construction can be accomplished much sooner.

12. At what age are the various stages of lip construction accomplished?

1. When the patients weighs 10 pounds, the Latham appliance is inserted, and the parents turn the screw daily until the segments are in alignment.

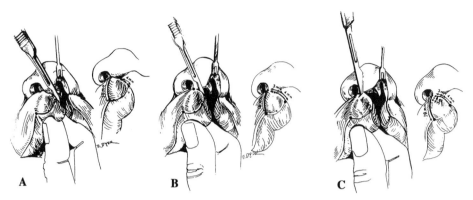

Millard rotation-advancement unilateral cleft lip repair. *A,* Points 1, 2, and 3 mark the residual Cupid's bow on the mucocutaneous junction. The rotation incision pares the edges of the cleft from point 3 to the base of the columella. This distance usually measures 4–5 mm compared with 10 mm on the normal (noncleft) side. *B,* The rotation incision hugs the columella and is carried two-thirds of the way across the base of the columella to gain an additional 3 mm. Flap C, attached to the columella, is released from the lip. *C,* The backcut is placed in the lip at 90°, running medial and parallel to the normal philtrum column. When carried through the skin, muscle, and mucosa, this incision releases another 3 mm. This maneuver achieves the total of 10 mm required to match the normal side and places the Cupid's bow in balanced position. (From Millard DR Jr: Cleft lip. In McCarthy JG (ed): Plastic Surgery. Philadelphia, W.B. Saunders, 1990, p 2637, with permission.)

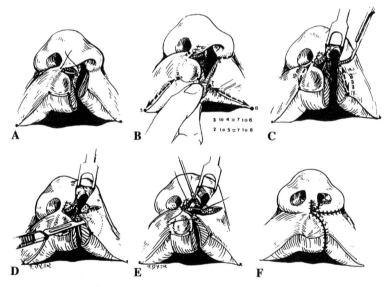

Millard rotation-advancement unilateral cleft lip repair. *A,* Flap C is transposed into the backcut and sutured to add length to the columella. *B,* The highest point of the lateral lip is marked at point 6, where a transverse incision will free the lip from the flared alar base. Because the pared edge of the advancement flap must match the rotation incision (3 to 4), point 7 is marked along the free edge so that 6 to 7 = 3 to 4. The same distance from the height of Cupid's bow to the commissure on the normal side (2 to 5) should be marked on the cleft lip element. With the lateral lip under the tension necessary to close the lip, there is more running room from point 8 for positioning point 7 so that 2 to 5 = 7 to 8. *C,* Flap C has been sutured into the backcut. The alar base is released from the lip. The height of the lateral lip (10 mm) equals the rotation of 10 mm, thus matching the bow peak-to-columella base of 10 mm on the noncleft side. *D,* The bunched muscle of the lateral lip element is freed generously from the skin and mucosa so that with muscle approximation across the cleft there is no residual muscle bulge. The tip of the alar base is denuded of epithelium. *E,* The denuded tip of the alar base is sutured to the septum near the anterior nasal spine to cinch the alar flare. The key suture first picks up the muscle in the tip of the advancement flap and then crosses into the backcut of the rotation. *F,* After the alar cinch suture and the key lip suture have been tied, the tissues are in correct position and require only three-layer closure of the mucosa, muscle, and skin. (From Millard DR Jr: Cleft lip. In McCarthy JG (ed): Plastic Surgery. Philadelphia, W.B. Saunders, 1990, p 2638, with permission.)

2. When segments are in alignment and 2–3 mm apart (after 2–4 weeks), the appliance is removed. Two to three days later the gingivoperiosteoplasty and lip adhesion are performed.

3. At 6–7 months of age the rotation-advancement of the lip is carried out; the nasal correction is done at the same time.

4. At 18 months the remaining cleft of the hard and soft palate is closed with the von Langenbeck method or in some cases a Wardill-Kilner V-Y or unilateral V-Y method, depending on the defect. Minor lip and nose deformities can be improved at this time.

13. Why is the lip adhesion used?

Before the development of presurgical orthodontics, lip adhesion served as a crude orthodontic molding action. After alignment of the alveolar segments and closure of the alveolar cleft, the lip adhesion provides a gentle dressing with the least tension during healing. It also turns a wide complete cleft into an easier-to-correct incomplete cleft.

14. What are the key deformities in the unilateral cleft lip nose? How are they corrected?

1. A unilateral short columella is lengthened with a C-flap.

2. Deviation and distortion of the septum are corrected during presurgical orthodontics.

3. Dislocation and slumping of the alar cartilage are corrected by dissecting the medial two-thirds of the alar cartilage and then constructing the medial crus with sutures to the normal side.

4. Flaring of the alar base is corrected with the alar cinch procedure.

15. Why is the rotation-advancement lip operation the method of choice?

1. The actions of rotation and advancement place normal tissues into normal positions, creating a symmetrical Cupid's bow.

2. Rotation and advancement position the scar of union along the philtrum column line and preserve the integrity of the philtrum dimple.

3. The actions of rotation and advancement aid in the nasal correction.

4. A well-executed rotation-advancement is capable of producing an aesthetic result.

5. When the method is not done correctly, it is still possible to achieve a satisfactory secondary result without great difficulty. The rotation-advancement method avoids the interlocking of little flaps that are impossible to unscramble.

BILATERAL CLEFTS

16. What are the specific deformities in a bilateral cleft?

1. In the complete bilateral cleft the premaxillary vomer segment has not fused with the lateral maxillary segments so that the premaxillary vomer segment grows forward unimpeded to jut far ahead of the lateral segments.

2. There is a shortage of skin tissue in the vertical length of the frontonasal component as measured from the nasal tip to the inferior border of the prolabium, particularly in the columella. This shortage is due to lack of stretch during normal embryogenesis.

3. Patients have no important muscle in the prolabium, no philtrum columns or dimple, and no Cupid's bow.

4. The alae are spread wide; the alar cartilages are dislocated from their mates in the tip and slump along the alae; and the columella is short to nonexistent, which causes the nasal tip to be depressed.

17. What one aspect of the bilateral cleft is sometimes an advantage?

Symmetrical bilateral clefts at least have symmetry. Asymmetric bilateral clefts vary in their symmetry.

18. Summarize the evolution of bilateral cleft surgery.

1. To ease bilateral cleft lip closure, early surgeons amputated the premaxilla, which produced an oral cripple.

2. Early surgery by Brophy used a circumferential wire to encircle the three maxillary elements and crunch them together to facilitate cleft lip closure. This technique affected normal maxillary

growth—a problem discovered and criticized by Pruzansky. Berkowtiz, a student of Pruzansky, still harbors fear of early surgery.

3. Closure of the lip over the premaxillary prominence caused ventroflexion of the septum.

4. Modern alignment of these segments is designed to ease the premaxilla back into the arch, much like sliding a drawer. Many surgeons use presurgical orthodontics to align the maxillary segments. Georgiade and Latham devised a method of retracting the premaxilla. Latham later refined the method with two-pin and chain traction on the projecting premaxilla, along with bilateral spreading of the collapsed lateral maxillary segments, to achieve a reasonable atraumatic alignment of the arch.

19. How is maxillary alignment maintained?

A bilateral gingivoperiosteoplasty creates a mucoperiosteal tunnel across each side of the cleft as the alveolar clefts and the floor of the nose are closed. This technique allows bone to grow across the cleft and avoids the need for later secondary bone grafting.

20. What is the major risk of early alveolar construction?

In a few cases some retrusion of the premaxilla has been noted.

21. Can this risk be avoided?

As experience with this orthopedic approach increases, the premaxillary retrusion can be prevented, reduced, and certainly corrected, often with mere orthodontic treatment.

22. What are the advantages of early orthodontic manipulation and gingivoperiosteoplasty of the alveolar cleft?

1. Obliteration of fistulas.

2. Creation of a bony bridge across the cleft that later will accept teeth and avoids the need for secondary bone grafting.

3. Construction of a stable symmetric platform that enables earlier definitive correction of the lip and nose. This technique enables the surgeon to correct the deformity by 4 years, before the age of memory.

23. How are the soft tissues treated in bilateral clefts?

1. Some methods focus entirely on joining the lateral lip elements to the prolabium with no concern for the nose (Manchester).

2. Some methods treat both lip and nose.

24. What is the key to correction of the nose?

1. Some surgeons acknowledge that the columella is short and requires skin lengthening (Carter, Cronin).

2. Some surgeons have devised methods to achieve columella length from above (Mulliken, Trott, Mohan).

25. What is the best method of action?

1. In patients in whom some columella is present and in races that require minimal columella length, it may be possible to get by without introducing new skin.

2. About 50 years ago Gensoul took a V-Y flap from the center of the prolabium to lengthen the columella, but this technique made three vertical scars in the lip.

3. In patients with little or no columella, a forked flap taken from excessive prolabium skin and scar will provide the extra skin to release the depressed nasal tip.

26. How is the forked flap used?

1. The forked flap can be used as a secondary procedure to narrow a wide prolabium, to revise bilateral lip scars, and to construct a columella.

2. The flap can be taken from the prolabium after 1–2 years of stretching and banked in whisker position under the alae before it is advanced into the columella. This advancement is best done at about 4 years of age. At this time the alar cartilages can be freed and joined to each other in the tip to reconstruct the medial crura. The alar bases can be cinched for final correction of the bilateral nasal deformity.

27. How is the lip of a bilateral cleft closed?

At the time of gingivoperiosteoplasty, the lip adhesion involves approximating the sides of the freshened prolabium to the lateral lip elements. The lateral lip elements are freshened by the turndown of mucocutaneous flaps from their sides. The lateral mucocutaneous flaps are used to overlap the turndown of inferior prolabium vermilion. This technique provides several bonuses. The unnatural prolabium vermilion is turned out of view, and a natural looking Cupid's bow is created that helps to camouflage the bilateral deformity.

At the time of palate closure at 18 months the prolabium has usually stretched enough to spare easily a forked flap that is banked in the whisker position beneath the alae. At the time of advancement of the banked forked flap from whisker position at 4 years, the nasal tip is released, the alar cartilages are freed and sutured to reconstruct the medial crura, and the columella is lengthened.

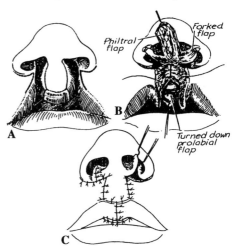

Millard bilateral cleft lip repair. *A*, The philtrum is outlined with a turndown flap of prolabial vermillion; the lateral prolabial tissues become the forked flaps. Circumalar marks design the alar base flaps; lateral lip marks show the turndown of vermillion flaps, carrying the white roll of the mucocutaneous junction. *B*, The lateral mucosa and muscle are sutured together behind the prolabium, which has been elevated temporarily. *C*, The lip has been approximated, a slight excess of vermillion flaps creating a tubercle. The fork flaps are sutured end-on to the alar base flaps; their raw surfaces are approximated to form a mound in the floor of the nose for future columella lengthening. (From Millard DR Jr: Cleft lip. In McCarthy JG (ed): Plastic Surgery. Philadelphia, W.B. Saunders, 1990, p 2684, with permission.)

28. What is important to the future treatment of clefts?

Genetic engineering probably will have more impact in preventing the deformity than in utero surgery in correcting the deformity.

BIBLIOGRAPHY

Unilateral Clefts
1. Blair VP, Brown JB: Mirault operation for single harelip. Surg Gynecol Obstet 51:81, 1930.
2. Brown JB, McDowell F: Small triangular flap operation for the primary repair of single cleft lips. Plast Reconst Surg 5:392, 1950.
3. Hagedorn W: Die Operation der Hasenscharte mit Zickzachnaht. Zentralbl Chir 19:281, 1892.
4. Kilner TP: Cleft lip and palate repair. St. Thomas Hosp Rep 2:127, 1937.
5. Langenbeck B von: Die uranoplastik mittelst Abloesung des mucoesperiostalen Gaumeneuberzuges. Arch Clin Chir 2:205–287, 1861. [Also Plast Reconstr Surg 49:326–330, 1972.]
6. Latham RA: Orthopedic advancement of the cleft maxillary segment. A preliminary report. Cleft Palate J 17:277, 1980.
7. LeMesurier AB: Method of cutting and suturing lip in complete unilateral cleft lip. Plast Reconstr Surg 4:1, 1949.
8. Millard DR Jr: A primary camouflage of the unilateral harelook. Transactions of the First International Congress of Plastic Sugery, Stockholm. Baltimore, Williams & Wilkins, 1957, pp 160–166.
9. Millard DR Jr: Cleft Craft. Boston, Little, Brown, 1976.
10. Millard DR Jr: Earlier correction of the unilateral cleft lip nose. Plast Reconstr Surg 70:64, 1982.
11. Millard DR Jr, Latham RA: Improved primary surgical and dental treatment of clefts. Plast Reconstr Surg 86:856, 1990.
12. Millard DR Jr: Combining the von Langenbeck and the Wardill-Kilner operations in certain clefts of the palate. Cleft Palate J 1991.
13. Millard DR Jr: Embryonic rationale for the primary correction of classical congenital clefts of the lip and palate. Hunterian Lecture delivered during the meeting of the British Association of Plastic Surgeons held at Oxford on July 7, 1994. Ann R Coll Surg 1994, pp 150–160.

14. Millard DR Jr: A Rhinoplasty Tetralogy. Boston, Little, Brown, 1996.
15. Mirault G: Deux lettres sur operation du bec-de-lievre considere dans ses divers etats de simplicite et de complication. J Chir (Paris) 2:257, 1844; 3:5, 1845.
16. Randall P: A triangular flap operation for the primary repair of unilateral clefts of the lip. Plast Reconstr Surg 23:331, 1959.
17. Tennison CW: The repair of the unilateral cleft lip by the stencil method. Plast Reconstr Surg 9:115–120, 1952.
18. Wardill WBM: Cleft palate. Br J Surg 16:127–148, 1928.

Bilateral Clefts
 1. Brophy TW: The radical cure of congenital cleft palate. Dent Cosmos 41:882, 1899.
 2. Carter WW: N Y State J Med Nov. 1914.
 3. Cronin TD: Lengthening the columella by the use of skin from the nasal floors and alae. Plast Reconstr Surg 21:417, 1958.
 4. Gensoul JJ: J Hebd Med Chir Pratique 1833, p 29.
 5. Georgiade NG, Latham RA: Maxillary arch alignment in bilateral cleft lip and palate repair using the pinned coaxial screw appliance. Plast Reconstr Surg 56:52, 1975.
 6. Manchester WM: The repair of double cleft lip as part of an integrated program. Plast Reconstr Surg 45:207, 1970.
 7. Millard DR Jr. Columella lengthening by a forked flap. Plast Reconstr Surg 22:454–457, 1958.
 8. Millard DR Jr: Adaptation of the rotation-advancement principle in bilateral cleft lip. In Wallace AB (ed): Transactions of the Second International Congress of Plastic Surgery, London, 1959. Edinburgh, Churchill-Livingstone, 1960.
 9. Millard DR Jr: A primary compromise for bilateral cleft lip. Surg Gynecol Obstet 111:557, 1960.
10. Millard DR Jr, Berkowitz S, Latham RA, Wolfe SA: A discussion on pre-surgical orthodontics in patients with clefts. Cleft Palate J 25:403, 1988.
11. Millard DR Jr, Latham RA: Improved primary surgical and dental treatment of clefts. Plast Reconstr Surg 45:207, 1990.
12. Mulliken JB: Bilateral complete cleft lip and nasal deformity: An anthropometric analsyis of staged to synchronous repair. Plast Reconstr Surg 96:9–23, 1995.
13. Pruzansky S: Factors determining arch form in cleft lip and palate. Am J Orthod 41:827–851, 1955.
14. Trott JA, Mohan N: A preliminary report on one-stage open tip rhinoplasty at the time of lip repair in bilateral cleft lip and palate. The Alor Setar experience. Br J Plast Surg 46:215–222, 1993.

13. CLEFT PALATE

*Peter Randall, M.D., Don La Rossa, M.D., Marilyn Cohen, B.A.,
and Ghada Afifi, M.D.*

1. What is a cleft palate?
It is a failure of the two halves of the roof of the mouth, or palatal shelves, to join in the midline and fuse. The cleft may involve the soft palate or both soft and hard palates.

2. Explain the terms *primary* and *secondary* palate, *prepalatal* and *palatal* structures.
The **incisive foramen**, which is located behind the incisor teeth, is the site where the lateral maxillary bones meet the midline premaxilla. A cleft lip usually involves structures anterior to the incisive foramen, such as the alveolus, lip, and nasal tip cartilages, as well as the floor of the nose. These structures usually are referred to as the structures of the **primary** palate or **prepalatal** structures. They may be cleft unilaterally or bilaterally.

The structures posterior to the incisive foramen, including the hard palate, soft palate, and uvula, are usually referred to as the **secondary** palate or **palatal** structures. Thus, the incisive foramen separates the primary (prepalatal) and secondary (palatal) structures.

3. What is the premaxilla?
The premaxilla is the alveolar segment of the maxilla that includes the nasal spine and four incisor teeth. It is located centrally and anterior to the incisive foramen.

4. When is a cleft palate associated with a cleft lip? What is the overall incidence?

The most frequent combination is a unilateral cleft of the lip and palate, which is seen more often in boys than girls, predominantly on the left side. The hereditary incidence is fairly high. The next most frequent cleft—of the palate alone—is seen more frequently in girls; the hereditary incidence is fairly low. In Caucasians, the incidence is approximately 1.4 per 1,000 live births; in blacks, it is approximately 0.43/1,000; and in Asians, it may be as high as 3.2/1,000. Actually, the most common cleft is a cleft uvula, or bifid uvula, which has an incidence of about 2%. Most cases are asymptomatic; however, as many as 20% of patients may have some degree of velopharyngeal incompetence.

5. How can clefts be classified?

Clefts can be described as complete (i.e., penetrating all the way through the structures) or incomplete. Prepalatal clefts or clefts of the primary palate also should be described as unilateral (right or left) or bilateral; they may be described even further as involving one-third, two-thirds, or three-thirds (complete) of the lip. Similarly, palatal clefts may be described as involving one-third, two-thirds, or three-thirds of the soft palate and one-third, two-thirds, or three-thirds of the hard palate, extending up to the incisive foramen.

A **submucosal cleft palate** is not an overt cleft. The levator muscle fibers fail to fuse completely in the midline, usually leading to velopharyngeal incompetence. A thin area, called a **zona pellucida**, is often seen centrally at the site where the muscle is lacking. A notch often can be palpated at the posterior edge of the hard palate, which normally has a palpable prominence or posterior nasal spine. Patients often have a bifid uvula, which may be a simple bilobed uvula or a completely split uvula.

A **bifid uvula**, seen in 2% of the normal American population, may be associated with palatal incompetence; patients should be followed for possible speech problems. A congenital absence of the muscularis uvulae also may occur with or without a bifid uvula and is often associated with palatal incompetence.

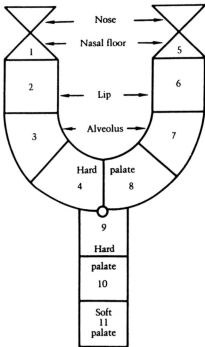

Millard's modification of Kernahan's and Elsahy's striped Y classification for cleft lip and palate. The small circle indicates the incisive foramen; the triangles indicate the nasal tip and nasal floor. (From Randall P: Cleft palate. In Smith JW, Aston SJ (eds): Grabb and Smith's Plastic Surgery, 4th ed. Boston, Little, Brown, 1991, p 291, with permission.)

6. What is the etiology of cleft palate?

Cleft palate is believed to be a multifactorial defect; a cleft can be caused in many different ways. A high incidence of clefts in some families suggest a genetic etiology. Clefts may be associated with syndromes such as Stickler's syndrome, velocardiofacial syndrome, fetal alcohol syndrome, DiGeorge syndrome, and trisomies. Experimentally, clefts have been induced by a number of agents, including alcohol, insulin, tretinoin, corticosteroids, anticonvulsants, phenobarbital, carbon monoxide, salicylates, oxygen deficiency, arabasine, and possibly smoking. Other factors probably exist. In any one case, it is usually difficult to identify one cause.

7. How does a primary or prepalatal cleft form?

Primary clefts result from a lack of mesenchymal development. The mesenchymal islands—one central and two lateral—normally develop and fuse. Lack of development of one of the three islands results in an unstable condition with ectoderm of the skin in contact with ectoderm of the oral mucosa; complete or incomplete breakdown occurs at this point.

8. Why are left-sided secondary or palatal clefts more common than right-sided clefts?

In the 7-week-old embyro, the two palatal shelves lie almost vertically. Normally, the neck straightens from its flexed position, the tongue drops posteriorly, and the shelves rotate superiorly to the horizontal position; they fuse from anterior to posterior to form the intact palate by 12 weeks. In rodents, the right palatal shelf reaches the horizontal position before the left one, leaving the left side susceptible to developmental interruption for a greater period than the right side. This may account for the greater incidence of left-sided clefts.

9. What is Simonart's band?

A cleft of the primary palate is often bridged by a band of lip tissue—Simonart's band. Some regard this band of tissue as the result of a healing process after breakdown of the lip elements. Others propose that Simonart's band may result from partial formation of the epithelial wall.

10. Which muscles are the most important for achieving velopharyngeal closure?

The levator palatini muscles pull the middle third of the soft palate superiorly and posteriorly to produce firm contact with the posterior pharyngeal wall at about the level of the adenoidal pad.

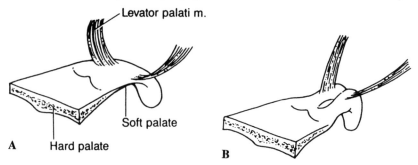

The levator muscles pull approximately 45° superiorly and posteriorly. *A,* At rest. *B,* After contraction. (From Randall P, LaRossa D: Cleft palate. In McCarthy JG (ed): Plastic Surgery. Philadelphia, W.B. Saunders, 1990, p 2727, with permission.)

11. Do any other muscles contribute to velopharyngeal closure?

Absolutely. The paired palatopharyngeus muscles pull the soft palate posteriorly; the muscularis uvulae cause the uvula to thicken centrally with contraction, and the superior pharyngeal constrictor muscles move the lateral pharyngeal walls medially or the posterior pharyngeal wall anteriorly with contraction.

12. What is the most important anatomic abnormality seen with a cleft palate?

Disorientation of the levator palatini muscles, which normally join in the midline with a transverse orientation and insert into the palatal aponeurosis at approximately the middle third of the soft palate. In the case of a cleft, the muscles are much more longitudinally oriented and insert into the posterior edge of the palatal bone and along the bony cleft. (See figure, top of next page.)

13. What is an intravelar veloplasty?

Kriens first emphasized the abnormal orientation of the levator palatini muscles and the need to detach them from their abnormal insertion and reorient them in a transverse direction. Suturing the muscles in an overlapping fashion rather than end to end produces a tighter levator sling.

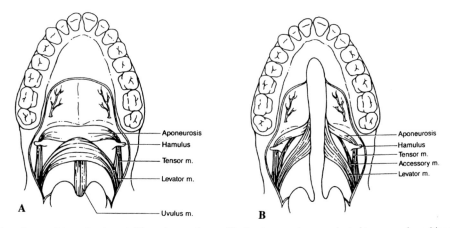

Musculature of the soft palate. *A,* Normal musculature. The levator muscles are oriented transversely and insert in the palatine aponeurosis in the midportion of the soft palate. *B,* Cleft musculature. The levator muscles are oriented more lontigudinally and insert on the posterior edge of the palatal bone and along the bony cleft edges. (From Randall P, LaRossa D: Cleft palate. In McCarthy JG (ed): Plastic Surgery. Philadelphia, W.B. Saunders, 1990, pp 2726 and 2730, with permission.)

14. What is Passavant's ridge?

During gagging, the forceful contraction of both the levator palatini muscles and the superior pharyngeal constrictors may produce a bulge or ridge on the posterior pharynx above the arch of the atlas—Passavant's ridge. This ridge also may be associated with velopharyngeal incompetence as a compensatory mechanism to assist with velopharyngeal closure.

15. How can a mother know if her child has a cleft palate?

The cleft was probably first identified by the obstetrician or pediatrician. The mother may or may not directly observe the cleft; instead, her only clues may be the child's poor-to-absent ability to build suction along with regurgitation of milk into the nose. Some clefts also may be detected prenatally by ultrasound even before 18 weeks' gestation.

16. How should a mother feed a child with a cleft palate if the child cannot suck?

Most children born with a cleft demonstrate normal sucking motions, but the mother should know that the prime difficulty is inability to build up adequate suction. Usually the ability to swallow is not impaired. The child should be held in a head-up position at about 45° and usually can be bottle-fed with a preemie nipple that has additional cross-cuts in the end. A plastic bottle that can be squeezed or a bulb syringe with a nipple can deliver too much milk and cause choking. The baby can be expected to swallow more air and to need more burping, but with good delivery of milk a long time should not be required for each feeding. Regurgitation through the nose may be expected because of the deficiency of the palatal midline tissues.

17. Who should evaluate a newborn with a cleft palate?

Ideally, a newborn with a cleft should be seen by the surgeon who will ultimately repair the cleft so that he or she can discuss the entire spectrum of care with the parents. Introduction to key people on the cleft palate team is also advisable so that parents may identify the respective roles of each; hence early intervention is facilitated. Instructions for adequate feeding and airway protection are most important. Introduction to parental support groups is also helpful.

18. What disciplines should be available on a cleft palate team?

The team should include a pediatrician, a surgeon experienced in cleft management, a speech pathologist, a pediatric otolaryngologist, a well-versed orthodontist, a pediatric dentist, and an audiologist. The team also should have access to a geneticist, a prosthodontist, an ophthalmologist, a clinical psychologist and/or psychiatrist, a physical anthropologist, a social worker, and a nurse experienced in cleft problems.

19. What are the major sequelae of an unrepaired cleft palate?

Initially, the main problems are an inability to build up suction and nasal regurgitation. The patient usually has poor eustachian tube function, which may lead to fluid in the middle ear space, and is prone to recurrent otitis media. Breathing may be a major problem, particularly if the chin is short and the tongue falls backward, causing inspiratory obstruction as in Pierre Robin sequence. Speech may be significantly affected in the unrepaired or repaired incompetent palate, including hypernasality with vowel sounds and distortion of the pressure consonants. With involvement of the alveolar ridge, the adjacent teeth are usually angled into the cleft and may be malformed or absent. Dental caries and severe malocclusion may be present or develop.

20. At what age should the palate be surgically repaired?

Most authorities concur that repair is best performed between 6 and 9 months of age. Some data indicate a slight improvement with closure at 3–6 months of age, although other reports show no additional benefit. Most agree that closure should be complete before 18 months of age.

21. What is the benefit of earlier closure?

The greatest benefit is better speech. Even with babbling, a child is learning to articulate. If speech develops before closure of the palate is complete, the child usually has difficulty in building up pressure for the production of sounds such as P and T. He or she will have even more trouble controlling sustained pressure for the production of sounds such as S and SH. As a result, the child may develop speech in which these sounds are missing or distorted. Alternatively, the child may develop what is called **compensatory articulation**, such as the glottal stop and pharyngeal fricative.

22. What is the von Langenbeck operation?

Described in 1859, the von Langenbeck operation remains a reliable method of cleft palate repair. It involves elevation of large mucoperiosteal flaps from the hard palate with midline approximation of the cleft margins of both hard and soft palates with long, relaxing incisions laterally. The levator muscles are completely detached from their abnormal bony insertion, and the soft palate musculature is repaired in the midline. A palatal lengthening procedure is not included in this operation.

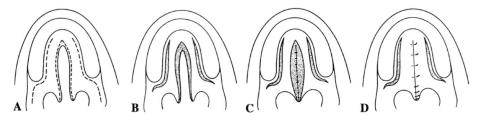

The von Langenbeck operation. *A*, Flap design. *B*, The lateral relaxing incisions are made, and the mucoperiosteal flaps are elevated. *C*, The nasal mucosa is closed and the muscles sutured together after detachment from their insertion. *D*, The oral closure. (From Randall P, LaRossa D: Cleft palate. In McCarthy JG (ed): Plastic Surgery. Philadelphia, W.B. Saunders, 1990, p 2743, with permission.)

23. What is the Furlow double-reversing Z-plasty technique?

This procedure consists of two Z-plasties of the soft palate, one on the oral mucosa and the other in the reverse orientation on the nasal mucosa. The levator muscle on one side is included in the posteriorly based **oral** mucosal Z-plasty, whereas the levator muscle from the opposite side is included in the posteriorly based **nasal** mucosal Z-plasty flap (see figure, top of next page). The hard palate cleft is closed using a vomer flap (see question 25). This procedure reorients the malpositioned levator muscles, permits overlap of the muscles, and produces some degree of palatal lengthening.

24. What is the Wardill-Kilner-Veau operation?

The Wardill-Kilner-Veau operation is a V-Y advancement of the mucoperiosteum of the hard palate, designed specifically to lengthen the palate in the anteroposterior plane at the time of primary palatoplasty. As a result of the V-Y lengthening, bare membranous bone is left exposed in the area

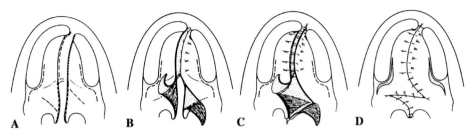

The Furlow double Z-plasty operation. A, Flap design. B, Oral and nasal mucosal Z-plasty flaps are elevated. C, The nasal mucosal closure. D, The oral mucosal closure. The soft palate has been lengthened and the levator muscles properly oriented. (From Randall P, LaRossa D: Cleft palate. In McCarthy JG (ed): Plastic Surgery. Philadelphia, W.B. Saunders, 1990, p 2740, with permission.)

from which the flaps were advanced. These areas granulate and epithelialize within 2–3 weeks but remain areas of fibrous scar and may contribute to subsequent maxillary growth disturbances.

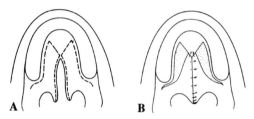

The Wardill-Kilner-Veau operation. A, Flap design. B, V-Y lengthening leaves an exposed bare area of bone after closure. (From Randall P, LaRossa D: Cleft palate. In McCarthy JG (ed): Plastic Surgery. Philadelphia, W.B. Saunders, 1990, p 2744, with permission.)

25. What is a vomer flap?

Hard palate closure can be performed by elevating a wide superiorly based flap of nasal mucosa from the vomer. With bilateral clefts, vomer flaps can be obtained from each side of the vomer. This technique avoids the need for elevating large mucoperiosteal flaps from the hard palate and the potential risk of resultant maxillary growth disturbances.

26. Is there an alternative to surgical repair?

In rare instances in which the patient has a medical condition that makes surgery or general anesthesia too risky, a dental prosthesis is a possible alternative. Older children (age 15 years and older) in developing countries, for example, can be managed with a prosthesis if dental services are available.

27. What is velopharyngeal incompetence (VPI)? How soon after surgery should a child be evaluated for VPI?

VPI is the inability of the soft palate to make contact with the posterior pharyngeal wall (i.e., velopharyngeal closure) during speech, resulting in hypernasality. Evaluation of palatal function is an ongoing process that should begin as speech development occurs and continue through puberty. Usually, incompetence can be diagnosed by 4 or 5 years of age and occasionally earlier.

28. Who should decide to operate on an incompetent palate?

This decision is usually made by a competent speech pathologist in conjunction with the surgeon. Even though the trained ear is probably the most accurate way to assess incompetence, if surgery is contemplated, dynamic assessment of palatal function is usually advisable. Assessment can be done through multiplane videofluoroscopy or nasoendoscopic examination. Additional studies of pressure flow or objective nasal resonant measurement also may be helpful.

29. What can be done about residual speech problems after cleft palate repair?

A number of approaches may be used. With minor incompetence or inconsistent incompetence, speech therapy alone may succeed in improving speech. More often, a secondary operation is necessary, such as a posterior pharyngeal flap or lateral pharyngoplasty. With minimal incompetence, a palatal lengthening operation or a procedure to advance the posterior pharyngeal wall may be advised. Some cases may be managed with a prosthesis that simply lifts the palate into a more competent position to permit velopharyngeal closure or obturates the defect.

30. Why do children with palatal clefts have ear problems?
The levator veli palatini and tensor veli palatini muscles insert to some extent on the eustachian tube. Both are probably responsible for competence of the tube in preventing reflux from the nasopharynx into the eustachian tube as well as for opening the tube to equalize pressure in the middle ear. With impaired ability to equalize middle ear pressure, infants with clefts usually have fluid in the middle ear space, which soon becomes thick and viscous. Untreated, this condition leads to an increase in the incidence and severity of otitis media. Treatment consists of myringotomies, evacuation of the fluid, and insertion of indwelling ventilating tubes as well as vigilance for otitis media. Palate repair seems to reduce ear problems, but children whose ear problems have been neglected frequently have a high incidence of permanent hearing loss.

31. What is the likelihood of a cleft in another child from the same parents?
The likelihood depends on a number of factors, but generally, if there is no known teratogen or first-degree relative with a cleft, the likelihood in the Caucasian population is about 0.14%. If a first- or second-degree relative has a cleft, the likelihood increases to about 5%; if two first- or second-degree relatives have a cleft, it increases to 15–25%.

32. Is there a way to decrease the incidence of clefts?
Other than avoiding exposure to known teratogens, the answer is not clear. Folic acid taken during pregnancy has been shown to decrease the incidence of spina bifida, and some believe that it also decreases the incidence of clefts. However, this theory has not been generally accepted and remains an area of investigation.

BIBLIOGRAPHY

1. American Cleft Palate–Craniofacial Association: Parameters for Evaluation and Treatment of Patients with Cleft Lip–Palate or Other Craniofacial Anomalies. In Phillips BJ, Warren DW (eds): The Cleft Palate and Craniofacial Team. Chapel Hill, NC, American Cleft Palate Association, 1993.
2. Bartlett SP, Yu J: Congenital disorders. In Ruberg RL, Smith DJ (eds): Plastic Surgery. St. Louis, Mosby, 1994, pp 271–277.
3. Berkowitz S: Team Management in Cleft Lip and Palate. San Diego, Singular Publishing Group, 1996.
4. Burdi AR: Epidemiology, etiology, and pathogenesis of cleft lip and cleft palate. Cleft Palate J 14:262–269, 1977.
5. David DJ, Bagnall AD: Velopharyngeal incompetence. In McCarthy JG (ed): Plastic Surgery. Philadelphia, W.B. Saunders, 1990, pp 2903–2921.
6. Johnson MC: Embryology of the head and neck. In McCarthy JG (ed): Plastic Surgery. Philadelphia, W.B. Saunders, 1990, pp 2451–2495.
7. Johnson MC, Bronsky PT, Millicorsky G: Embryogenesis of cleft lip and palate. In McCarthy JG (ed): Plastic Surgery. Philadelphia, W.B. Saunders, 1990, pp 2515–2552.
8. Kernahan DA: The striped Y-A symbolic classification for cleft lip and palate. Plast Reconstr Surg 47:469, 1971.
9. McCarthy JG, Cutting C, Hogan VM: Introduction to facial clefts. In McCarthy JG (ed): Plastic Surgery. Philadelphia, W.B. Saunders, pp 2437–2450.
10. McWilliams BJ, Randall P, LaRossa D, et al: Speech characteristics associated with the Furlow palatoplasty as compared with other surgical techniques. Plast Reconstr Surg 98:610–619, 1996.
11. Millard DR: Wide and/or short cleft palate. Plast Reconstr Surg 29:41–57, 1962.
12. Millard DR: Classification. In Millard DR (ed): Cleft Craft. Boston, Little, Brown, 1977, p 52.
13. Randall P, LaRossa D: Cleft palate. In McCarthy JG (ed): Plastic Surgery. Philadelphia, W.B. Saunders, 1990, pp 2723–2752.
14. Randall P, LaRossa D, Fakhraee SM, Cohen MA: Cleft palate closure at three to seven months of age: A preliminary report. Plast Reconstr Surg 71:624–628, 1983.
15. Sando WC, Jurkiewicz MI: Cleft palate. In Jurkiewicz MJ, Krizek TJ, Mathes SJ, Ariyan S (eds): Plastic Surgery: Principles and Practics. St. Louis, Mosby, 1990, pp 81–97.
16. Shaw WC, et al: A six-center international study of treatment outcome in patients with clefts of the lip and palate. Parts I–V. Cleft Palate J 29:393–413, 1992.

14. ORTHODONTICS FOR ORAL CLEFT CRANIOFACIAL DISORDERS

John L. Spolyar, D.D.S., M.S.

PASSIVE PROSTHETICS (NEONATAL PERIOD)

1. What is a passive infant oral prosthesis?

An infant oral prosthesis is a passive device much like a denture without teeth that covers and follows the anatomic outline of the hard palate and its defect. To maintain position and to resist displacement, the margins of the prosthesis usually extend over the lateral alveolar segments and may extend into and over the lateral surfaces of the nasal cavity and vomer. The prosthesis is routinely made from polymerized methyl methacrylate (acrylic).

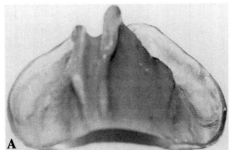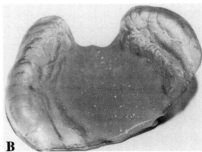

Passive infant oral prosthesis. *A,* Prosthesis on anatomic side shows nasal extension for retention. *B,* Oral side of prosthesis.

2. What does the prosthesis do?

A palatal prosthesis divides the oral and nasal cavities into functional spaces while providing a tactile reference for the tongue. Function is then segregated with the nose for airway and the oral cavity for feeding and proper tongue posturing. This segregation aids feeding and breathing and facilitates proper physiologic resting posture for the tongue with tip forward.

3. Does a prosthesis affect growth?

After surgical lip repair in cases of complete unilateral cleft lip/palate (UCLP) and bilateral cleft lip/palate (BCLP), medial displacement of the cleft segments is inevitable. A passive prosthesis, especially with proper nasal extension, prevents medial relocation of the cleft segments and provides normalized maxillary displacement growth in width achievement. Preventing medial collapse and promoting maxillary transverse growth have positive effects and serve to optimize oral volume, nasal respiration, dentoalveolar segment alignment, facial development, and overall anatomic balance. Perhaps the best potential growth and facial skeletal development is achieved by integrating passive prosthesis stabilization with rehabilitation protocols.

4. When is the prosthesis worn?

A prosthesis is best used as early as possible in the neonate's life—perhaps before the initial repair to facilitate feeding. If provided in coordination with the initial repair, a prosthesis is best left in place for 1–2 weeks before daily removal for cleaning. The appliance is best used on a full-time basis until a few weeks before palatoplasty, when it is used only during feeding. Appliance cleaning more frequent than daily may be indicated during upper respiratory tract infections that obstruct the nasal port because of mucous drainage.

5. How long does it take before a prosthesis is outgrown?

Facial growth occurs most in the vertical and least in the transverse plane. The prosthesis must be adjusted about every 6 weeks to reduce retentive undercuts and to broaden alveolar contacts. Generally, once the weight of the infant doubles, effective appliance retention is lost, and the appliance is no longer useful.

6. Does extension of the prosthesis over the alveolar structures restrict normal development of the lateral dental segments?

The "pressure" of alveolar remodeling growth easily exceeds the passive resistance of the appliance. With appliance adjustments over the alveolar extensions, normal development should proceed without restriction.

PRESURGICAL ORTHOPEDIC CORRECTION (NEONATAL PERIOD)

7. What is presurgical orthopedic correction (POC)?

POC is a procedure used to correct an anatomically abnormal bony relationship before any primary reconstructive surgery is performed.

8. How does POC apply to oral cleft patients?

In neonates with complete BCLP and UCLP, cleft maxillary components are distorted and abnormally positioned. The overlying soft tissue mirrors the skeletal deformity and gives the recognizable pattern of deformity in UCLP and BCLP. The objectives of POC are to reposition displaced basal segments and to realign soft tissue margins of like kind before corrective surgery is performed.

9. What problems attend oral cleft treatment without POC?
- Lip closure alone does not reposition the maxilla and premaxilla in BCLP or pull the cleft maxillary segment forward in UCLP well enough for closure of the cleft.
- Lip repair alone does not reposition the maxilla forward in BCLP to provide a full midface or pull the cleft maxillary segment forward in UCLP to balance the malar and alar bases or reduce the stigmatizing "crooked face."
- A protruded premaxilla at the base of the columella makes columellar lengthening and nasal tip correction impossible until the patient reaches adolescence.
- Persistent fistulas and residual clefts in the alveolus require the difficult surgery of bone grafting when the patient is between 6 and 8 years old.

10. What are the benefits of POC?
- A better platform is produced for the lip and nose as well as for the alveolus.
- Primary surgical closure can be performed without tension.
- A more precise method controls the cleft components without dependence on simple closure of the lip over the deformity to mold the distorted parts.
- Dissection of mucoperiosteum at the edge of the cleft facilitates a two-layer closure without tension.
- Alveolar integrity established to facilitate dental development.
- Closure of the hard and soft palate is facilitated.
- An intact primary palate is achieved at an early age.
- Gingivoperiosteoplasty can be done with or without primary bone grafting.
- A normal maxillary arch without fistulas is achieved with early secondary palate closure. Early "fork-flap" columellar surgery is possible in BCLP and may produce a good nose and lip.
- An intact oral cavity without fistulation is routinely established well within the first year of life with a clearly improved possibility for intelligible speech to follow.

11. What are the various techniques used in POC?

The techniques are best grouped by type of device retention as either passive or fixed (pinned).

12. What techniques use passive retention?

1. In the 1950s McNeil and Burston used a passive oral prosthesis and external facial or head straps to effect segment repositioning and remodeling.

2. A T-shaped extraoral traction device is applied to the nostril on the normal side in UCLP cases. The design tactic is to use transverse traction to correct the midfacial asymmetry and to minimize the posterior retraction forces on the developing maxilla.

3. Another technique for BCLP uses a passive oropalatal prosthesis as an anchor, and a Latex rubber retraction strip is looped over the prolabium to reposition the maxilla and premaxilla.

13. How effective are passive techniques?

The results are variable in regard to achieving treatment objectives. All of these early techniques share the following disadvantages:
- Inconsistency and difficulty with patient compliance
- Incomplete control of directional mechanics best directed at the orthopedic deformity
- Unpredictable and partial achievement of treatment objectives.
- Extended treatment time
- Labor intensive
- More expensive than non-POC treatment protocols

Their advantages include:
- Less invasive than pinning techniques, which require general anesthesia for placement
- Less expensive than pinning techniques

14. What techniques use pinned retention?

1. In 1957 Hagerty first reported the use of pins to retain an expandable stainless steel bar in cleft palate treatment.

2. In 1965 Hagerty et al. reported the use of an expandable acrylic palatal prosthesis with intraosseous pinning for anchorage.

3. Contemporary techniques were reported during the 1970s and 1980s by Georgiade and Latham. BCLP was treated with a coaxial mechanism that expanded the maxillary base and repositioned the premaxilla at the same time. Latham et al. reported on the design and use of this extraorally activated expansion device that applied elastic traction to the premaxilla.

4. In 1980 Latham reported the treatment of UCLP with a device for orthopedic advancement of the cleft maxillary segment. It was much like the maxillary base device used today.

15. How effective are pinned techniques?

Results are highly consistent in achieving treatment objectives with the attending benefits and advantages described above. The disadvantages include the following:
- Device placement requires a hospital operating room (OR).
- Pinned techniques are more expensive than passive retention POC.

16. How is POC used in UCLP and BCLP treatment?

1. Soon after birth an impression is obtained, and the maxillary POC device is fabricated on a stone model.

2. OR placement of the device is coordinated with myringotomy and pressure-equalizing (PE) tube procedures.

3. The maxillary base device is retained by four channel-locking pins, two on each side, which pass through the acrylic base material into the palate for intraosseous fixation.

4. For cases of BCLP, a staple is placed through the bony septal structure of the premaxilla to connect respositioning chains.

17. How does the UCLP device produce orthopedic correction?

1. Once the device is in place, a drive screw is activated one-half turn (0.25-mm displacement), and activation is continued once or twice a day by the parent at home.

2. The patient is observed on a regular basis. Activation continues until, by design, no further turning of the screw is possible. The segments should be well aligned with 1–3 mm of space (defect) between the nearly abutting segments.

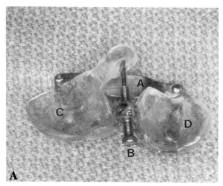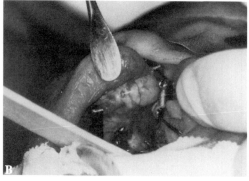

UCLP POC device. *A*, Viewed from its anatomic side. A coplanar double hinge (A) allows rotation and translation of the greater (GS) and lesser segment (LS) to one another. Turning screw (B) against GS (C) pulls LS (D)
forward. The principal action is LS advancement with outward rotation and GS advancement with inward rotation. *B*, With device in place, the drive screw lies adjacent to the cleft segment and is easily accessed at the front
of the cleft defect.

18. How long does it take before a patient with UCLP is ready for reconstructive surgery?

1. Screw activation takes from 3–6 weeks to complete, depending on the size of the cleft, rate
of activation, and amount of correction designed into the device (up to 14 mm).

2. A resting period of 2–3 weeks allows dissipation of any residual load (strain) that builds up
after applying the active force (stress).

3. If the device is applied by age 4 weeks, the first reconstructive surgery can be done at age
3 months.

19. How does the BCLP device produce orthopedic correction?

1. Once the device is in place, as the case demands, an expansion screw can be activated one-
quarter turn (0.25-mm expansion at the anterior cleft segment) at a time. As instructed, activation
once or twice a day by the parent at home or, perhaps better, one full revolution by the physician
during weekly follow-up well achieves proper lateral segment placement.

2. The elastic chain tension is checked for possible adjustment on a weekly basis. The pressure
should not exceed 2 ounces per side. Excessive force causes undue septal staple translation without
orthopedic effect and possible failure.

3. The patient is observed on a regular basis until the case is fully corrected with proper max-
illa-premaxilla segment alignment and 0–2 mm of space at each cleft defect.

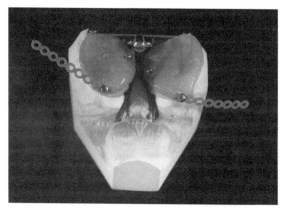

BCLP pinned POC base device can be expanded, enabling lateral segment placement to fit the premaxilla. The expansion
screw at the drive box is activated from the
front of the mouth. The device also acts as
a base appliance for maxillary protraction
in response to the coupling force for premaxillary retraction. Bilateral elastic chains
attached to the premaxilla pass around a
roller (not shown) under the drive box and
then proceed forward and laterally to hook
onto buttons for tensioning at the head of
each segment.

20. How long does it take before a patient with BCLP is ready for reconstructive surgery?

1. Elastic chain repositioning takes from 4–7 weeks to complete, depending on amount of premaxillary protrusion, size of the premaxilla, age of patient, and rate of activation.

2. A resting period of 2–3 weeks allows dissipation of any residual load to reduce rebound.

3. If the device is applied by age 4 weeks, the first reconstructive surgery can be done at age 3–4 months.

21. What are the significant treatment effects in BCLP?

The single most important response is forward maxillary repositioning to achieve premaxillary-maxillary alignment. The premaxilla shows less orthopedic adjustment and the vomer the least. This response is apparently age-dependent.

22. What is the incidence of postalveolar cleft palate fistulation (CPF) in patients treated with and without POC?

CPF is reported in 20–25% of patients treated without POC . The incidence may be as high as 50% in one-stage neonatal protocols. CPF was reported to be less than 8% in UCLP and BCLP treated with POC.

23. Do pinned POC devices stimulate maxillary growth?

Yes, in BCLP treatment. Maxillary forward translation in BCLP is about twice normal during the active phase of treatment.

24. Does pinned POC treatment adversely affect maxillary growth?

No.

ORTHODONTIC MANAGEMENT

Primary Dentition (Age 3–6 Years)

25. What is the primary dentition?

The first teeth to erupt, also known as milk teeth and baby teeth. Because the primary dentition is completely replaced by the adult dentition, **deciduous dentition** is a proper designation. Most children complete their primary dentition at the age of 2.5–3.0 years.

26. Why is orthodontic treatment important at this age?

Treatment positively influences postural and vegetative functions, occlusal function, facial growth, speech, eustachian tube and middle ear effusion, and reconstructive efforts.

27. What is achieved with orthodontic treatment?

Early treatment offers an opportunity for greater ease and efficacy of orthopedic procedures to increase space and optimize conditions for eruption and root formation; to attain proper occlusion; to increase oronasal volume; and to change the maxillary facial platform.

28. What physical signs are most important?

- Severe dental crossbites, both bilateral and anterior occlusal
- Very narrow maxillary dental arch
- Anterior (incisal) openbite
- Shallow or narrow palate
- Shifting of the bite, usually to one side, causing functional or postural mandibular asymmetry (functional shifts)

Other important related problems are encumbered speech, oral respiration with noisy sleeping pattern, bad oral habits (thumb [digit] sucking, tongue thrusting, bruxism, and severe attrition), and recurrent otitis media.

29. What procedures are undertaken at this age?

Principally, orthopedic with transverse maxillary distraction (expansion) and anterior repositioning (protraction).

30. What kinds of devices are used for maxillary expansion?

Expansion devices are either removable or fixed. **Removable** devices use a slow continuous expansion rate of 2 mm/month until completed. **Fixed** devices, either attached by stainless steel bands or directly bonded to posterior segment teeth, may use rapid continuous expansion at a rate of 0.5 mm/day or less to completion of expansion.

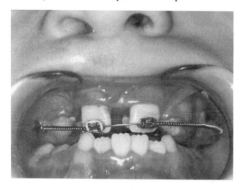

Intraoral view of rapid palatal expansion device directly bonded to the dentition with simultaneous orthodontic treatment for incisor alignment and decompensation for anterior crossbite correction. Note the separation of central incisors—a rare event in complete oral cleft patients—well after alveolar bone graft.

31. How long of a rest period is needed after expansion?

A bonded fixed device is used with expansion over a 2-week period in a regimen of 4–5 mm segments followed by a 4–6-week period of rest. This sequence is repeated until expansion is completed. Accumulation of residual load during rapid expansion is dissipated during the rest periods. Research has shown that residual load accumulating during rapid palatal expansion completely dissipates in 5–7 weeks, depending on patient age. Many orthodontists prefer a 3-month rest period after rapid palatal expansion. Such long periods of rest are unnecessary after slow expansion.

32. How much expansion is necessary?

The amount of appliance expansion varies from as little as 7 mm to as much as 20 mm with use of two devices. In certain cases expansion beyond that necessary for occlusal balance may be desirable to increase nasal airway volume.

33. When was maxillary expansion first used?

No one knows. But it was first reported in the literature in 1859 for the correction of constricted maxillary dental arches over a period of 2 weeks.

34. What other use do expansion devices have?

A fixed expansion device or retained removable device is a handle to the maxilla. This handle of opportunity is realized in maxillary protraction for correction of maxillary midfacial deficiency and anterior dental crossbite.

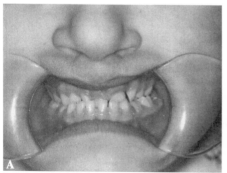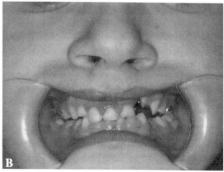

A, Intraoral view before maxillary protraction. *B*, Same view after maxillary protraction.

35. During primary dentition, when is the best time for maxillary protraction?

The best time is determined by the eruption of the permanent central incisors, which secure the repositioned maxilla with a proper bite. This translates to a dental age of at least 5 years to begin protraction treatment, which continues for 12 months. In general, the best time is before age 7 years.

Mixed Dentition (Age 7–11 Years)

36. What is mixed dentition?
    The period when both primary and permanent teeth are present in the mouth. It is referred to as the "ugly duckling stage" and represents a period of marvelous complexity in dental arrangements and numbers. At inception (before incisors erupt) there is a total of 48 teeth; this number is reduced to 28 over a period of about 5 years.

37. What are the succedaneous or successional teeth?
    The incisors, cuspids, and bicuspids occupy a place in the arch once held by a primary tooth.

38. What are the accessional teeth?
    All teeth that erupt posterior to the primary teeth (e.g., first, second, and third molars).

39. What is achieved by orthodontic treatment of mixed dentition?
    During this period there is, perhaps, one last opportunity for segment alignment of the maxillary components, dental alignment, and space definition at sites of agenic teeth (almost always lateral incisors). In a nutshell, it is a most important opportunity to define maxillary dental arch perimeter.

40. What treatment procedures are used?
 • Maxillary expansion and protraction   • Orthodontic treatment
 • Preparatory extractions   • Tooth straightening
    Preparatory extractions often include supernumerary teeth (teeth not present in a normal dentition and, in oral cleft patients, associated with cleft margins by the alveolar defect). Supernumerary teeth are commonly ectopic. If multiple, the additional supernumerary teeth are usually unerupted (impacted) and elevated within the anterior maxillary cleft segment. Orthodontic treatment is used to remove incisor irregularities, to create space for the agenic lateral incisor(s) and prospective graft sites, and to define buccal segment dental arch length. The decision to extract permanent teeth to reduce excessive dental crowding is often made during this period.

41. Why is this period critical for the alveolar bone graft?
    With the canine root 25–50% formed, success rates for grafting are high during this age range.

42. Why is it important to graft the alveolar defect when the canine root is less than 50% formed?
    Canine teeth may erupt and migrate through the bone graft. With root formation beyond 50%, teeth begin eruptive bodily relocation in excess of root lengthening, and the cuspid may penetrate from its intraosseous crypt into the void of the alveolar defect.

Adolescent and Adult Dentition (Age 12–17 Years and Beyond)

43. What is adolescent dentition?
    The first 6 years after onset of full eruption of succedaneous teeth during the period of accelerated adolescent growth in stature and facial development.

44. What orthodontic appliances are used during this period?
    Occasionally, maxillary expansion may be indicated for a second time or, less often, primarily. Rigidly bonded or banded jackscrew appliances are most effective, but often spring wire-type expansion devices attached to two molars may be used successfully for buccal segment dental expansion. However, the principal procedures are carried out with comprehensive orthodontic appliances and complete bracing of all clinically erupted permanent teeth. This technique gives virtual control over the six possible bodily movements in space for each tooth.

Controversy

45. Is alveolar bone grafting a definitive procedure?
    Bone grafting is not a definitive procedure even when it is entirely successful. The first graft may not compensate for vagaries of cleft type and individual variation, and results may be impossible to

predict. A fuller alveolus for an osseointegrated implant or multiunit fixed prosthesis or elevation at the ala base is often a legitimate indication for a second graft during adolescence and adulthood.

FACIAL GROWTH IN ORAL CLEFT PATIENTS

46. Is craniofacial morphology of parents related to susceptibility for oral cleft in offspring?
Yes. Good evidence from cephalometric studies in parents of children with cleft lip (CL) and/or cleft palate (CP) supports this hypothesis. In the **lateral view**, all such parents have significantly shorter upper facial height compared with lower facial height. A larger cranial base saddle angle was found in parents of children with CLP and CP. In the **frontal view**, all parents had a significantly narrower head (skull) width (HW) and smaller cephalic index. There were also greater ratios of HW to interorbital, interzygomaticofrontal suture, nasal, bizygomatic, and alar width. Parents of children with CLP also showed asymmetries in nasal alveolar shelf. In summary, shorter height and greater width in the upper face characterize all parent types.

47. How is the craniofacial status of adult patients with isolated unilateral cleft lip/alveolus (UCLA) surgically treated in childhood different from that of normal samples?
Facial height is greater than in controls, and the maxilla-mandibular relationship demonstrates a flat facial angle. Patients with UCLA have a balanced retrognathic-apertognathic profile. With the least severe deformity, UCLA craniofacial status is closer to the normal population than to the remaining oral cleft population.

48. How is the craniofacial status of adult patients with isolated UCLP surgically treated in childhood different from that of normal samples?
Facial height tends to be larger than in controls. The facial angle demonstrates a retrusive configuration with midfacial deficiency. The maxillofacial abnormality is explained by the severity of the deformity of patients with UCLP, manifest as a long-face, backward-divergent, and midfacial-deficient profile. Mandibular deformity is independent of severity of UCLP deformity.

49. How is the craniofacial status of adult patients with isolated BCLP surgically treated in childhood different from that of normal samples?
A similar deformity pattern to UCLP is found in BCLP with bimaxillary dentofacial retrusion, clockwise facial rotation, lower facial height enlargement, and retrocheilia (reduced upper lip thickness).

50. How is the craniofacial status of infants with isolated CP different from that of the CLA sample?
The structures that are shorter in infants with CP compared with CLA (an acceptable normal standard) are maxillary length, posterior maxillary height, mandibular length in both corpus and ramus, nasopharyngeal depth and height, and anterior cranial base length. Larger structures are mandibular angle (gonial), palatal plane angle, and open facial rotation. In summary, infants with CP represent a different population from infants with isolated clefts of primary palate.

51. How is the craniofacial status of adult patients with isolated CP treated and untreated in childhood different from that of normal samples?
Whether surgically treated in childhood or not, the craniofacial status is about the same in adults with CP. The maxilla is shorter in length and retruded in position. The mandible is more posterior and retrognathic and smaller, with an increased plane angle; it is like the mandible found in patients with complete oral cleft and primary cleft palate. The facial angle, however, is not unlike that of controls. Differences are also found among the different types of CP. Patients with clefts of only the soft palate have the least affected maxilla but the most retrognathic profile. Patients with soft and partial hard palate cleft have the most retruded maxilla. Cases with soft and complete hard palate cleft have the best overall facial balance, nearly normal mandibular form, and profiles that are not retrognathic.

52. How does a pharyngeal flap affect facial development?
Done rather early in life, a pharyngeal flap contributes mechanical, functional, and tissue factors affecting facial growth. The flap causes a greater reduction in forward maxillary growth than what

ordinarily occurs. The maxillary vertical dimension is unaffected. A greater facial opening rotation maintains facial balance. In general, restraint, scar, and increased nasal impedance to airflow disturb maxillary growth.

BIBLIOGRAPHY

1. Bishara SE: Cephalometric evaluation of facial growth in operated and non-operated individuals with isolated clefts of the palate. Cleft Palate J 10:239–246, 1973.
2. Bishara SE, Krause CJ, Olin WH, et al: Facial and dental relationships of individuals with unoperated clefts of the lip and/or palate. Cleft Palate J 13:238–252, 1976.
3. Bishara SE, Staley RM: Maxillary expansion: Clinical implications. Am J Orthod Dentofacial Orthop 91:3–14, 1987.
4. Blechschmidt E: Principles of biodynamic differentiation. In Bosma JF (ed): Development of the basicranium. Bethesda, MD, U.S. Department of Health, Education, and Welfare, 1976, pp 54–80.
5. Dahl E, Kreiborg S, Jensen BL, Fogh-Andersen P: Comparison of craniofacial morphology in infants with incomplete cleft lip and infants with isolated cleft palate. Cleft Palate J 19:258–266, 1982.
6. El Deeb M, Messer LB, Lehnert MW, et al: Canine eruption into grafted bone in maxillary alveolar cleft defects. Cleft Palate J 19:9–16, 1982.
7. Farkas LG, Lindsay WK: Morphology of the adult face after repair of isolated cleft palate in childhood. Cleft Palate J 9:132–142, 1972.
8. Hayashi I, Sakuda M, Takimoto K, Miyazaki T: Craniofacial growth in complete unilateral cleft lip and palate: A roentgenocephalometric study. Cleft Palate J 13:215–237, 1976.
9. Isaacson RJ, Wood JL, Ingram AH: Forces produced by rapid maxillary expansion. Angle Orthod 34:256–270, 1964.
10. Moyers RE: Handbook of Orthodontics, 2nd ed. Chicago, Year Book, 1963.
11. Nakasima A, Ichinose M: Characteristics of craniofacial structures of parents of children with cleft lip and/or palate. Am J Orthod 84:140–146, 1983.
12. Rosenstein SW: Early maxillary orthopaedics and appliance fabrication. In Kernahan DA, Rosenstein SW (ed): Cleft Lip and Palate: A System of Management. Baltimore, Williams & Wilkins, pp 120–127, 1990.
13. Rune B, Jacobsson S, Sarnas KV, Selvik G: A roentgens stereophotogrammetric study of implant stability and movement of segments in the maxilla of infants with cleft lip and palate. Cleft Palate J 16:267–278, 1979.
14. Smahel Z: Craniofacial morphology in adults with bilateral complete cleft lip and palate. Cleft Palate J 21:159–169, 1984.
15. Smahel Z, Brejcha M: Difference in craniofacial morphology between complete and incomplete unilateral cleft lip and palate in adults. Cleft Palate J 20:113–127, 1983.
16. Spolyar JL: The design, fabrication, and use of a full-coverage bonded rapid maxillary expansion appliance. Am J Orthod 86:136–145, 1984.
17. Spolyar JL: Growth comparison of cases with and without presurgical or orthopaedic correction. Proceedings of the 9th Annual Cleft Lip and Palate Symposium. Atlanta, Scottish Rite Children's Medical Center, 1996, pp 339–340.
18. Spolyar JL, Jackson IT, Phillips RJL, et al: The Latham technique: Contemporary presurgical orthopedics for the complete oral cleft technique and preliminary evaluation—A bone marker study. Perspect Plast Surg 6:179–210, 1992.
19. Subtelny JD, Nieto RP: A longitudinal study of maxillary growth following pharyngeal-flap surgery. Cleft Palate J 15:118–131, 1978.
20. Tindland RS: Skeletal response to maxillary protraction in patients with cleft lip and palate before age 10 years. Cleft Palate Craniofac J 31:295–308, 1994.
21. Tindland RS, Rygh P, Boe OE: Orthopedic protraction of the upper jaw in cleft lip and palate patients during the deciduous and mixed dentition periods in comparison with normal growth and development. Cleft Palate Craniofacial J 30:182–194, 1993.
22. Tindland RS, Rygh P, Boe OE: Intercanine widening and sagittal effect of maxillary transverse expansion in patients with cleft lip and palate during the deciduous and mixed dentitions. Cleft Palate Craniofac J 30:195–207, 1993.
23. Zilberman Y: Observations on the dentition and face in clefts of the alveolar process. Cleft Palate J 10:230–238, 1973.

15. CEPHALOMETRICS

Prasanna-Kumar Shivapuja, D.D.S., M.S., and John L. Spolyar, D.D.S., M.S.

1. What is cephalometrics?

Cephalometrics is the science of measurement of the skull, which began in the early 18th century. After the introduction of X radiation, measurements were made on standardized radiographs. The technique of radiographic cephalometrics was introduced by Hofrath in Germany and Brodbent in 1934. The initial purpose was to do research in growth and development of skeletal structures and to establish a quantitative method for obtaining descriptive information about dentofacial patterns.

2. How is cephalometric analysis performed?

By acquiring a standardized lateral view of the skull. A tracing is made of the skull film, and measurements are taken between points and planes constructed from anatomic landmarks.

3. How is a standard cephalogram obtained?

There are two specific requirements for obtaining a true standardized lateral head film. The distance from the x-ray source to the object should be 60 inches. The distance from the object to the film should be 6 inches. The central beam is directed through the center of the ear rods to strike the x-ray film at right angles. To limit parallax distortion due to shifting, the head should be stabilized with a head holder called a cephalostat. When these constants are maintained, a standardized lateral cephalogram is obtained with 10% magnification of the head. The lateral cephalogram must be made with the mandible in centric position and lips relaxed.

4. Why is a cephalostat used?

The cephalostat provides a means to standardize image and magnification distortions of the cephalograph with standard positioning of the x-ray source.

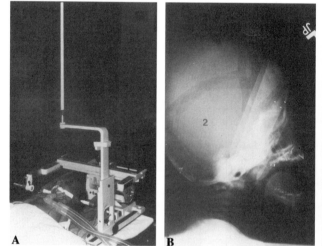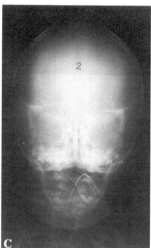

A

B

C

A, Portable cephalostat (Porta-Stat) used in the operating room to secure lateral (B) and frontal (C) cephalometric radiographs. (From Spolyar JL: Design evaluation and use of a portable cephalometric cephalostat: The Porta-Stat (an x-ray subsystem). Spec Care Dent March–April 1988, pp 64–70, with permission.)

5. How do you trace a cephalogram?

Tracing is done on a 0.003-in acetate paper with a 0.05-mm lead pencil. The side closest to the film is traced. In tracing the mandibular structures, the superior part of the body and distal part of the ramus should be traced (the side closest to the film). Whenever there is a double image, the contours of the image can be traced by bisecting the two images. The diagram at the right indicates the representative landmarks that need to be traced.

Landmarks for cephalogram tracing. (From Salzman JA: Practice of Orthodontics, Vols. 1 and 2. Philadelphia, Lippincott-Raven, 1966, with permission.)

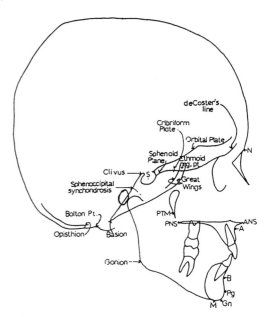

6. What are the requirements for a landmark?
1. The landmarks should be easily seen on a radiograph, uniform in outline, and easily reproducible.
2. Lines and planes should have significant relationship to the vectors of growth of specific areas.
3. Landmarks should permit valid quantitative measurements of lines and angles projected from them.
4. Measure points and measurements should have significant relationship to the information sought.
5. Measurements should be amenable to statistical analysis.

7. What are the most commonly used landmarks?

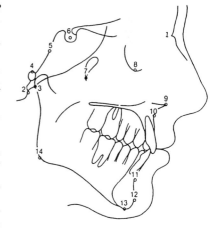

1. Nasion (N): the anteriormost point on the fronto-nasal suture.
2. Basion (Ba): the lowermost point on the anterior point of the foramen magnum.
3. Articulare (Ar): the point of intersection of the cranial base and the posterior border of the mandibular ramus.
4. Porion (Po): the midpoint of the upper contour of the external auditory canal.
5. Spinooccipital synchondrosis (SO): the junction between the occipital bone and basisphenoid.
6. Sella (S): the center of the sella turcica.
7. Pterygomaxillary fissure (PTM): the point on the base of the fissure where the anterior and posterior walls meet.
8. Orbitale (Or): the lowest point on the inferior margin of the bony orbit.
9. Anterior nasal spine (ANS): the tip of the anterior nasal spine (sometimes modified as the point on the upper or lower contour of the spine where it is 3 mm thick).
10. Point A (A): the innermost point on the contour of the premaxilla between the anterior nasal spine and incisor tooth.
11. Point B (B): the innermost point on the contour of the mandible between the incisor and the bony chin.
12. Pogonion (Pog): the anteriormost point on the contour of the bony chin.
13. Menton (Me): the most inferior point on the mandibular symphysis.
14. Gonion (Go): point on the angle of the mandible obtained by bisecting the angle formed by intersection of a tangent drawn to the lower and posterior borders of the ramus.
15. Gnathion (Gn): a constructed point located between the pogonion and menton.
    (From Proffit WR, Thomas PM, Camilla-Tulloch JF: Contemporary Orthodontics. St. Louis, Mosby, 1986, with permission.)

8. What is a cephalometric plane?

A plane by definition connects three or more points. A line by definition connects two or more points. These two terms are often used synonymously. The commonly used planes are as follows:

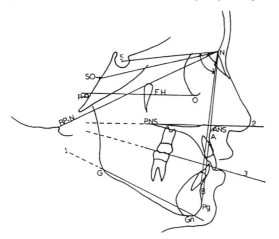

Cranial base planes
1. Basion-nasion (Ba-N)
2. Sella-nasion (S-N)
3. Frankfort horizontal plane (Po-Or)

Maxillary planes
1. Palatal plane: constructed by joining the anterior nasal spine to the posterior nasal spine
2. Occlusal plane: plane extending between the mesial cusp of the maxillary molar through the point that bisects the overbite
3. Nasion-point A plane
4. Long axis of maxillary incisor

Mandibular planes
1. Mandibular plane: line drawn tangent to the lower border of the mandible and passing through the menton
2. Nasion-point B
3. Nasion-pogonion facial axis plane
4. Long axis of mandibular incisor

(From Salzman JA: Practice of Orthodontics, Vols. 1 and 2. Philadelphia, Lippincott-Raven, 1966, with permission.)

9. What are the components of cephalometric analysis?

Skeletal analysis, profile analysis, and dental analysis.

10. What is the purpose of the skeletal analysis?

The main purpose is to classify facial types and to establish the relative anteroposterior relation of the basal arches. Angle SNA indicates the anteroposterior positioning of the maxilla in reference to the cranial base. The normal angle for a Caucasian is 82°. An angle that exceeds 82° indicates maxillary protrusion, and an angle less than 82° indicates maxillary retrusion. Angle SNB indicates anteroposterior relation of the mandible in reference to the cranial base. The mean is 80°. The basal arch analysis indicates the relation between the maxilla and mandible (ANB angle). The normal value is 2°.

An important factor in skeletal analysis is analysis of the vertical relation of the maxilla and mandible to the cranial base. The first of these measurements is the ratio of total facial height (measured from nasion to menton). If this value is considered as 100%, the upper part of the face (nasion to anterior nasal spine) should be 45%, and the lower part (anterior nasal spine to menton) should be 55%, although men tend to be slightly longer in the lower one-third of the face. The second measurement is to relate the anterior maxilla to the cranial base by evaluating tooth exposure on the cephalogram (with lips relaxed) and frontal facial picture. Both should show tooth exposure of approximately 2 mm. The third measurement is to relate the posterior maxilla to the cranial base by measuring the distance from the palatal plane to S-N. The fourth measurement is of the mandibular plane angle, which, when measured to the Frankfort plane, should be 25°.

11. What does the dental analysis indicate?

It indicates anteroposterior positioning of the teeth in relation to their basal bones. The long axis of the maxillary incisor should be angled at 104° to the cranial base. The long axis of the mandibular incisor should be angled at 90° to the mandibular plane.

12. What does the profile analysis assess?

Profile analysis permits appraisal of the soft tissue that covers the skeletal facial profile. Remember that the soft-tissue profile is related to facial skeletal dimensions, tonicity of the soft tissue, and habitual posture of the face in the head in space. An easy way to evaluate the profile is to relate the face to Ricketts' aesthetic plane (the line extending from the soft tissue nose tip to the soft tissue chin). The upper lip should lie 2 mm behind the plane; the lower lip should lie on the plane.

The nasolabial angle is formed at the base of the nose by a line drawn parallel to the base of the nose and a tangent drawn to the upper lip. It is also an important factor in establishing the anteroposterior position of the maxilla. The nasolabial angle should be 102° in both men and women with a standard deviation of 8°. An acute nasolabial angle may be a reflection of maxillary dentoalveolar protrusion. To rule out the influence of the nose on this angle, the upper lip should be evaluated in relation to the vertical orientation of the face. The tangent drawn to the upper lip should be 8° in men and 14° in women with the nasion perpendicular. An obtuse nasolabial angle or a decreased cant of the upper lip is an indication of a retrusive maxilla.

Normal Values for Commonly Used Measurements

MEASUREMENT	MEAN VALUE (CAUCASIAN)	MEAN VALUE (AFRICAN-AMERICAN)
SNA	82	85
SNB	80	81
ANB	2	4
U1-NA	22	23
	4 mm	7 mm
L1-NB	25	34
	4 mm	10 mm
U1-L1	131	111
L1-MP	90	—
FMA	25	25
Facial axis	0–2	—

13. What is holdaway ratio?

Holdaway ratio, which is used to evaluate lip retrusion or prominence, is an orthodontic method that relates the prominence of the mandibular incisor to the NB line and the pogonion to the NB line. For an ideal holdaway ratio, the lower incisor and the pogonion should be the same distance from the NB line. The ratio is depicted as 1:1. Per cephalometric standards, the lower incisor should be 4 mm in front of the line NB and therefore the chin should also be 4 mm in front of the NB line. It is important that the surgeon not advance the chin beyond the confines of the mandibular incisor teeth.

14. What are the applications of cephalometrics?

(1) Diagnosis, (2) growth prediction, (3) visual treatment objective, and (4) surgical treatment objective (STO).

15. How is the STO carried out?

The STO is carried out on a lateral cephalogram taken in centric position with the lips relaxed. A frontal facial picture with the lips relaxed and a picture with a wide smile on are also helpful in deciding the vertical positioning of the maxilla.

16. How do you evaluate the effect of treatment?

It can be evaluated by the process called superimposition. There are three basic types:

1. **Overall superimposition** is usually done by superimposing the anterior cranial base on de Caster's plane. After the age of 7 years, the sphenoethmoidal synchondrosis is fused, after which the anterior cranial base is a stable structure that can be used for superimposition. This form of superimposition indicates the overall change in the maxilla and mandible in reference to the cranial base.

2. **Maxillary superimposition** is done by superimposing the anterior nasal spine on the palatal plane (ANS-PNS). It reveals the dental changes in the maxilla.

3. **Mandibular superimposition** is done by superimposing on the lingual aspect of the symphysis parallel to the lower border of the mandible or mandibular plane. It indicates the changes in the mandibular dentition due to treatment.

Cephalometrics is a valuable tool in the diagnosis and treatment planning of orthodontic and surgical cases, but it must be used only as an adjunct to clinical diagnosis. After all, we treat patients and faces, not x-rays.

BIBLIOGRAPHY

1. Grayson B, Cutting C, Bookstein FL, et al: The three-dimensional cephalogram: Theory, technique and clinical applications. Am J Orthod 94:327, 1988.

2. Profitt WR, Thomas PM, Camilla-Tulloch JF: Contemporary Orthodontics. St. Louis, Mosby, 1986.
3. Riolo ML, et al: An Atlas of Craniofacial Growth: Cephalometric Standards from the University School Growth Study. Ann Arbor, MI, Center for Human Growth and Development, University of Michigan, 1979.
4. Salzman JA: Practice of Orthodontics, Vols. 1 and 2. Philadelphia, Lippincott-Raven, 1966.
5. Spolyar JL: Design, evaluation, and use of a portable cephalometric cephalostat: The Porta-Stat (an x-ray subsystem). Spec Care Dent March–April 1988, pp 64–70.
6. Wolfe AA, Berkowitz S: Plastic Surgery of the Facial Skeleton. Boston, Little, Brown, 1989.
7. Wolfe AA, Spiro SA, Wider TM: Surgery of the jaws. In Aston SJ, Beasley RW, Thorne CHM (eds): Grabb and Smith's Plastic Surgery, 5th ed. Philadelphia, Lippincott-Raven, 1997.
8. Zide B, Grayson B, McCarthy JG: Cephalometric analysis. Part I. Plast Reconstr Surg 68:816, 1981.
9. Zide B, Grayson B, McCarthy JG: Cephalometric analysis for upper and lower midface sugery. Part II. Plast Reconstr Surg 68:961, 1981.
10. Zide B, Grayson B, McCarthy JG: Cephalometric analysis for mandibular surgery. Part III. Plast Reconstr Surg 69:155, 1982.

16. CRANIOSYNOSTOSIS

Jeffrey Weinzweig, M.D., Jhonny Salomon, M.D., and Patrick K. Sullivan, M.D.

1. What is craniosynostosis? Who first described it?

Craniosynostosis designates premature fusion of one or more sutures in either the cranial vault or cranial base. Hippocrates provided the first description of this anomaly in 100 B.C. He noted the variable appearance of the calvarial deformities and correlated it with the pattern of cranial suture involvement.

2. What structure is currently believed to be primary site of abnormality responsible for craniosynostosis?

The cranial suture. Three theories of the pathogenesis of craniosynostosis are:
1. The suture is the site of abnormality, and the cranial base is the secondary deformity.
2. The cranial base is the primary site of abnormality, resulting in secondary cranial deformities.
3. The defect is in the mesenchymal blastema of both the cranial base and cranial sutures.

The first theory is the most widely accepted. Cultured sagittal suture synostotic cells demonstrate higher alkaline phosphastase levels, thought to be related to osteoblastic cell activity. In addition, the doubling time is longer for synostotic cells than for both normal suture and bone, revealing a potential for growth deficiency.

3. What structure is critical to suture patency?

The dura. Its importance is not related to the tension transferred from the underlying growing brain to the dura but more to a substance that diffuses across a semipermeable membrane and keeps the suture patent. Osteoprogenitor cells within the dura may synthesize locally acting osteogenic-inhibiting factors that regulate suture patency. Proficiency of these factors or a suppressor substance may result in synostosis.

4. How are cranial bones formed?

1. **Intramembranous ossification** begins at the end of the second month of gestation. A center of osteogenesis develops directly in vascularized mesenchyme. Expansion of the ossification center proceeds radially via appositional growth. Initially cancellous bone forms, but as trabeculae thicken and the bone becomes less porous, it becomes compact bone. Eventually each intramembranous cranial bone has enlarged to the point at which it articulates with an adjacent bone via a syndesmosis or suture. Growth then proceeds at the sutures. Until about 8 years of age, the intramembranous cranial bones are single plates of compact bone. After this time, they become two plates of compact bone, separated by marrow and cancellous bone, or diploë.

2. **Endochondral ossification** is the method by which the majority of the bones of the cranial base form. This method of ossification is more complex and proceeds by the replacement of preexisting cartilaginous models. Endochondral ossification is also the mode of ossification for the axial

and appendicular skeleton. Cranial base articulations differ from those of the vault in that they are synchondroses—bones connected by cartilage instead of syndesmoses.

5. What are the two regions of the skull?
1. The **viscerocranium** or **splanchnocranium** is the facial skeleton.
2. The **neurocranium** houses the brain. The neurocranium consists of the vault, which forms its roof and walls, and the cranial base, which forms its floor.

6. What is the primary stimulus for growth at the cranial suture?
Growth at the suture area is a secondary, compensatory, and mechanically obligatory event following the primary growth of the enclosed brain and ocular globes. The bones of the calvaria are displaced outward by the enlarging brain. Each bone of the domed skull roof responds to the expansion of the brain by depositing new bone at the contact edges of the sutures.

7. At what age are brain volume and cranial capacity approximately 50% that of the adult?
At 6 months of age. Brain volume in the normal child almost triples within the first year of life. By 2 years, the cranial capacity is 4 times that at birth. For this rapid brain growth to proceed normally, the open cranial vault and base sutures must spread during phases of rapid growth. Craniosynostosis thus presents an obstacle to normal cranial vault growth.

8. In which direction does cranial growth occur with relation to a synostotic suture? What is Virchow's law?
In 1851, Virchow noted a cessation of growth in a direction perpendicular to that of the affected suture. As a result, growth proceeds (with or without overcompensation) in a direction parallel to the affected suture. This is Virchow's law.

9. What is the incidence of craniosynostosis?
It is approximately 343 in 1,000,000 live births. Most cases of nonsyndromic, single-suture synostosis are sporadic, whereas syndromic cases are usually inherited in an autosomal dominant or recessive pattern with variable penetrance, depending on the syndrome.

10. What is syndromic synostosis? How common is it?
It often consists of a constellation of congenital abnormalities, including craniosynostosis, commonly coronal, as in Cruzon's and Apert's syndromes. Syndromic synostosis accounts for only 6% of all cases of craniosynostosis (approximately 2 in 100,000 live births).

11. What is the incidence of increased intracranial pressure (ICP) with single- and multiple-suture involvement?
Using an epidural sensor device to monitor 121 patients with craniosynostosis, Marchac and Renier documented intracranial hypertension (ICP >15 mmHg) in 42% of patients with involvement of multiple sutures and 13% of patients with only single-suture involvement. A progressive reduction of ICP over time was noted in patients who underwent cranial vault remodeling.

12. What is the pathognomonic ophthalmologic sign of increased ICP?
Papilledema.

13. What does "thumb-printing" or a "copper-beaten" finding indicate?
Both terms describe the classic radiographic evidence of increased intracranial pressure on skull films. Imagine the craterlike surface of a golf ball. Transfer that image to the inner surface of the cranium and voilà—thumb-printing!

14. What is the most common isolated single-suture synostosis?
Sagittal synostosis, or scaphocephaly, which is characterized by a narrow, elongated cranial vault and reduced bitemporal dimension (the basic "toaster head").

15. Which type of craniosynostosis is most often associated with hypotelorism?
Metopic synostosis. In addition to the more common finding of a palpable, midline forehead ridge, this type of craniosynostosis is also associated with a decreased distance between the bony orbits (hypotelorism).

16. What are the different types of nonsyndromic isolated craniosynostoses?

Head shape abnormality	Affected sutures
Frontal plagiocephaly	Unilateral coronal
Occipital plagiocephaly	Unilateral lambdoid
Frontal brachycephaly	Bilateral coronal
Occipital brachycephaly	Bilateral lambdoid
Scaphocephaly	Sagittal
Trigonocephaly	Metopic

17. To which multiple-suture synostoses do the terms "tower skull," "pointed head," and "cloverleaf skull" refer?

Acrocephaly and turricephaly ("tower skull") designate a type of untreated brachycephaly with an excess of skull height and vertical elongation of the forehead. There may be multiple-suture involvement in addition to bicoronal synostosis.

Oxycephaly ("pointed head") is characterized by a retroverted forehead, tilted posteroinferiorly on a plane with the nasal dorsum. The forehead is usually reduced in the horizontal dimension with elevation in the region of the anterior fontanel. There may be multiple-suture involvement in addition to bicoronal synostosis.

The Kleeblattschädel anomaly is characterized by a trilobed "cloverleaf skull" with bitemporal and vertex bulging. The spectrum of suture synostosis is broad; newborns with the deformity may show no evidence of sutural synostosis.

18. What characteristics differentiate Crouzon's syndrome from Apert's syndrome?

Crouzon's and Apert's syndromes are both characterized by craniosynostosis and a froglike facies secondary to exorbitism, hypertelorism, and midface hypoplasia, all of which tend to be more severe in Apert's syndrome. A number of additional features distinguish the two anomalies:

Characteristic	Crouzon's Syndrome	Apert's Syndrome
Affected sutures	Coronal (most common), sagittal, or lambdoid	Coronal (usually)
Calvarial deformity	Brachycephaly, scaphocephaly, trigonocephaly, or oxycephaly	Brachycephaly and turricephaly
Hand anomalies	None	Symmetric syndactyly of the hands and feet
Ocular findings	Nystagmus, strabismus, optic nerve atrophy	Ptosis, antimongoloid slant of palpebral fissure
Development	Normal	Retardation common

19. Name three syndromes associated with hand anomalies.

1. **Apert's syndrome** (acrocephalosyndactyly) is transmitted by an autosomal dominant mode of inheritance. It is characterized by craniosynostosis, exorbitism, midface hypoplasia, and symmetric syndactyly of the hands and feet. Although Tessier noted multiple additional characteristics of patients with Apert's syndrome, syndactyly essentially differentiates it from Crouzon's syndrome.

2. **Pfeiffer's syndrome** is autosomal dominant in transmission. It is characterized by craniosynostosis, exorbitism, midface hypoplasia, and enlarged thumbs and great toes.

3. **Carpenter's syndrome** is autosomal recessive in transmission. It is characterized by craniosynostosis, polysyndactyly of the feet, and short hands with variable soft tissue syndactyly.

20. What is secondary craniosynostosis?

Any pathologic condition interfering with the normal development of the cranial bones may cause a compensatory synostosis of the cranial sutures and secondary craniosynostosis. An abnormally high incidence of craniosynostosis has been seen in patients with hematologic disorders, malformations (microcephaly or encephalocele), metabolic disorders (hyperthyroidism, vitamin D-resistant rickets, mucopolysaccharidosis) and other disorders, such as Hurler's syndrome and achondroplasia, that affect generalized skeletal development.

21. How does one differentiate between deformational and synostotic plagiocephaly? Which is more common?

Synostotic frontal plagiocephaly, secondary to unilateral coronal synostosis, is an uncommon disorder that occurs in 1 of 10,000 live births. It is 0.2% as common as deformational plagiocephaly. Isolated unilateral lambdoidal synostosis is an extremely rare cause of synostotic occipital plagiocephaly, accounting for only 0.8–1.3% of all syndromic and nonsyndromic cases.

Deformational frontal plagiocephaly results in an ipsilateral narrow palpebral fissure and lower eyebrow, inferiorly positioned ipsilateral ear, and no angulation of the nasal root. The chin may deviate toward the involved side. From the vertex ("bird's eye") view, the deformational plagiocephalic cranium appears as though it has been compressed from forehead to opposite occiput ("parallelogrammic head"). The cheek and ear are retruded on the same side as the flattened forehead with bossing of the ipsilateral posterior parietal bone and minor contrecoup flattening of the opposite occipitoparietal region.

Synostotic frontal plagiocephaly results in an ipsilateral widened palpebral fissure, superiorly and posteriorly displaced supraorbital rim and eyebrow, higher ipsilateral ear, and deviation of the nasal root toward the flattened side. The chin often points to the contralateral side. The frontal fontanelle is displaced toward the normal side. Viewed from above, the ear and cheek are anterior on the same side as the flattened forehead. Sutural ridging is inconsistently found in coronal synostosis; its absence does not exclude the diagnosis.

Anatomic Feature	Synostotic	Deformational
Ipsilateral supraorbital rim	High	Low
Ipsilateral eyebrow position	High	Low
Ipsilateral ear	Anterior and high	Posterior and low
Ipsilateral cheek	Forward	Backward
Nasal root	Ipsilateral deviation	Midline
Chin deviation	Contralateral	Ipsilateral
Ipsilateral palpebral fissure	Wide and low	Narrow and high
Anterior fontanelle deviation	Contralateral	None

22. Once the diagnosis of deformational plagiocephaly is made in a 2-month-old infant with a pronounced posterior head shape abnormality, what is the appropriate management?

The parents should be advised to have the infant sleep prone, and a molding helmet should be fabricated and worn 23 hours each day until normal cranial shape has been restored. Close follow-up every 2–3 months is warranted.

23. What is the harlequin deformity?

The harlequin deformity is the characteristic radiographic finding in patients with synostotic frontal plagiocephaly. It describes the abnormal shape of the orbit due to ipsilateral superior displacement of the lesser wing of the sphenoid.

24. What is torticollis?

Torticollis, which literally means "twisted neck," results from shortening of the sternocleidomastoid muscle. It is characterized by a tilting of the head toward the affected side; the chin points up and toward the opposite side. The shoulder is higher on the affected side, and the external ear is sometimes more prominent on the affected side. When the condition persists beyond a few weeks in infancy, an asymmetry develops in which the face and skull on the affected side appear smaller.

25. Is there an association between deformational plagiocephaly and torticollis?

Definitely. True torticollis—in which the head tilts toward the abnormal side—is present in 64% of children with deformational plagiocephaly. Ocular torticollis, in which the child attempts to correct for strabismus-induced diplopia by tilting the head toward the normal side, is present in approximately 50% of children with synostotic plagiocephaly.

26. What are the two goals of surgery for patients with craniosynostosis?

1. Decompression of the intracranial space (to reduce ICP, to prevent visual problems, and to permit normal mental development)

2. Achievement of satisfactory craniofacial form

27. What is the ideal timing for correction of craniosynostosis?

The thickness of the calvarial bone between 3 and 12 months of age is usually adequate to permit reconstructive osteotomies yet soft enough to facilitate remodeling. Delayed reconstructions after 1½ years of age are usually technically more difficult.

28. Which reconstructive procedures are performed before 1 year of age? Which are performed after 1 year of age?

Frontal bone advancement with or without strip craniectomies, cranial vault remodeling, monobloc or craniofacial advancement, and shunt surgery for hydrocephalus are performed early, usually before 6 months of age. Late procedures include Le Fort III advancement with or without concomitant frontal bone advancement (usually at 3–4 years of age), monobloc advancement, and jaw surgery (usually in early adolescence), which may include a Le Fort I osteotomy and genioplasty.

29. Is a strip craniectomy sufficient treatment for sagittal synostosis?

No. Sagittal or parasagittal strip craniectomy has been used with limited success only in cases of mild isolated sagittal synostosis. Most cases of sagittal synostosis, however, require cranial vault remodeling, with removal of the affected suture and performance of frontal, parietal, and occipital "barrel-stave" osteotomies.

30. How is metopic synostosis corrected?

Except in the mildest cases of trigonocephaly, for which observation or burring of the midline forehead ridge may be sufficient, a more substantial procedure involving simultaneous supraorbital and frontal remodeling is usually necessary. Despite the fact that metopic synostosis is an uncommon form of craniosynostosis, with an incidence of less than 10% of all cases of craniosynostosis, it is the most obvious deformity associated with premature fusion of a single suture because of its prominent frontal keel, narrow forehead, and close-set eyes. Removal of the deformed supraorbital bar and flattening of the nasion angle, using either a midline fracture or osteotomy, results in a lateral canthal advancement with replacement on the midfacial segment.

With more severe cases of metopic synostosis, in which hypotelorism is present, a nasofrontal osteotomy is performed before attachment of the supraorbital bar to the inferior midfacial segment. The frontonasal junction is separated with an osteotome, and a bone graft is inserted. This procedure immediately increases the intercanthal distance and partially corrects the hypotelorism.

31. What is the appropriate treatment for an infant with bilateral coronal synostosis and a moderate degree of exorbitism? Is this approach useful in an infant with syndromic synostosis (Crouzon's or Apert's syndrome)?

The Tessier type of frontal bone advancement is advocated for the infant with bilateral coronal synostosis and a moderate degree of exorbitism as well as the infant with syndromic synostosis. The osteotomies are made across the nasofrontal junction, across the roof of the orbit, and along the lateral orbital wall. Osteotomy extensions are made into the temporal fossa to provide a tongue-in-groove arrangement that obviates the need for bone grafts for fixation purposes. The frontal bone flap is then wired to the advanced supraorbital bar. Advancement of the frontal bone as far as 20 mm can be performed in this manner, with significant expansion of the orbital volume. Closure of the scalp after significant frontal bone advancement can be facilitated by scoring of the galea (see figure, top of next page).

32. How does treatment for unilateral coronal synostosis (plagiocephaly) differ from treatment for bilateral coronal synostosis (brachycephaly)?

Early approaches to the treatment of plagiocephaly included simple coronal strip craniectomies and extended strip craniectomies with removal of the involved suture, but these procedures do not reliably produce upper craniofacial symmetry. Although plagiocephaly is a unilateral malformation, the preferred treatment usually consists of bilateral forehead remodeling along with removal and

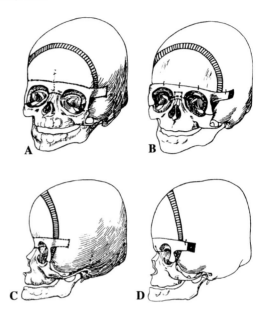

Frontal bone advancement or frontoorbital re-
modeling. *A, C,* Lines of osteotomy/osteotectomy.
B, D, Calvarium following frontal bone advance-
ment and remodeling. (From McCarthy JG,
Epstein FJ, Wood-Smith D: Craniosynostosis. In
McCarthy JG (ed): Plastic Surgery. Philadelphia,
W.B. Saunders, 1990, p 3028, with permission.)

modification of a single supraorbital bandeau (bar) extending across both orbits, as advocated by
Marchac. This technique permits simultaneous restoration of forehead symmetry as well as correction of the anteroposterior position and superoinferior discrepancy of the supraorbital rims.
Plagiocephaly reconstruction is very similar to brachycephaly correction in that a bilateral approach
is usually optimal; however, orbital symmetry presents a greater problem in the case of plagiocephaly, requiring anteroinferior and slight medial translocation of the affected supraorbital rim.

33. What is a Le Fort III advancement osteotomy?

A Le Fort III advancement osteotomy is performed for the purpose of advancing the midface in
the patient with severe midfacial retrusion. The bony framework of the nose is divided at the nasofrontal junction; the osteotomy line is continued backward across the medial wall of the orbit on
each side, then downward to the floor of the orbit. A narrow osteotome is used to section the delicate
lamina papyracea of the ethmoid, which forms the portion of the medial wall posterior to the
lacrimal bone. A transverse cut is made across the orbital floor and joins the inferior orbital fissure to
the lower end of the medial wall osteotomy.

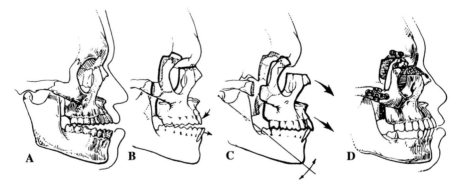

Le Fort III advancement. *A,* Maxillary hypoplasia with midface retrusion. *B,* Lines of osteotomy. *C,* Anteroinferior
translation of the osteotomized segment. *D,* Autogenous bone grafts are placed in the nasofrontal junction, lateral
orbital wall, zygomatic arch, and pterygomaxillary fissure defects. Fixation is achieved with miniplates. (From
McCarthy JG, Epstein FJ, Wood-Smith D: Craniosynostosis. In McCarthy JG (ed): Plastic Surgery. Philadelphia,
W.B. Saunders, 1990, p 3038, with permission.)

The lateral orbital wall is sectioned transversely in the region of the frontozygomatic suture line or above it. The orbital contents are retracted medially, and the lateral orbital wall is divided at its junction with the cranium. The zygomatic arch is similarly sectioned. The lateral orbital wall osteotomy is continued inferiorly and posteriorly through the pterygomaxillary fissure. Once the osteotomies have been performed, the midfacial skeleton can be loosened with the Rowe disimpacting forceps. Bone grafts are placed in the defects of the nasofrontal junction, lateral orbital wall, and pterygomaxillary fissure. After intermaxillary fixation, interosseous wires or miniplate fixation is used to stabilize the nasofrontal, zygomaticofrontal, and zygomaticotemporal osteotomies.

34. When should a Le Fort III advancement osteotomy be performed with a simultaneous Le Fort I osteotomy or frontal bone advancement ?

The combination of Le Fort III/Le Fort I osteotomies permits differential advancement of the midface and maxillary segments. This approach is indicated for patients in whom the deformity is restricted to the upper aspects of the midface (exorbitism and maxillary hypoplasia) and in whom dental occlusal relationships are within acceptable range. The Le Fort I osteotomy is performed superior to the apices of the teeth and below the infraorbital nerve. It is continued medially and superiorly to terminate at the upper margin of the piriform aperture. The osteotomy continues laterally to join the pterygomaxillary fissure.

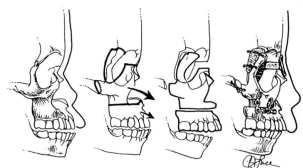

The Le Fort III/Le Fort I osteotomy combination permits differential advancement of the midface and maxillary segments. Autogenous bone grafts are placed in the defects and fixation is accomplished with wires or miniplates. (From McCarthy JG, Epstein FJ, Wood-Smith D: Craniosynostosis. In McCarthy JG (ed): Plastic Surgery. Philadelphia, W.B. Saunders, 1990, p 3044, with permission.)

The combination of Le Fort III/frontal bone advancement osteotomies permits simultaneous advancement of the midface as well as the frontal bone. This approach is preferred in patients with brachycephaly and midfacial retrusion. Once the frontal bone flap is removed, the supraorbital osteotomy is extended horizontally to the region of the temporal fossa and continued in stepwise fashion inferiorly toward the base of the skull. The step design of this osteotomy permits bony contact after advancement of the frontal bandeau. The osteotomy is continued in a horizontal fashion through the lateral orbital wall and roof posteriorly. The procedure is completed by performing the Le Fort III osteotomy. This combination permits simultaneous advancement of the frontal bone, part of the roof, and the lateral wall of the orbits.

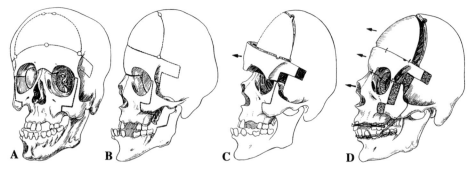

The Le Fort III/frontal bone advancement osteotomy combination permits simultaneous advancement of the midface as well as the frontal bone. *A, B,* Lines of osteotomy. *C,* Frontal bone segment advanced. *D,* Final position after advancement of all bony segments with bone grafts in place and skeletal fixation completed. (From McCarthy JG, Epstein FJ, Wood-Smith D: Craniosynostosis. In McCarthy JG (ed): Plastic Surgery. Philadelphia, W.B. Saunders, 1990, p 3042, with permission.)

CONTROVERSY

35. What is a monobloc advancement? Is it safe?

Twenty years ago Ortiz-Monasterio popularized a method of increasing orbital volume for the correction of severe exorbitism by the simultaneous advancement of the forehead, orbits, and midface. The lines of osteotomy for the monobloc advancement are similar to those for the combined Le Fort III / frontal bone advancement except that the nasofrontal junction and frontozygomatic suture are not osteotomized. The Le Fort III segment also incorporates the roof of the orbits. In doing so, the extent of orbital volume expansion is limited.

Although this procedure is advocated by a number of highly experienced surgeons, including Tessier, the increased risk of infection and associated CSF leak remains a significant concern. This risk is due to the communication created between the nasal and intracranial cavities by the osteotomy design. Despite the use of pericranial flaps to separate these cavities, the increased risk associated with their potential persistent communication remains.

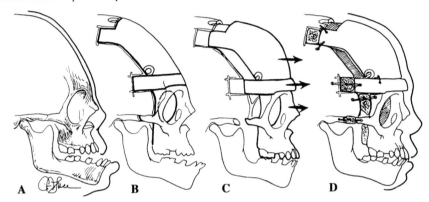

A   B   C   D

Monobloc advancement. *A*, Hypoplastic midface and orbitofrontal region. *B*, Lines of osteotomy. The Le Fort III segment incorporates the roof of the orbits; the frontal bone is remodeled in two segments. *C*, The three bony segments can be advanced to varying degrees. *D*, Final position after advancement of all bony segments with bone grafts in place and skeletal fixation completed. (From McCarthy JG, Epstein FJ, Wood-Smith D: Craniosynostosis. In McCarthy JG (ed): Plastic Surgery. Philadelphia, W.B. Saunders, 1990, p 3045, with permission.)

BIBLIOGRAPHY

1. Bruneteau RJ, Mulliken JB: Frontal plagiocephaly: Synostotic, compensational or deformational. Plast Reconstr Surg 89:21, 1992.
2. Eppley BL, Sandove AM: Surgical correction of metopic suture synostosis. Clin Plast Surg 21:555–562, 1994.
3. Marchac D: Radical forehead remodeling for craniostenosis. Plast Reconstr Surg 61:823, 1978.
4. Marchac D, Renier D: Craniofacial Surgery for Craniosynostosis. Boston, Little, Brown, 1982.
5. McCarthy JG, Epstein FJ, Wood-Smith D: Craniosynostosis. In McCarthy JG (ed): Plastic Surgery. Philadelphia, W.B. Saunders, 1990, pp 3013–3053.
6. Ocampo RV, Persing JA: Sagittal synostosis. Clin Plast Surg 21:563–574, 1994.
7. Ortiz-Monasterio F, Fuente Dell Campo A, Carrillo A: Advancement of the orbits and the midface in one piece, combined with frontal repositioning, for the correction of Crouzon's deformities. Plast Reconstr Surg 61:507, 1978.
8. Ortiz-Monasterio F, Fuente Dell Campo A: Refinements on the bloc orbitofacial advancement. In Caronni EP (ed): Craniofacial Surgery. Boston, Little, Brown, 1985, pp 263–274.
9. Posnick JC: The craniofacial dysostosis syndromes: Current reconstructive strategies. Clin Plast Surg 21:585, 1994.
10. Tessier P: Relationship of craniostenoses to craniofacial dysostoses, and to faciostenoses: A study with therapeutic implications. Plast Reconstr Surg 48:224, 1971.
11. Tessier P: The definitive plastic surgical treatment of the severe facial deformities of craniofacial dysostoses, Crouzon's and Apert's disease. Plast Reconstr Surg 48:419, 1971.

17. ORBITAL HYPERTELORISM

Joseph L. Daw, Jr., M.D., D.D.S., and Louis Morales, Jr., M.D.

1. What anatomic dimension is used to identify orbital hypertelorism?
Interorbital distance (IOD) defines the presence or absence of orbital hypertelorism. It is the distance between the medial walls of the orbits at dacryon (junction of the frontal and lacrimal bones and the maxilla). IOD should not be confused with intercanthal distance (ICD), which is the distance between the medial canthal tendon insertions. An increase in the ICD but not the IOD is referred to as pseudoorbital hypertelorism. Interpupillary distance (IPD) should not be used to determine orbital hypertelorism because many patients may have exotropia or esotropia.

2. What is considered a normal interorbital distance?
The average IOD in men is 28 mm and in women 25 mm. By age 2 years, 70% of the IOD has been attained. At birth, the IOD is approximately 16 mm.

3. How is orbital hypertelorism classified?
There are two methods of classification. The most commonly used system, described by Tessier, is based on the IOD. Patients are divided into type I (30–34 mm), type II (35–39 mm), and type III (≥ 40 mm). Munro classified orbital hypertelorism according to the shape of the medial orbital wall. Type A medial orbital walls are parallel. In type B, the anterior interorbital tissues show a ballooning out. In type C, the central portion of the medial wall balloons out. The posterior ethmoidal cells are widest in type D. Types C and D are more difficult to correct.

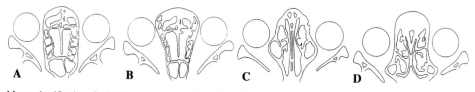

Munro classification of orbital hypertelorism. *A,* Parallel medial orbital walls. *B,* Ballooning out of anterior inferorbital tissue. *C,* Ballooning out of central portion of medial wall. *D,* Widening of posterior ethmoid cells. (From Munro IR, Das SK: Improving results in orbital hypertelorism correction. Ann Plast Surg 2:499–507, 1979, with permission.)

4. Where is the level of the cribriform plate located?
Normally, the cribriform plate is positioned 10 mm below the level of the orbital roof. However, with orbital hypertelorism, the cribriform plate may be located up to 20 mm below the orbital roof.

5. What anatomic structures are altered in patients with orbital hypertelorism?
The primary deformity is widening of the ethmoid sinuses transversely. The axis of orbits is more divergent (normal = approximately 25°). The lateral orbital wall, therefore, may be foreshortened. The crista galli may be enlarged or duplicated. The glabella is usually flatter, and the frontal sinuses, once developed, are often enlarged. The nose is usually short and wide. Specifically, the nasal bones may be short, whereas the upper lateral and lower lateral cartilages may be larger and bifid. In addition, the nasal septum may be duplicated or unusually wide. Structures that usually are not affected or affected to a lesser degree include the cribriform plate, greater and lesser sphenoid wings, and optic canals.

6. What causes orbital hypertelorism?
Orbital hypertelorism is not a syndrome but rather a physical finding that is associated with a great variety of congenital malformations. It may be seen in midline or paramedian craniofacial clefts, craniofacial syndromes (e.g., Apert and Crouzon syndromes), and sincipital encephaloceles. Other causes include amniotic banding syndromes, dermoid cysts, glial tumors, and teratomas. Patients with cleft lip and palate also may have a mild degree of hypertelorism.

7. What are the types of sincipital encephaloceles?

A cephalocele is a herniation of intracranial contents through a cranial defect. When it contains the meninges and cerebrospinal fluid, it is referred to as a meningocele; when both meninges and cerebral tissue are present, it is called a meningoencephalocele. Cephaloceles are classified by anatomic location: sincipital (also referred to as frontal or frontoethmoidal), parietal, basal, and occipital. Sincipital encephaloceles are found between the bregma and the anterior margin of the ethmoid bone. They are further classified by the direction of herniation: nasofrontal, nasoethmoidal, and nasoorbital. Sincipital encephaloceles show great geographic and ethnic variation. Among European and North American Caucasians, sincipital encephaloceles are rare, whereas in Southeast Asia and Nigeria they are much more common.

8. What surgical methods are used to correct orbital hypertelorism?

The most commonly used method is a combined intracranial/extracranial approach to provide access to create the osteotomies. Osteotomies are made in all walls of the orbit circumferentially, resulting in total mobilization of the orbits. Resection of structures within the interorbital space, including enlarged ethmoidal air cells and nasal septum, is required. Resection of bone anteriorly and in the anterior cranial fossa may be accomplished as either median or paramedian segments.

In patients with orbital hypertelorism and significant transverse constriction of the maxillary dental arch, facial bipartition may be performed. This procedure simultaneously narrows the interorbital distance, expands the transverse width of the maxillary dental arch, and levels the maxillary occlusal plane.

A subcranial approach may be used in less severe forms of orbital hypertelorism, in which the cribriform plate has not prolapsed inferiorly. A U-shaped osteotomy of the orbits is developed, involving only the medial wall, floor, and lateral wall.

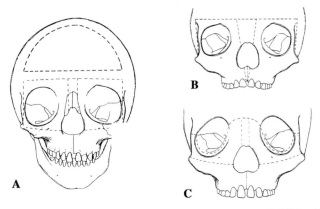

Surgical correction of orbital hypertelorism. *A,* Intracranial/extracranial approach. *B,* Facial bipartition. *C,* Subcranial approach. (From Dufresne CR: Complex Craniofacial Problems. New York, Churchill Livingstone, 1992, with permission.)

9. What effect does the intraorbital/intranasal exenteration have on future growth of the midface?

According to the experience of McCarthy and others, normal development of the midface can be expected when correction of orbital hypertelorism is performed in a growing child. However, Mulliken and others demonstrated an adverse effect on anterior facial growth in young children who underwent correction of hypertelorism.

10. What steps must be taken to preserve olfactory function during surgical correction of orbital hypertelorism?

Preservation of olfactory function depends on avoidance of injury to the cribriform plate and maintenance of the continuity of the mucosa of the upper nasal septum and superior turbinates. The olfactory nerve end organs are located within this mucosa.

11. What ancillary procedures are usually required in conjunction with primary correction of orbital hypertelorism?

Nasal reconstruction is one of the most important steps in the correction of orbital hypertelorism. The nasal dorsum is reconstructed using a bone graft (calvarial, rib or ilium), which is secured as a cantilever. If excessive nasal skin is present, it must be excised if the dorsal augmentation does not completely fill the soft tissue envelope. The excision of the dorsal nasal skin is designed as an hourglass shape. Besides tightening the skin transversely, a lengthening of the nasal soft tissue is created with closure. This technique is of additional benefit because the nose in patients with orbital hypertelorism is usually short. If the nasal cartilages are bifid, they should be corrected as well.

Medial canthoplasties are usually necessary at completion of the procedure, because often the insertion of the medial canthal tendons has been detached during the intraorbital dissection. Medial canthoplasty may be accomplished with transnasal wiring from one medial canthal tendon to the other.

12. What deformities may persist or become apparent after correction of orbital hypertelorism?

The most common residual deformity is canthal drift, which results in the production of epicanthal folds. This deformity may give a false impression of relapse of the medial translocation of the orbits. Bony relapse is likely to result from inadequate exenteration of intraorbital or intranasal structures or inadequate translocation of the orbits. Other postoperative sequelae include enophthalmos, ptosis, strabismus, nasolacrimal dysfunction, shortened palpebral fissures, and temporal depression.

BIBLIOGRAPHY

1. David DJ, Simpson DA: Frontoethmoidal meningoencephaloceles. Clin Plast Surg 14:83–89, 1987.
2. Dufresne CR: Orbital hypertelorism. In Dufresne CR, Carson BS, Zinreich SJ (eds): Complex Craniofacial Problems. New York, Churchill Livingstone, 1992, pp 227–249.
3. McCarthy JG, Thorne CHM, Wood-Smith D: Principles of craniofacial surgery: Orbital hypertelorism. In McCarthy JG (ed): Plastic Surgery. Philadelphia, W.B. Saunders, 1990, pp 2982–3002.
4. Mulliken JB, Kaban LB, Evans CA, et al: Facial skeletal changes following hypertelorbitism correction. Plast Reconstr Surg 77:7–16, 1986.
5. Munro IR, Das SK: Improving results in orbital hypertelorism correction. Ann Plast Surg 2:499–508, 1979.
6. Ortiz-Monasterio F, Molina F: Orbital hypertelorism. Clin Plast Surg 21:599–612, 1994.
7. Simpson DA, David DJ, White J: Cephaloceles: Treatment, outcome, and antenatal diagnosis. Neurosurg 15: 14–20, 1984.
8. Tessier P, Tulasne JF: Stability in correction of hypertelorbitism and Treacher Collins syndromes. Clin Plast Surg 16: 195-199, 1989.
9. van der Meulen JCH, Vaandrager JM: Surgery related to the correction of hypertelorism. Plast Reconstr Surg 71:6–17, 1983.

18. CRANIOFACIAL SYNDROMES

Salvatore Lettieri, M.D., and Craig A. Vander Kolk, M.D.

1. What exactly is a syndrome?

A syndrome is a set of symptoms that occur together. A particular syndrome may have three, four, or ten manifestations, but a key sequence of symptoms leads to the diagnosis of a particular syndrome. For example, an infant who presents with midface hypoplasia and exorbitism may be diagnosed with Crouzon syndrome. However, with one other symptom (i.e, syndactyly of the middle digits of the hands and feet), the patient is diagnosed with Apert's syndrome.

2. What is the difference between a malformation and a deformation?

A **malformation** is a defective or abnormal formation that is acquired during development. A **deformation** occurs secondary to extrinsic forces. Posterior flattening of one side of the head may be secondary to intrinsic or extrinsic forces. If an infant is laid in the same position, the young, membranous bones of the cranium are subject to flattening; the morphologic diagnosis is plagiocephaly. Unilateral lambdoidal synostosis may cause a similar finding. Removal or redirection of the external forces often corrects deformational abnormalities.

3. What is the difference between penetrance and expression?

Both terms relate to an inheritable trait as manifested in relation to the principal gene or affected genes. Penetrance relates to frequency, whereas expression relates to extent. Patients may have a particular gene or trait that does not manifest fully (i.e., variable expression). Genetic relationships may involve a continuum of effect with variable expression. A theoretic example is the difference between Crouzon syndrome and Apert syndrome. The two have similar craniofacial features; however, patients with Apert syndrome have syndactyly. In addition, the midface hypoplasia seems to be a bit more severe, and the incidence of mental deficiency is greater. Although two distinctive genetic abnormalities may distinguish Apert syndrome and Crouzon syndrome, sometimes a patient diagnosed with Crouzon syndrome may indeed be a patient with Apert syndrome and minimal expression of the involved traits. Such problems are common with syndromic classifications as opposed to genetic diagnoses.

4. What is the difference between trigonocephaly and metopic synostosis?

This classic question invites a differentiation between morphologic and pathologic diagnosis. **Trigonocephaly** refers to the morphologic shape, whereas **metopic synostosis** is a pathologic entity. Synostosis is the premature closure of a suture; metopic synostosis refers to premature closure of the metopic suture. Because the classification of craniosynostosis is based on the involved suture, the anatomy of the sutures must be known. The involved sutures are usually the coronal (unilateral or bilateral), metopic, sagittal, and lambdoid. The morphologic shapes of the head include trigonocephaly, scaphocephaly, plagiocephaly, brachycephaly, or turricephaly. Trigonocephaly, which refers to a triangle-shaped forehead, is related to premature fusion of the metopic suture. Scaphocephaly results from premature fusion of the sagittal suture and gives an enlongated look to the head because of limited growth perpendicular to the suture. Plagiocephaly, which refers to flattening of the affected site, results from unilateral coronal suture synostosis or unilateral lambdoid suture synostosis. Torticollis, or repeated positioning of the head to one side, also may cause posterior flattening of the head. The deformational abnormality of the skull entails a morphologic diagnosis of plagiocephaly without a clinical or pathologic diagnosis of synostosis. This distinction is an important element for differentiation of cause, treatment, and outcome.

5. How does growth occur in relationship to an affected suture?

Traditionally, because synostosis is premature fusion, it is thought that no growth occurs at the suture site. Growth, therefore, occurs parallel to the affected suture with restriction perpendicular to the suture. For example, a patient with sagittal synostosis has an enlongated head with anterior and posterior growth but restricted growth in the lateral direction. A patient with unilateral coronal synostosis on the right side has restricted growth in the right anterior to left posterior direction with compensatory enlongation in the left anterior to right posterior direction. This pattern, first described by Virchow in the 19th century, continues to be the classic depiction of growth. Theories of cause and treatment continue to change.

6. Which syndrome also affects the limbs?

Several syndromes affect the limbs. Among the more common is Apert syndrome, which involves syndactyly of the feet and hands. Crouzon Syndrome, which has similar facial features to Apert syndrome, does not involve hand anomalies. Other syndromes in which the limbs are affected include Saethre-Chotzen syndrome (brachydactyly), Pfeiffer syndrome (large, broad great toes and thumbs), Carpenter syndrome (short hands and polysyndactyly of the feet), and Nagar syndrome (missing digits, syndactyly, and either hypoplastic or aplastic thumbs and/or radius).

7. Are all syndromic children destined to develop a learning deficiency?

This is one of the most difficult questions to address. The only way to be certain is to leave all affected children unoperated and then assess subsequent development. Patients with Crouzon syndrome have had a normal adult life without surgical intervention. Many patients who present in infancy undergo surgery. Mental retardation occurs in less than 5% of patients with Crouzon syndrome. Apert syndrome, which is similar to Crouzon in its craniofacial abnormalities, has a much higher rate of mental retardation (over 50% of patients). Timing of surgical intervention to improve the incidence or severity of mental retardation is controversial. To date, no evidence proves or disproves any theory.

8. Who was Pierre Robin? Why is he important?

Pierre Robin (1867–1950) was a French dental surgeon who contributed greatly to orthodontics. He called attention to problems associated with glossoptosis and airway obstruction—a congenital anomaly consisting of micrognathia, cleft palate, and prominent tongue. In later publications, he claimed that many ailments were related to the enlarged tongue, including acrocyanosis, flat feet, cryptorchidism, constipation, gastroenteritis, and even appendicitis. Affected children have classic facies with partial or complete airway obstruction and difficulty with feeding. They may or may not have a cleft palate; they usually have retrognathia or micrognathia. The prone position is best because it facilitates breathing. Many patients require a tracheostomy and often a feeding tube to facilitate breathing and nutrition. Various treatments have been tried, including partial glossectomy and mandible advancement. Other mechanical treatments include suturing the tongue forward or placing a K-wire through the mandible to try to keep it in a forward position. More recently distraction osteogenesis has been used with some early success. We should remember that the Pierre Robin anomaly is a *sequence* and not a *syndrome*.

9. Which syndrome has a built-in metabolic disorder?

Albright syndrome (pseudohypoparathyroidism). Craniofacial manifestations include a rounded and low nasal bridge and short neck. Patients often have cataracts and short metacarpals and metatarsals. They also may have hypocalcemia and hyperphosphatasemia. This autosomal dominant disorder seems to be associated with a deficiency in a regulatory protein required to couple membrane receptors to adenyl cyclase. This action stimulates cyclic adenyl cyclase monophosphate.

10. With which syndrome do you see lower lip pits?

Van der Woude's syndrome (lip pit-cleft lip syndrome). Lower lip pits are present in 80% of patients, who may be missing the central and lateral incisors, canines, or bicuspids. In addition, patients often have a cleft lip but may or may not have a cleft palate or cleft uvula. Van der Woude's syndrome is an autosomal dominant disorder, whereas just about everything else is autosomal recessive. So it is easier to remember the few dominant disorders and guess recessive for the rest.

11. What differentiates Klippel-Trénaunay-Weber from Parkes-Weber syndrome?

Both are neoplastic syndromes, but arteriovenous fistulas are present in Parkes-Weber syndrome. The syndrome without arteriovenous fistulas was first reported by Klippel and Trénaunay. The craniofacial manifestations include asymmetric facial hypertrophy, hemangiomatta, and microcephaly; intracranial calcifications also may be present. Other interesting findings include enlarged abdominal viscera and disturbed major blood vessels. Patients are usually mentally impaired and may be prone to seizures. The limb hypertrophy can be quite devastating, and the soft tissue surrounding the limb may be several times the diameter of an unaffected limb. Once the diagnosis is made, the abdominal viscera, brain, eyes, urinary, and gastrointestinal tracts should be checked for evidence of hemangiomatta with early intervention as indicated.

12. What is telorbitism?

Tessier coined this term, which describes a condition in which the orbits are far apart. Most craniofacial syndromes involve varying degrees of telorbitism. Some, such as Apert and Crouzon syndromes, have shallow orbits and the appearance of telorbitism. Most procedures that are performed do not readily address the extent of the telorbitism unless it is associated with a specific reduction of the midfacial bones and movement of the orbits. Correction can be extremely difficult and challenging. The important corollary to this question is which patients may have hypotelorism. Hypotelorism is associated with Binder's syndrome, Down syndrome, trigonocephaly, holoprosencephaly, and arhinocephaly. All other syndromes have either normal or widened orbits.

13. Are all craniosynostoses associated with a syndrome?

Not really. Syndromes are present only in 10–20% of patients with primary craniosynostosis. Cohen reported a total of 64 diagnoses that involved craniosynostosis. At this point certainly more have been discovered or reported. Usually single-suture synostoses are isolated, sporadic anomalies, whereas multiple-suture synostoses are syndromic.

14. Does surgery always correct the craniofacial deformity?

We certainly try. The amount of correction is directly related to the degree of the problem. Craniosynostosis may be simple and straightforward, such as sagittal synostosis, which leads to scaphacephaly. Patients may have a single sagittal strip craniectomy with removal of a 3–4-cm width of bone overlying the sagittal suture and removal of portions of the coronal sutures. Patients often do very well if surgery is done early (3–4 months of age). A patient with midfacial hypoplasia and mild exorbitism may be treated with a frontal advancement as the first stage and a possible LeFort III advancement at a later age. Corrective surgery of a craniofacial deformity is largely static, whereas the growing intracranial and extracranial tissues are dynamic. The intent is to predict the amount of needed growth and to overcome the potential deficiency in bony growth caused by either surgery or the underlying disorder.

15. What is the most common craniofacial cleft?

When talking about craniofacial clefts, one must distinguish between the typical cleft lip and palate and facial clefts. None of the various classification schemes is perfect, but the easiest to remember is the Tessier classification. Basically, the face is cut in half with a right and a left side, and each side is considered a clock with 14 hours instead of 12. The clock runs from 0 to 14, both of which occur in the midline. Zero is in the facial region, whereas 14 is in the midcranial region. For example, a number 0 cleft is directly through the midnose, and a number 14 cleft is through the nasal-frontal suture and midfrontal region. Extending laterally, cleft numbers 1, 2, and 3 pass through the pyriform aperture. The next three clefts (numbers 4, 5, and 6) involve the lower eyelid and can be easily remembered as the medial, middle, and lateral thirds of the lower eyelid. Cleft number 7 is outside the lower eyelid and involves the lateral oral commissure. Bilateral number 7 clefts have the appearance of a broad smile. The Tessier number 7 facial cleft is the most common craniofacial cleft and occurs in approximately 1 of 3,000 births. Usually the clefts occur in pairs that total 14 (e.g., a number 0 cleft usually occurs with number 14, and a number 1 cleft usually occurs with a number 13). The Tessier number 7 cleft is usually not associated with any other cleft, although it may be bilateral. The Tessier number 8 cleft begins at the lateral commissure of the palpebral fissure and extends into the temporal region. It often is present with a Tessier cleft number 6 (the two total 14). Expression is variable, and only one craniofacial cleft may be present. Of note, Treacher Collins syndrome also may be described as cleft numbers 6, 7, and 8. Numbers 8–14 can be remembered as the cranial extensions of their midfacial counterparts (see chapter 19).

BIBLIOGRAPHY

1. Cohen MM Jr (ed): Craniosynostosis: Diagnosis, Evaluation, and Management. New York, Raven Press, 1986.
2. Firkin BG, Whitworth JA: Dictionary of Medical Eponyms. New York, Parthenon, 1987.
3. Goodrich JJ, Hall CD: Craniofacial Anomalies: Growth and Development from a Surgical Perspective. New York, Thieme Medical Publishers, 1995.
4. Jones KL: Recognizable Patterns of Human Malformation, 5th ed. Philadelphia, W.B. Saunders, 1997.
5. McCarthy J (ed): Plastic Surgery. Philadelphia, W.B. Saunders, 1990.
6. Renier D, Marchac D: Discussion of longitudinal assessment of mental development in infants with nonsyndromic craniosynostosis with and without cranial release and reconstruction. Plast Reconstr Surg 92:831, 1993.

19. CRANIOFACIAL CLEFTS

Jeffrey Weinzweig, M.D.

1. When does the embryologic development of the face take place?

Embryogenesis of the face takes place between the fourth and eighth weeks of gestation, during which the crown-rump length (CRL) of the fetus enlarges from 3.5 mm to 28 mm.

2. When does the most rapid phase of facial development occur?

The most dramatic changes in facial development occur in the extraordinarily brief period between 17 and 27 mm CRL (seventh and eighth weeks of gestation). In embryos with a 17-mm CRL the facial processes have fused, marking the end of the transformation phase.

3. Morphogenesis of the craniofacial skeleton begins with the formation of which bone?

The sphenoid body and its extensions. Morphogenesis continues with the formation of the middle and anterior cranial fossae and a reduction of the interorbital distance. Evolution proceeds with the union of the two nasal halves and the development of the nasomaxillary complex, which expands forward, downward, and laterally. In embryos with a 27-mm CRL the skeleton is completed with a lengthening of the mandibular ramus, which adapts itself to the formation of the nasomaxillary complex.

4. Why do craniofacial clefts occur?

Embryogenesis of the craniofacial region is extremely complex. Significant demands are placed on the coordination of cell separation, migration, and interaction during a brief 4-week period. The proper amount of tissue must be present at an exact moment in the correct three-dimensional relationship for normal craniofacial development to occur. Any mishap in this intricate program can lead to disastrous consequences. Evidence from animal and clinical studies supports a multifactorial etiology. Factors such as infection with influenza A_2 virus, infestation with toxoplasmosis protozoan, maternal metabolic disorders, and exposure to teratogenic compounds, including anticonvulsants, antimetabolic and alkylating agents, steroids, and tranquilizers, are believed to play a role in the etiopathogenesis of craniofacial clefts.

5. What are the two leading theories of facial cleft formation?

1. **Failure of fusion.** This classic theory, proposed by Dursy (1869) and His (1892), contends that the central region of the face is the site of union of the free ends of the facial processes. The face takes form as the various processes fuse. After epithelial contact is established by these processes, penetration by the mesoderm completes the fusion. Disruption of this sequence results in cleft formation.

2. **Mesodermal migration and penetration.** This theory, proposed by Pohlman (1910) and Veau and Politzer (1936), contends that separate processes are not found in the central portion of the face; therefore, free ends of the facial processes do not exist. Instead, the central portion of the face is composed of a continuous sheet of a bilamellar membrane of ectoderm known as the primary plate, which is demarcated by epithelial seams that delineate the principal "processes." Into this double layer of ectoderm, referred to as the epithelial wall, mesenchyme migrates and penetrates to smooth out the seams. The lower face and neck are formed by a series of branchial arches that consist of a thin sheet of mesoderm lying between the ectoderm and endoderm. The craniofacial mesoderm is augmented by neuroectoderm brought in by the migrating neural crest cells, from which the craniofacial skeleton is believed to be principally derived. If penetration by the neuroectoderm does not occur, the unsupported epithelial wall breaks down to form a facial cleft. The severity of the cleft is inversely proportional to the degree of penetration by the neuroectoderm. If penetration fails altogether, a complete cleft is formed as the epithelial wall dehisces. Partial penetration results in the development of an incomplete cleft.

6. What is the incidence of craniofacial clefts?

The exact incidence of craniofacial clefts is unknown because cases are rare and series tend to be small. However, extraction of cases of rare facial clefts from larger series of common clefts of the lip and palate provides a comparative incidence of 9.5 to 34 rare facial clefts per 1000 common clefts. As common clefts of the lip and palate occur with an overall incidence of approximately 1.5 per 1000 live births, the extrapolated incidence of rare facial clefts would be approximately 1.4–5.1 per 100,000 live births.

7. Who was the first to recognize the three-dimensional complexity of craniofacial clefts ?

Paul Tessier, who stated that "a fissure of the soft tissues corresponds as a general rule with a cleft of the bony structures."

8. How is the Tessier classification of craniofacial clefts structured?

The orbit, nose, and mouth are key landmarks through which craniofacial clefts follow constant axes. The clefts are numbered from 0 to 14, with the lower numbers (0–7) representing the facial clefts and the higher numbers (8–14) representing their cranial extensions. Multiple and bilateral clefts may occur in the same patient. When a malformation crosses both hemispheres, a craniofacial cleft is produced that generally follows a set "time zone." Examples of these combinations include the no. 0-14, 1-13, 2-12, 3-11, and 4-10 clefts.

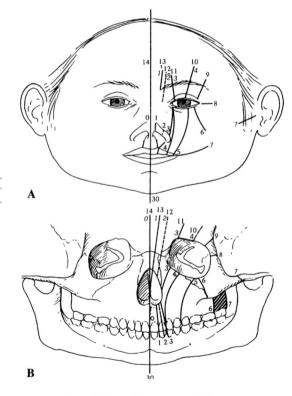

Tessier classification of craniofacial clefts. A, Path of various clefts on the face. B, Location of the clefts on the facial skeleton. (Courtesy of Dr. P. Tessier.)

9. What is internasal dysplasia? To which Tessier cleft does this term apply?

Internasal dysplasia is a developmental arrest in the groove separating the two nasal halves before union has occurred. This anomaly is known as the Tessier no. 0 cleft. Depending on the time of developmental arrest, a wide spectrum of anomalies is seen. In less severe cases, the anomaly is characterized by bifidity of the columella, nasal tip, dorsum, and distal part of the cartilaginous septum. Occasionally, a median cleft of the lip, a median notch in the Cupid's bow, or a duplication of the labial frenulum is found. In more severe cases, the nasal halves are widely separated and orbital hypertelorism is present (see figure A, next page). The premaxilla may be bifid, and the maxilla may demonstrate a keel-shaped deformity in which the incisors are rotated upward in each half of the alveolar processes. A medial cleft of the palate may extend upward to the cribriform plate. The wider the cleft, the greater the interorbital distance, the shorter the nose, and the more arched the maxillary vault. At the other extreme, the nose may be totally absent or represented by a proboscis. The median bony defect in such cases extends into the ethmoids to produce orbital hypotelorism or cyclopia (see figure B below). The associated brain malformation usually limits the life span to infancy.

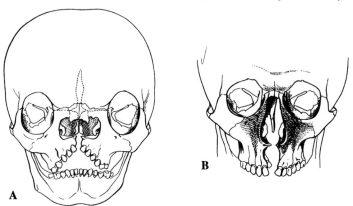

No. 0 cleft. *A*, The osseous cleft passes between the central incisors, resulting in broadening of the nasal frame-work and orbital hypertelorism. *B*, Portions of the premaxilla and nasal septum are absent and the supporting structures of the nose are hypoplastic with resultant orbital hypotelorism. (Courtesy of Dr. P. Tessier.)

10. Which craniofacial clefts begin at Cupid's bow?
   Tessier no. 1, 2, and 3 clefts begin at Cupid's bow. In addition, no. 4 and 5 clefts, and, rarely, no. 6 clefts may involve Cupid's bow. Therefore, all common cleft lips must be evaluated closely for additional structural anomalies.

11. What is nasoschizis? To which clefts does this term refer?
   Nasoschizis is related to clefts of the lateral aspect of the nose. These clefts are commonly referred to as Tessier no. 1 or 2 clefts. The no. 1 cleft begins at Cupid's bow. The common cleft of the lip is an example of this malformation. The spectrum of these anomalies ranges from a small notch in the alar rim to a wide defect involving one or both nasal halves. Clefting of the alveolar arch between the central and lateral incisors is commonly seen. The piriform aperture is violated lateral to

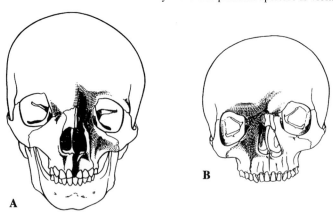

No. 1 cleft (*A*). The osseous location of this malformation is paramedian with compensatory lateral displacement of the orbit in the noncleft side. No. 2 cleft (*B*). Clefting of the alveolar arch occurs in the region of the lateral incisor. The piriform aperture is involved at its base as the cleft passes through the broadened frontal process of the maxilla to produce orbital hypertelorism. (Courtesy of Dr. P. Tessier.)

the anterior nasal spine. The no. 2 cleft also begins in Cupid's bow and crosses the alveolus in the region of the lateral incisor. The piriform aperture is divided at its base, and the nasal septum is intact but deviated by the maxillary distortion.

12. What is an oronasoocular cleft?

Also referred to as an oblique facial cleft, the oronasoocular cleft is a no. 3 cleft that begins at Cupid's bow, undermines the base of the nasal ala, and continues cephalad into the lower eyelid (see figure A below). This is the first of the Tessier clefts to involve the orbit directly. The osseous component of the cleft passes through the alveolus between the lateral incisor and canine (see figure B below). The cleft continues cephalad through the piriform aperture and the frontal process of the maxilla and terminates in the lacrimal groove. The underlying nasolacrimal system is disrupted, producing an obstructed nasolacrimal duct and a sac that is prone to recurrent infections. The lower canaliculus is malformed and irreparable. This cleft is seen more commonly than the no. 1 and 2 clefts.

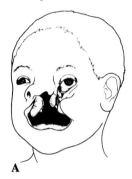
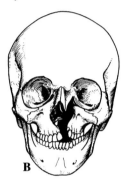

No. 3 cleft. *A,* This cleft begins at Cupid's bow, undermines the base of the nasal ala, and continues cephalad into the lower eyelid, where a coloboma is found medial to the punctum. *B,* The no. 3 cleft is the first cleft to involve the orbit directly. The osseous component of the cleft passes through the alveolus between the lateral incisor and canine, then continues cephalad through the piriform aperture and the frontal process of the maxilla to terminate in the lacrimal groove. (From Stratoudakin AC: An outline of craniofacial anomalies and principles of their correction. In Georgiade GS, Georgiade NG, Riefkol R, Barwick WJ (eds): Textbook of Plastic, Maxillofacial and Reconstructive Surgery, 2nd ed. Baltimore, Williams & Wilkins,1992, p 343, with permission.)

13. What are colobomas? Where are they found in relation to the punctum in the no. 3 cleft?

Colobomas, which are notches (clefts) of the eyelid of varying degrees, involve the lower eyelid and are found medial to the punctum.

14. Why is the no. 4 cleft also called meloschisis?

First described by von Kulmus in Latin in 1732, the no. 4 cleft represents a departure of the deformity from the median facial structures. The cleft moves onto the cheek and, therefore, is also referred to as meloschisis. This oroocular or oculofacial cleft begins lateral to the Cupid's bow and philtrum. It passes lateral to the nasal ala, which is largely uninvolved, and onto the cheek. The cleft terminates in the lower eyelid, medial to the punctum (see figure A, top of next page). The osseous component of the cleft starts between the lateral incisor and canine. The piriform aperture, nasolacrimal canal, and lacrimal sac are spared as the cleft courses medial to the infraorbital foramen to terminate in the medial aspect of the inferior orbital rim and floor (see figure B, top of next page).

15. Which of the oblique facial clefts may permit orbital content prolapse into the maxillary sinus?

Prolapse of orbital contents into the maxilla occurs most commonly with no. 4 clefts and to a lesser degree with no. 5 clefts. The no. 5 cleft is rare; it originates in the lip just medial to the oral commissure. This cleft courses cephalad across the lateral portion of the cheek (meloschisis) into the area of the medial and lateral thirds of the lower eyelid (see figure A, next page). The vertical distance between the mouth and lower eyelid is decreased, and the upper lip and lower lid are drawn toward each other. The eye may be microophthalmic. The alveolar portion of the cleft is found posterior to

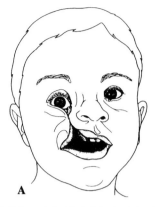 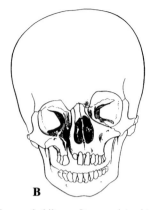

A   B

No. 4 cleft. *A,* This oculofacial cleft begins lateral to Cupid's bow and philtrum. It passes lateral to the nasal ala and onto the cheek, then terminates in the lower eyelid, medial to the punctum. (From Stratoudakin AC: An outline of craniofacial anomalies and principles of their correction. In Georgiade GS, Georgiade NG, Riefkol R, Barwick WJ (eds): Textbook of Plastic, Maxillofacial and Reconstructive Surgery, 2nd ed. Baltimore, Williams & Wilkins, 1992, p 343, with permission.) *B,* The cleft passes between the infraorbital foramen and the piriform aperture. The orbit, maxillary sinus, and oral cavity are united by the cleft. (Courtesy of Dr. P. Tessier.)

the canine in the premolar region. The cleft then passes lateral to the infraorbital foramen and enters the orbit through the middle third of the orbital rim and floor (see figure B below). The orbital contents may prolapse through the gap into the maxillary sinus.

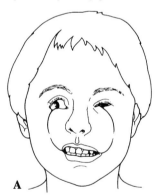 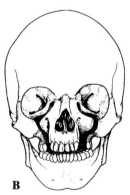

A   B

No. 5 cleft (bilateral). *A,* This cleft begins just medial to the oral commisure and courses cephalad across the lateral cheek into the area of the medial and lateral thirds of the lower eyelid. *B,* The bony cleft begins posterior to the canine, then passes lateral to the infraorbital foramen and enters the orbit through the middle third of the orbital rim and floor. (From Stratoudakin AC: An outline of craniofacial anomalies and principles of their correction. In Georgiade GS, Georgiade NG, Riefkol R, Barwick WJ (eds): Textbook of Plastic, Maxillofacial and Reconstructive Surgery, 2nd ed. Baltimore, Williams & Wilkins, 1992, p 343, with permission.)

16. Which cleft represents an incomplete form of the Treacher Collins anomaly?

The no. 6 cleft. A coloboma of the lateral third of the eyelid marks the cephalic end of the cleft as it descends lateral to the oral commissure toward the angle of the mandible. The palpebral fissures have an antimongoloid slant. The bony cleft passes through the zygomatico-maxillary suture and involves the lateral third of the infraorbital rim. The zygoma is present but hypoplastic.

17. Which is the least rare of the craniofacial clefts? With which more familiar anomaly is it associated?

The no. 7 cleft, the least rare of the craniofacial clefts, is more commonly referred to as hemifacial microsomia. Additional descriptive terms include first and second branchial arch syndrome, otomandibular dysostosis, craniofacial microsomia, intrauterine facial necrosis, oromandibuloauricular syndrome, and lateral facial clefts. The incidence of this malformation is between 1 in 3000 and 1 in 5642 births.

Clinical expression is highly variable. A skin tag may represent the "forme fruste" or microform of the malformation. A severe no. 7 cleft begins as a macrostomia at the oral commissure and continues as a furrow across the cheek toward a microtic ear. The fifth and seventh cranial nerves and the muscles that they supply also may be involved. The osseous component of the no. 7 cleft is centered in the region of the zygomaticotemporal suture with hypoplasia of the zygoma and temporal bone. The zygomatic arch is disrupted and represented by proximal and distal stumps; varying degrees of mandibular deficiency, including complete absence of the ramus, are seen on the affected side.

18. When was hemifacial microsomia first described?
The earliest description of the malformation is the cuneiform inscriptions on the teratologic tables written by the Chaldeans of Mesopotamia about 2000 B.C.

19. What syndrome is closely related to hemifacial microsomia but has the additional features of epibulbar ocular dermoids and vertebral anomalies?
Goldenhar syndrome. However, as less than 5% of hemifacial microsomia cases actually demonstrate the findings that distinguish them as Goldenhar syndrome, many do not recognize this as a distinct entity.

20. Which craniofacial cleft is often occupied by a dermatocele?
The no. 8 cleft. The bony component of this cleft is centered at the frontozygomatic suture. It begins at the lateral commissure of the palpebral fissure and extends into the temporal region.

21. The bilateral combination of nos. 6, 7, and 8 clefts represents the complete form of which syndrome? (Hint: the zygomas are absent.)
Treacher Collins syndrome. The three clefts involve the maxillozygomatic, temporozygomatic, and frontozygomatic sutures and are responsible for the absence of the zygoma in this malformation, the hallmark of the complete form of Treacher Collins syndrome. The no. 6 cleft is responsible for the coloboma of the lower eyelid. The no. 7 cleft is responsible for the absence of the zygomatic arch. The no. 8 cleft completes the malformation by contributing to the absence of the lateral orbital rim.

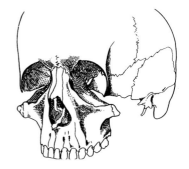

Nos. 6, 7, and 8 clefts (bilateral). These three clefts are responsible for the absence of the zygoma in this malformation, the hallmark of the complete form of Treacher Collins syndrome. (Courtesy of Dr. P. Tessier.)

22. Which is the rarest of the craniofacial clefts and the first to involve the superior hemisphere of the orbit?
The no. 9 cleft, which is found in the superolateral angle of the orbit and affects the underlying superior orbital rim and orbital roof. The eyelid is divided in its lateral third, as is the eyebrow, because the cleft extends into the temporal hairline.

23. Which cleft is the cranial extension of the no. 4 facial cleft and is often occupied by a frontoorbital encephalocele?
The no. 10 cleft, which traverses the middle third of the orbit, upper eyelid, and eyebrow. The osseous component of the cleft involves the midportion of the superior orbital rim, the adjacent orbital roof, and the frontal bones. A frontoorbital encephalocele frequently displaces the entire orbit in an inferior and lateral direction to produce orbital hypertelorism.

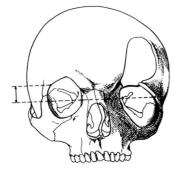

No. 10 cleft. The osseous cleft involves the midportion of the superior orbital rim, adjacent orbital roof, and frontal bones. A frontoorbital encephalocele frequently displaces the entire orbit infralaterally to produce orbital hypertelorism. (Courtesy of Dr. P. Tessier.)

24. Which cleft is usually found in combination with the no. 3 cleft? When is it associated with orbital hypertelorism?

The no. 11 cleft is the cranial extension of the no. 3 facial cleft and has not been reported as an isolated deformity. The cleft traverses the medial third of the upper eyelid and eyebrow as it courses into the frontal hairline. The osseous cleft may pass lateral to the ethmoid bone to create a cleft in the medial third of the superior orbital rim. Alternatively, the cleft may course through the ethmoidal labyrinth, in which case orbital hypertelorism is produced.

25. Why is orbital hypertelorism usually associated with the no. 12 cleft?

The no. 12 cleft, which is the cranial extension of the no. 2 facial cleft, disrupts the eyebrow just lateral to the medial border. The bony cleft passes through the frontal process of the maxilla or between this structure and the nasal bone. The ethmoidal labyrinth is increased in its transverse dimension to account for the associated hypertelorism.

26. Which cleft is associated with transverse widening of the cribriform plate?

The hallmark of the no. 13 cleft, which is the cranial extension of the no. 1 facial cleft, is widening of the olfactory groove with concomitant transverse widening of the cribriform plate. The cleft lies medial to the eyebrow, which is usually displaced inferiorly. Orbital hypertelorism is a constant finding with the cleft traversing the nasal bone, ethmoidal labyrinth, and olfactory groove.

27. "The face predicts the brain." Explain.

Because of the intimate association of the frontonasal prominence with the development of the forebrain, the severity of centrally located craniofacial malformations appears to parallel that of forebrain defects. Therefore, the extent of facial deformity provides a clue to the severity of the developmental arrest of the forebrain.

28. In addition to the no. 0 cleft, which other cleft is associated with both hypotelorism and hypertelorism?

The no. 14 cleft, which is the cranial extension of the no. 0 facial cleft, may result from structural agenesis or tissue overabundance. When the cleft is secondary to agenesis, orbital hypotelorism is usually seen. The holoprosencephalic malformations, in which embryologic division of the prosencephaly into two parts is disrupted, fall into this group of anomalies. When frontonasal dysplasia (medial cleft face syndrome) or a frontonasal encephalocele occurs, orbital hypertelorism is seen (see figure, top of next page). The basic fault in embryogenesis lies in the malformation of the nasal capsule. The developing forebrain thus remains in its lowlying position. As a result of morphokinetic arrest of the normal medial movement of the eyes, the orbits remain in their widespread fetal position. In such cases, the crista galli may be widened, duplicated, or absent, and the cribriform plate may be caudally displaced as much as 20 mm.

29. Which structures must be considered in the reconstruction of a craniofacial cleft?

Reestablishment of facial integrity in patients with median or paramedian clefts involves all disrupted structures—the skeleton, facial muscles, and skin. Reconstruction is based on the following principles:

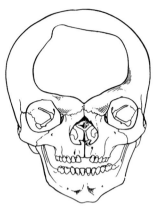

No. 14 cleft. When this cleft is associated with a frontonasal encephalocele, orbital hypertelorism is seen (From Tessier P: Anatomical classification of facial, cranio-facial and latero-facial clefts. J Maxillofac Surg 4:69, 1976, with permission.)

1. Reconstruction of the skeleton is accomplished by removal of abnormal elements, transposition of skeletal components, and use of bone grafts.

2. Reinsertion of the facial muscles is achieved by transposition and fixation of dystopic remnants. An intact muscular layer serves to establish and maintain form, to animate the face, and to stimulate growth.

3. Restoration of the skin is performed by transposition of local flaps. The cutaneous layer provides protection for the underlying structures and preserves facial contour by its attachment to the skeleton.

30. What is a no. 30 cleft?
Median clefts of the lower lip and mandible represent the caudal extension of the no. 0 cleft. The cleft of the lower lip may be limited to the soft tissue and present, in its most minor form, as a lip notch. More frequently, however, the cleft extends into the bony mandibular symphysis. As the severity of the malformation increases, the neck structures, hyoid bone, and even sternum are progressively involved. This group of deformities is classified as no. 30 clefts. (Take a closer look at the figure in question 8.)

BIBLIOGRAPHY

1. DeMyer W, Zeman W, Palmer CA: The face predicts the brain: Diagnostic significance of median facial anomalies for holoprosencephaly. Pediatrics 34:256, 1964.
2. Kawamoto HK Jr: The kaleidoscopic world of rare craniofacial clefts: Order out of chaos [Tessier classification]. Clin Plast Surg 3:529, 1976.
3. Kawamoto HK Jr: Rare craniofacial clefts. In McCarthy JG (ed): Plastic Surgery. Philadelphia, W. B. Saunders, 1990, pp 2922–2973.
4. Kawamoto HK Jr: Craniofacial anomalies. In Smith JW, Aston SJ (eds): Grabb and Smith's Plastic Surgery, 4th ed. Boston, Little, Brown, 1991, pp 143–170.
5. Marchac D, Renier D: Craniofacial Surgery for Craniosynostosis. Boston, Little, Brown, 1982.
6. McCarthy JG, Cutting CB, Hogan VM: Introduction to facial clefts. In McCarthy JG (ed): Plastic Surgery. Philadelphia, W. B. Saunders, 1990, pp 2437–2450.
7. Stratoudakis AC: An outline of craniofacial anomalies and principles of their correction. In Georgiade GS, Georgiade NG, Riefkohl R, Barwick WJ (eds): Textbook of Plastic, Maxillofacial and Reconstructive Surgery, 2nd ed. Baltimore, Williams & Wilkins, 1992, pp 333–362.
8. Tessier P: Fente orbito-faciales verticales et obliques (colobomas) completes et frustes. Ann Chir Plast 14:301, 1969.
9. Tessier P: Colobomas: Vertical and oblique complete facial clefts. Panminerva Med 11:95, 1969.
10. Tessier P: Anatomical classification of facial, cranio-facial, and latero-facial clefts. J Maxillofac Surg 4:69, 1976.
11. Van der Meulen JC, Mazzola R, Vermey-Keers C, et al: A morphogenetic classification of craniofacial malformations. Plast Reconstr Surg 71:560, 1983.
12. Van der Meulen JC: Oblique facial clefts: Pathology, etiology and reconstruction. Plast Reconstr Surg 71:6, 1983.
13. Van der Meulen JC: The classification and management of facial clefts. In Cohen M (ed): Mastery of Plastic and Reconstructive Surgery. Boston, Little, Brown, 1994, pp 486–498.

20. CRANIOFACIAL MICROSOMIA

M. Rusen Kapucu, M.D., and H.Wolfgang Losken, M.D., F.R.C.S.(Edin)

1. What is craniofacial microsomia?

Craniofacial microsomia is a spectrum of morphogenetic anomalies involving the skeletal, soft tissue, and neuromuscular structures derived from the first and second branchial arches.

2. Do craniofacial microsomia and hemifacial microsomia represent the same entity?

Yes—as do the first and second branchial arch syndrome, oculoauriculovertebral spectrum, otomandibular dysostosis, and lateral facial dysplasia. The variety of names reflects an incomplete understanding of the pathogenesis as well as the wide spectrum of clinical deformities included in this category.

3. How frequently does craniofacial microsomia occur?

Craniofacial microsomia is the second most common congenital facial anomaly after cleft lip and palate with an incidence of 1 in 5,600 live births. The anomaly is unilateral in 80% of cases. The male-to-female ratio is 3:2, and the anomaly has a 3:2 preference for the right side.

4. Is there a genetic predisposition to craniofacial microsomia?

Most cases are sporadic, although both autosomal dominant and autosomal recessive inheritance have been reported. It has been estimated that the recurrence rate in first-degree relatives is 3%.

5. What does a typical patient with craniofacial microsomia look like?

Hypoplasia of the mandibular ramus, which is usually accompanied by hypoplasia of the zygoma, maxilla, and temporal bone, causes flattening of the lateral part of the face. In unilateral cases, the chin is deviated to the affected side and the occlusal plane is tilted upward on the affected side. Varying forms of microtia are found, and soft tissue hypoplasia contributes to the asymmetry of the face.

6. Which deformities are frequently present in craniofacial microsomia other than skeletal hypoplasia and microtia?

Macrostomia, facial paralysis, palate paralysis, and hypoplasia or paralysis of the masseter, temporalis, and pterygoid muscles.

7. What is Goldenhar syndrome?

Bilateral craniofacial microsomia with epibulbar dermoids and vertebral anomalies.

8. Where are the skin tags found in craniofacial microsomia?

In the preauricular area and between the first (maxillary) and second (mandibular) branchial arches.

9. Classify the mandibular malformation in craniofacial microsomia.

In type I, the mildest form, all components of the mandible are present but hypoplastic to varying degrees. The temporomandibular joint is present, but cartilage and joint space are reduced. In type IIA, the condylar process is cone-shaped and forms an articulation that allows hinge but not translatory movement. In type IIB, no condylar process articulates with the temporal bone, but a coronoid process of varying size is present. The entire mandibular ramus is absent in type III.

10. What are the goals of surgical treatment in craniofacial microsomia?

The goals are construction and reshaping of the craniofacial skeleton, augmentation of soft tissue, and treatment of associated conditions such as auricular malformations and facial paralysis.

11. What orthodontic treatment is used in patients with craniofacial microsomia?

An intraoral functional appliance is constructed to hold the affected mandible in a lowered, forward position that stimulates an increase in the size of both the abnormal condyle and the short coronoid process. It is used in young children during the presurgical phase and may be particularly beneficial in patients with type I deformities. It is also used in the postoperative period to prevent relapse of the mandibular deformity and to stimulate growth of the maxilla.

12. What surgical methods are available to construct the mandibular ramus and increase the size of the mandible?

The procedure depends on the extent of bony deficiency. In children with type I and type II malformations, in which a mandibular ramus is present, available bone may be increased in size and lengthened by distraction osteogenesis. In type III malformations, the mandibular ramus and condyle need to be constructed with costochondral and/or iliac bone grafts.

13. What is distraction osteogenesis?

Distraction osteogenesis is bone formation in the gap between the gradually distracted bone ends on each side of a corticotomy. Because new bone is generated in the treated location, use of this method obviates the need for harvesting bone grafts from other body parts, avoiding donor site morbidity.

14. How is distraction osteogenesis used for lengthening the mandible?

A corticotomy (or osteotomy) is performed in the mandible. Pins inserted into the bone on each side of the corticotomy are connected to a fixator device. The fixator is manipulated by turning a screw, which causes distraction of the callus between the bone segments at a rate of 1 mm per day. When the desired amount of lengthening is achieved, distraction is stopped. The fixator and pins are removed when radiologic evidence of satisfactory bone formation is seen, usually 6–9 weeks after the end of distraction.

15. What are the aims of distraction of the hypoplastic mandible?

(1) To lengthen the mandibular ramus; (2) to lengthen the mandibular body; (3) to reduce the gonial angle; and (4) to increase the intergonial distance.

16. How is mandibular distraction planned?

By measuring the ramus and body length on cephalometric radiographs or three-dimensional CT scans, and comparing this measurement with the unaffected side and the normal length for a child of the same age and sex, the necessary amount of lengthening can be determined.

17. How do you know when mandibular distraction is adequate?

When the distance between the lateral canthus and lateral commissure of the mouth is the same as the unaffected side and when the mandibular occlusal midline is overcorrected by 3–4 mm.

18. Describe the skeletal construction in children with type III mandibular malformation.

The absent mandibular ramus, condyle, glenoid fossa, and often deficient zygoma need to be constructed with bone grafts. Costochondral grafts are preferred for condylar reconstruction to provide an optimal joint surface and growth from the costochondral junction. Costal, iliac, and calvarial bone grafts are used to reconstruct the other structures.

19. What is the sequence of reconstructive surgery in children with craniofacial microsomia?

1. Excision of preauricular skin tags in the first year of life
2. Mandibular distraction at 2 years of age
3. Costochondral grafts at 4 years of age
4. Ear reconstruction at 6 years of age
5. Soft tissue augmentation after adolescence

20. Does the maxillary deformity require surgery?

In children with mild-to-moderate malformations, early construction of the mandibular ramus produces a posterior open bite and allows space for the maxilla to grow downward. Orthodontic appliances can facilitate this growth, and the oblique occlusal plane may gradually be corrected. In patients who present late for treatment or in whom the maxilla does not grow satisfactorily, a Le Fort I maxillary osteotomy is needed.

21. How is the soft tissue deficiency treated?

The method of choice depends on the amount of soft tissue deficiency. Mild deficiency usually can be corrected by dermal and/or fat grafts. In patients with more significant soft tissue hypoplasia, de-epithelialized fasciocutaneous free flaps, such as the scapular flap, are preferred.

BIBLIOGRAPHY

1. Horgan JE, Padwa BL, LaBrie RA, Mulliken JB: OMENS-Plus: Analysis of craniofacial and extracraniofacial anomalies in hemifacial microsomia. Cleft Palate Craniofac J 32:405–412, 1995.
2. Losken HW, Patterson GT, Lazarou SA, Whitney T: Planning mandibular distraction: Preliminary report. Cleft Palate Craniofac J 32:71–76, 1995.
3. McCarthy JG: The role of distraction osteogenesis in the reconstruction of the mandible in unilateral craniofacial microsomia. Clin Plast Surg 21:625–631, 1994.
4. Murray JE, Kaban LB, Mulliken JB: Analysis and treatment of hemifacial microsomia. Plast Reconstr Surg 74:186–199, 1984.
5. Siebert JW, Anson G, Longaker MT: Microsurgical correction of facial asymmetry in 60 consecutive cases. Plast Reconstr Surg 97:354–363, 1996.
6. Vargervik K, Hoffman W, Kaban LB: Comprehensive surgical and orthodontic management of hemifacial microsomia. In Turvey TA, Vig KWL, Fonesca RJ (eds): Facial Clefts and Craniosynostosis. Philadelphia, W.B. Saunders, 1996.

21. SKULL BASE SURGERY

Stephen P. Beals, M.D., F.A.C.S., Ramon Angel S. Robles, M.D., and Kerry A. Golden, M.P.T.

1. What are the anatomic divisions of the cranial base?

Anterior cranial fossa—formed *anterolaterally* by the frontal bone, *inferiorly* by the orbital plates and the anterior portion of the body of the sphenoid, *medially* by the cribriform plate of the ethmoid bone, and *posteriorly* by the lesser wings of the sphenoid bone.

Middle cranial fossa—formed *anteriorly* by the posterior margins of the lesser wings of the sphenoid bone, the anterior clinoid processes, and the ridge forming the anterior margin of the chiasmatic groove; *laterally* by the temporal squamae, the parietal bones, and the greater wings of the sphenoid; and *posteriorly* by the petrous portion of the temporal bone and dorsum sellae.

Posterior cranial fossa—formed *anteriorly* by the dorsum sellae and the clivus of the sphenoid, *inferiorly* by the basal part of the occipital bone, *anterolaterally* by the petrous and mastoid portions of the temporal bone and the mastoid angles of the parietal bones, and *posteriorly* by the occipital bone.

2. List the foramina found in each segment of the cranial base and their contents.

Foramen	*Contents*
Anterior cranial fossa	
Foramen cecum	Vein from nasal cavity to superior sagittal sinus
Anterior ethmoidal foramen	Anterior ethmoidal vessels and nasociliary nerve
Posterior ethmoidal foramen	Posterior ethmoidal vessels and nerve
Foramina for olfactory nerves	Olfactory nerves
Middle cranial fossa	
Optic foramen	Optic nerve
Superior orbital fissure	Cranial nerves III, IV, VI, V_1
Foramen rotundum	Cranial nerve V_2
Foramen ovale	Cranial nerve V_3
Foramen spinosum	Middle meningeal artery

Table continued on next page.

Foramen	Contents
Anastomotic foramen	Branch from middle meningeal artery to lacrimal artery
Emissary foramen	Vein from cavernous sinus to pterygoid plexus
Innominate canal	Lesser petrosal nerve to otic ganglion
Foramen lacerum	Small nerve of the pterygoid canal and a small meningeal branch from the ascending pharyngeal artery
Posterior cranial fossa	
Jugular foramen	Inferior petrosal sinus, lateral sinus, meningeal branches from the occipital and ascending pharyngeal arteries, glossopharyngeal nerve, pneumogastric nerve, and spinal accessory nerve
Foramen magnum	Medulla oblongata and its membranes, spinal accessory nerves, vertebral arteries, anterior and posterior arteries, and occipitoaxial ligaments
Internal auditory meatus	Facial nerve, auditory nerve and artery
Anterior condyloid foramina	Cranial nerve XII and a meningeal branch from the ascending pharyngeal artery

3. What tumors (malignant and benign) are commonly found in the cranial base?

Malignant extracranial tumors: squamous cell carcinoma, adenoid cystic carcinoma, rhabdomyosarcoma, hemangiopericytoma, esthesioneuroblastoma, malignant schwannoma

Malignant intracranial tumors: esthesioneuroblastoma, malignant schwannoma

Malignant primary basicranial tumors: chondrosarcoma, osteogenic sarcoma, metastatic disease

Benign extracranial tumors: inverted papilloma, angiofibroma, salivary gland pleomorphic adenoma, paraganglioma, mucocele, cholesteatoma

Benign intracranial tumors: pituitary adenoma, craniopharyngioma, meningioma, schwannoma, ossifying fibroma

Benign primary basicranial tumors: fibrous dysplasia, osteoma, osteoblastoma, chordoma, congenital dermoid

4. What are the common clinical findings associated with tumors of the skull base?

History and physical examination provide valuable information about location and extent of a tumor. Presenting signs and symptoms may be vague and varied, depending on the type, size, and location of the tumor in the skull base. A skull base tumor may even remain silent until it has grown to a compromising size when symptoms then become evident. Signs of benign tumors are usually due to the compression of adjacent tissues, causing in the orbital region, for instance, proptosis, diplopia, epiphora, and conjunctival exposure. Symptoms of malignant tumors, which are invasive, are often headaches, focal seizures, and loss of cranial nerve function (i.e., blindness, anosmia, diplopia, ptosis, altered facial sensation and/or animation, altered speech and/or swallowing, tinnitus and/or hearing loss).

5. How has the development of transfacial approaches to the cranial base enabled skull base surgery to be performed more successfully?

Access to the midline skull base has always been difficult because of the complex anatomy of the vital structures. Transfacial approaches, developed over the past two decades, offer safe avenues of skull-base exposure, often allowing single-stage resection, which shortens operating time and reduces morbidity. The simultaneous advancement of medical technology in neurosurgery, radiographic techniques, anesthesia, and intraoperative and postoperative monitoring has further aided in the success of transfacial techniques. (See figures, top of next page.)

6. What are the advantages of transfacial approaches?

1. Separation of facial units with minimal traumatic displacement due to the embryonic fusion of the facial units in the midline or in the paramedian region

2. Viability of displaced facial units because the primary blood supply has a lateral-to-medial direction of flow

3. Relative ease of surgical access to the central skull base due to the multiple hollow anatomic spaces of the midface

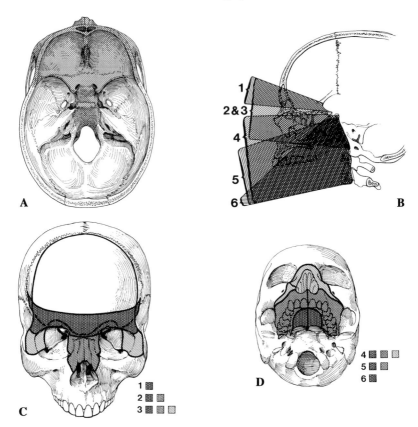

A, Scope of tumor sites in the anterior skull base and clivus that can be exposed by transfacial routes. *B*, Summation of the six different levels of approach demonstrating that the anatomic site of the tumor and direction of growth determine the level of transfacial exposure. The overlapping exposure shared by these approaches allows flexibility in choosing the best angle of surgical approach. *C*, The upper three approaches (levels I, II, III) are derived from the supraorbital bar. *D*, The lower three approaches provide exposure through the maxilla. (Reprinted with permission of the Barrow Neurological Institute, Phoenix, AZ.)

    4. Greater tolerance to postoperative swelling with displacement of facial units as opposed to similar displacement of the contents of the neurocranium
    5. Ability to reconstruct the facial units and maintain functional as well as aesthetic goals

7. What are the disadvantages of transfacial approaches?
    1. Contamination of the surgical wound with oropharyngeal bacterial flora
    2. Occasional need for facial incisions and subsequent scar development
    3. Emotional consideration for the patient related to surgical facial disassembly
    4. Potential need for tracheostomy or endotracheal intubation postoperatively

8. Why is the team approach important in conducting cranial base surgery?
    A multidisciplinary team approach is essential. It facilitates concentration of experience and promotes good communication and coordination of the treatment plan and projected outcomes. The integral specialties are neurosurgery, head and neck surgery, plastic surgery, and neurotology. Specialists in the field of endovascular radiology, radiation oncology, chemotherapy, ophthalmology, neurology, and neurorehabilitation also make critical contributions to the skull base team.

9. What diagnostic tests are most commonly used in the diagnosis of skull base tumors?
    • **CT scan with contrast** provides information about bony involvement. Displacement of bone is generally seen with benign tumors, whereas malignant lesions show invasion and lysis.

- **MRI with T1- and T2-weighted images** provides details about soft tissue and extent of tumor margins.
- **Angiography** provides information about tumor vascularity and involvement of the carotid artery and/or other critical vascular structures.
- **Nasoendoscopy** provides information about tumor presence in the nasal and paranasal regions.

10. What is the role of tumor biopsy in diagnosing lesions of the skull base?

A direct biopsy is desirable before the final treatment plan is determined for accessible tumors. For inaccessible lesions, it is sometimes feasible to use CT-guided fine-needle aspiration to obtain a biopsy before surgery. When a specimen cannot be obtained preoperatively, a biopsy with frozen section is taken during surgery before full exposure of the tumor.

11. How do you prepare a patient for cranial base surgery?
   1. Complete history and physical examination along with informed consent
   2. Clinical photographs
   3. Cephalometric x-rays, dental models, and splint fabrication if occlusion will be interrupted
   4. Routine laboratory tests and type and crossmatch for 4–6 units of blood
   5. Cryoprecipitate, in anticipation of use in fibrin glue
   6. CT scan or MRI on the way to surgery for immune serum globulin wand referencing
   7. Prophylactic antibiotics given in meningicidal doses

12. What transfacial surgical approach is used to access tumors of the anterior cranial fossa and tumors that extend into the superior orbital region?

The transfrontal approach–level I is performed through a bicoronal scalp incision. The radix and upper orbits are exposed, and the temporalis muscles are reflected so that a bicoronal craniotomy can be done. The incision must be posterior enough to provide an adequate frontogaleal flap. The dura is then dissected from the exposed anterior cranial fossa and cribriform plate. This procedure is facilitated by removal of the supraorbital bar. Watertight reconstruction, maintaining separation between the nasopharynx and cranial fossa, is achieved with local flaps, cranial autografts, and fibrin glue where indicated.

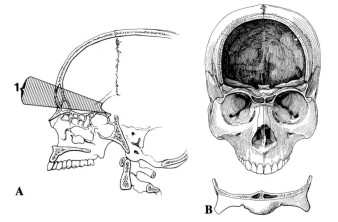

A, Level I transfrontal exposure for anterior cranial fossa and cribriform lesions. *B*, Level I exposure requires osteotomy of the supraorbital bar. (Reprinted with permission of the Barrow Neurological Institute, Phoenix, AZ.)

13. What transfacial surgical approach is used to expose the anterior cranial fossa, nasopharynx, clivus, orbit, and tumors that grow anteriorly?

The transfrontal nasal approach–level II is performed through a bicoronal incision. The radix, nasal bones, and nasal process of the maxilla are exposed, and the periorbita are stripped by reflecting the flap anteriorly. The medial canthal ligaments are taken down, the upper lateral cartilages are detached from the nasal bones, and the nasolacrimal ducts are exposed and preserved. A bifrontal craniotomy is performed, and dural dissection is completed. The supraorbital bar and nasal orbital complex are osteotomized and removed. After tumor resection, the frontal nasal fragment is affixed in its anatomic position with rigid fixation. The upper lateral cartilages are reattached to the nasal bones, and the medial canthal ligaments are repaired by transnasal wiring. Skull base reconstruction is achieved with local flaps and cranial autografts as needed.

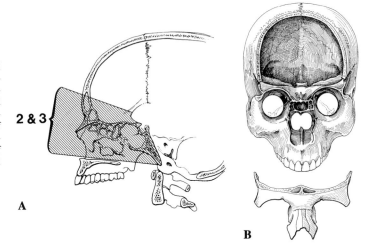

A, Level II transfrontal nasal exposure for anterior approach to the anterior cranial fossa and clivus. *B*, Level II exposure requires removal of the frontonasal unit. (Reprinted with permission of the Barrow Neurological Institute, Phoenix, AZ.)

A

B

14. What transfacial surgical approach is used for resection of large anterior cranial fossa or nasopharyngeal lesions and clival lesions with anterior extension?

The transfrontal nasal-orbital approach—level III is done with dissection identical to that used in the level II approach. The osteotomy includes the lateral orbital walls from the level of the infraorbital fissure as part of the supraorbital fragment. Most of the superior orbital roof also can be included in the fragment to facilitate the lateral retraction of the globes and greater midline exposure.

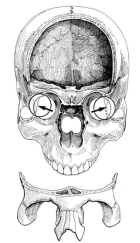

Level III transfrontal nasal-orbital exposure for larger anterior cranial fossa, nasopharyngeal, and clival lesions. This approach is similar to level II, except that it provides a wider exposure by allowing lateral retraction of the globes. Level III exposure requires inclusion of the lateral orbital walls on the frontonasal fragment. (Reprinted with permission of the Barrow Neurological Institute, Phoenix, AZ.)

15. What transfacial surgical approach is used for wide exposure of the entire midline skull base region and large nasopharyngeal and clival lesions that extend in all four directions?

The transnasomaxillary approach—level IV is done through a modified Weber-Ferguson incision, which is directed across the radix and along the opposite subciliary margin of the lower lid. After exposing the skeletal components, a Le Fort II osteotomy is performed. The osteotomy crosses just medial to the infraorbital foramen and nasolacrimal duct where the nasal fragment is divided into two fragments. It is done at the nasal process of the maxilla on one side and at the midline of the palate. The nasolacrimal duct often can be preserved if caution is used not to retract the nasal fragment excessively. The nasal soft-tissue complex remains intact and is also retracted with the fragment. (See figure, top of next page.)

16. What transfacial surgical approach is used for small clival lesions with superior, posterior, and inferior extensions and small-to-moderate nasopharyngeal lesions?

The transmaxillary approach—level V is performed through an intraoral approach in which an upper buccal sulcus incision is made. The anterior maxilla is prepared for a Le Fort I osteotomy and

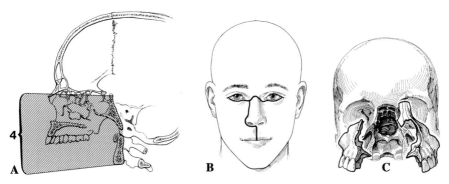

A, Level IV transnasomaxillary exposure yields a wide exposure of the entire central skull base from the radix to the cranial cervical junction. A similar degree of exposure usually can be obtained with a combination of level III and level V exposures. *B*, Incisions for the transnasomaxillary approach. *C*, Level IV exposure requires a Le Fort II osteotomy, then splitting of the maxillary fragment. (Reprinted with permission of the Barrow Neurological Institute, Phoenix, AZ.)

if a midline palatal split is required the soft palate is incised to one side of the uvula. The Le Fort I osteotomy is then performed and split through the midline. The two maxillary fragments can then be rotated laterally to expose the clivus. If greater exposure is needed, the pterygoid plates can be included on the fragments. A watertight reconstruction of the skull base is performed at closure.

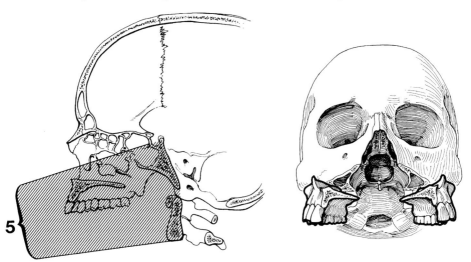

Left, Level V transmaxillary approach provides exposure of the clivus and nasopharyngeal area. *Right*, The level V approach requires a Le Fort I osteotomy and splitting of the palate for further exposure. (Reprinted with permission of the Barrow Neurological Institute, Phoenix, AZ.)

17. What transfacial surgical approach is used to expose the lower clival and upper cervical region for resection of small tumors?

The transpalatal technique—level VI is approached through the palate by incising both the nasal floor and oral mucosa. An incision is also made in the upper buccal sulcus, allowing the nasal floor to be approached extramucosally. The soft palate is incised to one side of the uvula and continued around the alveolar margin. The mucoperiostial flaps are then elevated, and the bony palate is osteotomized. The septum and nasal groove are separated along the nasal floor and cuts are made in the lateral nasal wall into the antra with an osteotome. The bony palate is removed, and the soft tissue portions are retracted. For further exposure, the vomer and perpendicular plate of the ethmoid are removed with a rongeur. After tumor resection, the bony palate is secured with rigid fixation, and the soft tissue is repaired.

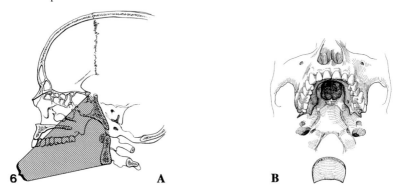

A, Level VI transpalatal exposure provides access to the lower clivus and upper cervical region. *B*, Level VI exposure requires removal of the hard palate. (Reprinted with permission of the Barrow Neurological Institute, Phoenix, AZ.)

18. What are the important aspects of closure and reconstruction of the cranial base?
- Watertight separation from the nasopharynx with local flaps and cranial autografts
- Fibrin glue to seal suture lines
- Rigid fixation of bone fragments
- Use of an occlusal splint and preregistered plates when osteotomies involve occlusion

19. What are the options for flap reconstruction?
1. **Local** (see figure below)
   - Pericranial flap: anteriorly based or laterally based on the temporalis muscle. This long flap extends the entire length of the anterior skull base but is very thin. It is best for the midline area.
   - Temporalis muscle: substantial but short muscle flap that usually cannot reach past the midline. It is best for lateral and orbital areas.
   - Frontogaleal flap: last resort for secondary reconstruction. It leaves the forehead skin very thin and vulnerable to breakdown and radiation.

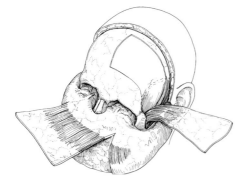

Scalp incisions must be planned and dissected to preserve and maximize the use of the pericranial, temporalis, and frontogaleal flaps. (Reprinted with permission of the Barrow Neurological Institute, Phoenix, AZ.)

2. **Regional:** the pectoralis major, latissimus dorsi, and trapezius muscles are useful for lateral skull defects (see figure at top of next page).

3. **Distant flaps:** the rectus abdominis free flap is versatile for closure of skull base defects. It can be used as a composite flap with the peritoneum and posterior rectus sheath as a vascularized dural graft. The latissimus dorsi and omentum also have been used to fill dead space and to cover the surface of the skull and upper face.

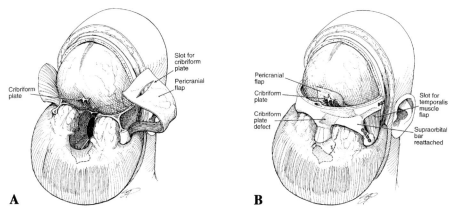

A, The osteotomy around the preserved cribriform plate is sealed with a perforated, laterally based pericranial flap. The cribriform plate is dropped through the flap (*B*) and wired in place, then sealed with fibrin glue. The flap courses through a lateral defect in this level II transfrontal nasal approach. (Reprinted with permission of the Barrow Neurological Institute, Phoenix, AZ.)

20. What is the postoperative management of a patient who has undergone skull base surgery?
    1. ICU monitoring
    2. Postoperative CT scans or MRIs to evaluate the brain, tumor site, and presence of any dead space and/or intracranial air
    3. Endotracheal intubation until adequate resolution of swelling to ensure airway protection
    4. Continuation of prophylactic antibiotics
    5. Lumbar drain for CSF management
    6. Close surveillance for infection, bleeding, and neurologic and/or medical complications

21. What complications may occur after skull base surgery?

Neurologic complications	Malocclusion	Epiphora
Systemic complications	Palatal fistula	Bleeding
Wound infection	Speech abnormalities	Flap or graft failure
CSF leak		

22. What improvements in survival rates after skull base surgery have been seen over the past four decades?
    In a 1995 study, O'Mally and Janecka demonstrated an increase in survival rates from 52% and 49% for 3 and 5 years after surgery (1960s and 1970s) to 57–59% for 3-year and 49% for 5-year survival in the 1970s and 1980s. A 5-year survival rate of 56–70% has been achieved in the 1980s and 1990s. The advances of skull base surgery over the past 40 years have allowed the decline in mortality rates and improved resectability of tumors once thought to be inoperable.

BIBLIOGRAPHY

1. Anderson JE: Grant's Atlas of Anatomy, 7th ed. Baltimore, Williams & Wilkins, 1978.
2. Beals SP, Joganic EF: Transfacial approaches to the craniovertebral junction. In Dickman CA, Sonntag VLJ, Spetzler RF (eds): Surgery of the Craniovertebral Junction. New York, Thieme, 1998.
3. Beals SP, Joganic EF, Hamilton MG, Spetzler RF: Posterior skull base transfacial approaches. Clin Plast Surg 22:491–511, 1995.
4. Beals SP, Joganic EF, Holcombe TC, Spetzler RF: Secondary skull base surgery. Clin Plast Surg 24:565–581, 1997.
5. Goss CM: Gray's Anatomy, 28th ed. Philadelphia, Lea & Febiger, 1966.
6. Janeka IP, Tiedemann K: Skull Base Surgery, Anatomy, Biology and Technology. Philadelphia, Lippincott-Raven, 1997.
7. O'Malley BWJ, Janeka IP: Evolution of outcomes in cranial base surgery. Semin Surg Oncol 11:221–227, 1995.

22. PRINCIPLES OF ORTHOGNATHIC SURGERY

Mitchell A. Stotland, M.D., and Henry K. Kawamoto, Jr., M.D., D.D.S.

1. What is the Angle classification?
The universally accepted system for describing dental occlusion was developed by the orthodontist Edward Angle. The Angle classification regards the upper first molar as its point of reference and describes the anterior-posterior (mesial-distal) relationship between the maxillary and mandibular arches.

In **class I occlusion (neutroocclusion)** the mesiobuccal cusp of the maxillary first molar articulates within the buccal groove of the lower first molar.

In **class II malocclusion** the lower arch is in a distal or posterior position relative to the maxillary arch. Thus, the mesiobuccal cusp of the maxillary first molar articulates with the distal portion of the mandibular second bicuspid and the mesial cusp of the first molar. Class II occlusion is sub-classified into divisions 1 and 2, in which the anterior teeth are flared labially or palatally, respectively.

In **class III malocclusion** the mandibular dentition is positioned mesially in relation to the maxillary dentition. Thus, the mesiobuccal cusp of the first upper molar intercuspates with the distobuccal groove of the lower first molar.

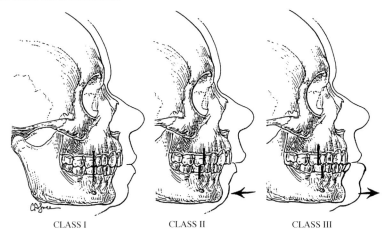

CLASS I   CLASS II   CLASS III

Angle classification of dental occlusion. (From McCarthy JG, Kawamoto HK Jr, Grayson BH, et al: Surgery of the jaws. In McCarthy JG (ed): Plastic Surgery. Philadelphia, W.B. Saunders, 1990, p 1193, with permission.)

2. What do the terms centric occlusion and centric relation mean?
Centric occlusion refers to a position of maximal, bilateral, balanced contact between the cusps of the maxillary and mandibular arches.

Centric relation is the most retruded, unstrained position of the mandibular condyle within the temporomandibular joint (TMJ)—i.e., within the glenoid fossa. Ideally, in centric occlusion the condyle sits anatomically within the glenoid bilaterally, reflecting simultaneous centric occlusion and centric relation. A number of problems, however, can result in asymmetric, premature dental contact upon closure with an unbalanced slide into occlusion that distracts the condyle and destroys its unstrained position. With prolonged loss of centric relation the distracting forces may lead to muscular, soft tissue, and bony pathologic changes in and around the TMJ. In repositioning the maxillary and/or the mandibular arches, it is critical not to overlook the concept of centric relation while focusing primarily on achieving centric occlusion. When repositioning the jaws, therefore, the orthognathic surgeon must make certain that the condyle is properly seated within the TMJ before initiating rigid bony fixation.

3. What is meant by overjet and overbite?

Overjet refers to the horizontal distance from the labial incisal edge of the lower central incisor to the labial incisal edge of the upper central incisor when the jaws are in centric occlusion (normal: upper incisal edge approximately 2 mm anterior to lower edge).

Overbite reflects the distance from the incisal edge of the upper central incisor to the incisal edge of the lower central incisor in centric occlusion (normal: upper incisal edge approximately 2 mm caudal to lower edge).

4. What do the cephalometric relationships SNA, SNB, and mandibular plane angle signify?

Cephalometry is a scientific measure of the dimensions of the head. Based on a standardized technique, a lateral radiogram (cephalogram) is obtained and used for analysis of facial proportions. Some of the more commonly used landmarks include:

Sella (S): the center of the pituitary fossa.

Nasion (N): the most anterior point at the nasofrontal junction.

Point A (Pt.A): the deepest midpoint on the maxillary alveolar process between the anterior nasal spine and the alveolar ridge.

Point B (Pt.B): the deepest midpoint on the mandibular alveolar process between the crest of the ridge and the most anterior point along the contour of the symphysis (pogonion [Pg]).

SNA: the angle that relates the maxilla to the cranial base (mean: 82 ± 3°).

SNB: the angle that relates the mandible to the cranial base (mean: 80 ± 3°).

The **mandibular plane angle** relates the posterior facial height to the anterior facial height. It is derived from the angle between the Frankfort horizontal plane and the mandibular plane. The mean mandibular plane angle is 21 ± 3° and is more obtuse in patients with an anterior-open bite and/or micro- or retrognathia. Patients with a deep-bite and/or the short-face syndrome tend to have a more acute mandibular plane angle.

The **Frankfort horizontal plane** is formed by the line joining the point located at the most superior extent of the external auditory meatus (Porion [Po]) with the lowest point on the inferior bony border of the left orbital cavity (Orbitale [O]).

The **mandibular plane** is formed by the line joining the most inferoposterior point at the mandibular angle (gonion [Go]) with the lowest point on the contour of the mandibular symphysis (menton [Me]).

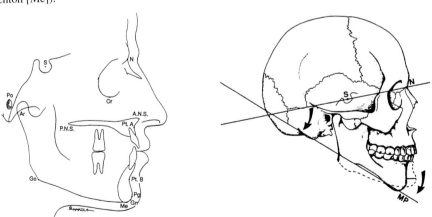

Cephalometric relationships. (*Left*, from Ferraro JW: Cephalometry and cephalometric analysis. In Ferraro JW (ed): Fundamentals of Maxillofacial Surgery. New York, Springer Verlag, 1997, p 236; *Right*, from McCarthy JG, Kawamoto HK Jr, Grayson BH, et al: Surgery of the jaws. In McCarthy JG (ed): Plastic Surgery. Philadelphia, W.B. Saunders, 1990, p 1196, with permission.)

5. What is the normal amount of incisor show with the lips in repose and during smiling?

With the lips in repose 2–3 mm of upper central incisor exposure is considered attractive. Up to 4–6 mm of show may be attractive in women as long as mentalis strain (manifested by chin dimpling) is not needed to achieve lip competence. With smiling, the full length of the upper incisors ideally should be visible with little or no evidence of gum exposure.

6. Describe the classic vertical proportions of the face in profile.

The proportions derived from the so-called classic canons are used only as a point of reference. Variation is the norm. What is considered "ideal" proportion has changed somewhat over the centuries and certainly differs with race and culture. It is often useful to evaluate the face in terms of vertically equal thirds. The hairline (trichion) to supraorbital rims represents the upper third; supraorbital rim to subnasale is the middle third; and subnasale to menton is the lower third. The lower third is often further subdivided: subnasale to stomion represents the upper third and stomion to menton the lower two-thirds of the facial lower third. The upper lip in profile usually sits at the level of the lower lip or slightly anterior. The labiomental groove is approximately 4 mm deep in women and 6 mm deep in men. Changes in lip position, labiomental groove depth, and vertical dimension of the facial thirds can be key indicators of facial disproportion that may be corrected by orthognathic surgery.

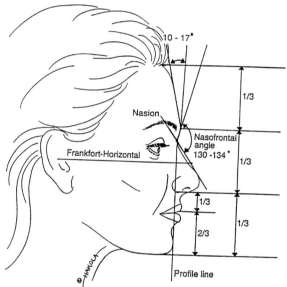

Vertical proportions of the face in profile. (From Guyuron B, Cohen SR: Facial evaluation for orthognathic surgery. In Ferraro JW (ed): Fundamentals of Maxillofacial Surgery. New York, Springer Verlag, 1997, p 227, with permission.)

7. What is the value of a surgical splint in an orthognathic procedure? How are splints made?

Precise control of three-dimensional movements is necessary for surgically repositioning tooth-bearing segments of bone. This principle is critical in the achievement of a balanced, stable, and aesthetically pleasing bimaxillary relationship. However, after mobilizing an osteotomy segment, exact control of three-dimensionality can be difficult. Surgical splints are used to guide the movements of the osteotomized segments before performing rigid fixation. Preoperatively one obtains dental impressions of both jaws. From these impressions stone models of the upper and lower dental arches are prepared. It is also necessary to acquire an occlusal registration from the patient (e.g.. a wax bite). The models are then mounted together in their occlusal relationship onto an articulator. Based on a cephalometric and facial profile evaluation, the exact movements required at surgery are determined and performed on the stone models in a mock procedure. Then, with the model arches resting together in their final position of maximal intercuspation, a thin wafer of acrylic is allowed to harden along the occlusal surfaces. This represents the guiding splint that is used at the time of surgery to help determine bony repositioning.

8. What is the rationale behind orthodontic preparation prior to orthognathic surgery?

The objective of presurgical orthodontics is to align the teeth properly over basal bone (i.e., max-
~nd mandible) and to coordinate the two arches so that they fit together ideally at the time of sur-
ıobilization. Dental models are serially obtained during the period of orthodontia to determine

precisely the dental movements that will result in a stable, class I occlusal relationship after surgery. In many patients dental compensations develop in response to long-standing skeletal deformity (eg., flared lower incisors in class II cases, retroclined lower incisors in class III cases). Such compensations usually need to be corrected preoperatively to allow maximal postoperative dental intercuspation. This orthodontic correction results in a temporary, preoperative worsening of the deformity but ultimately leads to a more stable postoperative outcome.

9. **What are the most common osteotomies used to perform mandibular repositioning?**

(1) Vertical and oblique ramus osteotomy, (2) inverted L osteotomy, and (3) sagittal-split osteotomy. All three techniques can be used to perform a mandibular set-back procedure for the treatment of mandibular prognathism. The sagittal-split osteotomy is generally the procedure of choice for mandibular advancement in the treatment of micrognathia.

10. **Classify chin deformities.**

A chin deformity may exist independently of an overall maxillary or mandibular deformity. A patient exhibiting class I occlusion and otherwise pleasing facial proportions may suffer aesthetically from an abnormally proportioned chin. Osseous genioplasties, therefore, may be performed alone or in conjunction with orthognathic procedures to improve facial harmony. A useful classification breaks down chin deformities into seven categories. Appreciation of the exact nature of the chin deformity helps to determine the specific method of skeletal or soft tissue correction required.

1. **Macrogenia:** horizontal, vertical, or combination bony excess.
2. **Microgenia:** horizontal, vertical, or combination bony deficiency.
3. **Combined micro- and macrogenia:** combination deformity; excess and deficiency in different planes.
4. **Asymmetric chin.**
5. **Pseudomacrogenia:** normal bony volume with excessive soft tissue.
6. **Pseudomicrogenia:** normal bony volume with retrogenia secondary to excessive maxillary growth and associated mandibular clockwise autorotation.
7. **Witch's chin deformity:** secondary to a soft tissue ptosis.

11. **What is the long face syndrome? Suggest a basic surgical approach.**

This appearance is associated with vertical maxillary excess. Physical findings may include excessive lower-third facial height, narrowed alar base, obtuse nasolabial angle, anterior-open bite with associated mentalis strain or lip incompetence, excessive gingival show and upper incisor display in repose and with smiling, and retrognathia associated with a backward autorotation of the mandible (clockwise rotation and obtuse mandibular plane angle, as seen on the lateral cephalogram). After prior orthodontic preparation, surgical treatment typically includes a Le Fort I osteotomy with maxillary impaction. A baseline class II malocclusion may not be corrected by a combination of maxillary impaction and mandibular autorotation. Correction of occlusion is achieved either by incorporating a posterior movement of the maxilla or by adding a mandibular advancement to the maxillary impaction. If a true microgenia exists (i.e., separate from the retrogenia caused by backward mandibular rotation), an osseous genioplasty may be added to achieve desired facial harmony. Decisions are based on an overall assessment of the patient's facial profile and balance.

12. **What is the short face syndrome? Suggest a basic surgical approach.**

This appearance is associated with vertical maxillary deficiency. Physical findings may include decreased lower-third facial height, lack of incisor show with an edentulous appearance, widened alar bases, acute nasolabial angle, deep bite with excessively protruding chin, and an acute mandibular plane angle. Surgical treatment includes a Le Fort I osteotomy with down-fracture. The procedure often necessitates an interposition bone graft to enhance stability and to prevent relapse. Often a horizontal maxillary advancement is also needed. A downward and/or backward movement of the chin is frequently required to address residual lower-third facial deficiency or chin protrusion.

13. **Describe the vascular supply of the mobilized Le Fort I maxillary segment.**

(1) The descending palatine artery (which divides into greater and lesser palatine vessels), (2) posterior superior alveolar artery, (3) infraorbital artery, (4) ascending palatine branch of the facial

artery, which arises directly from the external carotid artery, and (5) palatine branch of the ascending pharyngeal artery, a branch of the external carotid artery. **Note:** The descending palatine, posterior superior alveolar, and infraorbital arteries arise from the internal maxillary artery.

The posterior superior alveolar and infraorbital arteries perfuse the maxillary buccal alveolus, periodontium, and teeth. The other vessels listed above, which provide palatal contribution, supply the majority of blood to the mobilized Le Fort I maxillary segment. In fact, anatomic studies indicate that the descending palatine artery is commonly sacrificed during Le Fort I pterygopalatine disjunction. As as result, the major vascular supply of the mobilized Le Fort segment relies on the ascending palatine branch of the facial artery and the palatine branch of the ascending pharygeal artery.

14. What are the risks of nerve injury during orthognathic surgery?
   1. **Sagittal split mandibular osteotomy**
      • Neurosensory disturbance of the inferior alveolar nerve occurs in the vast majority of cases immediately after sagittal split osteotomy. However, long-term deficits (not all of which are symptomatic) occur in 10–15% of patients under 40 years of age.
      • Lingual nerve sensory disturbances are not common. Immediate postoperative tongue paresthesia secondary to lingual nerve injury probably occurs in less than 10% of patients. Long-term deficit occurs in < 1%.
      • Facial paralysis or paresis secondary to facial nerve injury is extremely rare and is typically associated with mandibular set-back procedures. Facial nerve disturbances associated with sagittal split osteotomies have resolved spontaneously in all reported cases.
   2. **Vertical ramus mandibular osteotomy** involves an extremely low incidence of injury to either the inferior alveolar or lingual nerves. With an intraoral approach to this procedure, facial nerve injury is also uncommon.
   3. **Genioplasty:** Long-term dysfunction of the distal inferior alveolar nerve (mental nerve) should occur in < 5% of cases.
   4. **Le Fort I osteotomy**
      • Temporary sensory disturbance resulting from traction injury to the infraorbital nerve and to the greater palatine neurovascular bundle is common immediately after Le Fort I osteotomy. Fortunately, these changes almost always resolve spontaneously over the ensuing weeks or months.
      • During down-fracture of the maxillary segment the nasopalatine nerve is necessarily severed. This results in a sensory loss to the region of the premaxillary palatal mucosa that is typically self-limited or nonsymptomatic.

15. What is the normal range of vertical mandibular opening in adults? Describe the normal motion of the TMJ.
   The average interincisal opening is 40–50 mm. The first 20–25 mm of opening is provided for by a hinge action of the TMJ. The remaining 15–20 mm of opening occurs through an anteroinferior translation of the condyle along the articular eminence. Vertical mandibular opening of 10–24 mm is severely limiting. An opening of 25–35 mm is functional but not ideal. Excessive mandibular opening may be associated with laxity of the TMJ capsule and may result in joint subluxation or dislocation.

CONTROVERSIES

16. Does orthognathic surgery improve TMJ symptoms?
   The relationship between TMJ dysfunction and malocclusion has been a subject of long-standing debate. Some patients with skeletal malocclusion habitually assume a convenient bite, sliding the mandible out of a centric relation position to approximate more closely a neutral class I dental relationship. With time, the associated strain on the TMJ may lead to symptomatic pathologic changes. By attempting to achieve a simultaneous correction of both skeletal and dental occlusion (i.e., combining centric relation with centric occlusion), orthognathic surgery may relieve some of the abnormal forces applied to the joint. Overall, however, although it may prove beneficial in any given case, clinical reports are conflicting and do not suggest that orthognathic surgery reliably

leads to an improvement in TMJ symptoms, probably because of the complex nature of TMJ disease in general.

17. What is progressive condylar resorption? What is its cause? How is it treated?

Condylar resorption occurs in adults and results in progressive retrusion of the mandible (high-angle mandibular deficiency). Progressive condylar resorption (PCR) occurs mainly in young females. The multiple theories about its cause include condylar avascular necrosis, increased TMJ estrogen responsiveness, and joint loading. Although some consider PCR to be a one-time event without recurrence, clinical reports have demonstrated multiple episodes of condylar resorption separated by intervals of quiescence. In respect to orthognathic surgery, TMJ loading after mandibular advancement may lead to postoperative PCR and clinical relapse. Opinion differs as to the treatment of PCR after orthognathic surgery. The application of maxillomandibular fixation is advocated by some to rest the condyles before allowing them to adapt gradually to the increased stress following mandibular advancement. Others believe that early and active TMJ function is indicated to promote optimal pericondylar blood flow and nutrition. Reoperation for relapse secondary to PCR has been disappointing with evidence of renewed flare-ups of condylar resorption leading to further clinical relapse.

BIBLIOGRAPHY

1. Crawford JG, Stoelinga PJ, Blijdorp PA, et al: Stability after reoperation for progressive condylar resorption after orthognathic surgery: Report of seven cases. J Oral Maxillofac Surg 52:460, 1994.
2. Ferraro JW (ed): Fundamentals of Maxillofacial Surgery. New York,Springer-Verlag, 1997.
3. Frydman WL: Nerve injuries. Oral Maxillofac Surg Clin North Am 9:207, 1997.
4. Guyuron B, Michelow BJ, Willis L: A practical classification of chin deformities. Aesth Plast Surg 19:257, 1995.
5. McCarthy JG, Kawamoto HK Jr, Grayson BH, et al: Surgery of the jaws. In McCarthy JG (ed): Plastic Surgery. Philadelphia, W.B. Saunders, 1990, p 1187.
6. Onizawa K, Schmelzeisen R, Vogt S: Alteration of temporo-mandibular joint symptoms after orthognathic surgery: Comparison with healthy volunteers. J Oral Maxillofac Surg 53:117; discussion, 122, 1995.
7. Siebert JW, Angrigiani C, McCarthy JG, Longaker MT: Blood supply of the Lefort I maxillary segment: An anatomic study. Plast Reconstr Surg 100:843, 1997.

23. DENTAL BASICS

Cynthia L. Rosenberg, D.D.S., M.S.D.

1. How are teeth identified?

The most common notation system for permanent teeth is the Universal system. The maxillary teeth are numbered 1–16, starting with the upper right third molar (no. 1) and proceeding to the upper left third molar (no. 16). The mandibular teeth are numbered 17–32, starting with the lower left third molar (no. 17) and preceding to the lower right third molar (no. 32). Thus, the maxillary left central incisor is no. 9.

$$\text{Right} \quad \frac{1\quad 2\quad 3\quad 4\quad 5\quad 6\quad 7\quad 8\ |\ 9\quad 10\quad 11\quad 12\quad 13\quad 14\quad 15\quad 16}{32\quad 31\quad 30\quad 29\quad 28\quad 27\quad 26\quad 25\ |\ 24\quad 23\quad 22\quad 21\quad 20\quad 19\quad 18\quad 17} \quad \text{Left}$$

The 20 deciduous or primary teeth are noted in the same manner, using letters A–T. The upper right second primary molar is A, and, proceeding around the arches, the lower right second primary molar is T.

$$\text{Right} \quad \frac{A\quad B\quad C\quad D\quad E\ |\ F\quad G\quad H\quad I\quad J}{T\quad S\quad R\quad Q\quad P\ |\ O\quad N\quad M\quad L\quad K} \quad \text{Left}$$

The Palmer notation system, used mostly by American orthodontists, numbers the teeth 1–8 in each quadrant, starting with the central incisor (no. 1) and proceeding to the third molar (no. 8). The quadrant is indicated by a bracket around the number. Thus, the maxillary left central incisor is |1 .

$$\text{Right} \quad \frac{8\ 7\ 6\ 5\ 4\ 3\ 2\ 1\ |\ 1\ 2\ 3\ 4\ 5\ 6\ 7\ 8}{8\ 7\ 6\ 5\ 4\ 3\ 2\ 1\ |\ 1\ 2\ 3\ 4\ 5\ 6\ 7\ 8} \quad \text{Left}$$

A two-digit system introduced in 1970 by the Federation Dentaire Internationale (FDI) has been adopted by the International Standards Organization (ISO). The ISO/FDI system identifies each of the 32 permanent teeth with a two-digit number. The first digit identifies the quadrant (1–4), and the second digit identifies the tooth type (1–8). Thus, the maxillary left central incisor is 21 (pronounced "two-one").

$$\text{Right} \quad \frac{18\ 17\ 16\ 15\ 14\ 13\ 12\ 11\ |\ 21\ 22\ 23\ 24\ 25\ 26\ 27\ 28}{48\ 47\ 46\ 45\ 44\ 43\ 42\ 41\ |\ 31\ 32\ 33\ 34\ 35\ 36\ 37\ 38} \quad \text{Left}$$

The 20 deciduous or primary teeth are represented in similar fashion: quadrant (5–8) and tooth type (1–5). Thus, the primary maxillary left central incisor is 61 (pronounced "six-one").

$$\text{Right} \quad \frac{55\ 54\ 53\ 52\ 51\ |\ 61\ 62\ 63\ 64\ 65}{85\ 84\ 83\ 82\ 81\ |\ 71\ 72\ 73\ 74\ 75} \quad \text{Left}$$

2. How are the surfaces of the teeth described?

The surfaces of the teeth that face the central incisors (toward the midline) are the **mesial** surfaces. Those that face away from the midline (toward the mandibular condyles) are the **distal** surfaces. The **labial** and **buccal** surfaces of teeth indicate areas that face either the lip or the cheek, respectively.

3. What is the Angle classification?

The Angle classification of malocclusion, developed in 1890 by Edward Angle, is based on the position of the upper first molar. In class I occlusion, the mesiobuccal cusp of the maxillary first molar occludes in the mesiobuccal groove of the mandibular first molar, producing a normal anteroposterior relationship. In class II malocclusion, the lower first molar is distal to the upper first molar, usually one-half to one full cusp distance. Angle divided class II malocclusion into two divisions. In class II, division 1, the upper anterior teeth are flared forward. In class II, division 2, the anterior teeth of both the maxilla and mandible are retruded with a deep overbite. In class III malocclusion, the lower first molar is mesial to the upper first molar, usually one-half to one full cusp distance. The lower incisors may be edge to edge or labial to the upper incisors, producing an anterior crossbite or underbite. Angle's classification of malocclusion provides a description only of the anteroposterior tooth relationship.

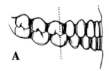

A

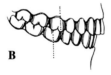

B

Angle classification of occlusion. *A*, Class I, normal occlusion. *B*, Class II malocclusion. *C*, Class III malocclusion. (From Manson P: Facial fractures. In Aston SJ, Beasley RW, Thorne CHM (eds): Grabb and Smith's Plastic Surgery, 5th ed. Lippincott-Raven, Philadelphia, 1997, p 386, with permission.)

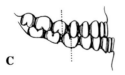

C

4. Describe the anatomy of a tooth.

A tooth consists of a crown, the portion one sees in the oral cavity, and a root, which is attached to the bony walls of the alveolar socket by periodontal membrane fibers. The crown is covered by enamel, and the root is covered by cementum. Their junction is called the cervical line. Beneath the enamel and cementum is the dentin, which makes up the bulk of the tooth. In the center of the crown is the pulp chamber, which continues as the pulp canal in the root. The pulp tissue furnishes the nerve and blood supply to the tooth through the apical foramen.

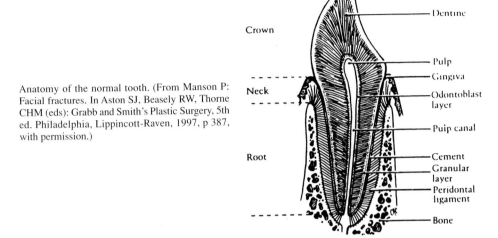

Anatomy of the normal tooth. (From Manson P: Facial fractures. In Aston SJ, Beasely RW, Thorne CHM (eds): Grabb and Smith's Plastic Surgery, 5th ed. Philadelphia, Lippincott-Raven, 1997, p 387, with permission.)

Crown

Neck

Root

Enamel

Dentine

Pulp

Gingiva

Odontoblast layer

Pulp canal

Cement

Granular layer

Peridontal ligament

Bone

5. What are the names of the teeth?

The 32 permanent teeth are divided into 4 quadrants. Starting at the midline, each quadrant has a central incisor, lateral incisor, canine (cuspid), first premolar (bicuspid), second premolar (bicuspid), and first, second, and third molars. The 20 deciduous or primary teeth are divided into 4 quadrants. Starting at the midline, each quadrant has a central incisor, lateral incisor, canine, first molar and second molar.

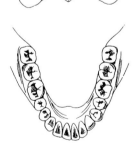

Normal adult dental arches contain 32 teeth, 16 in each arch. There are 3 molars, 2 bicupsids, 1 cuspid, and 2 incisors on each half of both maxillary and mandibular dental arches. (From Manson P: Facial fractures. In Aston SJ, Beasley RW, Thorne CHM (eds): Grabb and Smith's Plastic Surgery, 5th ed. Lippincott-Raven, Philadelphia, 1997, p 386, with permission.)

6. What is the nerve supply to the teeth?

The only nerve supply to the mandibular teeth is the inferior alveolar branch of the mandibular division of the trigeminal nerve. The maxillary teeth are supplied by the maxillary division of the trigeminal nerve, which divides into the posterior superior alveolar branch from the pterygopalatine portion and the middle and anterior superior alveolar branches from the infraorbital nerve. The three superior alveolar branches form a plexus that directly supplies the maxillary teeth.

7. What are natal and neonatal teeth?

Natal teeth are found in the oral cavity at birth. Neonatal teeth erupt during the first month of life. They are most common in the mandibular anterior region and are usually shells of enamel without roots. Neonatal teeth are commonly seen in cleft palates, often in eruption cysts.

8. What is a supernumerary tooth?

A supernumerary tooth is an extra tooth in excess of normal dentition. It is more common in permanent dentition, occurs more often in males, and may or may not erupt. They are most frequently found in the maxilla. Multiple supernumerary teeth are seen in a number of syndromes such as cleidocranial dysplasia and accompanying cleft lip and palate. A supernumerary tooth located between the maxillary central incisors is called a mesiodens.

9. What is the most common congenitally missing tooth?

The most common missing tooth is the third molar, followed by the mandibular second premolar, maxillary lateral incisor, and maxillary second premolar. Agenesis of numerous teeth (oligodontia) or failure of all of the teeth to develop (anodontia) is often associated with ectodermal dysplasia and oral-facial-digital syndrome.

10. What is the difference between overbite, overjet, and anterior openbite?

Overbite is the amount of vertical overlap measured between the upper and lower incisal edges when the teeth are in occlusion. **Overjet** is the horizontal overlap measured from the labial surface of the lower incisor to the labial surface of the upper incisor, parallel to the occlusal plane, when the teeth are in occlusion. **Anterior openbite** is a negative overbite in which the upper and lower incisors do not make contact.

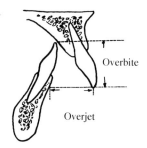

Relationship of the incisal edges. Overbite is the vertical overlap and overjet the horizontal overlap of the incisal edges. (From McCarthy JG, Kawamoto HK, Grayson BH, et al: Surgery of the jaws. In McCarthy JG (ed): Plastic Surgery. Philadelphia, W.B. Saunders, 1990, p 1194, with permission.)

11. What is a crossbite?

A crossbite is an abnormality in the buccolingual relationships of the teeth. In neutral occlusion, the buccal cusps of the upper teeth overlap those of the lower teeth. A **buccal crossbite** results from tilting of the maxillary teeth toward the cheek. A **lingual crossbite** results from lingual displacement (toward the tongue) of the upper teeth in relation to the lower teeth. The buccal cusps of the upper teeth no longer overlap those of the lower teeth.

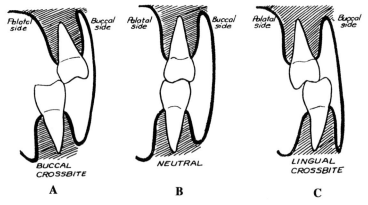

Buccolingual relationship of the teeth. A, Buccal crossbite. B, Neutral (centric) occlusion. C, Lingual crossbite. (From McCarthy JG, Kawamoto HK, Grayson BH, et al: Surgery of the jaws. In McCarthy JG (ed): Plastic Surgery. Philadelphia, W.B. Saunders, 1990, p 1194, with permission.)

12. What is the occlusal plane?

When teeth erupt to meet each other, they form the occlusal plane. The anteroposterior curve of the occlusal plane is called the curve of Spee. An occlusal curve also exists in the transverse plane, called the curve of Wilson. The teeth are not positioned straight up and down in the mouth but align along a spherical, three-dimensional curve.

13. What is the difference between centric relation and centric occlusion?

Centric relation is a position determined by maximal contraction of the muscles of the jaw. It is considered a stable, reproducible position that relates bone to bone through the temporomandibular joint. It does not depend on interdigitation of the teeth. **Centric occlusion** is a position determined by the way the teeth fit best together with the greatest amount of interdigitation. It is related to tooth occlusion and not muscle or bone. Wear facets or abraded surfaces of teeth are a function of centric occlusion.

14. What are the most common traumatic injuries to teeth?

Traumatic injuries to teeth include fractures, subluxation, and avulsion. Tooth fractures are the most common injury to permanent teeth and may involve the enamel, dentin, pulp, and/or root. Fracture involving the pulp requires endodontic treatment. Treatment of a root fracture depends on its location. The prognosis for repair and maintenance of tooth vitality is most favorable if the fracture is in the apical third of the root. Subluxation is either intrusion or extrusion. An intruded primary tooth will erupt on its own. An intruded permanent tooth requires orthodontic treatment to reposition. If a primary tooth is extruded, it should be removed. An extruded permanent tooth should be repositioned in the socket with gentle pressure and splinted for 3–4 weeks. The critical factor for successful reimplantation of an avulsed tooth is the physiologic status of the periodontal ligament cells on the root surface and not the length of extraoral time.

15. When do teeth erupt?

The primary teeth begin to erupt at approximately age 6 months in the following order:
- Central incisors, 6–7mo
- Canines, 16-18 mo
- Lateral incisors, 7–9 mo
- Second primary molars, 20–24 mo
- First primary molars, 12–14 mo

Roughly four teeth erupt every 4 months in the primary dentition. The eruption sequences of the maxillary and mandibular teeth are approximately the same.

The mandibular permanent teeth tend to erupt before the maxillary permanent teeth. The first permanent tooth to erupt is the first molar at approximately age 6 years. It erupts distal to the primary second molar. The remaining permanent teeth erupt in the following order:
- Mandibular central incisors, 6 yr
- Mandibular canines, 10 yr
- Mandibular lateral incisors, 7 yr
- Second premolars, 11 yr
- Maxillary central incisors, 7 yr
- Maxillary canines, 11 yr
- Maxillary lateral incisors, 8 yr
- Second molars, 12 yr
- First premolars, 10 yr
- Third molars, 17 yr

The permanent incisors, canines, and premolars are called succedaneous teeth because they replace (succeed) the primary teeth.

16. What is a mamelon?

A mamelon is a rounded protuberance found on the incisal edges of newly erupted incisor teeth. Each tooth has three mamelons. They are soon worn down through normal attrition. Mamelons will remain if the teeth are malaligned and there is no opposing incisal contact, as in an openbite.

17. Describe the embryology of teeth.

As early as 28 days in utero, odontogenic epithelium is recognized on the mandibular and maxillary processes. This tissue proliferates and forms the dental laminae from which tooth buds develop. Each tooth goes through a series of stages as cells differentiate and proliferate. Odontoblasts give rise to dentin, a process called dentinogenesis, and ameloblasts form enamel, a process called amelogenesis. As enamel and dentin are deposited, the crown is formed from the cusp tips to the cervical region. After enamel formation is nearly completed, root development begins.

A knowledge of tooth embryology is helpful in understanding oral pathology. Ameloblastoma, for example, is an aggressive odontogenic tumor that is thought to form from ameloblasts that do not differentiate to the stage of enamel formation.

18. What is the process of dental decay?

The earliest clinically recognizable stage of dental decay is a white-spot lesion, which results from oral bacteria that proliferate in the presence of fermentable carbohydrates and form acids that cause tooth demineralization. At this point the surface of enamel is still intact, and the lesion is reversible. Once the decay process goes through the enamel and reaches the dentin, it spreads laterally and quickly inflames the pulp tissue. Pulp tissue is not capable of healing. Severe pain is usually present by this time, and a periapical abscess may form in the surrounding bone. Dental decay may be difficult to see clinically. Dental radiographs show a decayed area of a tooth as more radiolucent than the unaffected area.

19. What are the muscles of mastication?

The masticatory muscles concerned with mandibular movement include the masseter, medial pterygoid, lateral pterygoid, and temporalis muscles. These muscles are paired.

20. How do the muscles of mastication move the mandible?

The lateral pterygoid is divided into two heads. The superior head is active during jaw-closing movement; the inferior head is active during jaw-opening and protrusion movement. The masseter muscle is the most powerful muscle of mastication; it elevates the mandible and assists in protrusion. The medial pterygoid muscle, like the masseter, elevates the mandible and is active during protrusion. It also helps in lateral positioning of the jaw. The temporalis muscle is divided into two parts. It is the principal positioner of the mandible during closing. The posterior part retrudes the mandible; the anterior part is active in clenching.

21. What are the average measurements of mandibular movement in an adult?

The maximal mandibular opening is 50–60 mm as measured from the incisal edges of the anterior teeth. A person should be able to open the equivalent width of three fingers. The maximal lateral movement is 10–12 mm, approximately the width of the maxillary central incisor. The maximal protrusive range is 8–11 mm. The retrusive range is 1–3 mm. Retrusive movement is the discrepancy between centric occlusion and centric relation. Age, size, and skeletal morphology of the individual must be taken into consideration in evaluating these measurements.

BIBLIOGRAPHY

1. Ash MM: Wheeler's Dental Anatomy, Physiology and Occlusion, 7th ed. Philadelphia, W.B. Saunders, 1993.
2. Avery JK (ed): Oral Development and Histology. Baltimore, Williams & Wilkins, 1987.
3. McCarthy JG (ed): Plastic Surgery. Philadelphia, W.B. Saunders, 1990.
4. Peck S, Peck L: Tooth numbering progress. Angle Orthod 66(2):83–84, 1996.
5. Ranly DM: A Synopsis of Craniofacial Growth, 2nd ed. Norwalk, CT, Appleton & Lange, 1988.
6. Thaller SR, Montgomery WW (eds): Guide to Dental Problems for Physicians and Surgeons. Baltimore, Williams & Wilkins, 1988.

IV. *Craniofacial Surgery II—Traumatic*

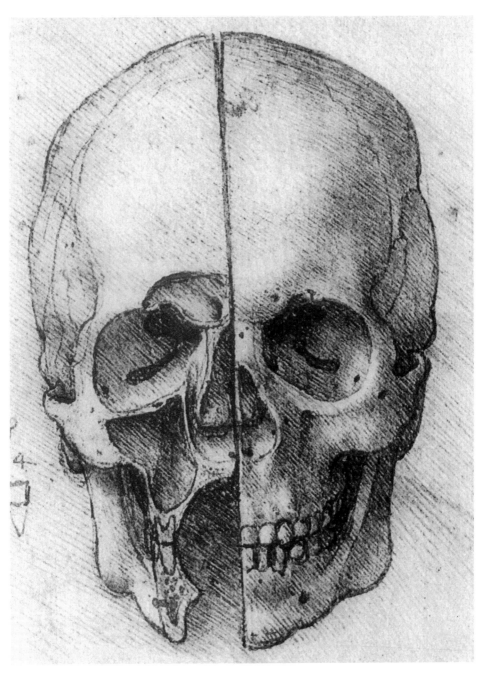

The Skull Sectioned
Leonardo da Vinci
1489
Pen and ink over traces of black chalk
The Royal Library at Windsor Castle, Windsor
The Royal Collection
© 1998 Her Majesty Queen Elizabeth II

24. ASSESSMENT AND MANAGEMENT OF FACIAL INJURIES

Paul N. Manson, M.D.

1. What are life-threatening facial injuries?

1. **Hemorrhage:** Occasionally, profuse hemorrhage results from maxillofacial injuries. Such injuries are either upper Le Fort fractures or nasal ethmoidal fractures in which nasal and sinus wall vessels are transected. Usually, hemorrhage is controlled by anterior-posterior nasal packing. A posterior nasal pack acts as an obturator against which the anterior packing can be placed. Failure to control bleeding should prompt re-packing. In the case of Le Fort fractures, placement of the patient in intermaxillary fixation often dramatically limits blood loss. If these measures are not successful, hemorrhage may be occurring from the cranial base, where lacerations of the carotid or jugular systems are possible with skull base fractures. Angiography should be performed, and embolization of appropriate bleeding areas may be attempted. If these measures fail, ligation of the external carotid *and* superficial temporal arteries will limit blood flow in the common area of maxillofacial artery transection (generally the internal maxillary artery and nasal and sinus branches) by up to 90%.

2. **Airway:** Airway obstruction is seen with fractures of the nose or upper and lower jaws or with swelling in the floor of the mouth. Either jaw may displace posteriorly to partially obstruct the pharynx.

3. **Aspiration:** Aspiration occurs when patients are unable to manage their airway. Fractures of the upper and lower jaw commonly permit aspiration. Neck swelling, pharynx and tongue swelling and obtundation, and floor of mouth swelling disturb swallowing mechanisms.

2. The presence of fat in a periorbital laceration should mandate what examination?

It implies the possibility of a globe-penetrating injury, and the globe should be carefully examined, both externally and fundoscopically, for the presence of a laceration. As a baseline, visual acuity should be recorded in every patient with a facial injury, as should the presence of double vision. In comatose patients, the pupillary reaction is noted.

3. The presence of a Marcus Gunn pupil implies what cranial nerve injury?

Injury to the optic nerve, if partial, may present as a Marcus Gunn pupil. The Marcus Gunn pupil implies a paradoxical pupillary dilatation when a light is swung between the intact and injured eyes. Normally, the light causes constriction on the side of the injured and normal eyes eye as it is swung back and forth between the opposite eye and the eye in question. When the optic nerve is injured, paradoxical dilatation rather than alternating constriction occurs. This finding implies a partial lesion of the optic nerve. Optic nerve lesions are first detected by a change in the rapidity of the response of the pupil to light. Thereafter, visual acuity deficits occur, including the Marcus Gunn pupil. Any diminished vision should prompt treatment for an optic nerve injury and/or evaluation of the cause, such as retinal detachment, hyphema, or other intraocular problem.

4. The presence of nasal bleeding implies fracture of what craniofacial structure?

Nasal bleeding is a nonspecific event that accompanies many craniofacial fractures. Frontobasalar fractures present as nasal bleeding, as do fractures of the frontal sinus. Medial orbital fractures commonly produce ipsilateral epistaxis, as do fractures of the inferior orbit (floor) and zygoma. Bilateral epistaxis is seen in bilateral midface fractures, such as those of the Le Fort type, the naso-ethmoidal region, and the nose.

5. Numbness in the infraorbital division of the trigeminal nerve is consistent with what fracture?

It is consistent with a fracture of the floor of the orbit or the zygoma. The absence of numbness should place the diagnosis of these fractures in question. The presence of numbness in an orbital floor fracture is not a prognostic sign that implies the necessity for operative intervention. Numbness following a zygoma fracture, when the zygoma fracture is medially impacted into the nerve canal, affects the prognosis of sensory recovery if the fracture displacement is not corrected. Decompression of the infraorbital foramen by fracture reduction is indicated. The infraorbital nerve travels from the posterior margin of the inferior orbital fissure anteriorly and medially across the floor of the orbit. In the proximal ⅔ of the orbit the nerve is in a groove; in the distal third it is in a canal. The canal exits the maxilla about 10 mm below the infraorbital rim parallel to the lateral margin of the cornea in straight-forward gaze. A branch of the nerve travels in the anterior wall of the maxilla to reach the anterior incisor and cuspid teeth. Other branches enter the soft tissue to innervate the upper lip, ipsilateral nose, and skin of the medial cheek. Numbness in either of these areas implies damage to the nerve from crushing within fracture sites. Symptoms may be partial or total in each set of branches. Therefore, numbness of the teeth and lip implies that the fracture affects one or more branches of the nerve.

6. The presence of cyanosis, drooling, and hoarseness implies damage to what structures and the necessity for operative intervention in what area?

Such symptoms indicate impending complete respiratory obstruction. Fractures of the upper and lower jaws, fracture of the larynx, or swelling in the floor of the mouth produce respiratory obstruction. If possible, a tracheostomy should be performed under operative conditions that permit careful identification of the trachea. A tracheostomy should be performed through a horizontal incision in the skin and a vertical incision between the strap muscles, dissecting down to the trachea. A vertical incision is made into the second and third tracheal rings and a tube can be inserted. In urgent situations, a cricothyroidotomy may be performed between the cricoid and the hyoid cartilages. Cricothyroidotomy is meant to be a rapid, life-saving maneuver and should be converted to a tracheostomy as soon as possible.

7. Cervical spine fractures accompany what maxillofacial injury?

Cervical spine fractures commonly accompany maxillofacial soft tissue or bony injuries, and are frequently seen in frontal impact and mandibular fractures. An association with mandibular fractures has been both confirmed and denied in separate studies. Several studies have shown a slight association of mandibular fractures with upper cervical spine fractures. Generally the upper and lower cervical areas are the most difficult to image radiologically and if they cannot be cleared, the patient must be treated as if he or she has a cervical spine fracture until the injury is excluded. The presence of a cervical spine fracture may dictate that standard approaches to facial injuries must be converted to alternative approaches that do not require rotation or extension of the neck.

8. Which maxillofacial fractures are more difficult to localize in CT scans?

The presence of a nondisplaced fracture (classically of the ramus of the mandible) is one of the most difficult to identify in CT scans. Axial and coronal imaging is preferred with appropriate bone windows. Soft tissue windows often miss nondisplaced maxillofacial fractures; proper imaging, proper slice thickness, and combining physical examination findings with CT scan data help to prevent "missed" injuries.

9. The Panorex exam of the mandible is likely to miss fractures in what mandibular region?

The Panorex radiograph generally requires patient cooperation and is a flat view taken by a movable x-ray beam that displays the entire mandible as a flat structure. Some overlap and blurring is usually seen in the symphysis-parasymphysis region; therefore, injuries in this area are frequently missed. The combination of Panorex exam and CT scan detects almost all mandibular fractures.

10. Split palate and alveolar fractures have what symptoms in contrast with a Le Fort fracture?

Fractures of the palate and alveolus generally present with mucosal and palatal lacerations. These are not the usual symptoms of Le Fort fractures and imply damage to the dental alveolar structures. Both Le Fort fractures and palatal alveolar fractures present with nasal bleeding and may present with numbness in the teeth. Alveolar fractures and fractures of the palate allow mobility of the maxillary dentition. Le Fort fractures have a mobile maxilla, but the segments of the dental arch are not mobile. Segments of the arch in palate fractures often are displaced laterally and are mobile, whereas the Le Fort fracture displays mobility at the Le Fort I, II or III levels. In Le Fort fractures, the maxillary dental arch moves as a one-piece unit. The presence of a palatal alveolar fracture demands additional reduction techniques and/or splinting in combination with techniques used to stabilize Le Fort fractures.

11. Which nasal ethmoidal fractures do not display telecanthus?

Nasoethmoidal orbital fractures, which are greensticked or incomplete at the junction of the internal angular process of the frontal bone with the frontal process of the maxilla, are usually rotated posteriorly and medially at the inferior orbital rim and piriform aperture. Therefore, they tend to tense the medial canthal attachment and lengthen the palpebral fissure. A "bowstringing" effect on the palpebral fissure is created, along with an ipsilateral depression along the side of the nose and the inferior orbital rim. The presence of a complete fracture at the internal angular process of the frontal bone allows the attachment of the medial canthal ligament to the frontal process of the maxilla to move laterally, which produces the classic telecanthus seen in complete nasoethmoidal orbital fractures.

12. Cerebrospinal fluid fistulae can be detected by what examinations?

Cerebrospinal fluid fistulae are detected by suspicion. If nasal drainage is examined, the presence of a double ring on absorption of the nasal drainage on a paper towel implies that the blood is separate from another component. The blood ring is internal, and the lighter fluid ring is external, implying the presence of another substance (cerebrospinal fluid). The cerebrospinal fluid contains glucose, whereas nasal mucous or drainage does not. The location of a cerebrospinal fluid fistula is often suspected on a carefully performed CT scan. Alternatively, dye or radiographically active material may be placed in the spinal fluid with a lumbar puncture and collected in the nose to identify the presence of cerebrospinal fluid rhinorrhea. Dyes also may be imaged as they pass through the site of the fistula.

13. Subcondylar fractures of the mandible generally present with what occlusal disturbance?

Subcondylar fractures of the mandible usually present with a contralateral open bite in the anterior dentition and premature contact on the ipsilateral side. The ramus is shortened by the fracture on the affected side; therefore, a premature contact in the molar dentition on the injured side opens the bite in the contralateral anterior dentition.

14. Untreated Le Fort II and III fractures generally present with what changes in facial structure and occlusion?

Untreated fractures of the Le Fort variety generally present with bilateral eyelid ecchymosis, bilateral infraorbital nerve numbness, bilateral nasal bleeding, and dramatic facial swelling. A malocclusion is present. Generally the maxilla has dropped inferiorly in its posterior aspect, creating premature contact in the posterior dentition and an anterior open bite. The maxillary dental arch is usually rotated. The facial features are flattened and elongated, producing the so-called donkey facies of maxillary and zygomatic retrusion, nasal retrusion, and an increase in the length of the middle third of the facial region.

15. Incomplete or greenstick Le Fort fractures present with what symptoms and are characteristically found at what level?

Incomplete Le Fort fractures present with minimal signs of facial injury. Often they masquerade as an isolated zygomatic fracture. Incomplete fractures are more common in upper (Le Fort II and Le Fort III) fractures. Maxillary mobility is normally the hallmark of a Le Fort fracture; however, it is absent in incomplete injuries. Displacements are usually slight, and the malocclusion is easily missed. Often there is a slight rotation or a slight malocclusion. The malocclusion can be ascribed, therefore, to swelling and is easily missed. The fracture is also easily missed in radiographs, because there is no displacement between fragments, and the CT scans do not image undisplaced fractures with clarity. Therefore, the diagnosis must be suspected in any patient with minor malocclusion and periorbital bruising. The injury is usually treated satisfactorily by the application of arch bars and traction elastics for a short (3-week) period. Missing the fracture generally requires a maxillary Le Fort I osteotomy as an elective corrective procedure.

16. The presence of an anterior cranial fossa fracture is suspected by what clinical signs?

Generally, fractures of the anterior cranial fossa are not only easily missed in radiographs (they generally require carefully taken CT scans), but they may be missed on physical examination. The presence of a forehead bruise or laceration is common. The patient may demonstrate a "spectacle" hematoma—a hematoma in the upper lid confined to the distribution of the orbital septum. Therefore, the bruise abruptly stops where the orbital septum attaches to the superior orbital rim and produces a classic hematoma of the upper eyelid. Such hematomas are diagnostic of a fracture within the superior orbit; therefore, it is an anterior cranial fossa fracture. Disturbances of olfaction and a cerebrospinal fluid leak also may accompany these injuries. The most common cerebral symptom is a slight disturbance of memory or consciousness. Even brief periods of unconsciousness imply brain contusion.

17. What is the difference between enophthalmos and ocular dystopia?

Fractures of the lower two-thirds of the orbit commonly produce changes in eye position by expansion of the orbit. Fractures of the superior portion of the orbit generally are displaced inward and downward and cause the globe to be driven forward and downward by orbital volume constriction. Fractures of the inferior portion of the orbit may either constrict or expand the orbital cavity. Constriction is most commonly produced by a medially displaced zygoma fracture, which may cause exophthalmos of the globe. In fractures of the zygoma, orbital floor, or medial orbit that expand the volume of the orbit, the globe is displaced posteriorly and medially. The posterior displacement of the globe is termed enophthalmos. Generally, an increase of 1 cc in orbital volume is required for each millimeter displacement of the globe. Inferior globe displacement is called ocular dystopia. Displacement is permitted by expansion of the floor, medial orbital wall, and, in cases of the zygoma, the inferior orbital rim.

18. How are injuries of the parotid duct detected?

Parotid duct injuries should be suspected on the basis of a physical examination. Lacerations in the vicinity of the duct (which travels on a line between the ear canal and the base of the nose and exits into the mouth opposite the second maxillary bicuspid-first molar area) are suspect for parotid duct injury. Because the buccal branch of the facial nerve and the parotid duct run close to each other, injury to either structure alone is less common than injury to both. Therefore, lacerations that present with buccal branch facial nerve weakness should raise suspicion for parotid duct injuries. The duct can be cannulated with an angiocath intraorally. If saline is flushed into the duct, the appearance of saline in the wound is diagnostic of a duct or anterior glandular laceration. Such injuries benefit from operative exploration and repair of the duct. Repair is conducted over a fine "stent" catheter with nonabsorbable sutures.

19. Blunt craniofacial injuries accompanied by facial nerve palsy are generally due to fracture of what structure?

Fractures of the temporal bone are common skull-base fractures. They may be longitudinal or transverse. High-dose steroids and decompression are considered for certain injuries. The prognosis varies with the site of the fracture.

20. Subluxation of the condylar head anterior to the glenoid fossa produces what symptom?

It produces an open bite and inability to close the mouth. The mandible is "locked" open. The joint is usually anesthetized to relax the muscles; then finger pressure is delivered downward to the posterior maxillary dentition to ease the condylar head back into the fossa. Limited mouth opening is prescribed. Occasionally, surgical intervention is necessary to prevent recurrent dislocations.

21. Transection of the lacrimal system is suggested by what physical signs?

It is usually heralded by a laceration in the vicinity of the medial canthus. The lacrimal punctum may be dilated and saline squirted through the punctum into the system. Appearance of saline in the wound is diagnostic of a canalicular laceration. Both upper and lower canalicular lacerations should be repaired. Tubes are placed into the nose, through the lacerated canniculus to splint the repair. Damage to the lacrimal system commonly accompanies Le Fort III and nasoethmoid fractures. However, such damage usually produces compromise or obstruction of the lacrimal system within the nasal lacrimal duct; repair and repositioning of the fracture fragments often permit adequate function of the system. Repair of a chronically obstructed nasal lacrimal duct is accomplished with a dacryocystorrhinostomy.

22. Facial lacerations rarely require debridement because the blood supply is good and the tissue will usually heal. True or false?

Most facial lacerations benefit from debridement. The facial blood supply is excellent, and often contused bits of tissue will heal but with increased scarring. Therefore, the zone of contusion should be excised, if permitted by flexibility and availability of soft tissue, to prevent distortion. Excision should not be performed in the upper and lower eyelid areas because the eyelids may not be able to close completely over the globe. In general, excision also should not be performed in eyelid or eyelid margin lacerations, nostril rim lacerations, or lacerations of the lip margins or ear because distortion may be noticeable. In other areas, resection of the contused skin allows conversion to a primary surgically created wound with more predictable healing and generally improved appearance. A layered repair of the facial soft tissue, including the fat mimetic muscle system and the skin dermal and epidermal components, should be performed.

23. Three-dimensional CT scans are indicated in what kind of fracture evaluation?

Three-dimensional CT scans are helpful for an overall picture of the fracture and are most useful for comparing symmetry between the sides or displacement of the zygoma or mandible. They are not as useful in the orbit because they are not sensitive to orbital wall displacement. The combination of axial and coronal CT scans with both bone and soft tissue windows provides the most accurate facial injury assessment.

24. What potentially lethal facial fracture emergency is commonly overlooked?

Aspiration often accompanies fractures of the upper and lower jaws. It is easily missed and accounts for pulmonary complications that may have severe consequences. It is prevented by recognition, patient positioning, and intubation.

25. What disastrous complications result from instrumentation of unrecognized fractures of the anterior cranial fossa?

Disastrous complications may occur if instrumentation procedures are performed in carelessly unrecognized fractures of the anterior cranial fossa. Fractures of the anterior cranial fossa produce a bony discontinuity that allows penetration of nasogastric tubes, nasal fracture reduction instruments, and nasal packing into the anterior cranial fossa. One must be aware of the usual location of the cribriform plate, and instruments must be angled away from this region specifically. Both instruments and nasogastric tubes have been inadvertently introduced into the anterior cranial fossa with disastrous consequences.

26. Numbness of the lower lip usually accompanies what type of mandibular fracture?

The inferior alveolar nerve enters the mandible in the upper ramus and travels through the angle region and the body of the mandible until it reaches the mental foramen opposite the first bicuspid tooth. It then exits the jaw and travels in the soft tissue. Fractures of the angle and body region, therefore, may produce numbness by displacement of fragments impinging on the nerve and/or transecting it. The presence of numbness should prompt a thorough examination for mandibular fracture. Generally, such fractures are also accompanied by malocclusion and bleeding from a tooth socket.

27. Acutely, orbital floor fractures present with what symptoms? What criteria should be used to establish the need for operative reduction?

Orbital fractures generally present with numbness in the distribution of the infraorbital nerve, double vision, periorbital and subconjunctival hematoma, and perhaps a visual acuity deficit. The visual acuity deficit is not specific to the orbital fracture, but implies damage to the globe or the optic nerve. Generally orbital fractures present with exophthalmus due to swelling. Enophthalmus is present within 1–3 weeks if the orbital cavity is significantly enlarged and appears as the swelling resolves. An orbital volume enlargement of more than 5–10% justifies open reduction. Generally, orbital fractures are accompanied by diplopia when the patient looks upward or downward. Diplopia in downgaze is quite disabling and is due most commonly to muscular contusion. Diplopia that is due to interference with the excursion of the extraocular muscle system, by virtue of entrapment of fat that is tethered to the muscles by fine ligaments or, less commonly, entrapment of the muscle itself, should be treated with operative intervention. Diplopia due to muscle contusion usually improves significantly without operative intervention.

BIBLIOGRAPHY

1. Dufresne C, Manson PN: Facial fractures in children. In McCarthy JG, May J, Littler W (eds): Plastic Surgery. Philadelphia, W.B. Saunders, 1990, pp 1143–1187.
2. Evans G, Manson PN, Clark N: Identification and management of minimally displaced nasoethmoidal orbital fractures. Ann Plastic Surg 35:469–471, 1995.

3. Manson PN: Maxillofacial injuries. In Siegel J (ed): Management of Trauma. New York, Churchill-Livingstone, 1986.
4. Manson PN (ed): Bone Grafts and Rigid Fixation in Craniofacial Surgery. Clin Plast Surg 16(1), 1989 [entire issue].
5. Manson PN: Facial fractures. In Aston SJ, Beasley RW, Thorne CHM (eds): Grabb and Smith's Plastic Surgery, 5th ed. Philadelphia, Lippincott-Raven, 1997, pp 383–412.
6. Manson PN: Midface fractures. In Georgiade N, Riefhohl R, Barwick W (eds): Plastic, Maxillofacial and Reconstructive Surgery, 2nd ed. Baltimore, Williams & Wilkins, 1992, pp 409–433.
7. Manson P: Facial fractures. In Grotting J (ed): Re-operative Aesthetic and Reconstructive Surgery. St. Louis, Quality Medical Publishing, 1994.
8. Manson P, Clark N, Robertson B, Crawly W: Comprehensive management of pan facial fractures. J Craniomaxillofac Trauma 11:43–56, 1995.
9. Manson P, Iliff N: Management of blow-out fractures of the orbital floor: Early repair of selected injuries. Surv Ophthalmol 35:280–291, 1991.
10. Manson P, Iliff N, Vander Kolk C, et al: Rigid fixation of orbital fractures. Plast Reconstr Surg 86:1103–1109, 1990.
11. Manson P, Markowitz B, Mirvis S, et al: Toward CT-based facial fractures of the maxilla and palate. Plast Reconstr Surg 85:202–212, 1990.
12. Markowitz B, Manson P, Sargent L, et al: Management of the medial canthal tendon in nasoethmoid orbital fractures: The importance of the central fragment in treatment and classification. Plast Reconstr Surg 87:843–853, 1991.
13. Paskert JP, Manson PN: The bimanual examination for assessing instability in naso-ethmoidal orbital injuries. Plast Reconstr Surg 83:165–167, 1989.
14. Romano JJ, Manson PN, Mirvis WE, et al: LeFort fractures without mobility. Plast Reconstr Surg 85:355–362, 1990.

25. PEDIATRIC FACIAL FRACTURES

Richard C. Schultz, M.D., F.A.C.S.

1. What are the four most common causes of nasal fractures in children?
Auto accidents (40%), sports injuries (25%), intended injuries (15%), and home injuries (10%).

2. What type of anesthesia is used most frequently during the reduction of nasal fractures?
In children over the age of 6 years, displaced nasal fractures can readily be reduced under local anesthesia using intranasal packs of cocaine and epinephrine and external block using 1% or 2% Xylocaine solution with epinephrine. Total nasal anesthesia can be achieved in this manner, but most patients benefit from the use of intravenous sedation for additional comfort.

3. What three surgical instruments are routinely used to reduce displaced nasal fractures?

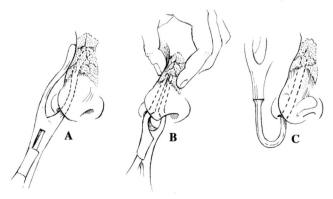

A, Walshan forceps; *B*, Asch septal forceps; and *C*, Salinger reduction instrument. (From Schultz RC (ed): Facial injuries, 3rd ed. Chicago, Year Book Medical Publishers, 1988, with permission.)

4. What are the three most common facial fractures in children?
Nasal fractures, fractures of the zygoma, and mandibular fractures.

5. What are the most serious facial fractures in children? Why?
Fractures of the upper third of the face (supraorbital and glabellar fractures) are the most serious. These fractures are frequently associated with fractures of the frontal and temporal bones, extend intracranially, and are associated with intracranial injury.

6. What are the four standard approaches to open reduction of fractures of the upper third of the face?

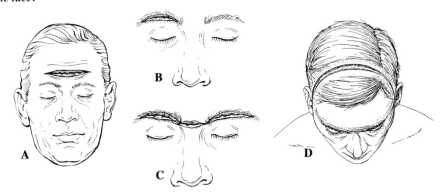

A, Through an existing forehead laceration or a transverse forehead line. *B,* Through or just above the eyebrow. *C,* A gull-wing approach through both eyebrows and across the nasal bridge. *D,* The classic bitemporal (coronal) forehead flap. (From Schultz RC (ed): Facial injuries, 3rd ed. Chicago, Year Book Medical Publishers, 1988, with permission.)

7. What is the most frequently used surgical approach to reduction of depressed fractures of the zygoma in children?

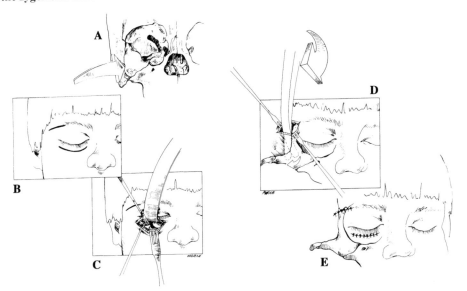

A, Force involved in causing a depressed fracture of the zygoma. *B,* Proposed incisions in the lower eyelid and lateral aspect of the brow. *C,* Incision and dissection of the periosteum covering the inferior orbital rim and exploration of the orbital floor. *D,* Elevation of the depressed zygoma through the lateral orbital incision by reversing the forces causing the depressed fracture. *E,* Restoration of the malar contour and repair of the small incisions in the lower eyelid and lateral orbital rim. (From Schultz RC (ed): Facial injuries, 3rd ed. Chicago, Year Book Medical Publishers, 1988, with permission.)

8. What are the bony structures that support the vertical dimensions of the facial bones in children?

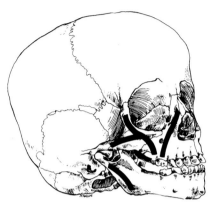

Location of the thickened bony buttresses that support the vertical and oblique dimensions of the face. (From Schultz RC (ed): Facial injuries, 3rd ed. Chicago, Year Book Medical Publishers, 1988, with permission.)

9. What are the most complex facial fractures in children?

Fractures of the middle third of the face are the most complex, because they involve not only the vertical and horizontal dimensions of the face but also the interdental occlusion.

10. How are fractures of the maxilla classified?

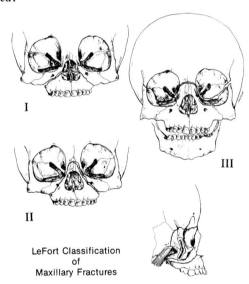

I, Transverse (Le Fort I). *II*, Pyramidal (Le Fort II). *III*, Craniofacial dysjunction (Le Fort III). (From Schultz RC (ed): Facial injuries, 3rd ed. Chicago, Year Book Medical Publishers, 1988, with permission.)

LeFort Classification of Maxillary Fractures

11. How are displaced maxillary fractures reduced? What instruments are used?

Surgeons first attempt to reduce maxillary fractures by closed means, using maxillary disimpaction forceps to disimpact and reduce the fractures (see figure, top of next page). The blades of these instruments lie within the nostril floor and along the hard palate. The blades are curved in such a fashion as to follow the anatomic contours. A rocking motion is sometimes necessary to reestablish the maxillary position both vertically and horizontally. This maneuver does not provide fixation. The various forms of fixation available to the craniomaxillofacial surgeon involve wiring mini- or micro-plates (usually titanium or Vitallium) in conjunction with the use of bone grafts.

12. Describe the most common fracture of the mandible in children.

Greenstick fractures of the mandible, particularly in the condylar region, are relatively common in children. Fractures with dislocation are seen less often but are more apt to occur in the body of the mandible.

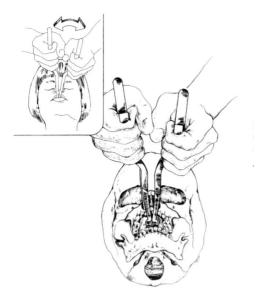

Reduction of maxillary fracture by closed means, using maxillary disimpaction forceps to disimpact and reduce the fracture. (From Schultz RC (ed): Facial injuries, 3rd ed. Chicago, Year Book Medical Publishers, 1988, with permission.)

13. What is the major growth center of the mandible?

The condyle is the major growth center. Growth occurs at the periosteal surface by apposition of bone to the superoposterior surfaces of the condylar head, contributing to downward and forward mandibular growth. During the first three years of life the condyle consists of a delicate vascular sponge with a covering of thin cortical bone. Within this period a severe blow applied to the long axis of the mandible can result in a crushing and mushrooming of this delicate structure. Crushing may cause intrascapular hemorrhage and hemarthrosis in the glenoid fossa, which in turn may lead to ankylosis of the joint and growth disturbances.

14. What type of condylar fracture is seen most often in children?

Subcondylar greenstick fractures are more common than intracapsular fractures. Subcondylar greenstick fractures are usually displaced medially and cause a temporary lateral crossbite. They sometimes go unnoticed but rarely result in permanent disability or deformity unless they are bilateral. Bilateral fracture dislocation in the condylar region with telescoping of the fragments is a serious threat to growth and normal occlusion. The treatment of choice is closed reduction and intermaxillary fixation for 3–4 weeks. Unless occlusion is otherwise unattainable, open reduction should not be attempted, because some degree of arthrosis and growth disturbance may result from the procedure.

15. Why are mandibular fractures in children so complicated to treat?

Fractures through the body of the mandible in children are complicated by mixed dentition with teeth in various stages of eruption. Radiographs can be misleading when undisplaced fractures are covered by developing tooth buds. Panorex x-ray examination may provide additional information in such cases. In the mandible filled with developing deciduous and permanent teeth, the ratio of tooth structure to alveolar bone is high. The fractures, therefore, are likely to follow the lines of developing teeth. Unerupted teeth in the line of fracture may result in loss or maleruption of the developing tooth. Fractures through the body of the mandible, particularly parasymphyseal fractures, are likely to be accompanied by a condylar fracture on the opposite side.

16. Describe the methods and problems of treating mandibular fractures in children.

During the period of mixed dentition, deciduous teeth may be exfoliating and permanent teeth just erupting. This process may interfere with the use of interdental wires and arch bars. The use of interdental wires is further complicated because primary teeth are conically shaped and thus hold wire ligatures poorly. In this situation conventional methods such as open interosseous wiring, arch bar fixation, and Blair-Ivy loops are inappropriate. A custom-made acrylic trough splint can be used instead. After reduction of the fracture, the splint is fit into position over the teeth having first incorporated hooks in the acrylic anteriorly for wire fixation. The splint can be held in position by circumandibular wiring. This latter form of treatment is particularly indicated in patients with displaced fractures of both the body and condyle, because immobilization of the body fracture is essential but immobilization of the condylar fracture is contraindicated. When intermaxillary fixation is indicated, the circumandibular wires can be ligated by wire intraorally to the piriform aperture. The bony ridge making up the piriform aperture in a child is bordered by a substantial bony lip; it is approached through a small incision in the upper labiodental sulcus over the lateral incisor tooth.

CONTROVERSY

17. Which is preferable in the management of pediatric facial fractures: closed or open reduction?
Whether to use closed or open reduction of facial fractures has always been controversial. It is well known that open reduction and direct exposure result in greater anatomic reduction of any fracture. Such treatment usually leads to internal wire or miniplate fixation. Although such treatment is intellectually and anatomically satisfying, the problems of dissection, periosteal elevation, and interference with growth centers are controversial issues. In general, closed reduction is always preferable if reasonable anatomic positioning can be achieved, thus avoiding extensive dissection. As growth continues, remodeling of bony contour may be anticipated in children. In addition, the intermaxillary occlusion in children can be more forgiving, and the use of orthodontia for a more precise occlusion becomes an option at a later age.

BIBLIOGRAPHY

1. Enlow DH: Facial Growth. Philadelphia, W.B. Saunders, 1990.
2. Kaban LB, Mulliken JB, Murray JE: Facial fractures in children: An analysis of 122 fractures in 109 patients. Plast Reconstr Surg 59:15, 1977.
3. McCoy FJ, Chandler RD, Crow ML: Facial fractures in children. Plast Reconstr Surg 37:209, 1966.
4. Panker HG, Lehman JA Jr: Management of facial fractures in children. Perspect Plast Surg 3:1, 1989.
5. Rowe NL: Fractures of the facial skeleton in children. J Oral Surg 26:505, 1968.
6. Rowe NL: Fractures of the jaws in children. J Oral Surg 27:497, 1969.
7. Schultz RC: Supraorbital and glabellar fractures. Plast Reconstr Surg 42:227, 1970.
8. Schultz RC: Nasal fractures. J Trauma 15:319, 1975.
9. Schultz RC: Pediatric facial fractures. In Kernahan DA, Thomas H (eds): Symposium on Pediatric Surgery. St. Louis, Mosby, 1982.
10. Schultz RC (ed): Facial Injuries, 3rd ed. Chicago, Year Book Medical Publishers, 1988.
11. Schultz RC: Complications of facial fractures. In Goldwyn RM (ed): Unfavorable Results in Plastic Surgery. Boston, Little, Brown, 1984.
12. Schultz RC, de Camera D: Athletic facial injuries. JAMA 252:3395, 1984.

26. FRONTAL SINUS FRACTURES

J. Gerald Minniti, M.D., and Raymond Harshbarger, M.D.

1. What are the most common causes of frontal sinus injury?
The great majority of injuries (60–80%) result from automobile accidents. Assaults run a distant second (approximately 20–30%), and the rest are due to falls from a height.

2. How common are fractures of the lower frontal bone compared with other facial bones?
Although fractures occur at the sutures between the frontal and zygomatic bones in the malar complex fracture, it is much less common for the lower frontal bone to fracture (5–15% of all maxillofacial injuries). This portion of the frontal bone represents the anterior table of the frontal sinus and is extremely thick; the forces required to fracture it are 2–3 times greater than the forces needed to fracture the zygoma, maxilla, or mandible. Such fractures typically occur with a direct blow to the glabella region or supraorbital rims; most glabellar fractures involve the frontal sinuses.

3. Is frontal sinus injury typically associated with other maxillofacial injuries?

Yes. Because of the great energy required to fracture this portion of the frontal bone, other significant maxillofacial injuries are the rule, not the exception. Frontal sinus fractures are most frequently associated with nasoorbitoethmoidal (NOE) fractures .

4. Is frontal sinus injury typically associated with other bodily injuries?

Yes. In one large series of patients who suffered frontal sinus injury, approximately 75% had other bodily injuries, 50% presented in shock, and 25% died within the first 2 weeks of presentation to the hospital.

5. Who is at a much higher risk for involvement of the frontal sinuses in craniofacial fractures—children or adults?

The frontal sinus starts as merely an ethmoidal anlage at birth and begins pneumatic expansion at age 7 years; development is complete by 18–20 years. The remnants of this embryonic connection between sinuses are the nasofrontal ducts, a bilateral structure that drains the frontal sinus from its posteromedial aspect, through the ethmoidal air cells and out to the nasal cavity, usually at the middle meatus (below the middle turbinate). The small or nonexistent sinuses in the frontal bone in children and young adolescents make the frontal bone less likely to be involved in a fracture in this area.

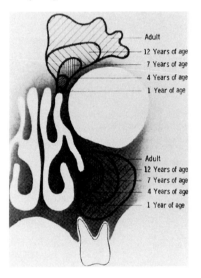

The developing frontal sinus. (From Naumann HH (ed): Head and Neck Surgery of the Paranasal Sinuses. Philadelphia, W.B. Saunders, 1980, p 357, with permission.)

6. What are the initial signs of frontal sinus fracture?

Any blow to the forehead causing lacerations, contusions, or hematoma heralds a possible injury of the frontal sinus. Such findings associated with cerebrospinal rhinorrhea or palpable bony depression of the brow evoke strong suspicion of frontal sinus involvement. (**Caution:** a visible or palpable depression is not always appreciated in the initial days after injury because of swelling or hematoma.) Supraorbital anesthesia, subconjunctival hematoma, and subcutaneous air crepitus are other associated findings. A great majority of people presenting with frontal sinus fractures have associated eye injuries. Initial signs of fracture may range from minimal to none; complications may develop years later due to lack of treatment.

7. What radiographic modality best detects and delineates the presence and extent of frontal sinus fractures?

Plain radiographs may pick up large, displaced frontal sinus fractures by depicting cortical malalignment or air fluid levels but frequently miss smaller fractures. Furthermore, involvement of the nasofrontal duct is impossible to detect with plain radiographs. The Water's view of the skull shows a well-developed frontal sinus with its scalloped superior border. CT scan has become the standard for evaluation of craniofacial trauma and is most sensitive in determining frontal sinus fractures. Small, minimally displaced fractures of the floor, septum, or anterior or posterior tables (the posterior wall and roof) are easily seen. Unfortunately, direct visualization of the ducts and possible injury to the ducts is beyond the resolution of the CT scan. Fractures of the floor that run near the midline, cross the midline, run near the posterior wall, or involve the nasoethmoidal complex are indirect evidence of ductal injury.

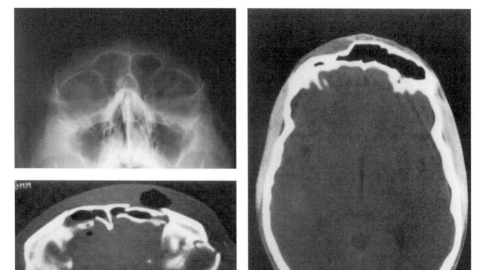

Top left, Water's view plain radiograph of the skull showing a normal, well-developed frontal sinus. *Right,* CT scan of the head showing a displaced fracture of the anterior table of the frontal sinus. *Bottom left,* CT scan of the head showing displaced fracture of both anterior and posterior tables of the frontal sinus. Note the small pneumocephaly behind the posterior table of the right frontal sinus. (From Rohrich RJ, Hollier LH: Management of frontal sinus fractures: Changing concepts. Clin Plast Surg 19:219–232, 1992, with permission.)

8. What are the anatomic boundaries of the frontal sinus?

The frontal sinus is typically a bilateral, air-filled cavity that in cross-section is triangular. A thick anterior table provides the contour of the glabella, brow, and lower forehead. A thin posterior table separates the air space from the frontal lobes in the anterior cranial fossa. The floor of the sinus overlies the ethmoidal air cells anteromedially and the orbits posterolaterally. The extent of the lateral and superior margins is variable. The supraorbital rims demarcate the lower anterior border.

9. What complications are associated with frontal sinus fractures? What causes them?

Most of the complications associated with frontal sinus injury are secondary to obstruction of the nasofrontal duct, entrapment of mucosa in the fracture lines, or dural tears. Early complications include epistaxis, cerebrospinal fluid leakage, meningitis, and intracranial hematomas. Complications occurring within weeks are sinusitis, mucoceles, cerebrospinal fluid leakage, and meningitis. Later complications (up to many years) include osteomyelitis, mucopyoceles, intracranial abscesses, and orbital abscesses. (See figure, top of next page.)

10. What is the function of the frontal sinuses?

Although the function of the paranasal sinuses is conjectural, it is certain that the frontal sinuses serve as a mechanical barrier to protect the brain. They are air-filled compressible cavities that absorb impact energy that otherwise would be imparted to brain parenchyma. Being in continuity with the upper respiratory tract, the paranasal sinuses are lined with columnar epithelium replete with cilia and mucus-secreting glands that drain through the nasofrontal ducts.

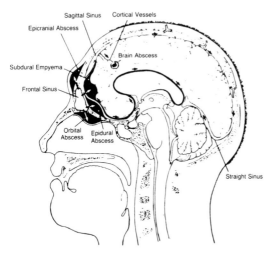

A midsagittal section through the frontal sinus depicting possible routes for spread of infection. (From Mohr RM, Nelson LR: Frontal sinus ablation for frontal osteomyelitis. Laryngoscope 92:1006–1015, 1982, with permission.)

11. Are frontal sinus fractures a surgical emergency?
Fractures of the frontal sinuses are not a surgical emergency unless other associated ophthalmologic or neurologic injuries require emergent surgery. Patients with suspected frontal sinus fracture should be placed on a broad-spectrum intravenous antibiotic as soon as possible to prevent early infectious sequelae.

CONTROVERSIES

12. What are the indications for surgery?
The status of the anterior and posterior tables and the nasofrontal ducts dictates the need for surgery. Nondisplaced anterior table fractures can be safely observed. Displaced anterior table fractures, however, may cause a cosmetic deformity and require surgery. The indications for management of minimally or nondisplaced posterior table fractures remain controversial. Most clinical studies and animal models show that such fractures can be observed if there is no cerebrospinal fluid leak or suspicion of nasofrontal duct injury. Displaced posterior table fractures greater than one wall thick merit surgical exploration and reduction. Suspicion of nasofrontal duct involvement also dictates the need for exploration.

13. What are the surgical approaches to exploration and repair of frontal sinus fractures?
Although exploration can be done in a preexisting wound or local incision, a coronal incision offers the greatest access to the whole frontal sinus as well as the ethmoidal, orbital, and intracranial regions and is the least conspicuous incision. Exploration and reduction of anterior table fractures alone usually can be performed through an osteoplastic bone flap, which is created by unroofing the remaining anterior table while keeping it in continuity with its periosteum for complete access to the sinus. Posterior table fractures that are significantly displaced in the presence of cerebrospinal fluid rhinorrhea require a frontal craniotomy in conjunction with a neurosurgical team to assess and repair dural or parenchymal injuries.

14. What methods are used for repair of frontal sinus fractures?
1. Fractures of the anterior table alone without injury to the nasofrontal duct can be simply reduced and stabilized with microplates or wires.
2. Fractures involving the nasofrontal duct rarely do well when repair of the duct is attempted with long-term Silastic catheters to promote drainage. The safest and surest procedure is obliteration of the sinus. This procedure entails removing all mucosa and inner cortex from the sinus and upper duct with a high-speed burr, then packing the duct and sinus with material that encourages scarring and ossification. Many materials have been used, including autologous tissue such as bone, muscle, fat, and periosteal flaps; foreign substances such as gelfoam (synthetic collagen); and nothing at all.

All methods have been shown to have comparable success, but cancellous iliac bone seems to have the lowest long-term complication rate.

3. Fractures that destroy the posterior table usually are associated with dural or parenchymal injury and require a craniotomy. The frontal sinus should then be cranialized. After any neurosurgical repair of the dura, the posterior table is removed, and the anterior table and floor are reduced and stabilized. The remaining mucosa and inner cortices of the sinus and duct are burred, and the duct is packed with bone. The brain is then allowed to resume its proper location in a newly enlarged anterior cranial fossa.

BIBLIOGRAPHY

1. Disa JD, Robertson BC, Metzinger SE, Manson PN: Transverse glabellar flap for obliteration/isolation of the nasofrontal duct from the anterior cranial base. Ann Plast Surg 36:453–457, 1996.
2. Hoffman HT, Krause CJ: Traumatic injuries to the frontal sinus. In Fonseca RJ, Walker RV (eds): Oral and Maxillofacial Trauma. Philadelphia, W.B. Saunders, 1991, pp 576–599.
3. Ioannides C, Freihofer HP, Friens J: Fractures of the frontal sinus: A rationale of treatment. Br J Plast Surg 46:208–214, 1993.
4. Rohrich RJ, Hollier LH: Management of frontal sinus fractures: Changing concepts. Clin Plast Surg 19:219–232, 1992.
5. Rohrich RJ, Mickel TJ: Frontal sinus obliteration: In search of the ideal autogenous material. Plast Reconstr Surg 95:580–585, 1995.
6. Wolfe SA, Johnson P: Frontal sinus injuries: Primary care and management of late complications. Plast Reconstr Surg 82:781–789, 1988

27. FRACTURES OF THE NOSE

Dennis E. Lenhart, M.D., and Rudolph F. Dolezal, M.D.

1. Which five bones make up the nose?
1. Maxilla: frontal process of maxilla
2. Frontal bone: nasal process of frontal bone
3. Nasal bones
4. Vomer: contributes to the septum
5. Ethmoid: perpendicular plate of the ethmoid also contributes to the septum

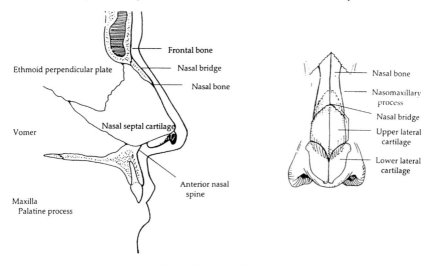

Structural anatomy of the nose.

2. A patient reports numbness of the nasal tip after a nasal fracture. Which nerve is injured?
Anterior ethmoidal nerve. The external branch of the anterior ethmoidal nerve emerges between the nasal bone and upper lateral nasal cartilage to supply sensation to the skin of the dorsum of the lower nose and tip. The innervation of the nose is as follows:
Trigeminal nerve (cranial nerve V)
  V_1 (ophthalmic division)
   • Infratrochlear nerve: skin of bridge and upper lateral area
   • Anterior ethmoidal nerve to internal and external nasal branches
  V_2 (maxillary division)
   • Infraorbital nerve: skin of lower lateral half
   • Nasopalatine nerve: nasal septum and anterior hard palate

3. Where is the rhinion? Why is it important in nasal fractures?
The nose is basically a pyramidal structure with two nasal passages separated by a midline septum. The upper third of the nose is supported by the nasal bones. The lower third of the nose is supported by the interrelationships between the paired lateral cartilages and septum; the septum is responsible for the major portion of the dorsal support. The rhinion is the junction of bony and cartilaginous nasal framework. The proximal portions of the upper lateral cartilages are overlapped by the caudal portion of the nasal bones. The distal portions of the upper lateral cartilages lie under the cephalic border of the lower lateral cartilages. The midline septum lies within the vomerine groove, solidly attached at its inferior border. Fractures at the rhinion may dislocate the upper lateral cartilage attachment under paired nasal bones, creating a saddle deformity.

4. After nasal trauma a patient develops severe nosebleed that fails to respond to nasal packing. Ligation of the maxillary branch of the external carotid artery also fails to control the bleeding, and speculum examination reveals that the source is superior to the middle turbinate. What is the likely source of the bleeding?
The blood supply to the nose is from both internal and external carotid arteries. The main blood supply is from the external carotid artery via the maxillary artery (sphenopalatine, greater palatine, and infraorbital branches). The facial artery off the external carotid also supplies the anterior portion via the superior labial branch. The external carotid artery supplies the nose inferior to the middle turbinate.
The internal carotid artery contributes via anterior and posterior ethmoidal branches and ophthalmic branches. The internal carotid contributes to the nose superior to the middle turbinate and is the likely source of bleeding in this patient. It is also the likely source of bleeding in patients with aggressive osteotomies as the chisel approaches the glabella.

5. Where do nasal bones usually fracture?
The paired nasal bones articulate in the midline with each other; they are supported laterally by the frontal processes of the maxilla and superiorly by the nasal processes of the frontal bone. The proximal nasal bones are stronger and thicker and relatively resistant to fracture. Fractures occur more commonly in the distal nasal bones, which are broader and thinner. Direct frontal blows over the nasal dorsum usually result in fracture of the thin lower half of the nasal bones. Only when the force of the blow is more severe does the fracture involve the more proximal nasal bones, possibly with extension into the frontal process of the maxilla and frontal bone.

6. Why may persistent epiphoria result after nasal fractures?
Fractured bone segments in more severe injuries may be driven into the nasolacrimal system at various levels, resulting in obstruction producing permanent epiphoria.

7. How can nasal fractures change the interorbital distance?
Violent blows to the nose result in fracture and comminution of the nasal bones, frontal processes of the maxilla, lacrimal bones, septal cartilage, and ethmoid. Displacement of these fragments and the attached medial canthal ligaments results in broadening and widening of the nasal dorsum and widening of the interorbital distance.

8. What is the role of radiographs in the diagnosis and treatment of nasal fractures?

Radiographs are of limited value in the treatment of nasal fractures. Standard facial radiographs may not clearly demonstrate nasal fractures. A nasal series that includes a 45° occipitomental view and a low-density soft tissue technique on profile usually demonstrate nasal fractures, if present. Although radiographs serve as a physical record of a nasal fracture, they are not absolutely necessary to diagnose the injury. In addition, the presence of a fracture on a radiograph is not an indication for surgery. CT scans accurately image nasal fractures but should be used only to rule out suspected injuries to the orbitoethmoid region. Therefore, the decision to operate depends on the physical findings; radiographs only assist in this process. Although radiographic documentation is recommended for medical legal reasons, physical examination of the nose determines whether surgical intervention is indicated.

9. When may nasal packing be used after nasal fracture?

After fracture reduction, intranasal packing may be used for the following purposes:
1. To control bleeding and prevent septal hematoma
2. To splint the nasal septum into position and to keep the septal mucosa approximated to the septal cartilage
3. To prevent synechiae if large areas of mucosa are abraded
4. To treat comminuted nasal fractures
5. To provide internal support for reduced bone fragments

10. What are the indications for septoplasty at the time of closed reduction?

The septum plays an important role in determining the eventual position of the nasal bones and appearance of the external nose. If septal injury is not identified and corrected, the reduction of the nasal bones may not be adequate and eventual functional and cosmetic results may be unsatisfactory. The indications for septoplasty are as follows:
1. Inability to obtain reasonable alignment by closed method
   • Dislocation of the caudal septum from the vomerine groove usually does not reduce with repositioning of the bony nasal pyramid. Manipulative reduction may be attempted; if it is unsuccessful, open reduction (septoplasty) should be performed. The procedure may involve repositioning the caudal septum or removing a small strip of cartilage along the inferior border.
   • Septal fractures may be severely displaced and irreducible. Local or limited submucosal resection of the area of septal overlap releases the locked septal displacement and provides better alignment, appearance, and function of the nose.
2. Patients with a preinjury history of nasal airway obstruction.
3. Septal deformity due to undetected or late treatment of a septal hematoma.

11. What is the treatment of a severely comminuted nasal fracture?

Severely comminuted nasal fractures usually can be reduced primarily and supported with intranasal packing and externally applied splints. External splints include standard nasal casts and splints, as well as the small padded metal splints applied to the lateral sides of the nose over the nasal bones, and are held in place by transnasal wires or nonabsorbable sutures. Packing is placed underneath the nasal bones so that the bone fragments are sandwiched between and supported by internal and external support mechanisms. The combination of internal and external splinting function helps (1) to prevent hematoma and later skin thickening, (2) to compress and narrow the splayed nasal dorsum, and (3) to conserve nasal height.

Some comminuted injuries may require open reduction with direct wiring of fragments, and some may require bone grafting. However, open reduction early after injury risks loss of bone fragments with little soft tissue attachment and should be used with caution.

12. What is the cause of the saddle deformity?

Saddle deformities result from loss of support of the nasal dorsum. They are usually composite injuries that involve both bone and cartilage, allowing the nasal bones and upper lateral cartilages to drop into the piriform aperture. Such injuries include telescoping septal fractures and fractures at the rhinion that dislocate the upper lateral cartilage attachments. Septal hematomas also may create a saddle deformity by causing necrosis of the septum and subsequent loss of dorsal support.

13. When is secondary treatment of nasal fractures indicated?

It is indicated for patients with either functional or cosmetic problems. Even with adequate reduction, late deformity may still occur, and patients should be warned. Late deformities may include a nasal hump or deviation, loss of dorsal height, septal deviation, and nasal obstruction. Most authors recommend early closed reduction followed by late correction of residual cosmetic deformities or functional problems with formal rhinoplasty.

14. Why are septal hematomas a problem?

The mucoperichondrium of the nose has a rich blood supply, and bleeding is common with nasal trauma. Hematomas of the septum are frequently bilateral, because fractures of the septal cartilage allow passage of blood from one side to the other. Blood is trapped between the mucoperichondrial sleeves and may cause two problems:

1. Untreated septal hematomas may organize and fibrose to form a thickened section of cartilage that may obstruct the nasal airway.

2. If the hematoma exerts excessive pressure, necrosis of the septum may result, ending in a septal perforation.

Loss of a significant portion of the septum is usually associated with complete collapse of the cartilaginous dorsum of the nose and results in a saddle deformity.

15. What is the treatment of an acute septal hematoma?

Septal hematomas are treated with an incision along the base or most inferior portion of the hematoma to allow dependent drainage and prevent refilling of the cavity with blood or serum. Bilateral hematomas can be treated with bilateral incisions, maintaining an intact septal cartilage, or with a unilateral incision and resection of a window of cartilage to create a bilateral communication. A light nasal packing is recommended as well as prophylactic antibiotics.

16. What are the late complications of nasal fractures?

1. Nasal airway obstruction may develop from septal hematomas, malunited fractures, or scar contractures. Septal hematomas may organize and fibrose, calcify, or chondrify, forming a thickened portion of the nasal septum that obstructs the airway. Malunited fractures of the piriform margin and scar contracture of vestibular lining also may result in obstruction.

2. Saddle deformity due to shortening and collapse

3. Dorsal hump due to periosteal reaction to hematoma

4. Nasal deviation due to malunion

5. Synechiae may form between the septum and turbinates in areas where soft tissue lacerations occur and the tissues are in contact.

6. Osteitis associated with compound fractures or infected hematomas

7. Epistaxis

8. Headaches

17. During initial examination, what should the examiner specifically look for inside the nose?

Be sure that the inside of the nose is examined and palpated so that a septal hematoma or large mucosal rent is not missed. Immediate or persistent nasal obstruction after trauma may indicate septal hematoma, which should be drained to prevent late sequelae. Large rents in the mucosa should be repaired to avoid late synechiae.

18. In adults, reduction of a nasal fracture may be performed up to 3–4 weeks after the injury. What about pediatric patients?

Nasal fractures in pediatric patients should be reduced within the first few days after injury because the rapid healing of the facial bones in children may make later reduction difficult.

19. A patient was treated for a nasal fracture with involvement of the septum 6 months ago and now presents with complaints of difficulty in breathing through his nose. What happened?

Despite adequate septal reduction after fracture, some patients have symptoms of nasal obstruction months or years after treatment because of the inherent forces in the cartilage that have a memory for relapse deformation.

20. Can a septoplasty be performed in pediatric patients in either early or late treatment of nasal-septal fractures without affecting later growth?

A septoplasty can be safely performed in pediatric patients as long as the growth center at the nasal spine of the maxilla is avoided.

BIBLIOGRAPHY

1. Colton JJ, Beekhuis GJ: Management of nasal fractures. Otolaryngol Clin North Am 19:73, 1986.
2. Fry HJH: Nasal skeletal trauma and the interlocked stresses of the nasal septal cartilage. Br J Plast Surg 20:146, 1967.
3. Harrison DH: Nasal injuries: Their pathogenesis and treatment. Br J Plast Surg 32:67, 1979.
4. Hollinshead WH: Anatomy for Surgeons, 3rd ed. New York, Harper & Row, 1982.
5. Illum P: Long-term results after treatment of nasal fractures. J Laryngol Otol 100:273, 1986.
6. McCarthy JG: Plastic Surgery. Philadelphia, W.B. Saunders, 1990.
7. Mayell MJ: Nasal fractures. Their occurrence, management, and some late results. J R Coll Surg Edin 18:31, 1973.
8. Murray JB, Maran AG, Mackenzie IJ, Raab G: Open versus closed reduction of the fractured nose. Arch Otolaryngol 110:797, 1984.
9. Pollock RA: Nasal trauma: Pathomechanics and surgical management of acute injuries. Clin Plast Surg 19:133, 1992.

28. FRACTURES OF THE ORBIT

Jeffrey Weinzweig, M.D., and Scott P. Bartlett, M.D.

ANATOMY

1. The orbit is composed of how many bones?

Seven. The zygoma, lesser and greater wings of the sphenoid, frontal bone, ethmoid bone, lacrimal bone, palatine bone, and maxilla articulate to form each orbit. The paired structures are separated in the midline by the nasal bones and interorbital space.

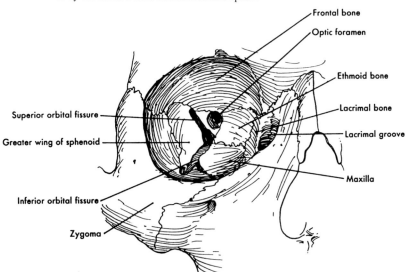

Anatomy of the orbit. (From Whitaker LA, Bartlett SP: Craniofacial anomalies. In Jurkiewicz MJ, Krizek TJ, Mathes SJ, Ariyan S (eds): Plastic Surgery: Principles and Practice. St. Louis, Mosby, 1990, p 104, with permission.)

2. What is the relationship between the anterior cranial fossa and the orbit?
The orbits are situated immediately below the floor of the anterior cranial fossa, the lateral portion of which is formed by the roof of the orbits. The medial portion of the anterior cranial fossa is formed by the roof of each ethmoid sinus laterally and by the cribriform plate medially.

3. Which bony structures surround the orbit and protect its contents?
Superiorly: the supraorbital rim is formed by the supraorbital arch of the frontal bone.
Inferiorly: the thick infraorbital rim is formed by the zygoma laterally and the maxilla medially.
Medially: the nasal spine of the frontal bone and the frontal process of the maxilla constitute the anteromedial orbital wall.
Laterally: the frontal process of the zygoma and the zygomatic process of the frontal bone constitute the lateral orbital rim.

4. The orbital walls are composed of which bones?
The **roof** is composed mainly of the orbital plate of the frontal bone. Posteriorly it receives a minor contribution from the lesser wing of the sphenoid.
The **orbital floor** is composed of the orbital plate of the maxilla, the zygomatic bone anterolaterally, and the orbital process of the palatine bone posteriorly. The orbital floor is equivalent to the roof of the maxillary sinus.
The **lateral wall** is formed primarily by the orbital surface of the zygomatic bone and the greater wing of the sphenoid bone. The sphenoid portion of the lateral wall is separated from the roof by the superior orbital fissure and from the floor by the inferior orbital fissure.
The **medial wall** is quadrangular in shape and composed of four bones: (1) the ethmoid bone centrally; (2) the frontal bone superoanteriorly; (3) the lacrimal bone inferoanteriorly; and (4) the sphenoid bone posteriorly. The medial wall is quite thin; the ethmoidal portion has been termed the lamina papyracea (paper-like), which is the largest component of the medial wall.

5. Which is the only bone that exists entirely within the orbital confines?
The lacrimal bone.

6. Which nerve traverses the floor of the orbit?
The infraorbital nerve. The infraorbital groove courses forward from the inferior orbital fissure. Anteriorly, the groove becomes a canal within the maxilla, finally forming the infraorbital foramen on the anterior surface of the maxilla. The groove and canal transmit the infraorbital nerve and artery.

7. The bony orbit is cylindrical. True or false?
False. It is described as conical or pyramidally shaped, but neither term is completely accurate. The widest diameter of the orbit is located just behind the orbital rim approximately 1.5 cm within the orbital cavity. From this point posteriorly, the orbit narrows dramatically in its middle and posterior thirds. The orbital rim is an elliptically shaped structure, whereas the orbit immediately behind the rim is more circular in configuration. The floor of the orbit has no sharp demarcation with the medial wall but proceeds into the wall by tilting upward in its medial aspect at a 45° angle. The medial wall has a quadrangular rather than a triangular configuration.

8. Which bone is the keystone of the orbit?
The sphenoid bone. All neurovascular structures to the orbit pass through this bone.

9. How deep is the orbit?
Orbital depth measured to the optic strut (the bone between the optic foramen and superior orbital fissure) varies from 45–55 mm. At the entrance orbital height measures approximately 35 mm and orbital width approximately 40 mm.

10. Where is the optic foramen located? What about the optic canal?
The **optic foramen** is situated medial to the superior orbital fissure within the substance of the lesser wing of the sphenoid. It is found at the junction of the lateral and medial walls of the orbit in its far posterior position. It is close to the posterior portion of the ethmoid sinus, not at the true apex

of the orbit. The posterior ethmoidal vessels are found within 5 mm of the optic nerve. The optic nerve is usually located 40–45 mm behind the infraorbital rim.

The **optic canal** is 4–10 mm in length. The optic nerve and ophthalmic artery pass through the optic canal from an intracranial to an intraorbital position. The canal is formed medially by the body of the sphenoid and laterally by the lesser wing. The bony optic canal forms a tight sheath around the optic nerve; fractures with swelling predispose to vascular compression of the nerve in the canal.

11. Where is the superior orbital fissure located? Which structures pass through it?

The superior orbital fissure is a 22-mm cleft that runs outward, forward, and upward from the apex of the orbit. This fissure, which separates the greater and lesser wings of the sphenoid and lies between the optic foramen and the foramen rotundum, provides passage to the three motor nerves to the extraocular muscles of the orbit—the oculomotor nerve (CN III), trochlear nerve (CN IV), and abducens nerve (CN VI). The ophthalmic division of the trigeminal nerve (CN V_1) also enters the orbit through this fissure.

12. Nothing passes through the inferior orbital fissure. True or false?

False. The inferior orbital fissure, which separates the greater sphenoid wing portion of the lateral wall from the floor, permits passage of (1) the maxillary division of the trigeminal nerve (CN V_2) and its branches (including the infraorbital nerve); (2) the infraorbital artery; (3) branches of the sphenopalatine ganglion; and (4) branches of the inferior ophthalmic vein to the pterygoid plexus.

13. What is Tenon's capsule?

Tenon's capsule is a fascial structure that subdivides the orbital cavity into two halves—an anterior (or precapsular) segment and a posterior (or retrocapsular) segment. The ocular globe occupies only the anterior half of the orbital cavity. The posterior half of the orbital cavity is filled with fat, muscles, vessels, and nerves that supply the ocular globe and extraocular muscles and provide sensation to the soft tissue surrounding the orbit.

14. What is the anulus of Zinn?

The anulus of Zinn, or common tendinous ring, is the fibrous thickening of the periosteum from which the recti muscles originate.

15. What are the functions of the extraocular muscles?

Lateral rectus muscle: abduction
Medial rectus muscle: adduction
Inferior rectus muscle: depression, adduction, and extorsion (extorsion—the superior pole of globe moves laterally)
Superior rectus muscle: elevation, adduction, and intorsion (intorsion—the superior pole of the globe moves medially)
Superior oblique muscle: depression, abduction, and intorsion
Inferior oblique muscle: elevation, abduction, and extorsion

16. Why is the medial canthal tendon so important?

The medial canthal tendon is a complex of fascial support mechanisms that includes anterior, posterior, and vertical components. They insert in the frontal process of the maxilla (the medial orbital margin) from the anterior lacrimal crest to the nasal bone. The orbicularis oculi muscle originates from the medial canthal tendon. In addition, branches of the canthal tendon divide to extend through the upper and lower eyelids and to attach to the medial margin of the tarsal plates. Therefore, release of this tendon, as with fractures of the medial orbital wall, may result in telecanthus (an increase in the distance between the medial canthi, which may create the illusion of hypertelorism when bilateral).

17. Distinguish between intraconal and extraconal fat. Which is important for globe support?

The orbital fat can be divided into anterior and posterior portions. The anterior, extraocular fat is largely **extraconal**, which means that it exists outside the muscle cone. Posteriorly, only fine fascial communications separate the extraconal from the intraconal fat compartments. **Intraconal** fat constitutes three-fourths of the fat in the posterior orbit and may be displaced outside the muscle cone, contributing to a loss of globe support from loss of soft tissue volume. The fat on the anterior portion of the orbital floor is extraconal and does not contribute to globe support.

PATHOLOGY

18. What physical findings suggest an orbital fracture?

Periorbital edema, ecchymosis, and subconjunctival hemorrhage are seen with most orbital fractures. Fractures of the anterior orbit are characterized by palpable bony step-offs and sensory nerve disturbances; fractures of the middle orbit by changes in the position of the globe, oculomotor dysfunction, and diplopia; and fractures of the posterior orbit by visual and oculomotor disturbances.

19. What is a Marcus Gunn pupil?

With lesions involving the retina or optic nerve back to the chiasm, a light shone in the unaffected eye produces normal constriction of the pupils of both eyes (consensual response). However, a light shone in the affected eye produces a paradoxical dilation rather than constriction of the affected pupil. This afferent pupillary defect is referred to as a Marcus Gunn pupil. Such lesions, as well as globe rupture, lens dislocation, and vitreous hemorrhage, are uncommon but may accompany orbital fractures and underscore the need for an ophthalmologic evaluation in all cases of orbital fractures upon presentation.

20. What is the best radiographic study for diagnosis of an orbital fracture?

CT scan. Axial scans at 3-mm intervals demonstrate abnormalities of the medial and lateral walls and identify fractures of the nasoethmoidal region. Coronal scans, obtained by direct or reformatted images, demonstrate fractures of the orbital floor, roof, and interorbital space. In the absence of a CT scan, a Waters view is often sufficient to diagnose an orbital floor fracture; it allows visualization of blood in the maxillary sinus as well as orbital floor depression and herniation of orbital contents. Other findings that may include disruption of the medial wall and separation of the zygomaticofrontal (Z-F) suture.

21. What is the most common orbital fracture?

Zygomaticoorbital or malar complex fractures are the most common. Moderately displaced zygomatic injuries are frequently associated with fractures of the lateral orbital wall with comminution of the orbital floor and infraorbital rim.

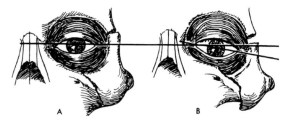

A   B

Fractures of the zygoma. *A*, Nondisplaced: the lateral canthus maintains normal position. *B*, Displacement of the zygoma and orbital floor: downward displacement of the globe and lateral canthus results. (From McCarthy JG (ed): Plastic Surgery. Philadelphia, W.B. Saunders, 1990, p 995, with permission.)

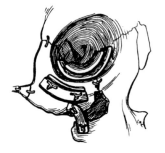

Zygomatic fractures may require orbital floor reconstruction, depending on the extent of the fracture. (From Smith JW, Aston SJ (eds): Grabb and Smith's Plastic Surgery, 4th ed. Boston, Little, Brown, 1991, p 364, with permission.)

22. What is the most common site of an isolated intraorbital fracture?

The most frequent intraorbital fracture involves the orbital floor just medial to the infraorbital canal and is usually confined to the medial portion of the floor and the lower portion of the medial orbital wall. Depressed fractures involving this portion of the orbit may allow the orbital soft tissue to be displaced into the maxillary and ethmoid sinuses, effectively increasing orbital volume.

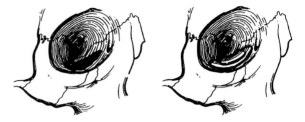

Orbital blow-out fracture (*left*). Orbital floor reconstruction with bone graft (*right*). (From Smith JW, Aston SJ (eds): Grabb and Smith's Plastic Surgery, 4th ed. Boston, Little, Brown, 1991, p 371, with permission.)

23. What is a "blow-out" fracture? What is the responsible mechanism?

A blow-out fracture is caused by a traumatic force applied to the orbital rim or globe and usually results in a sudden increase in intraorbital pressure. The incompressible intraorbital contents are displaced posteriorly, and the traumatic force is transmitted to the thin orbital floor and medial orbital wall, which are the first to fracture. The mechanism usually involves direct force transfer from the orbital rim to the orbital floor and medial wall, resulting in buckling and fracture. Force transfer through the globe occurs less frequently; otherwise, global injuries would accompany orbital fractures more often. Intraorbital contents often herniate through the fractured site and may become incarcerated by the edges of the fracture or by a "trapdoor" displacement of a segment of thin orbital bone.

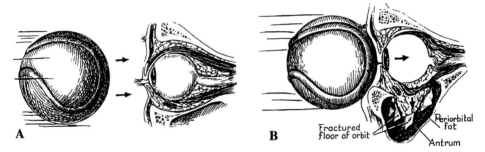

Mechanism of a blow-out fracture. A traumatic force applied to the rim or globe produces a fracture of the orbital floor with entrapment of orbital soft tissue contents. The inferior oblique and inferior rectus muscles and adjacent fat are often involved. (From Converse JM, Smith B: Enophthalmos and diplopia in fractures of the orbital floor. Br J Plast Surg 9:265, 1957, with permission.)

24. What is the difference between pure and impure blow-out fractures?

Pure blow-out fractures involve the thin areas of the orbital floor, medial wall, and lateral wall. The orbital rim, however, remains intact. **Impure blow-out fractures** are associated with fracture of the adjacent facial bones. The thick orbital rim is also fractured; its backward displacement causes comminution of the orbital floor. Transmission of the traumatic force to the orbital contents produces a superimposed blow-out fracture.

25. Hypoesthesia or anesthesia in the distribution of which nerve is seen in 90–95% of orbital floor fractures?

The infraorbital nerve.

26. How can entrapment of orbital contents be diagnosed in a comatose patient?

Diagnosis is made by performing a forced duction test. The insertion of a rectus muscle onto the ocular globe is grasped with a forceps approximately 7 mm from the limbus. The globe is then gently rotated in all four directions and any restriction noted. The inferior rectus muscle is usually used, although the superior, medial or lateral recti muscles may be used as well.

27. What are the goals of surgical treatment of orbital fractures?
The goals of surgical treatment are (1) reduction/release of any herniated or entrapped orbital contents and (2) restoration of normal orbital architecture. Intraorbital soft tissue contents must be freed from any fracture sites. Range of motion of the ocular globe after freeing of the orbital soft tissue should be confirmed by an intraoperative forced duction test. This test should be performed before the entrapped tissue is released, after release, and again after insertion of any material used to reconstruct the orbital floor.

28. What are the principles of orbital fracture management?
The principles of orbital fracture management are (1) stabilization and reconstruction of the orbital ring (medial orbital, lateral orbital, supraorbital, and infraorbital rims); (2) reconstruction of orbital floor defects; and (3) repair and redraping of orbital soft tissue, including the medial and lateral canthal tendons. Sufficient exposure of all fracture sites is necessary to permit adequate reduction and fixation of all fracture fragments. This goal is achieved either by interosseous wiring or microplate/miniplate and screw fixation of the fractures with or without the need for bone grafting. The integrity of the orbital floor is restored either with bone grafts or inorganic implants. The purpose of the orbital floor insert, whether a bone graft or an inorganic implant, is to reestablish the size of the orbital cavity. Occasionally, the depressed segment of orbital floor can be retrieved and, if of sufficient size and appropriate configuration, rotated 90° to provide coverage of the floor defect. Any material used for floor reconstruction should be anchored to prevent displacement or extrusion of the material. Medial and/or lateral canthopexies are performed, when necessary, to restore proper suspension of the orbital globe.

29. What materials are used to reconstruct the orbital floor?
- Autogenous bone grafts (split calvarial, iliac, or split rib) (see figures in questions 21 and 22)
- Allogenic bone grafts (radiated cadaveric tibia)
- Inorganic alloplastic materials (e.g, Medpor, Silastic, Vitallium, stainless steel, Teflon, Supramid, or titanium implants).

30. What are the most frequent sequelae of inadequately treated fractures of the orbital floor?
Diplopia and enophthalmos.

31. What is the principal mechanism responsible for post-traumatic enophthalmos?
Displacement of a relatively constant volume of orbital soft tissue into an enlarged bony orbital volume. Fat atrophy does not appear to play an etiopathogenic role. Enophthalmos in excess of 5 mm results in a noticeable deformity. Correction of enophthalmos involves correction of orbital cavity size and restoration of the shape of its walls to their original configuration.

32. What is diplopia? Is it always an indication for surgery?
Diplopia is a fancy term for double vision and is *rarely* an indication for surgery. It is usually transient and, if present only at the extremes of gaze rather than within a functional field of vision, is not a critical symptom. It is commonly attributed to hematoma or edema that causes muscular imbalance by elevating the ocular globe or to injury of the extraocular musculature and temporary effects on the oculorotary mechanism.

33. What are the major surgical indications for orbital fracture repair?
Muscle entrapment and increased orbital volume. Entrapment, which is confirmed by a forced duction test and CT scan demonstrating soft tissue incarceration, warrants early exploration. Increased orbital volume secondary to significant fractures that have an area > 2 cm² of displaced orbital wall may result in globe displacement (enophthalmos and globe dystopia) and also necessitates fracture repair. Enophthalmos secondary to a floor defect is managed with a lower lid or transconjunctival incision. Enophthalmos secondary to expansion of the medial wall can be approached from the floor if the enlargement is in the lower half of the medial orbital wall. Otherwise, a coronal incision is warranted. Enophthalmos secondary to lateral wall involvement usually requires a coronal incision.

34. What complications are associated with fractures of the orbital roof?

Fractures of the orbital roof usually involve the supraorbital ridge, frontal bone, and frontal sinus and frequently reduce orbital volume. Globe displacement occurs in an inferolateral direction and may result in proptosis. The trochlea of the superior oblique muscle is often damaged because of its proximity with the surface of the roof, resulting in transitory diplopia. CN VI may be traumatized with orbital roof fractures, resulting in paralysis of the lateral rectus muscle and limitation of ocular abduction. Additional complications include dural tears, anterior cranial base injuries, cerebrospinal fluid leaks, cerebral herniation, and pulsatile exophthalmos.

35. Which fracture may result in an antimongoloid slant of the palpebral fissure? Why?

Inferoposterior displacement of a malar complex or zygoma fracture causes an antimongoloid slant. This slant results from the inferior displacement of the lateral canthal tendon, which moves with the fractured lateral orbital wall.

36. How is the orbital floor approached surgically?

There are multiple approaches to the orbit. The **bicoronal incision**, popularized by Tessier, provides wide access to the orbits, nose, and zygomas as well as the cranium. It is the preferred incision for extensive surgery, especially when the orbital roof must be visualized and the orbital contents must be mobilized 360°.

The **subciliary lower eyelid incision** begins approximately 2–3 mm below the lash line and extends from the punctum to 8–10 mm lateral to the lateral canthus (see top figure, next page). This incision is made through the skin, and the dissection is continued to the inferior edge of the tarsus. A skin-muscle flap is then raised from the tarsus; the septum orbitale is followed below the tarsus until the rim of the orbit is reached. An incision is made through the periosteum on the anterior aspect of the orbital rim to avoid damaging the septum, which inserts on the anterolateral portion of the orbit at the recess of Eisler. The periosteum is then elevated from the rim and orbital floor. This approach allows easy access to the lateral and medial walls and floor of the orbit.

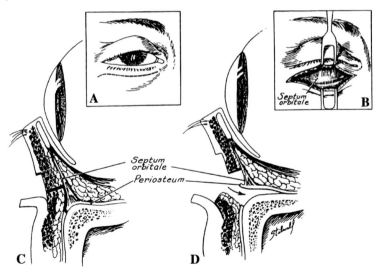

The subciliary eyelid incision. *A*, Incision design. *B*, Exposure of the septum orbitale. *C*, Sagittal section demonstrating the skin incision extended through the orbicularis oculi muscle and the path of dissection over the septum orbitale to the orbital rim. *D*, Periosteum of the orbit (periorbita) is elevated from the orbital floor. (From Converse JM, Cole JG, Smith B: Late treatment of blowout fractures of the floor of the orbit. A case report. Plast Reconstr Surg 28:183, 1961, with permission.)

The **mid-lid incision** is performed within the lid crease, 4–5 mm below the ciliary margin. This incision avoids many of the problems associated with the subciliary incision.

The **transconjunctival incision**, advocated by Tessier for correction of craniofacial anomalies and by Converse for posttraumatic deformities, is made through the conjunctiva, capsulopalpebral fascia (lid retractors), and periosteum to the orbital rim. This incision directly exposes the orbital fat without incising the septum orbitale and avoids an external scar. When combined with a lateral canthotomy incision, this approach provides exposure of all four walls of the orbit.

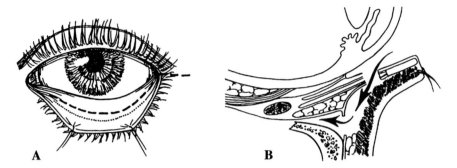

The transconjunctival incision combined with a lateral canthotomy. *A,* Incision design. *B,* Sagittal section demonstrating the incision through the conjunctiva, capsulopalpebral fascia, and periosteum to the orbital rim. The preseptal approach is used to prevent herniation of periorbital fat into the operative field. (From Manson PN, Markowitz BL: Fractures of the orbit and nasoethmoidal bones. In Cohen M (ed): Mastery of Plastic and Reconstructive Surgery. Boston, Little, Brown, 1994, p 1147, with permission.)

The **lateral brow incision** provides exposure of the frontozygomatic suture and part of the lateral wall and roof of the orbit.

Medial canthal incisions are usually made in a curvilinear direction. They provide excellent exposure of the medial canthus, medial wall of the orbit, and nasal bones.

The **intraoral approach** provides excellent exposure of the inferior orbital rim, maxilla, and zygoma.

37. Which incision has the greatest propensity for complications such as scleral show or ectropion?

The subciliary incision. Scleral show and ectropion are frequent sequelae after lower lid surgery due to lid retraction. Many of these conditions improve with time, but permanent scarring within the lower eyelid may result in permanent deformity that requires release of scar tissue and even grafting.

38. Is the Caldwell-Luc approach to the orbital floor a wise one?

Absolutely not. Reduction of orbital contents through a Caldwell-Luc transmaxillary approach is potentially dangerous because it is a blind approach. Complete reduction of herniated orbital contents is therefore not ensured, and thorough exploration of the orbital floor is not possible.

39. What is the superior orbital fissure syndrome?

Fractures involving the superior orbital fissure produce a combination of cranial nerve palsies known as the superior orbital fissure syndrome. The syndrome consists of ptosis of the eyelid, proptosis of the globe, paralysis of cranial nerves III, IV, and VI, and anesthesia in the distribution of the first (ophthalmic) division of the trigeminal nerve (CN V_1). Sensory disturbances of the forehead, upper eyelid, conjunctiva, cornea, and sclera are seen.

40. What is the orbital apex syndrome?

If blindness occurs in combination with the superior orbital fissure syndrome, the condition is referred to as the orbital apex syndrome.

41. What is an NOE fracture?

Medial orbital wall fractures often accompany orbital floor fractures and are sometimes an undiagnosed cause of residual postoperative enophthalmos. More severe medial orbital wall fractures usually involve the naso-ethmoidal structures and thus are referred to as nasoethmoidal-orbital fractures or nasoorbital-ethmoidal fractures—or simply NOE fractures.

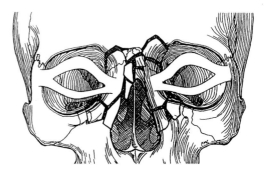

Bilateral comminuted nasoethmoidal-orbital fractures. Note displacement of the medial orbital wall fragments containing the attachment of the medial canthal tendons. (From Manson PN, Markowitz BL: Fractures of the orbit and nasoethmoidal bones. In Cohen M (ed): Mastery of Plastic and Reconstructive Surgery. Boston, Little, Brown, 1994, p 1150, with permission.)

42. What classic clinical findings are associated with an NOE fracture?

Telecanthus and a saddle nose deformity. NOE fractures consist of injury to one or both frontal processes of the maxilla and nose. The frontal process of the maxilla contains the attachment of the medial canthal ligament. If the medial orbital rim and its canthal attachment are dislocated, the result is telecanthus, which is an increase in the distance between the medial canthi (intercanthal distance). In contrast to orbital hypertelorism, the orbit itself is not displaced laterally. The pseudo-hyperteloric appearance of the orbits is accentuated by the flattening and widening of the bony dorsum of the nose. As a result, the eyes appear far apart. The most reliable clinical sign of an NOE fracture is movement of the frontal process of the maxilla on direct finger pressure over the medial canthal ligament.

43. How can the intercanthal distance be preserved after an NOE fracture?

The most important step in the management of an NOE fracture is performance of a transnasal canthopexy. The segment of bone to which the medial canthal tendon is attached is mobilized so that drill holes may be placed behind the canthal ligament for transnasal wires. Two parallel holes are placed in the most superior and posterior aspects of the bone fragment, above and posterior to the lacrimal fossa. Interosseous wires are used to link the medial orbital rim with the frontal bone, nasal bones, and inferior orbital rim. The bone fragments attached to the medial canthal ligament are then reduced and secured to the surrounding bone by interosseous wires. Two 26-gauge wires are then passed through the canthal ligament fragment from one frontal process to the other and tightened. This procedure preserves the intercanthal distance and corrects the telecanthus.

44. What is the surgical approach to the treatment of an NOE fracture?

Three incisions—coronal, subciliary or mid-lid, and maxillary gingivobuccal sulcus—are usually necessary to expose adequately the nasoethmoidal-orbital region. NOE fractures are complex and require specific reduction and fixation techniques based on the pattern and comminution of the fracture. A combination of interfragmentary wiring and plate and screw fixation is necessary to reconstruct the medial orbital wall, inferior orbital rim, nasofrontal junction, nasomaxillary buttress, and nasal bones. Despite interfragmentary wiring, the nasal dorsum almost always requires augmentation with a cantilever bone graft.

BIBLIOGRAPHY

1. Gruss JS: Naso-ethmoid-orbital fractures: Classification and role of primary bone grafting. Plast Reconstr Surg 75:303, 1985.
2. Jackson IT: Classification and treatment of orbito-zygomatic and orbito-ethmoid fractures: The place of bone grafting and plate fixation. Clin Plast Surg 16:77–91, 1989.
3. Kawamoto HK: Late post-traumatic enophthalmos: A correctable deformity? Plast Reconstr Surg 69:423–432, 1992.
4. Manson PN: Facial fractures. In Aston SJ, Beasley RW, Thorne CHM (eds): Grabb and Smith's Plastic Surgery, 5th ed. Philadelphia, Lippincott-Raven, 1997, pp 383–412.
5. Manson PN: Facial injuries. In McCarthy JG (ed): Plastic Surgery. Philadelphia, W.B. Saunders, 1990, pp 1043–1118.
6. Manson PN, Iliff N: Management of blow out fractures of the orbital floor. Surg Ophthal 35:280–292, 1991.

156

7. Markowitz B, Manson P, Sargent L, et al: Management of the medial canthal ligament in nasoethmoidal orbital fractures. Plast Reconstr Surg 87:843–853, 1991.
8. McCarthy JG, Jelks GW, Valauri AJ, et al: The orbit and zygoma. In McCarthy JG (ed): Plastic Surgery.
   Philadelphia, W.B. Saunders, 1990, pp 1574–1670.
9. Yaremchuk M: Changing concepts in the management of secondary orbital deformities. Clin Plast Surg
   19:113–124, 1992.
10. Whitaker L, Yaremchuk M: Secondary reconstruction of post-traumatic orbital deformities. Ann Plast Surg
    25:440–449, 1990.
11. Zide BM, Jelks GW: Surgical Anatomy of the Orbit. New York, Raven Press, 1985.

29. FRACTURES OF THE ZYGOMA

Gregory H. Pastrick, M.D., and Jack R. Bevivino, M.D.

1. Describe the anatomy of the zygoma.

The zygoma is a pyramidal bone of the midface. Its anterior convexity gives prominence to the malar eminence of the cheek, and its posterior concavity helps to form the temporal fossa. The zygoma forms the superolateral and superoanterior portions of the maxillary sinus. It articulates with the frontal, temporal, maxillary, and sphenoid bones. Superolaterally, the frontal process of the zygoma articulates with the zygomatic process of the frontal bone and forms the lateral orbital wall along with its intraorbital articulation with the sphenoid bone. The temporal process of the zygoma posterolaterally articulates with the zygomatic process of the temporal bone to create the zygomatic arch. The broad articulation inferiorly and medially with the maxilla forms the zygomaticomaxillary (ZM) buttress, the major buttressing structure between the midface and the cranium, as well as the infraorbital rim and lateral part of the orbital floor.

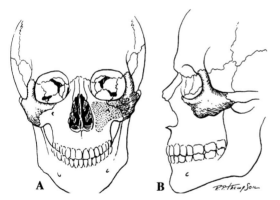

The zygoma and its articulating bones. *A,* The zygoma articulates with the frontal, sphenoid, maxillary, and temporal bones. The dots show the portion of the zygoma and the maxilla occupied by the maxillary sinus. *B,* Lateral view of the zygoma. (From Manson PN: Facial Injuries. In McCarthy JG (ed): Plastic Surgery. Philadelphia, W.B. Saunders, 1990, with permission.)

2. What is the pattern of the typical zygomatic or malar complex fracture?

Because of natural points of structural weakness in the area of the zygoma, a reproducible pattern of zygomatic complex fractures frequently occurs. Typically, the fracture line travels through the zygomaticofrontal (ZF) region and into the orbit at the zygomaticosphenoidal suture to the inferior orbital fissure. Anterior to the fissure, the fracture involves only the maxilla, where it traverses the orbital floor and infraorbital rim, goes through the infraorbital foramen, and continues inferiorly through the zygomaticomaxillary buttress. Posterior to the buttress, yet still in continuity, the lateral wall of the maxillary sinus is fractured. In addition, the zygomatic arch is fractured at its weakest point, about 1.5 cm posterior to the zygomaticotemporal suture, in the zygomatic process of the temporal bone. This typical fracture pattern is commonly encountered, but great variety exists depending on factors such as the direction and magnitude of the force, the density of the adjacent bones, and the amount of soft tissue covering the zygoma. Frequently, only isolated arch fractures occur.

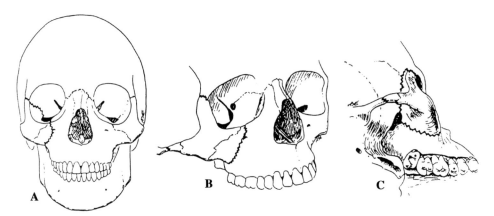

Common fracture pattern in zygomatic complex injury. *A*, Frontal view of skull showing fracture medial to zygomaticomaxillary suture and along zygomaticosphenoid suture within orbit. *B*, Oblique frontal view of skull showing fractures through frontozygomatic suture and posterior to zygomaticotemporal suture. *C*, Temporal view of skull showing fractures extending from the inferior orbital fissure both superiorly through the zygomaticosphenoid suture and inferiorly through the zygomatic buttress of the maxilla. (From Ellis E III: Fractures of the zygomatic complex and arch. In Fonseca RJ, Walker RV (eds): Oral and Maxillofacial Trauma. Philadelphia, W.B. Saunders, 1991, with permission.)

3. Why is the commonly used term *tripod fracture* a misnomer for zygomatic complex fractures?
Tripod fracture has been used to consolidate the typical fracture pattern of the zygomatic complex into a concise descriptive term that reflects the configuration of the complex as it relates to adjacent bones. It wrongly implies, however, that three legs, or processes, are involved. In reality the usual zygomatic complex fracture involves four major processes: the zygomaticofrontal region, infraorbital rim, zygomaticomaxillary buttress, and zygomatic arch.

4. How are zygomatic fractures classified?
Many classification systems can be found in the literature. Most are based on the anatomic position of the displaced bone as seen radiographically and are designed to guide the surgeon in treatment. The most commonly quoted classification system is that of Knight and North.

Classification of Malar Fractures

Undisplaced	Group I (7 cases) = 6%
Displaced	
Arch	Group II (12 cases) = 10%
Body	
Simple	
Depression without rotation	Group III (39 cases) = 33%
Depression with medial rotation	Group IV (24 cases) = 11%
Depression with lateral rotation	Group V (26 cases) = 22%
Complex	Group VI (23 cases) = 18%

From Knight JS, North JF: The classification of malar fractures: An analysis of displacement as a guide to treatment. Br J Plast Surg 13:325–339, with permission.

5. What are the signs and symptoms of zygomatic fractures?
- Pain
- Diplopia
- Periorbital ecchymosis and edema
- Subconjunctival ecchymosis
- Unilateral epistaxis due to tearing of the ipsilateral maxillary sinus mucosa
- Subcutaneous emphysema
- Flattening of the malar prominence or over the zygomatic arch
- Palpable bony step-off at the ZF suture, infraorbital rim, and ZM buttress

- Gingival buccal sulcus ecchymosis or hematoma
- Antimongoloid slant of the lateral palpebral fissure due to downward displacement of the attachment of the lateral palpebral ligament on Whitnall's tubercle of the zygoma
- Orbital dystopia from downward displacement of Lockwood's ligament
- Lower lid retraction from downward displacement of the orbital septum
- Enophthalmos
- Upward gaze lag secondary to entrapment of the orbital contents, including the inferior rectus muscle
- Infraorbital nerve sensory disturbance
- Trismus (see question 6)

The above list describes the spectrum of symptoms and physical findings due to fractures of the zygoma, yet in any patient only some of them may be found.

6. What is the mechanism of trismus caused by fracture of the zygoma?

The coronoid process of the mandible is closely associated anatomically with the zygoma. Displaced fractures of the body or arch of the zygoma may impinge on the coronoid process, thereby interfering with its movement. Trismus, however, also may be secondary to edema or muscle spasm of the temporalis or masseter muscles.

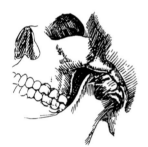 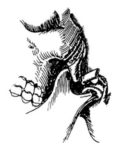

Fracture of the zygomatic arch with medial displacement against the coronoid process of the mandible, limiting mandibular motion. (From Manson PN: Facial injuries. In McCarthy JG (ed): Plastic Surgery. Philadelphia, W.B. Saunders, 1990, with permission.)

7. Which diagnostic images provide the most information in evaluating and formulating a treatment plan for zygomatic fractures?

A CT scan shows in detail the location of the fractures, displacement of the bones, and status of the soft tissues. Axial views are best to evaluate the lateral orbital wall and zygomatic arch, whereas coronal views are necessary to determine the extent of orbital floor involvement. Posteroanterior oblique (Waters) and submental vertex ("jughandle") roentgenograms are the two most useful plain films for evaluating these fractures, but CT scan is currently the diagnostic imaging tool preferred by most surgeons.

8. Which zygoma fractures require surgical intervention?

Surgical intervention should be based on both clinical and radiographic findings. Fractures that display significant displacement and/or instability require operative intervention to correct immediate problems or to prevent long-term sequelae such as facial dysmorphism, enophthalmos, or orbital dystopia. The long-term sequelae are much more difficult to correct once fracture healing is complete. Studies show that 9–50% of zygomatic fractures do not require operative treatment.

9. When is the optimal time to operate on zygomatic fractures?

There are important points to keep in mind in deciding when to operate on zygomatic fractures. Zygomatic fractures are not emergencies, and any associated life-threatening injuries must be addressed first. Initially soft tissue edema makes open reduction more difficult and may compromise the final result, but delay in intervention beyond the time for soft tissue fibrosis and fracture healing to occur (3–4 weeks) makes simple repositioning of the bones difficult. Ideally, open reduction should be performed on an otherwise uninjured patient before the onset of edema, but in reality this rarely occurs. Waiting several days for edema to resolve and, in the case of multitrauma, for the patient to stabilize does not compromise the surgical outcome and often results in better surgical results.

10. How does one determine that a displaced, noncomminuted zygomatic complex fracture has been properly reduced?

Of the four major processes (see question 3), at least three must be aligned under direct vision to ensure anatomic reduction of the entire complex. Integrity of the orbital floor also must be ascertained.

11. How are unstable zygomatic complex fractures stabilized after reduction?

Currently plate and screw fixation is used most frequently and is applied at the fractures at the ZF suture, infraorbital rim, and ZM buttress. Similarly, interfragment wiring may be used. Even stainless steel pins passed percutaneously from the zygoma to the maxilla or contralateral zygoma have been used for fixation.

12. Which zygoma fractures are unstable?

Many different opinions abound in the debate over which zygoma fractures are unstable and require fixation. Most agree that comminuted fractures are unstable. Some believe that the downward pull of the masseter muscle on the zygomatic body (its origin) makes a zygomatic complex fracture inherently unstable. However, some studies do not support this contention. Others say that wide separation at the ZF suture makes it unstable. The wide range (13–100% in a study of 21 surgical groups) in the percentage of zygomatic fractures requiring fixation after surgical reduction indicates the differences of opinion on this issue.

13. How are isolated displaced zygomatic arch fractures treated?

Zygomatic arch fractures displace medially. Probably the most popular approach to elevate a medially displaced zygomatic arch fracture is that described by Gillies (see question 14). Many surgeons believe that these fractures, once reduced, are stable because of the support of the underlying edematous temporalis muscle and require no fixation as long as no pressure is exerted to the ipsilateral face postoperatively. Fixation, if necessary, can be achieved by passing percutaneous sutures or wires around the arch fragments and tying them to an external device such as an aluminum finger splint or tongue blade. On occasion open reduction and fixation via a coronal or preauricular incision may be necessary.

14. Describe the "Gillies approach" to the zygoma.

A 2-cm incision is made obliquely in the temporal scalp about 2.5 cm anterior and 2.5 cm superior to the helix of the ear, avoiding injury to the branches of the superficial temporal artery. The incision is carried down to the glistening, white temporal fascia, which is then incised. The plane between the fascia and the underlying temporalis muscle is bluntly developed inferiorly with a periosteal elevator down to the zygomatic arch to which the fascia attaches. An elevator or other rigid instrument is then easily passed beneath (medial to) the arch or body of the zygoma to elevate it.

15. Name four standard approaches to the infraorbital rim and orbital floor.

The subciliary or blepharoplasty incision, the lower eyelid or subtarsal incision, the infraorbital incision, and the transconjunctival incision.

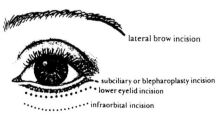

Common incisions to approach the zygoma. (From Ellis E III: Fractures of the zygomatic complex and arch. In Fonseca RJ, Walker RV (eds): Oral and Maxillofacial Trauma. Philadelphia, W.B. Saunders, 1991, with permission.)

16. What are the common approaches to the lateral orbital rim?

The lateral brow incision, lateral extension of the subciliary incision, and lateral extension of the upper eyelid blepharoplasty incision.

17. What are the advantages of the coronal incision for reduction of zygomatic fractures?

The coronal incision gives excellent exposure to the orbit, zygomatic body, and zygomatic arch. It is helpful in comminuted zygoma fractures, and the scar remains hidden in the hairline.

18. How can a displaced zygomatic complex fracture be reduced with no external scar?

Through a gingival buccal sulcus incision, access is gained to the infratemporal surface of the zygoma. A rigid instrument is then passed into this space to elevate and reduce the fracture. This incision also is commonly used to gain access to the ZM buttress for plating.

19. What is probably the most feared complication after surgical treatment of zygoma fractures?

Albeit rare, blindness may result from direct damage to the optic nerve due to displacement of a bony fragment or fracture of the optic canal; edema that causes compression of the nerve; or retrobulbar hematoma. Preoperative opthalmologic assessment of both eyes is imperative. Preexisting blindness in the contralateral, uninvolved eye is a relative contraindication to treatment because surgical reduction complicated by blindness in the eye on the involved side would be absolutely devastating to the patient (and surgeon).

20. How is malunion of the zygoma treated?

When minor deformity is present without orbital involvement or when comminution precludes repositioning of the zygoma en bloc, placement of subperiosteal implants may be used to restore normal malar contour. When more pronounced deformity exists along with functional deficits, zygomatic osteotomy to recreate the fracture, followed by bony repositioning, fixation, and possible bone grafting, is the only surgical option.

21. What is the treatment for fibroosseous ankylosis between the zygomatic arch and coronoid process of the mandible following zygoma fractures?

Coronoidectomy.

BIBLIOGRAPHY

1. Ellis E III: Fractures of the zygomatic complex and arch. In Fonseca RJ, Walker RV (eds): Oral and Maxillofacial Trauma. Philadelphia, W.B. Saunders, 1991, pp 435–514.
2. Knight JS, North JF: The classification of malar fractures: An analysis of displacement as a guide to treatment. Br J Plast Surg 13:325–339.
3. Manson PN: Facial injuries. In McCarthy JG (ed): Plastic Surgery. Philadelphia, W.B. Saunders, 1990, pp 991–1009.
4. Woodburne RT: Essentials of Human Anatomy. New York, Oxford University Press, 1988.

30. FRACTURES OF THE MAXILLA

Geoffrey C. Fenner, M.D., and S. Anthony Wolfe, M.D.

1. Who was Le Fort? What are Le Fort fractures?

René Le Fort was a French surgeon who at the end of the last century was interested in the patterns of midfacial fracture. He performed a number of experiments on cadaver heads, dropping them from the top floor of buildings onto a paved courtyard or striking them with a piano leg. He determined three basic fault lines along which the face fractured. In his initial description, the highest facial fracture was referred to as no. 1 and the lowest as no. 3.

In current parlance, the Le Fort I fracture refers to the transmaxillary fracture that goes through the maxilla at about the level of the piriform rim. The Le Fort II fracture occurs through the nasofrontal junction, and runs through the nasal processes of the maxilla and medial portion of the inferior orbital rim and then across the anterior maxilla, and extends back to and through the pterygoid plates. The Le Fort III fracture is a craniofacial disjunction with a separation at the frontozygomatic suture, nasofrontal junction, medial orbital wall, orbital floor, and zygomatic arch laterally. The maxilla below is intact in a pure Le Fort III fracture (see figure at top of next page).

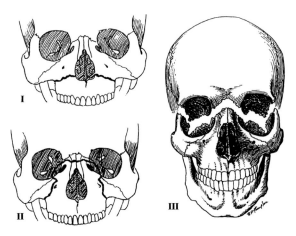

Le Fort I, II, and III fractures.

2. How do you clinically diagnose a midfacial fracture?

Diagnosis is reasonably easy in patients with displacement. Examine the occlusion. A displaced maxillary fracture is associated with malocclusion, and if the patient is awake, he or she usually can say that the bite relationship is altered. With the patient's mouth open, grasp the premaxilla and see if any movement can be elicited while holding the patient's head stable with the other hand. With impacted fractures it may not be possible to elicit movement. If movement is possible, the level of the fracture can easily be determined by palpation of the nasofrontal junction, lateral orbital rim, and infraorbital rims.

3. What is the difference between a Le Fort fracture and a Le Fort osteotomy?

In a Le Fort fracture, the fracture line usually extends through the pterygoid plates. In an osteotomy, one attempts to preserve the pterygoid plates by operative separation through the pterygomaxillary junction.

4. What would you do if you were operating on a patient with a displaced, impacted Le Fort I fracture that cannot be reduced?

The usual approach involves applying arch bars to the maxillary and mandibular dentition. If the maxilla is immobile at this point, Rowe forceps are inserted through the nose, and an effort is made to mobilize the maxilla by side-to-side and forward motion. If reduction is still not possible, one should proceed with a Le Fort I osteotomy using a reciprocating saw as in routine maxillofacial surgery.

5. What if loose teeth are associated with a maxillary fracture?

Teeth maintained by even a small blood supply can survive. The outlook depends on whether they are avulsed from their socket or whether alveolar bone is found around the tooth itself. In either event, the teeth should be placed carefully in occlusion and splinted not only with the arch bar but also with a methylmethacrylate interocclusal splint to immobilize the teeth as carefully as possible. The patient should receive antibiotics, maintain oral hygiene, and be referred to a dentist as soon as possible.

6. What should one do with a tooth that has been completely pulled out of its socket?

The tooth should be placed in either sterile saline or, if that is not available, milk. If replaced promptly (< 30 min) into the socket, a certain number of teeth will survive but will require subsequent root canal therapy because of loss of tooth vitality.

7. What are the buttresses of the maxilla?

The main vertical buttresses of the maxilla, which absorb the majority of forces, are the nasomaxillary, zygomaticomaxillary, and pterygomaxillary buttresses; another component, the vomer, connects the maxilla to the cranial base. The horizontal buttresses include the mandible, palate, orbital rims, and frontal bar.

8. When should bone grafts be used in the treatment of a maxillary fracture?

Primary bone grafts should be used along with rigid internal fixation when one of the major buttresses of the maxilla, excluding the pterygomaxillary and vomer, is substantially damaged. The bone grafts can be harvested from either the skull, ileum, or rib, depending on the surgeon's preference.

9. When is intermaxillary fixation required after a maxillary fracture?

If an isolated maxillary fracture was repaired with rigid internal fixation, resulting in stable occlusion at the end of the operation, the patient should not require prolonged intermaxillary fixation and may be maintained on light elastics at night, when not eating, and when not engaging in oral hygiene. This is the same approach used in orthognathic surgery. If multiple facial fractures involve the mandible, particularly both mandibular condyles, a course of intermaxillary fixation, ranging from 2–6 weeks, may be indicated. If this approach is used, we prefer an interocclusal splint to open up the bite at least 3–5 mm and to take the load off of the fractured condyles.

10. What imaging tests should be obtained in patients with a suspected maxillary fracture?

Whenever possible, a Panorex radiograph should be obtained in patients with suspected jaw fractures if they are able to undergo the procedure comfortably. This view provides the most information about the condition of the teeth and immediately adjacent bone. A CT scan, particularly including coronal cuts, is the most commonly obtained examination and gives much more information than any type of conventional radiographic examination. When a fracture of the orbit is suspected, it is almost mandatory to obtain a CT scan; again, the coronal views are the most useful.

11. What are the indications for exploration of the orbital floors in a Le Fort III or an orbito-zygomatic fracture?

In an occasional patient with hairline fractures without displacement, observation of an orbital fracture is acceptable. Most fractures involve substantial disruption of the orbital floors or medial orbital walls; exploration of the internal orbit is necessary, along with fixation of the fractures of the outer framework of the orbit, such as the frontozygomatic area and infraorbital rim. In rare cases, fractures require no additional material in the orbital cavity after reduction.

12. What material should be used for reconstruction of internal defects in the orbital cavity, such as the medial orbital wall and orbital floor?

Most inexperienced surgeons in North America still use various types of foreign substances for correction of orbital floor defects. Substances currently in use include silicone sheeting, Teflon sheeting, hydroxyapatite, polyethylene, and metallic mesh. Most experienced craniofacial surgeons use none of these materials and have a strong preference for autogenous bone grafts.

13. What incision should be used to explore the orbital floor?

In our experience, the subciliary incision, which is commonly used for lower lid blepharoplasty, should be avoided altogether for exploration of orbital fractures. It is associated with an unacceptably high incidence of lower lid retraction, which occurs even in the hands of experienced surgeons. Such lower lid retractions are quite difficult to correct with subsequent surgery. We prefer an incision that is lower on the eyelid, perhaps 5–7 mm below the ciliary margin, just below the tarsal plate of the lower lid, and located in a natural lower lid crease. Lower lid retraction is rare with this incision, and in our experience the cosmetic result is just as good, if not better, than with an incision higher on the eyelid. Alternatively, a transconjunctival approach may be used. This approach gives limited access for plating infraorbital rim fractures but acceptable exposure of the orbital floor. For further access to the infraorbital rim, it may be coupled with a lateral canthotomy. This procedure, however, requires precise canthal repositioning and leaves a scar that may be noticeable. For these reasons, we prefer the lower eyelid incision beneath the tarsus.

14. What are the preferred donor areas for bone grafts for the orbit and maxilla?

The answer depends on the surgeon's preference. The only important factor is that autogenous bone grafts must be fresh. Usually we prefer outer table calvarial grafts harvested from the nondominant parietooccipital area. Iliac bone is also excellent material. We find fewer indications for rib, although it is acceptable if the surgeon so prefers.

15. When miniplates and screws are used to obtain rigid internal fixation for maxillary and orbital fractures, should they be removed later?

The answer is generally no. If patients are bothered by the presence of the plates and can feel them or if low-grade infection is associated with the plates, the plates can be removed easily after sufficient time for bone healing (6–8 weeks). Biodegradable plates, made of a combination of polyglycolic and polylactic acid, are used in infant craniofacial surgery, and they may have some application in facial fractures in the future, although this use has not yet been studied carefully.

16. With which bones does the zygoma articulate?

Greater wing of the sphenoid, frontal, temporal, and maxillary bones.

17. What are the clinical signs of a zygoma fracture?

- Malar depression
- Circumorbital and subconjunctival ecchymosis
- Enophthalmos
- Deepening of the supratarsal fold
- Step deformity or tenderness along the infraorbital rim, frontozygomatic suture, arch or lateral buttress
- Diplopia
- Global dystopia
- Lateral canthal dystopia with an antimongoloid slant
- Infraorbital paresthesia
- Trismus (secondary to arch impingement on the coronoid process)

18. What is the preferred surgical approach for open reduction of a displaced zygomatic fracture?

A lateral brow or upper blepharoplasty incision, lower eyelid incision, and superior gingivobuccal sulcus incision adequately expose the zygomaticofrontal, infraorbital, and lateral zygomaticomaxillary buttress regions, respectively. Comminuted fractures of the zygoma are best approached through a coronal incision. Various lower eyelid incisions are reviewed in question 13.

19. What is the incidence of permanent diplopia after zygomatic fracture?

Initial transient diplopia is present in up to 10% of patients and is commonly evident on upward, downward, and lateral gaze. Permanent diplopia, evident on upward gaze, remains in 5% of patients. Causes of diplopia or mechanical globe restriction include entrapment and/or injury to the inferior oblique or inferior rectus muscle, Lockwood's ligament, Tenon's capsule, or periorbital fat. Restriction is confirmed by the forced duction or traction test. Nonrestrictive causes of diplopia include injury to extraocular muscles, neural injury, hematoma, and edema.

20. What are the causes of late enophthalmos?

Delayed enophthalmos occurs in 3% of cases and is due to inadequate fracture reduction with persistent volumetric orbital expansion, bone graft resorption, contraction of injured extraocular muscles, and intraorbital conal fat necrosis or atrophy.

21. What is the treatment for progressive loss of vision after blunt facial trauma?

Sight lost at the moment of injury is not likely to return. Conversely, progressive visual loss stands the best chance of recovery. Treatment includes megadose steroids (3–5 mg/kg/day). If the patient fails to regain or show improved vision within 12 hours, surgical decompression should be undertaken. The preferred approach in the United States is transethmoidal sphenoidotomy with removal of the medial wall of the optic canal.

22. What are the contraindications to immediate treatment of panfacial fractures?

- Uncontrolled intracranial pressure
- Systemic hemorrhage
- Coagulopathy
- Acute respiratory distress syndrome.

23. At what age does the maxillary sinus become mature?

The floor of the maxillary sinus remains above the level of the floor of the nose up to the age of 8 years. Eruption of the permanent maxillary dentition determines the inferior growth of the maxillary floor, which, therefore, is not complete until the age of 12–16 years.

BIBLIOGRAPHY

1. Anderson RL, Panje WR, Gross CE: Optic nerve blindness following blunt forehead trauma. Ophthalmology 89:445, 1982.
2. Andreasen JO: Luxation injuries. In Andreasen JO (ed): Traumatic Injuries of the Teeth. Philadelphia, W.B. Saunders, 1981, pp 151–202.
3. Barkley TL: Some aspects of the treatment of traumatic diplopia. Br J Plast Surg 11:147, 1963.
4. Dufresne CR, Manson PN: Pediatric facial trauma. In McCarthy JG (ed): Plastic Surgery. Philadelphia, W.B. Saunders, 1990, pp 1142–1187.
5. Kawamoto HK Jr: Late posttraumatic enophthalmos: A correctable deformity? Plast Reconstr Surg 69:423, 1982.
6. Le Fort R: Etude experimentale sur les fractures de la machoire superieure. Rev Chir Paris 23:208, 360, 479, 1901.
7. Manson P: Facial injuries. In McCarthy JG (ed): Plastic Surgery. Philadelphia, W.B. Saunders, 1990, pp 867–1141.
8. Manson PN, Su CT, Hoopes JE: Structural pillars of the facial skeleton. Plast Reconstr Surg 66:54, 1980.
9. Nguyen PN, Sullivan P: Advances in the management of orbital fractures. Clin Plast Surg 19:87, 1992.
10. Rowe NL, Killey HC: Fracture of the Facial Skeleton, 2nd ed. Baltimore, Williams & Wilkins, 1968.
11. Rowe LD, Miller E, Brandt-Zawadski M: Computed tomography in maxillofacial trauma. Laryngoscope 91:745, 1981.
12. Tessier P, Woillez M, Rougier J, et al: Maxillomalar fractures. In Wolfe SA (translator): Plastic Surgery of the Orbit and Eyelids. Chicago, Year Book, 1981, pp 42–57.
13. Wolfe SA: Treatment of post-traumatic orbital deformities. Clin Plast Surg 15:225, 1988.
14. Wolfe SA, Baker S: Facial Fractures. New York, Thieme, 1993.
15. Wolfe SA, Berkowitz S: Autogenous bone grafts versus alloplastic materials. In Plastic Surgery of the Facial Skeleton. Boston, Little, Brown, 1989, pp 25–38.
16. Wolfe SA, Berkowitz S: Maxilla. In Plastic Surgery of the Facial Skeleton. Boston, Little, Brown, 1989, pp 227–290.

31. FRACTURES OF THE MANDIBLE

John W. Polley, M.D., Jeffery S. Flagg, M.D., D.D.S.,
and Mimis Cohen, M.D., F.A.C.S.

1. What is the anatomy of the mandible?

The mandible is the largest and strongest of the facial bones; it consists of a basal bone and three processes. The basal bone extends from the symphysis at the chin to the lateral condyles on each side. In addition, it contains a horizontal portion, the body, and two perpendicular portions, the rami, which join the body nearly at right angles. The processes include the alveolar process, to which the teeth are attached; the coronoid process, to which the temporalis muscle is attached; and the angle, to which the masseter and medial pterygoid muscles attach. A cartilaginous disk completes the hinge joint known as the temporomandibular joint (TMJ), to which the transverse head of the lateral pterygoid muscle attaches.

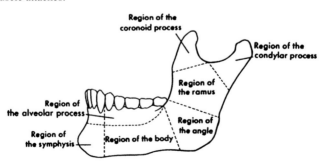

Regions of the mandible. (From Manson PN: Facial injuries. In McCarthy JG (ed): Plastic Surgery. Philadelphia, W.B. Saunders, 1990, p 931, with permission.)

2. How does the morphology of the mandible help it to resist forces such as those resulting from mastication or trauma?

The mandible is a U-shaped tubular bone consisting of an outer and inner cortex with bone marrow between them. The architecture in the trabeculae of spongy bone reflects the pattern of stress and strain within the region. Unidirectional forces result in bending. In these areas, the mandible is formed as a thick plate. When forces from all directions must be resisted, the bone has trabeculae. The trabeculae spring from the inner cortical layers like the flying buttresses of Gothic cathedrals and span the medullary spaces to the opposite side. As a result of trabeculae orientation, the stress of chewing is conveyed to the interior of the bone. The mandible forms several lines (trajectories) of equal pressure and equal tension that extend from the symphysis to the condyles. Stress that occurs from mastication or trauma is transferred from the interior of the mandible to the condyles via various trajectory lines. Here the condyles articulate with the glenoid fossa of the temporal bone. Nature has formed the mandible to withstand pressure and to transmit force to the base of the skull via the craniomandibular articulation.

3. What are the six Ps of mandibular fractures?

1. **Panorex.** Panoramic roentgenography produces a survey of the tooth-bearing portions of the maxilla and mandible. This information can be used to evaluate the fracture site(s), position of the fragments, and postoperative healing.

2. **Plain radiographs.** If the Panorex is inconclusive or not available, plain radiographs should include three views of the mandible (right or left lateral oblique, posteroanterior) and a skull series.

3. **Penicillin.** Drug of choice to combat the constant perculation of oral microorganisms. This, coupled with the continuous disruption of vascular ingrowth and osteolysis, is the most common and predictable source of fracture infection. The microorganisms most often encountered in the oral cavity are streptococci and *Bacteroides* sp.

4. **Peridex.** Peridex is an oral rinse containing 0.12% chlorhexidine gluconate. Approximately 30% of the microbial active ingredient is retained after rinsing. The retained drug is then slowly released into oral fluids.

5. **Preoperative work-up.** The physician who first examines a patient with a mandibular injury should examine all soft tissues thoroughly, evaluate the current status of dental hygiene, examine the teeth for evidence of trauma (chipped, mobile, displaced), evaluate the mandible for discontinuity with a bimanual exam, and look for ecchymosis in the floor of the mouth. Deviations in mandibular movements and malocclusion are the sine qua non of mandible fractures.

6. **Postoperative instructions.** Emphasize vigorous oral hygiene, oral antibiotics, mechanical soft diet, and the importance of follow-up examinations.

4. Describe the biomechanical response of the mandible to trauma.

The two principal components involved in fractures of the mandible are the dynamic factor (blow) and the stationary factor (jaw). The most common causes are altercations (47.5%) and automobile accidents (27.3%). The location, intensity, duration, and direction of the traumatizing force, with respect to the physical properties of the mandible, influence its biomechanical response. The condylar neck has the smallest cross-sectional area and the least ability to bend of any region of the mandible. Force applied to the point of the chin shows a high frequency of condylar neck fractures (72%). A severe force can push the condylar fragments out of the glenoid fossa. Body and angle fractures usually result from direct impact over these regions and are more often unilateral. Angle fractures are often associated with a parasymphyseal fracture on the contralateral side. The dynamic factor is characterized by the intensity of the blow, its duration, and its direction. Whereas a light blow may cause a greenstick fracture, a heavy blow may cause a compound, comminuted fracture. The direction of the force largely determines the location of the fracture.

5. How does the stationary component influence mandible fractures?

The stationary component is the jaw itself. The patient's age is important. With equal force a child may experience a greenstick fracture, whereas an elderly person with heavily calcified bone may sustain a complicated fracture. Mental and physical relaxation prevents fractures associated with muscular tension. A bone on which increased tension is placed by contractions of the attached musculature requires a lower threshold force for fracture. In contrast, an intoxicated patient may receive severe trauma to the mandible and suffer only bruises. The muscle masses serve as tissue cushions when relaxed but elicit strain patterns under tension.

6. What is the concept of favorable and unfavorable fractures?

A fracture is classified as favorable when the direction of the line of fracture does not allow independent muscular distractions. An unfavorable fracture occurs when the line of fracture permits the fragments to separate. The four muscles of mastication are the temporalis, masseter, medial pterygoid, and lateral pterygoid. After discontinuity of the mandible due to fracture, these muscles exert their actions on the fragments, leading to malocclusion. In the presence of teeth, it is important to restore occlusion.

At the mandibular angle, the posterior fragment is elevated and drawn forward by the action of the medial pterygoid and masseter muscles. The unfavorable oblique fracture is caused when the line of fracture runs from anterior-superior to posterior-inferior. However, if the inferior border fracture occurs further anteriorly and the line of fracture extends in a distal direction toward the ridge, a favorable fracture is seen. The angle of the anteroinferior portion locks the posterior fragment mechanically to withstand upward muscular pull. Most angle fractures are horizontally unfavorable fractures. Medial displacement may be considered in a similar fashion. Oblique fracture lines can form a large buccal cortical fragment that prevents medial displacement. A bird's-eye view reveals that a vertically unfavorable fracture line extends from a posterolateral point to an anteromedial point. No obstruction counters the action of the lateral pterygoid and mylohyoid muscles, and the posterior fragment is shifted medially. A vertically favorable fracture extends from an anterolateral to posteromedial point.

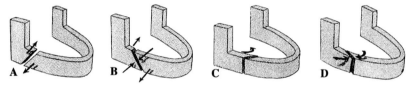

Favorable vs. unfavorable fractures. *A*, Horizontally unfavorable fractures extend downward and posteriorly. *B*, Horizontally favorable fractures extend downward and forward. *C*, Vertically unfavorable fractures extend forward and medially. *D*, Vertically favorable fractures extend from the lateral surface of the mandible posteriorly and medially. Arrows indicate the direction of muscle pull. With unfavorable fractures, the direction and bevel of the fracture line do not resist displacement by muscular action. With favorable fractures, the bevel and fracture line resist displacement and oppose muscular action. Fractures beveled in this direction tend to impact the fractured bone ends. (From Manson PN: Facial injuries. In McCarthy JG (ed): Plastic Surgery. Philadelphia, W.B. Saunders, 1990, p 940, with permission.)

7. Why is Angle's classification of malocclusion the standard in dentistry throughout the world?

Edward Angle, who presented his classification of dental malocclusion in 1898, recognized that facial balance was ideal when the midfacial position was in a harmonious relationship to the mandible. Angle noted that the most pleasing facial profile occurred when the supraorbital ridge, subnasal area, lower lip, and chin fall on a straight line. The engraving made by Angle illustrated how the normal occlusal relationships between the maxilla and mandible resulted in this profile.

8. How is malocclusion classified?

Normal occlusion occurs when the mesiobuccal cusp of the upper first molar is received in the buccal groove of the lower first molar (class I occlusion). An Angle class II malocclusion exists when the lower molars are displaced distally so that the mesiobuccal developmental groove fits under the distal cusp of the upper first molar or even further back, giving the profile of the classic retrognathic appearance. The class III occlusion is characterized by mandibular prognathism. The lower dental arch is carried forward so that the mesiobuccal developmental groove of the lower molar may be under the upper second bicuspid or even the first (see chapter 23).

9. Does mixed dentition play a role in mandible fractures?

The mixed dentition stage is the age at which both deciduous and secondary teeth have erupted in the oral cavity. In active children, the soft and hard tissues of the mouth are frequent recipients of trauma. As a rule, the lower first molars are the first permanent teeth to pierce the gum tissues. With children, fractures of the mandible are complicated by the presence of mixed dentition with teeth in various stages of eruption. Thus, the malocclusion cannot be easily evaluated. It should be emphasized that developing tooth buds may react in many unfavorable ways after disturbance. Roentgenograms may be misleading when undisplaced fractures are covered by developing tooth buds. Primary teeth lend themselves to wiring procedures for stabilization; however, only a few teeth may be present for attachment of fixation.

10. How do pediatric mandibular fractures differ from adult mandibular fractures?
Mandibular fractures are less common in children than in adults. Greenstick fractures of the mandible, particularly in the condylar region, are relatively common in children. The increased ossification capability of the juvenile periosteum allows faster healing and distinguishes it from the adult mandible. As a result, many mandibular fractures in children can be treated with immobilization for a short period. Direct osteosynthesis is reserved for displaced fractures. Problems with osteosynthesis in children include the need to avoid damage to developing tooth buds.

11. What is intermaxillary fixation (IMF)?
IMF refers to an era when the mandible was known as the inferior maxilla. Current terminology includes maxillomandibular fixation (MMF), IMF, and interdental fixation (which is used in the Current Procedural Terminology coding system). Intermaxillary fixation is obtained by applying wires or elastic bands between upper and lower jaws to which suitable anchoring devices can be attached. Arch bars are a common method for obtaining intermaxillary fixation. Thick gauge wire is used to secure molar teeth, whereas thinner wire is used for anterior teeth. Ivy loop wiring embraces only two adjacent teeth, to which elastics are secured. With one or two Ivy loops placed in each quadrant, traction is then placed between the jaws.

12. What are the advantages of rigid internal fixation in contrast with interosseous wiring for the repair of mandible fractures?
Open reduction of mandibular fractures with wire osteosynthesis requires 4–8 weeks of MMF for satisfactory healing. Rigid internal fixation (RIF) of mandibular fractures allows early mobilization of the jaws, reducing or eliminating the period of MMF. This is a significant benefit to patients, avoiding the potential sequelae of prolonged immobilization, including TMJ stiffness after removal of IMF, social inconvenience, phonetic disturbance, loss of effective work time, discomfort, and weight loss.

13. What is the spherical sliding principle in rigid osteosynthesis of mandible fractures?
Compressive forces are achieved with compression plates by a combination of factors. Dynamic and eccentric compression plates create interfragmental pressure by the spherical sliding principle. The practical application of this principle is based on clinical and experimental evidence that bone fragments immobilized with interfragment pressure greater than the forces tending to displace the fragments will mend by primary bone healing without callus formation. The compressive force results in greater stability of the fracture. The tension and pressure forces acting on the mandible during movement must be neutralized by the forces used to create interfragmental pressure. In the technique of rigid fixation, the vertical movement of the screw is changed to a horizontal compressive force vector as the screw head follows the incline of the screw hole in the compression plate. Thus, the fragments are reapproximated as the screw head is tightened.

14. What is the incidence of fractures in different areas of the adult mandible?

Angle	31%	Condyle	18%
Molar region	15%	Mental region	14%
Symphysis	8%	Cuspid	7%
Ramus	6%	Coronoid process	1%

15. What complications are associated with the repair of mandibular fractures?
Infection, malocclusion, tooth injury, delayed union, nonunion (pseudoarthrosis), osteomyelitis, inferior alveolar, and facial nerve injury. Of these, infection is one of the most problematic; it is the most frequent complication and is an important cause of nonunion.

16. How is the interocclusal distance measured?

The interocclusal distance is measured as the distance between the incisal edges of the maxillary and mandibular central incisors at the midline. Normal interocclusal distance is about 3.0–4.5 mm.

17. What percentage of patients with mandibular fractures present with concomitant cervical spine injury?

Associated injuries are present in 43% of all patients with mandibular fracture, most of whom were involved in vehicular accidents. Cervical spine fractures were found in 11% of this group of patients. It is imperative to rule out cervical neck fractures, especially in patients who are intoxicated or unconscious. Posteroanterior and lateral films should be reviewed with the radiologist before treatment is initiated.

18. What risk factors increase the possibility of infection with mandibular fractures?

Infected mandibular fractures are encountered in patients who sustain facial trauma and fail to seek immediate treatment. Mucosal tears and fractures extending through the periodontal ligament produce contamination of the fracture by oral flora. Fractures that occur through the tooth-bearing area, therefore, should be regarded as contaminated. Soft tissue injury also has been shown to be a key factor in infection rates. Bony sequestra, devitalized teeth, and hematoma also contribute to infection. Movement at the fracture site due to loose, mobile hardware, such as a loose screw in an otherwise stable plate, may cause infection in the presence of bacterial contamination. In some patients treatment must be delayed because of more serious injuries. Poor oral hygiene is also a major key to infection.

19. What techniques are used for treatment of alveolar bone fractures?

If teeth are present in the mobile fragment and stable part of the alveolus, an arch bar should be fixed to the teeth. After reduction, the fracture is stabilized by this fixation. If no teeth are present and the mobile fragment is still fixed to and nourished by the periosteum and mucosa, closing the wound by repair of the torn gingiva will suffice. If a removable prosthetic full or partial denture is present, it should be worn to readapt the bone.

20. What role does dentition play in mandibular fractures?

The body of the mandible (molar, mental, and cuspid regions) is involved frequently in mandible fractures (36%) because of the lines of trajectory that pass along the longitudinal axis of the teeth. Several factors influence the location of mandible fractures, including site, force, direction of impact, and presence of impacted teeth. When a force is distributed to the mandible, the mandible fractures at its weakest point. The weakest points are at the angle of the mandible (third molar) and canine region (tooth length—26 mm). One study found that patients with third molars were 3.8 times more likely to develop angle fractures and that the third molars weaken the mandibular angle via decreased area of bone. People at risk (e.g., contact sport athletes) may benefit from preventive removal of these teeth.

21. What treatments are ideal for symphyseal and parasymphyseal fractures?

Wire osteosynthesis alone may not provide rotational stability; thus, symphyseal and parasymphyseal fractures should be treated with compression plates. In addition, the bilateral posterior and lateral pull exerted by the mylohyoid and digastric muscles contributes to displacement of the fragments. Once MMF is obtained, the incision into the mucosa is made deep into the labial-alveolar sulcus, with care to leave sufficient attached gingival mucosa to enable closure without tension. The mandible is degloved with the utmost care not to injure the mental nerve. The bone fragments are then reduced with bone forceps and secured, if necessary. Next, a compression plate is contoured accurately; if this is not done, the screws may move the bone fragments and, after release of MMF, malocclusion results. Bony irregularities may be removed with a burr. Two screws are needed on each side of the bony plate to ensure compression and stability. Overbowing or overcontouring of the plate is often helpful in avoiding displacement of the fractured lingual cortical bone, which may lead to occlusal problems and displacement of the condyles.

22. What techniques are used for fractures of the condyles?

Condylar process fractures are common (18%) and are classified by fracture level, anatomic displacement, and position of the condyle. Generally, they are treated by MMF alone. Immobilization usually ranges from 2–4 weeks for isolated fractures. Duration depends on type of dentition, level of the condylar fracture, and degree of dislocation of the condylar head. Unilateral condylar fractures are often associated with a fracture in the mandibular body on the contralateral side. Bilateral condylar fractures usually are caused by a blow on the chin. Condylar fractures differ from mandibular body fractures in that MMF is of shorter duration to prevent pathologic changes in the TMJ. MMF may not be needed for unilateral condylar fractures in edentulous patients because small occlusal discrepancies can be corrected on renewal of the dentures.

Patients with condyles displaced from the glenoid fossa are candidates for open reduction. The main indications for open reduction are the inability to obtain adequate dental occlusion by closed reduction and deviation of mandibular movement by a displaced segment. This problem occurs when the condyle is subluxated almost completely in a medial direction so that it lies at right angles to the neck or when it is displaced in the opposite direction and projects laterally from the zygoma. Occasionally, the condyle is pushed through the external auditory canal or into the middle fossa.

23. How do you repair edentulous mandible fractures?
Occlusion cannot be achieved because of the lack of teeth for fixation and alveolar ridge atrophy. If wearable dentures are present, the mandible may be effectively fixed by the application of circumferential wires. Splints or fabricated acrylic saddles may ensure reduction and stabilization. Edentulous mandibular fractures may be good candidates for open procedures. Advantages include direct visualization, excellent stability of the fixed segments, early return of masticatory function, and stimulation of osteogenesis by the use of compressive forces. Open procedures also reduce the incidence of injury to the inferior alveolar nerve, located at the superior border of the atrophic mandible. Conservative periosteal stripping is paramount. A single plate on the lateral aspect of the mandible may lead to torsional instability and produce an unsatisfactory result. Therefore, if possible, a second plate is advisable. Lag screws also may be used for edentulous fractures. Generally, they are best suited for fractures of the symphyseal region, where both buccal and lingual cortices can be engaged.

24. List the clinical signs that may be associated with mandibular fractures.

1. Changes in occlusion	4. Ecchymosis of the floor of	8. Crepitation on manual
2. Changes in mandibular	the mouth, mucosa, or skin	palpation
excursions: limited	5. Soft tissue bleeding	9. Sensory disturbances
opening, deviation	6. Soft tissue swelling	10. Trismus
3. Step in occlusion	7. Palpable fracture line	11. TMJ disorders

25. What percentage of mandibular fractures are multiple?
More than 50% of mandibular fractures are multiple. For this reason, if one fracture is noted along the jaw, the patient should be examined closely for evidence of additional fractures. Radiographic films must be scrutinized carefully for discrete fracture lines.

26. Why does ecchymosis occur in the floor of the mouth in mandible fractures?
Bleeding caused by the fracture is trapped by the fanlike attachment of the mylohyoid musculature to the mandible. This condition presents clinically as ecchymosis in the floor of the mouth.

27. Before the application of maxillomandibular fixation, how do you establish a patient's pretraumatic occlusion?
Occlusal wear facets occur because of the constant action of the tooth cusps rubbing across one another. Occlusal wear patterns on the teeth should be noted because they relate to the normal movement of the mandible. By lining up the coinciding wear facets of the interdigitating maxillary and mandibular teeth for MMF, the surgeon can estimate the patient's normal occlusion.

28. What are the indications for removal of teeth involved in fracture lines in the mandible?
• Severe loosening of the tooth with chronic periodontal disease
• Fracture of the root of the tooth
• Extensive periodontal injury and broken alveolar walls
• Displacement of teeth from their alveolar socket

29. What muscle is primarily responsible for condylar displacement in patients with a subcondylar fracture?

The lateral pterygoid is the only muscle that inserts directly on the neck of the mandibular condyle. The forces of this muscle frequently result in anterior and medial displacement of the condyle in the presence of a subcondylar fracture.

30. What are the indications for open reduction and internal fixation of condylar fractures?
- Displacement into the middle cranial fossa
- Inability to obtain preinjury occlusion by closed reduction or awake manipulation
- Extracapsular lateral displacement of the condylar fragment(s)
- Presence of a foreign body thought to require removal (e.g., gunshot pellets)
- Severe angulation of the condyle
- Condyle outside the glenoid fossa

BIBLIOGRAPHY

1. Anderson T, Alpert B: Experience with rigid fixation of mandibular fractures and immediate function. J Oral Maxillofac Surg 50:555–560, 1992.
2. Angle EH: Treatment of Malocclusion of the Teeth and Fractures of the Maxillae: Angle's System. Philadelphia, S.S. White Dental Manufacturing, 1898.
3. Angle EH: Treatment of Malocclusion of the Teeth: Angle's System, 7th ed. Philadelphia, S.S. White Dental Manufacturing, 1907.
4. Bertz JE: Maxillofacial Injuries. Clin Symp 33(4):1–32, 1981.
5. Buchbinder B: Treatment of fractures of the edentulous mandible, 1943 to 1993: A review of the literature. J Oral Maxillofac Surg 51:1174–1180, 1993.
6. Calloway DM, Anton MA, Jacobs JS: Changing concepts and controversies in the management of mandibular fractures. Clin Plast Surg 19:67–68, 1992.
7. DuBrul EL: Sicher's Oral Anatomy, 7th ed. St. Louis, Mosby, 1980.
8. Ellis E, Walker LR: Treatment of mandibular angle fractures using one noncompression miniplate. J Oral Maxillofac Surg 54:864–871, 1996.
9. Fernandez JA, Mathog RH: Open treatment of condylar fractures with biphase technique. Arch Otolaryngol Head Neck Surg 113:262–266, 1987.
10. Fridrich KL, Pena-Velasco G, Olson RAJ: Changing trends with mandibular fractures: A review of 1,067 cases. J Oral Maxillofac Surg 50:586–589, 1992.
11. Gerald N, D'Innocenzo R: Modified technique for adapting a mandibular angle superior border plate. J Oral Maxillofac Surg 53:220–221, 1995.
12. Greenberg SA, Jacobs JS, Bessette RW: Temporomandibular joint dysfunction: Evaluation and treatment. Clin Plast Surg 16:707–724, 1989.
13. Gundlach KK: Fractures of the mandible. In Cohen M (ed): Mastery of Plastic and Reconstructive Surgery. Boston, Little, Brown, 1994.
14. Howard P, Wolfe SA: Fractures of the mandible. Ann Plast Surg 17:391, 1986.
15. Johansson B, Krekmanov L, Shomsson M: Miniplate osteosynthesis of infected mandibular fractures. J Craniomaxillofac Surg 16:22, 1988.
16. Kerr NW: Some observations on infection in maxillofacial fractures. Br J Oral Surg 4:132, 1966.
17. Koury M, Ellis III E: Rigid internal fixation for the treatment of infected mandibular fractures. J Oral Maxillofac Surg 50:434–443, 1992.
18. Kruger GO (ed): Textbook of Oral and Maxillofacial Surgery, 5th ed. St. Louis, Mosby, 1979.
19. Manson PN: Facial injuries. In McCarthy JG (ed): Plastic Surgery. Philadelphia, W.B. Saunders, 1990.
20. McDonald RE, Avery DR: Dentistry for the Child and Adolescent, 3rd ed. St. Louis, Mosby, 1978.
21. Oikarinen KS: Clinical management of injuries to the maxilla, mandible, and alveolus. Dent Clin North Am 39:113–130, 1995.
22. Rittmann WW, Perren SM: Cortical bone healing after internal fixation and infection. New York, Springer Verlag, 1974.
23. Reynolds FC, Zaepfel F: Management of chronic osteomyelitis secondary to compound fractures. J Bone Joint Surg 30A:331, 1948.
24. Schultz RC: Facial fractures in children and adolescents. In Cohen M (ed): Mastery of Plastic and Reconstructive Surgery. Boston, Little, Brown, 1994.
25. Strelzow VV, Strelzow AG: Osteosynthesis of mandible fractures in the angle region. Arch Otolaryngol 109:403, 1983.
26. Tevepaugh DB, Dodson TB: Are mandibular third molars a risk factor for angle fractures? A retrospective cohort study. J Oral Maxillofac Surg 53:646–649, 1995.
27. Theriot BA, Van Sickels JE, Triplett RG, Nishioka GJ: Intraosseous wire fixation versus rigid osseous fixation of mandibular fractures: A preliminary report. J Oral Maxillofac Surg 45:577–582, 1987.
28. Weinberg S: Surgical correction of facial fractures. Dent Clin North Am 26:631–658, 1982.

V. Head and Neck Reconstruction

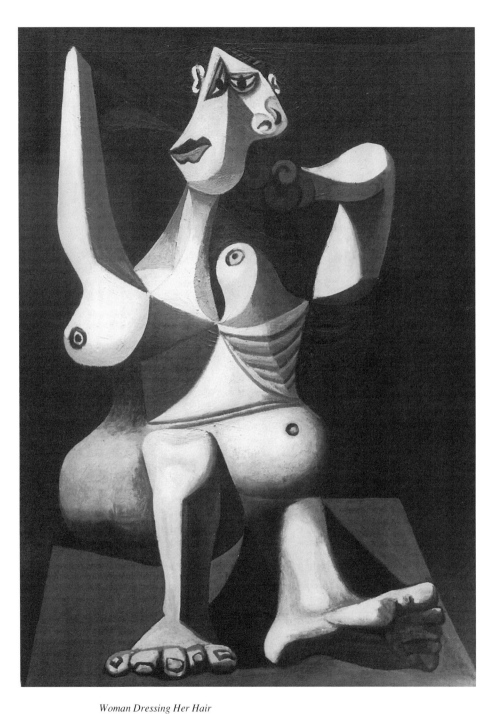

32. HEAD AND NECK EMBRYOLOGY AND ANATOMY

Charles D. Long, M.D., and Mark S. Granick, M.D.

1. What is a branchial arch?
Branchial arches form in the head and neck region of the developing embryo during the fourth week of gestation. Derived from migrating neural crest cells, these masses of tissue form the building blocks for later nerve, muscle, and skeletal structures.

2. Which muscles and nerves are derived from which arches?
- In general, the **first branchial arch** is the precursor for the muscles of mastication (e.g., temporalis, masseter, pterygoids). Also included are the mylohyoid, anterior belly of the digastric, tensor veli palatini, and tensor tympani. All of these muscles are innervated by the trigeminal nerve (cranial nerve [CN] V).
- The **second branchial arch** becomes the muscles of facial expression (e.g., orbicularis oris and oculi, frontalis, platysma) as well as the posterior belly of the digastric, stapedius, and stylohyoid muscles. All of these muscles are supplied by the facial nerve (CN VII).
- The stylopharyngeus muscle is derived from the **third branchial arch**, and is innervated by the glossopharyngeal nerve (CN IX).
- The **fourth, fifth, and sixth branchial arches** contribute to the formation of pharyngeal, laryngeal, and levator veli palatini muscles, all of which are supplied by the vagus nerve (CN X).

3. Where do branchial cysts come from?
Between the branchial arches are branchial clefts or grooves that are lined with surface ectoderm. The first cleft becomes the external auditory canal. The second, third, and fourth clefts usually are obliterated by the sixth week of gestation. Failure to do so or duplication of structures may result in fistulas, sinus tracts, or cysts, depending on how much remnant remains. Such anomalies can be found along the anterior border of the sternocleidomastoid muscle at any point from the external auditory canal to the clavicle.

4. Which branchial cleft anomaly is most common?
The second. The external component is found at the junction of the middle and lower thirds of the anterior border of the sternocleidomastoid muscle. The tract passes over the glossopharyngeal nerve and between the external and internal carotid arteries en route to the tonsillar fossa. The fossa must be excised under general anesthesia with a thorough understanding of the involved anatomy. Third branchial cleft anomalies, although rare, present in the same region as the second, but they course beneath the internal carotid. The surgeon must be aware of this possibility to avoid damaging vital structures. First branchial cleft cysts are less common but must be considered in excising masses above the hyoid bone, because their course may involve branches of the facial nerve. Preoperative patient counseling and planning are essential.

5. A young boy presents with a small mass in the midline of the neck below the hyoid bone. The mass has been present since birth. What is the most likely diagnosis?
A thyroglossal duct cyst. These cysts arise from remnant tissue left during the embryonic descent of the thyroid tissue from the base of the tongue to its pretracheal position by the eighth week of gestation. This "thyroglossal duct" usually disappears. However, duct remnants may be present as sinuses or cysts anywhere along the migration pathway. Usually identified by the second decade, thyroglossal cysts are most commonly in the midline at the level of the thyroid membrane.

6. What is the treatment?
Complete excision, including the entire duct remnant, which may pass through the hyoid bone and requires resection of the bone.

7. Are any preoperative tests important?

Because the mass may represent the patient's only thyroid tissue, it is necessary to demonstrate normal functioning thyroid tissue by thyroid scans and function tests.

8. A patient presents with a deep facial laceration in the emergency department. He cannot seem to close the ipsilateral eye, and saliva appears to be draining from the wound. Is anything wrong with this picture?

Yes. In performing routine laceration repairs in the emergency department, it is essential to understand the underlying anatomy before perfunctory closure. In this case, the patient has probably severed a branch of the facial nerve as well as the parotid duct or gland.

9. How can I find the facial nerve and parotid duct?

The **facial nerve (CN VII)** exits the styloid foramen and courses through the parenchyma of the parotid gland as it splits into five major branches: Temporal, Zygomatic, Buccal, Mandibular, and Cervical (Ten Zillion Bucks Means Cash). The temporal branch can be found along Pitanguy's line, which runs from 0.5 cm below the tragus to 1.5 cm above the lateral eyebrow. The facial nerve becomes more superficial as it heads medially, but is consistently deep to the superficial musculoaponeurotic system (SMAS). The muscles of facial animation are innervated on their deep surfaces, except the levator anguli oris, mentalis and buccinator muscles, which run deep to the plane of the nerve and are innervated on their superficial surfaces. In the midface, there are communications between branches (i.e., zygomatic and buccal); this is much less common in the frontal and mandibular regions, leading to increased chance of permanent deficits in injuries to terminal branches.

The **parotid (Stensen) duct** travels from the anteromedial border of the parotid gland to the anterior border of the masseter muscle, at which point it dives to emerge on the buccal mucosa opposite the maxillary second molar. A line drawn from the tragus of the ear to the middle of the upper lip approximates the path of the duct; a vertical line from the lateral canthus indicates the intraoral traverse.

10. A patient in the next emergency bed has a seemingly superficial wound to the neck but complains of numbness of the earlobe. What is the cause?

The great (not greater, since there is no lesser) auricular nerve is a sensory branch from the cervical plexus that crosses the anterior border of the sternocleidomastoid muscle consistently at a point 6.5 cm below the caudal edge of the bony external auditory canal. Because it is a superficial structure, it can be injured during parotid, facelift, carotid, and other neck dissections, leaving a bothersome numbness to the inferior ear.

11. Yet another patient has suffered a full-thickness injury to the scalp. What are the layers of the scalp?

S = Skin, C = subCutaneous tissue, A = Aponeurosis, L = Loose areolar tissue, and P = Pericranium.

12. The laceration is bleeding profusely. What is the blood supply to the scalp?

Five paired arteries comprise the vascular supply to the scalp: (1) supraorbital, (2) supratrochlear, (3) superficial temporal, (4) occipital, and (5) posterior auricular arteries.

13. Once you have repaired the laceration, the patient is so happy tears begin to flow. Where do the tears go?

Tears move on the eye from lateral to medial and are collected by the upper and lower puncta, which can be found 5–7 mm lateral to the canthal angle. They then travel in the cannaliculi 2 mm vertically, then 8 mm horizontally, to the common cannaliculus, which drains into the lacrimal sac. The lacrimal duct then transports the tears through the ethmoid bone to exit into the nose below the inferior nasal conchae.

14. What other structures empty into the nasal cavity? Where do they exit?

The nasal conchae (turbinates) are found on the lateral walls of the nasal cavity and help to humidify, purify, and warm the air by increasing surface area and turbulence. The conchae divide the lateral nasal wall into the inferior (below inferior concha), middle (below middle concha), superior (below superior concha), and supreme (above superior concha) meati. The frontal, maxillary, anterior ethmoid, and middle ethmoid sinuses drain into the middle meatus. The posterior ethmoid cells drain into the superior meatus, and the sphenoid sinus exits into the supreme meatus. The nasolacrimal duct empties below the inferior concha into the inferior meatus.

15. The trigeminal nerve supplies only sensory innervation for the face. True or false?

False. In addition to serving as the cutaneous nerve of the anterior and lateral face, the mandibular division of the trigeminal nerve (CN V_3) is also the motor nerve for the muscles of mastication. This group of four muscles acts directly on the mandible and traditionally includes the masseter, temporalis, medial pterygoid, and lateral pterygoid muscles. Accessory muscles, referred to as suprahyoid muscles because of their position superior to the hyoid bone, include the mylohyoid, digastric, and geniohyoid. Contraction of the masseter, temporalis, and medial pterygoid results in mandible elevation, whereas contraction of the lateral pterygoid and suprahyoid muscles result in mandible depression. Lateral and medial pterygoid contraction also results in mandible protrusion, whereas contraction of the suprahyoids and posterior portion of the temporalis also results in mandible retraction.

16. What are the contents of the carotid sheath?

Within the carotid sheath the vagus nerve (CN X) lies posterior to the common carotid artery and internal jugular vein.

17. How many branches does the external carotid artery give off? What are they?

The external carotid artery branches from the common carotid artery at the level of the upper border of the thyroid cartilage to give off eight of its own branches. It is the principal artery supplying the anterior aspect of the neck, face, scalp, oral and nasal cavities, bones of the skull, and dura mater. However, it does not supply the orbit or the brain. The main branches of the external carotid in the usual order of their appearance from inferior to superior are (1) the superior thyroid, (2) the ascending pharyngeal, (3) the lingual, (4) the facial, (5) the occipital, (6) the posterior auricular, (7) the superficial temporal, and (8) the maxillary.

17. What organ do both Arnold's nerve and Jacobsen's nerve supply? Where do they come from?

Both nerves provide sensory innervation to the ear. Arnold's nerve is a branch of the vagus nerve (CN X) and supplies the concha and auditory canal. Jacobsen's nerve is a branch of the glossopharyngeal nerve (CN IX) and supplies the concha, canal, and middle ear. The auriculotemporal nerve (CN V_3) supplies the root helix, crus, tragus, and canal, whereas the auricular branch off the facial nerve (CN VII) supplies the concha and canal. Thus, in all, four cranial nerves (V, VII, IX, and X) provide sensory innervation for the ear.

19. What are the foramina of the 12 cranial nerves?

Cranial Nerve		Foramen
Olfactory	(CN I)	Cribriform
Optic	(CN II)	Optic foramen
Oculomotor	(CN III)	Superior orbital fissure
Trochlear	(CN IV)	Superior orbital fissure
Trigeminal	(CN V_1)	Superior orbital fissure
Trigeminal	(CN V_2)	Foramen rotundum/inferior orbital fissure
Trigeminal	(CN V_3)	Foramen ovale
Abducens	(CN VI)	Superior orbital fissure
Facial	(CN VII)	Stylomastoid foramen
Vestibulocochlear	(CN VIII)	Internal acoustic meatus
Glossopharyngeal	(CN IX)	Jugular foramen
Vagus	(CN X)	Jugular foramen
Spinal accessory	(CN XI)	Jugular foramen
Hypoglossal	(CN XII)	Hypoglossal canal

20. What are the zones of the neck?

For use in the evaluation of penetrating neck trauma, the neck has been divided into three zones:

Zone I   Below a horizontal line 1 cm above the claviculomanubrial junction or inferior to the cricoid cartilage

Zone II   Between zone I and the angle of the mandible

Zone III   Between the angle of the mandible and base of the skull

Zones II and III are considered the neck proper; zone I is the base of the neck or thoracic inlet. Arteriography is often used to evaluate stable patients with overt signs of arterial injury, especially in zones I and III, because of the potential technical problems with exposure and vascular control in these regions.

BIBLIOGRAPHY

1. Johnston MC: Embryology of the head and neck. In McCarthy JG (ed): Plastic Surgery, vol 4. Philadelphia, W.B. Saunders, 1990, pp 2451–2495.
2. Langman J: Medical Embryology. Baltimore, Williams & Wilkins, 1981.
3. Netter FH: Atlas of Human Anatomy. Summit, NJ, CIBA-GEIGY Corp., 1991.
4. Pitanguy I, Silveria-Ramos A: The frontal branch of the facial nerve: The importance of its variation in face-lifting. Plast Reconstr Surg 38:352, 1966.
5. Ricciardelli E, Persing JA: Plastic surgery of the head and neck (anatomy/physiology/embryology). In Ruberg RL, Smith DJ (eds): Plastic Surgery: A Core Curriculum, vol 4. St. Louis, Mosby, 1994, pp 251–270.
6. Roth J, Granick MS, Solomon MP: Pediatric head and neck masses. In Bentz M (ed): Pediatric Plastic Surgery. East Norwalk, CT, Appleton & Lange, 1997.
7. Schwember G, Rodriguez A: Anatomic dissection of the extraparotid portion of the facial nerve. Plast Reconstr Surg 81:183, 1988.
8. Shestak KC, Ramasastry SS: Reconstruction of defects of the scalp and skull. In Cohen M (ed): Mastery of Plastic and Reconstructive Surgery. Boston, Little, Brown, 1994.
9. Zide BM, Jelks GW: Surgical Anatomy of the Orbit. New York, Raven Press, 1985.

33. HEAD AND NECK CANCER

David L. Callender, M.D., M.B.A., and Jeffrey N. Myers, M.D., Ph.D.

1. What is the appropriate evaluation of a lateral neck mass present in an adult for at least 3 weeks?

The differential diagnosis of a neck mass in an adult includes neoplastic or inflammatory disease, congenital anomalies, and other miscellaneous conditions. The likelihood of malignancy is increased in a patient with a history of tobacco or alcohol abuse, age greater than 40 years, chronic hoarseness, persistent dysphagia or odynophagia, persistent otalgia, or a history of malignancy of the skin or mucosal surfaces of the head and neck.

Diagnostic evaluation of a neck mass begins with a complete history and examination of the head and neck. Complete examination identifies a primary lesion in over 90% of patients who present with head and neck malignancy. After identification of a primary lesion, an imaging study of the head and neck (MRI or CT) is usually indicated to evaluate the extent of disease and to guide treatment planning. When a primary lesion is not found on examination, fine-needle aspiration (FNA) biopsy of the neck mass is indicated. If FNA biopsy demonstrates a benign lesion, treatment is tailored to the type and extent of disease. If malignancy is identified, an imaging study is performed to evaluate the extent of disease and to search for the occult primary lesion. Exam under anesthesia and endoscopy are also indicated. Directed biopsies of the nasopharynx, tonsil, tongue base, and pharyngeal wall may be performed if the primary lesion remains occult. When the FNA is nondiagnostic or equivocal for malignancy, open biopsy of the mass is usually indicated. Exams under anesthesia with endoscopy and neck mass biopsy are usually done concurrently. Incisions for open biopsy should be placed so that subsequent neck dissection can incorporate the biopsy incision.

2. What are the differences in radical, modified radical, and selective neck dissections?

Radical neck dissection is the classic procedure described by Crile in 1906 for management of metastatic cancer in cervical lymph nodes. The procedure consists of cervical dissection with removal of the sternocleidomastoid muscle, omohyoid muscle, internal jugular vein, spinal accessory nerve, cervical plexus nerves, submandibular salivary gland, tail of parotid gland, and all intervening lymphoareolar tissue containing lymph nodes (described as nodal levels I through VI). The principal indication for radical neck dissection is surgical management of bulky (N2 or greater) cervical nodal metastasis.

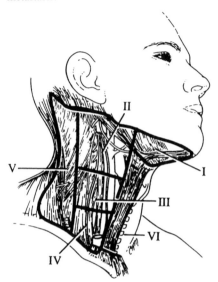

Lymph node levels in the neck. Level I indicates the submandibular and submental nodes; level II, upper jugular nodes; level III, middle jugular nodes; level IV, lower jugular nodes; level V, posterior triangle nodes; level IV, anterior compartment nodes. (From Robbins KT, Medina JE, Wolf GT, et al: Standardizing neck dissection terminology. Arch Otolaryngol Head Neck Surg 117:601–605, 1991, with permission.)

Modified radical neck dissection removes all of the same lymph node groups as the radical neck dissection but spares at least one of the nonlymphatic structures removed with the radical neck dissection. The indications for modified radical neck dissection are similar to those for radical neck dissection. The extent of metastatic disease usually determines the choice of radical vs. modified radical neck dissection. The so-called functional neck dissection, in which nodal levels I through VI are dissected but all nonlymphatic structures are spared, is a specific variation of the modified radical neck dissection.

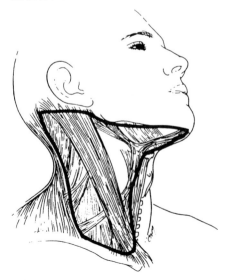

Area of nodes removed with radical and modified radical neck dissection. (From Robbins KT, Medina JE, Wolf GT, et al: Standardizing neck dissection terminology. Arch Otolaryngol Head Neck Surg 117:601– 605, 1991, with permission.)

Selective neck dissections remove the cervical lymph nodes considered to be at high risk for metastasis from a given primary site. Selective neck dissections are generally performed on an elective basis, although some patients with early nodal disease (N1) may be appropriately treated with selective neck dissection. The extent of selective neck dissection depends on the site and stage of the primary head and neck malignancy. The supraomohyoid neck dissection is an example of a selective neck dissection.

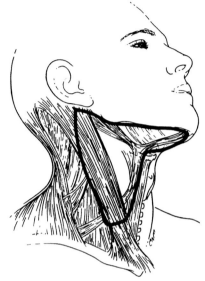

Area of nodes removed with supraomohyoid neck dissection. (From Robbins KT, Medina JE, Wolf GT, et al: Standardizing neck dissection terminology. Arch Otolaryngol Head Neck Surg 117:601–605, 1991, with permission.)

3. What are the principal indications for adjuvant postoperative external beam radiation therapy for patients with squamous cell carcinoma of the head and neck?

1. Close or positive surgical margins
2. Extracapsular extension of nodal disease
3. Perineural or vascular invasion
4. Multiple nodes containing metastatic cancer
5. High risk of occult disease in an undissected neck
6. Invasion of soft tissues or skin of the head and neck
7. Bone or cartilage invasion
8. Subglottic extension of laryngeal carcinoma

In these circumstances postoperative radiation therapy improves locoregional control rates and survival compared with surgery alone.

4. Describe the lymphatic drainage of the oral tongue.

The oral tongue has an extensive array of lymphatics that drain to the cervical nodes. The superior cervical (level II) lymph nodes are the most common site of cervical metastasis from oral tongue cancers. Lymph nodes in levels I and III are also at high risk for metastasis from early tongue cancer. Accordingly, surgical management of oral tongue cancers with clinically negative (N0) nodes frequently includes elective dissection of the nodes at highest risk for occult metastasis (levels I, II, and III). The supraomohyoid neck dissection removes nodes at high risk and provides staging information for patients with squamous cell carcinomas of the tongue.

5. Describe the staging of primary carcinoma in the oral cavity.

The American Joint Committee on Cancer Staging (AJCC) proposed the following system for staging of primary tumors (T):

TX   Primary tumor cannot be assessed
T0   No evidence of primary tumor
Tis   Carcinoma in situ
T1   Tumor ≤ 2 cm in greatest dimension
T2   Tumor > 2 cm but < 4 cm in greatest dimension

T3   Tumor > 4 cm in greatest dimension
T4   Tumor invades adjacent structures (e.g., through cortical bone, into deep muscle of tongue, maxillary sinus, skin. Superficial erosion of bone/tooth socket by gingival tumor is not sufficient to classify as T4.)

6. Describe the AJCC staging for regional lymph node metastasis (N) from oral cavity carcinoma.

NX   Regional lymph nodes cannot be assessed
N0   No regional lymph node metastasis
N1   Metastasis in a single ipsilateral lymph node, $\leq$ 3 cm in greatest dimension
N2   Metastasis in a single ipsilateral lymph node > 3 cm but < 6 cm in greatest dimension; in multiple ipsilateral lymph nodes, none > 6 cm in greatest dimension; or in bilateral or contralateral lymph nodes, none > 6 cm in greatest dimension
N2a   Metastasis in a single ipsilateral node > 3 cm but < 6 cm in greatest dimension
N2b   Metastasis in multiple ipsilateral lymph nodes, none > 6 cm in greatest dimension
N2c   Metastasis in bilateral or contralateral lymph nodes, none > 6 cm in greatest dimension
N3   Metastasis in a lymph node > 6 cm in greatest dimension

7. Describe the AJCC staging for distant metastasis (M) from oral cavity carcinoma.

MX   Distant metastasis cannot be assessed
M0   No distant metastasis
M1   Distant metastasis

8. Describe the TNM stage grouping for oral cavity carcinoma.

Stage	Primary Tumor	Node Metastasis	Distant Metastasis
0	Tis	N0	M0
I	T1	N0	M0
II	T2	N0	M0
III	T3	N0	M0
	T1	N1	M0
	T2	N1	M0
	T3	N1	M0
IVA	T4	N0	M0
	T4	N1	M0
	Any T	N2	M0
IVB	Any T	N3	M0
IVC	Any T	Any N	M1

9. What is the role of elective neck dissection in the management of patients with early (stages I and II) squamous cell carcinoma of the oral tongue?

Elective supraomohyoid neck dissection is usually recommended for patients with stages I and II oral tongue cancers. Patients with T1N0M0 and T2N0M0 oral tongue cancers have a substantial risk (30% and 50%, respectively) of occult metastatic disease in the neck. If elective supraomohyoid dissection identifies occult nodal metastasis in 2 or more lymph nodes or extracapsular nodal extension of disease, further treatment is warranted. Radiation therapy is the usual form of adjunctive treatment. If only one (or no) node from the supraomohyoid dissection contains occult cancer, the patient is at low risk for treatment failure and no additional treatment is indicated after supraomohyoid neck dissection.

No studies definitively establish that elective neck dissection improves survival for head and neck cancers at all sites. Prospective randomized trials are difficult to structure and perform. Compelling arguments, however, continue to prompt elective neck dissection for early tongue cancer:

1. The rate of occult metastasis is high in early tongue cancer. Elective dissection identifies patients with occult disease.

2. Salvage rates for patients with neck recurrence are low. Elective neck dissection should reduce the chance for recurrence in the neck by removing occult metastatic disease.

3. Survival after elective neck dissection is higher than after therapeutic neck dissection. Patients who develop neck recurrence have a markedly reduced chance for survival; thus the opportunity to remove nodal disease while still occult should improve survival.

On the other hand, only 30–50% of patients with early stage tongue cancer have true occult nodal disease. The remaining patients who undergo elective neck dissection for early stage tongue cancer will not have occult nodal disease. Unfortunately, no other method of evaluation and treatment identifies the patient with occult nodal disease. At present, supraomohyoid neck dissection functions as an appropriate staging procedure for patients with early squamous cell carcinoma of the tongue.

10. What is the role of elective radiation therapy?
Elective radiation therapy is also an effective option for treatment of the N0 neck for patients with squamous cell carcinoma of the oral tongue. No studies comparing elective radiation therapy with elective neck dissection have clearly demonstrated the benefit of one treatment modality over the other. Factors such as treatment choice for the primary lesion, health status of the patient, and patient preference determine the appropriate choice of treatment for the neck. Regardless of the choice of treatment, the prevailing opinion favors elective treatment of the N0 neck for patients with invasive squamous cell carcinoma of the oral tongue. When surgery is used to treat the primary tongue cancer, elective neck dissection of the N0 neck is indicated.

11. What methods are available for assessing mandibular bony invasion with carcinomas of the oral cavity?
Determination of the presence and extent of mandibular invasion is critical in formation of a treatment plan for the patient with oral cavity cancer. Various imaging studies are available for assessment of mandibular bone invasion, including plain films, orthopantography, CT, and MRI. The precise location and extent of the primary oral cavity tumor help determine the best choice of imaging study.

CT remains the most sensitive imaging study for assessing the integrity of the mandibular cortical bone. MRI more clearly demonstrates the presence of marrow involvement. An intact mandibular cortical line on MRI is believed to be an accurate indicator of an intact cortex, but an irregular cortical line and irregular marrow space are not specific indications of carcinoma because they also may be seen with infectious and inflammatory conditions of the mandible.

12. What surgical techniques are appropriate for management of oral cavity cancers that are adjacent to or invade the mandible?
Segmental mandibulectomy is indicated when carcinoma invades the mandible. The extent of the mandibulectomy depends on the extent of tumor invasion. An extraoral approach via the neck is often necessary to accomplish segmental resection with appropriate surgical margins. Choice of mandibular reconstruction procedure is based on the location of the defect. The most debilitating mandibular resections involve the anterior arch of the mandible. Reconstituting the bony arch after resection is necessary to provide good postoperative function of the oral cavity. Lateral mandibular defects, however, rarely require extensive reconstruction for the patient to function well following segmental mandibulectomy.

Mandibular-sparing techniques involving marginal (or rim) resections are appropriate when the tumor approaches or minimally erodes cortical bone. Marginal mandibulectomy is intended to provide a surgical margin that would be difficult to obtain with soft tissue resection alone. For example, marginal mandibulectomy is appropriate for surgical resection of a floor of mouth carcinoma that abuts but does not invade the inner surface of the mandible. Marginal mandibulectomy is oncologically sound when appropriately used. If direct invasion of the mandible is identified during the course of marginal mandibulectomy, the procedure should be converted into segmental mandibulectomy.

13. What are the most common sites for squamous cell carcinomas in the oropharynx?
Tonsils, tongue base, soft palate, and pharyngeal wall.

14. What is the role of surgery vs. radiation in treatment of early (T1 and T2) squamous cell carcinomas of the oropharynx?
Early cancers of the oropharynx are stage I and stage II lesions. Early oropharyngeal cancer is relatively uncommon because the patient does not often recognize symptoms of early disease. In a significant number of cases, a neck mass is the first presenting symptom. The presence of a neck mass increases the disease stage to at least stage III.

Surgery or radiation therapy provides effective control of early oropharyngeal cancers. The morbidity of surgical access can be considerable. Dysarthria, dysphagia, and aspiration often occur. Radiation therapy is also accompanied by complications. Xerostomia, dysgeusia, and dysphagia are frequently reported by patients after radiation therapy for head and neck malignancy. In general, the morbidity that follows radiation therapy is less severe than the morbidity after surgery. The possibility of tissue preservation and diminished morbidity after treatment persuades many patients and physicians to choose radiation therapy as the initial treatment for early oropharyngeal cancers.

15. How is the oropharynx accessed surgically?

The oropharynx is accessed transorally or through pharyngotomy. T1 cancers of the tonsil, soft palate, and superior pharyngeal wall usually can be managed with transoral excision. Larger tumors and tumors of the tongue base typically require broader exposure. Mandibulotomy with mandibular swing offers excellent exposure to the oropharynx and parapharyngeal space. More limited exposure to the lateral pharyngeal wall and inferior tongue base may be achieved with lateral and/or transhyoid pharyngotomy. Elective neck dissection frequently is appropriate when combined with surgical resection of the primary tumor. Neck dissection provides staging information about potential cervical metastasis and frequently facilitates surgical exposure to the oropharynx.

16. What surgical techniques provide adequate visualization for resection of advanced oropharynx cancers?

The traditional technique for resection of advanced oropharynx cancer is composite resection of the mandible and adjacent soft tissue containing the tumor. This procedure was formerly advocated because of the perceived need to remove mandibular cortex and periosteum that may harbor micrometastasis. A number of surgical anatomists previously theorized that lymphatic vessels from the oral cavity and oropharynx traversed through the mandibular cortex and periosteum before draining to the cervical lymph nodes. This theory has been disproved. Composite resection of the mandible may still be required when tumor involves the mandible. A significant advantage of composite resection is the broad exposure offered by the procedure.

A significant drawback of composite resection is the resulting cosmetic and functional deformity. When possible, resection of oropharynx cancers should preserve the mandible. Mandibular osteotomy with mandibular swing allows lateral retraction of the hemimandible. The combination of mandibulotomy and pharyngotomy provides good exposure to the oropharynx. A lip-splitting incision or mandibular visor flap is useful to access the mandible for composite resection or mandibulotomy. After mandibulotomy, an intraoral incision is made through the floor of mouth. Lingual, hypoglossal, and inferior alveolar nerves are preserved when possible. Various internal fixation methods may be used to reapproximate the mandible.

17. What are the principle advantages of radiation therapy for early cancers of the oropharynx and hypopharynx?

Radiation therapy is effective as a primary treatment for stages I and II cancers of the oropharynx and hypopharynx. Radiation offers treatment of the primary lesion as well as all draining cervical lymphatics. Bilateral and retropharyngeal lymph nodes are often at risk for occult metastasis with oropharynx and hypopharynx cancers. Aggressive bilateral neck dissection is necessary to remove these nodes. Dissection of retropharyngeal nodes is often problematic. Extensive bilateral nodal dissection is unnecessary with radiation therapy, which satisfactorily controls occult metastasis. In addition, as previously mentioned, surgical access and surgical resection for oropharynx cancer often leave the patient with significant functional morbidity. Resection of early hypopharynx cancers may require laryngectomy in some cases. Radiotherapy reduces posttreatment morbidity relative to surgery and offers equivalent control and survival.

18. What are the major differences in clinical behavior between cancers of the glottic and supraglottic larynx?

The **glottic larynx** includes the true vocal cords, anterior commissure, and posterior commissure. The glottic larynx is surrounded by ligamentous structures that act as anatomic barriers to extension of early glottic cancers. The anterior commissure, vocal ligament, thyroglottic ligament, and conus elasticus are the principal anatomic structures that surround the glottic larynx. The glottis is also poorly supplied with blood and lymphatic vessels. Accordingly, the risk of cervical metastasis with cancers confined to the glottis is low. The overall rate of cervical metastasis for T1 and T2 glottic cancers is less than 10%.

The **supraglottic larynx** is composed of the epiglottis, preepiglottic space, aryepiglottic folds, ventricular bands (false cords), and arytenoids. The supraglottic larynx is richly supplied with blood and lymphatic vessels. Like primary glottic cancer, early primary supraglottic cancers tend to stay confined to the supraglottis. Unlike glottic cancer, early cervical nodal metastasis is much more likely because of the extensive supraglottic lymphatic network. The overall cervical metastasis rate for T1 squamous cell carcinomas of the supraglottis is approximately 25%. The rate of cervical metastasis for T2 squamous cell carcinomas of the supraglottis may be as high as 70%. The risk for bilateral cervical metastasis is high because of the rich supraglottic lymphatic network. The risk for occult nodal disease with T1 and T2 supraglottic carcinomas is as high as 50%.

Behavioral patterns of early glottic and supraglottic cancers often allow function-sparing treatment. T1 and T2 glottic cancers are usually treated with conservation surgery or radiation therapy. Cervical lymph nodes do not usually require treatment with early glottic cancers because of the low rate of occult metastasis. The majority of T1 and T2 supraglottic cancers also may be treated with function-sparing surgery or radiation therapy. Because of the high risk for cervical metastasis, consideration should be given to elective treatment of bilateral cervical lymph nodes in all cases of supraglottic squamous cell carcinoma.

19. What is the role of a larynx preservation strategy using radiotherapy with or without chemotherapy in advanced laryngeal cancers?

Total laryngectomy is the accepted standard form of treatment for most patients with advanced laryngeal cancer. Larynx preservation strategies using radiation therapy for selected advanced cancers have been used for a number of years. More recently, chemotherapy has been used in combination with radiation therapy in an attempt to increase the effectiveness of laryngeal preservation protocols. The overall goal has been to preserve larynges and to match or exceed local control and survival rates achievable with conventional treatment. The well-known study by the Department of Veterans Affairs Laryngeal Cancer Study Group clearly demonstrated that a population of patients with advanced laryngeal cancer can be cured without laryngectomy, but several important questions remain to be answered. The contribution of chemotherapy to successful laryngeal preservation is unclear. Chemotherapy may have selected patients who would have responded to radiation therapy alone. Additional studies are needed to define more clearly which patients with advanced laryngeal cancer will benefit from laryngeal preservation attempts and to define appropriate combinations of treatment modalities.

20. What methods are currently available for speech rehabilitation in patients who undergo total laryngectomy?

Return of speech function is one of the most important determinants of quality of life after total laryngectomy. The three general methods of speech restoration after total laryngectomy are tracheoesophageal fistula (TEP) speech, esophageal speech, and use of a mechanical artificial larynx. Of the three, TEP speech has emerged as the favored method.

A **mechanical artificial larynx** is usually the first form of alaryngeal speech after laryngectomy. Most patients can use the artificial larynx in the first few postoperative days. The voice quality of the artificial larynx is mechanical and monotonic. Better voice quality is achievable with TEP or esophageal speech. Some patients, however, are not good candidates for the latter two methods because of anatomy, coexisting conditions, or preference; they can achieve satisfactory alaryngeal speech communication with a mechanical artificial larynx.

Esophageal speech requires the patient to force air into the neopharynx and esophagus. Controlled release of the air then generates vibration of the pharyngoesophageal segment and produces sound. The patient uses the normal articulation processes of the tongue and oral cavity to produce speech with the generated sound. The advantage of esophageal speech is that no specific procedures or devices are necessary. The significant disadvantage of esophageal speech is the difficulty in learning to inject and release air properly in the pharyngoesophageal segment. Only 10–25% of patients who undergo laryngectomy develop successful esophageal speech, despite intensive training efforts.

TEP speech requires surgical creation of a small fistula between the esophagus and trachea. The fistula is created with tracheoesophageal puncture (usually abbreviated as TEP) at the time of laryngectomy or as a secondary procedure. A prosthesis consisting of a one-way valve is then placed into the fistula within several days of TEP. To produce sound, the tracheostoma is occluded on exhalation forcing air into the pharyngoesophageal segment. As in esophageal speech, vibration of the pharyngeal and esophageal walls creates sound. Injection of air via TEP is much easier than with the esophageal speech method. Successful vocalization occurs in up to 95% of patients who have primary or secondary TEP. As with other methods of alaryngeal speech, patient selection is important to maximize the chance for success. Fortunately, most laryngectomy patients are now candidates for TEP, and significant complications of the procedure are rare. The simplicity of the procedure and high success rates make TEP speech the current standard of care for alaryngeal speech rehabilitation.

21. What is the appropriate treatment for a patient with metastatic squamous cell carcinoma of the neck when a primary malignancy has not been identified?

The best method for managing patients with metastatic unknown primary squamous cell carcinoma of the neck has not been determined in randomized prospective trials. Debate about most appropriate treatment ranges from radical neck dissection to aggressive radiation therapy aimed at the site of metastasis and likely primary sites. Unfortunately, studies are often difficult to compare because patient populations are defined differently in the various studies. Published 3- and 5-year survival rates range from 40–55% and 25–54%, respectively. Of interest, survival rates are substantially better when the primary tumor remains occult.

The clinical presentation and biopsy method often define the options for treatment of the metastatic unknown primary carcinoma in the neck. In the patient with an N1 neck and FNA biopsy diagnosis of malignancy, neck dissection is most appropriate as an initial staging and therapeutic procedure. Selective neck dissection is frequently possible. The pathologic findings in the neck dissection specimen are often helpful in planning further treatment. The identified locations of cervical metastasis usually suggest one or more primary sites. Postoperative radiation therapy may then be directed at the neck, most likely primary sites, and contralateral neck to improve locoregional control rates.

Some N1 patients may have open excisional biopsy of the metastatic node and no gross residual disease after biopsy. In such cases, therapeutic radiation treatment is appropriate. The fields are extended to cover potential primary sites. In the patient with N2 or N3 neck disease, radical or modified radical neck dissection is necessary. Radiation therapy may precede or follow neck dissection. The choice of preoperative vs. postoperative radiation therapy depends on the initial resectability of the neck disease and physician and patient preferences. Regardless of the clinical presentation, aggressive treatment of metastatic unknown primary squamous cell carcinoma of the neck is warranted considering the potential survival benefit.

22. What is the role of fine needle aspiration (FNA) biopsy in management of salivary gland masses in adults?

Over 90% of persistent salivary gland masses in adults are neoplastic. The appropriate treatment for all salivary neoplasms, benign or malignant, is surgical resection. Most patients with salivary gland masses do not benefit from FNA biopsy because surgical resection is required and FNA provides little information that will change the need for surgery.

Interpretation of FNA biopsy of salivary gland masses is difficult. Up to 20% of all salivary gland FNA attempts yield nondiagnostic material. Up to 20% of salivary gland FNA biopsies are falsely negative for malignancy. In addition, salivary gland masses are rare. Few pathologists have substantial experience in interpretation of cytologic material from salivary glands. Therefore, results of FNA biopsy of salivary gland masses are often open to question. Clinical impressions, regardless of FNA results, should serve as the principal determinant for choice of treatment.

FNA biopsy is useful for confirming clinical impressions in certain circumstances. Patients who are poor surgical risks and probably have benign tumors should have FNA in an attempt to characterize the lesion. Some benign salivary neoplasms, such as Warthin's tumor, have fairly characteristic FNA findings. If the lesion appears convincingly benign by cytologic exam, surgery usually may be safely deferred in patients with high risk for perioperative complications.

Patients who present with salivary masses and have a history of malignancy at another site also may have benefit from FNA. Confirmation of metastasis in the salivary gland may dramatically affect plans for treatment. Likewise, patients with lymphoma who have salivary gland masses can benefit from FNA. Otherwise, when the clinical impression is salivary gland neoplasm, FNA biopsy does little to confirm or deny the need for surgical resection.

23. What are the major indications for facial nerve sacrifice during surgery for parotid gland neoplasms?

The only indications for sacrifice of all or portions of the facial nerve during parotid gland surgery for neoplasm are direct nerve invasion and inability to remove the tumor without nerve sacrifice. Histologic diagnosis (e.g., adenoid cystic carcinoma) and proximity of tumor to nerve without direct invasion are not appropriate indications for facial nerve resection. Rates of locoregional control and survival after nerve preservation when direct invasion is absent are at least equal to more radical procedures that sacrifice the nerve in the absence of direct invasion.

24. What is the role for neck dissection in the management of parotid cancers?

Therapeutic neck dissection is clearly indicated in the treatment of parotid gland cancers that present with clinically apparent cervical metastases. The role for elective neck dissection in patients with parotid cancer and an N0 neck is much less clear. Parotid cancers rarely (10–15%) present with cervical metastasis. In addition, metastases rarely occur in the neck when the primary cancer is controlled. Furthermore, patients who would otherwise benefit most from elective neck dissection typically have indications for postoperative radiation to the primary tumor site. Occult cervical metastasis from salivary gland cancer is controlled with radiation therapy. Extension of the postoperative radiation therapy fields to the neck makes neck dissection unnecessary.

Elective neck dissection, however, may be useful in selected cases to provide better exposure for resection of the primary tumor. An example is a deep lobe parotid tumor with extension to the parapharyngeal space. Neck dissection allows access to the parapharyngeal space from the neck and facilitates tumor resection.

25. What is the appropriate initial management of patients with a thyroid nodule?

Initial evaluation of a thyroid nodule should determine which patients will benefit from a surgical procedure and which patients require medical management before or in lieu of surgery. One of the first appropriate diagnostic steps is determination of the serum level of thyroid-stimulating hormone (TSH). Clinical suspicion also may prompt evaluation of thyroxine (T4) and triiodothyronine (T3) levels. If the patient is determined to be hyperthyroid, a radionuclide scan is indicated to distinguish a hyperfunctioning nodule from a cold nodule. Identification of a hyperfunctioning nodule negates the need for further evaluation, because the risk of malignancy is extremely low.

Most patients with a thyroid nodule have a normal serum TSH level. FNA biopsy of the nodule is indicated in such patients. Most FNA attempts yield adequate material. The rate of nondiagnostic FNA biopsy of thyroid nodules is approximately 15%. This rate may be further substantially reduced with repeated aspiration. All patients who have identifiable malignancy on FNA should be considered candidates for surgical resection of thyroid malignancy. Only about 5% of patients, however, have lesions identified as malignant or suspicious for malignancy. The vast majority (at least 60%) have benign lesions identified by FNA. Solitary benign thyroid nodules are usually treated initially with thyroid suppression therapy.

FNA biopsy of the remaining patients identifies follicular epithelium with varying degrees of atypia. Patients above the age of 50 are typically considered to be candidates for surgical resection because the risk of malignancy is relatively high. Younger patients who are otherwise asymptomatic usually may be safely treated with thyroid suppression. If the nodule does not resolve, surgical resection is recommended.

26. What are the major prognostic factors that predict clinical outcomes for patients with differentiated thyroid (papillary and follicular) cancers?

Various classification and staging schemes attempt to predict outcomes for patients with differentiated thyroid cancers. Important prognostic factors are age at diagnosis, tumor size, histologic grade, extrathyroidal extension, cervical nodal metastasis, and distant metastasis. Different classification systems weight each of the factors in a slightly different manner. Thus far, no single system functions significantly better than any of the others.

Despite the fact that no system satisfactorily predicts prognosis for any individual patient, some general conclusions can be drawn about prognostic factors. Low risk for recurrence and disease-related mortality is correlated with younger age at time of diagnosis, smaller size of the primary tumor, absence of extrathyroidal extension, absence of regional or distant metastasis, and complete surgical resection.

27. What is the appropriate surgical margin for resection of cutaneous melanomas in the head and neck region?

Precise recommendations for appropriate surgical resection margins for cutaneous melanomas of the head and neck are difficult to make. General recommendations about margins for head and neck melanoma are extrapolated from data about melanomas of the trunk and extremities and from a limited number of clinical studies about specific subsites of head and neck melanoma.

Recommendations for surgical resection margins for melanoma are based on tumor thickness. All melanomas should be widely excised. The definition of wide excision depends on tumor thickness and subsite. For thin melanomas (< 1.0 mm in thickness), a 1-cm margin of normal skin around the melanoma and into the underlying subcutaneous tissue is adequate. Intermediate thickness melanomas (1.0–4.0 mm in thickness) should be excised with a 2-cm margin whenever possible. A principal problem with head and neck melanomas is that a 2-cm circumferential margin is often not possible without inflicting major cosmetic or functional deformity. The general rule is that the wide excision is carried to the anatomic margin of the cosmetic or functional unit. Supporting structures such as nasal cartilage, perichondrium and periosteum can often be preserved. Partial rhinectomy is rarely necessary for cutaneous melanomas of the nasal skin unless melanoma extends to the deeper supporting structures. Melanomas of the external ear can often be appropriately managed with wedge resection of the external ear and primary closure. Using this philosophy, local control of melanoma in the head and neck can be expected in greater than 90% of cases. Improvement in survival has not been clearly associated with more extensive local resections for cutaneous melanomas of the head and neck.

28. What is the role for elective neck dissection in the management of melanomas of the head and neck?

The value of elective neck dissection for all patients with cutaneous melanoma of the head and neck is still uncertain in terms of promoting improved survival. The recently published interim analysis of the Intergroup Melanoma Surgical Program suggests a survival benefit in selected subgroups of patients, but results are not final and subgroup classification and analysis have been questioned. The most significant benefit of elective dissection currently appears to be identification of patients with occult metastatic disease. Given the recent results of the Eastern Cooperative Oncology Group trials of adjuvant interferon-alpha-2b, identification of occult nodal disease and subsequent treatment with adjuvant interferon should provide survival benefit. Other methods for identification of occult cervical metastasis, such as lymphoscintigraphy and sentinel node biopsy, may prove to be more cost-effective means of identifying patients who will benefit from postoperative adjuvant treatment. The lymph node drainage patterns of the head and neck are generally more complicated than those of the trunk and extremities. Initial studies seem to indicate the utility of lymphoscintigraphy and sentinel node biopsy, although further studies are needed to establish efficacy and cost-effectiveness relative to elective node dissection for patients with cutaneous melanomas of the head and neck.

BIBLIOGRAPHY

1. Amdur RJ, Parsons JT, Mendenhall WM, et al: Postoperative irradiation for squamous cell carcinoma of the head and neck: An analysis of treatment and complications. Int J Radiat Oncol Biol Phys 16:26–36, 1989.
2. Batsakis JG, Sniege N, el-Naggar AK: Fine needle operation of salivary glands: Its utility and tissue effects. Ann Otol Rhinol Laryng 102:483–485, 1992.
3. Balch CM, Soong SJ, Bartolucci AA, et al: Efficacy of an elective regional lymph node dissection of 1 to 4 mm thick melanomas for patients 60 years of age and younger. Ann Surg 224:255–263, 1996.
4. Blalock D: Speech rehabilitation after treatment of laryngeal carcinoma. Otolaryngol Clin North Am 30:179–188, 1997.

5. Callender DL, Sherman SI, Gagel RF, et al: Cancer of the thyroid. In Myers EN, Suen JY (eds): Cancer of the Head and Neck, 3rd ed. Philadelphia, W.B. Saunders, 1996, pp 485–515.
6. Callender DL, Weber RS: Modified neck dissection. In Shockley WW, Pillsbury HC (eds): The Neck: Diagnosis and Surgery. St. Louis, Mosby, 1994, pp 413–430.
7. Department of Veterans Affairs Laryngeal Cancer Study Group: Induction chemotherapy plus radiation compared with surgery plus radiation in patients with advanced laryngeal cancer. N Engl J Med 324:1685–1690, 1991.
8. Fleming ID, Cooper JS, Henson DE, et al (eds): AJCC Cancer Staging Manual. Philadelphia, Lippincott-Raven, 1997.
9. Frankenthaler RA, Luna MA, Lee SS, et al: Prognostic variables in parotid gland cancer. Arch Otolaryngol Head Neck Surg 117:1251–1256, 1991.
10. Weber RS, Callender DL: Laryngeal conservation surgery. Semin Radiat Oncol 2:149–157, 1992.

34. LOCAL FLAPS OF THE HEAD AND NECK

Gregory R. D. Evans, M.D.

GENERAL PRINCIPLES

1. What are the advantages of using local flaps in the head and neck?
   1. Similar color and texture of the skin for the site of the defect.
   2. Donor sites frequently can be closed directly.
   3. Skin grafts do not always have 100% survival and appear pale or more pigmented than surrounding skin.
   4. There is frequently little or no scar contracture with the use of local flaps.

2. Full-thickness defects up to what width can be repaired with composite grafts?
   1.0–1.5 cm. In practicality, the color and texture mismatch precludes the use of grafts. One should make every attempt to use local tissue, when available, for reconstruction.

3. What are the major problems with the use of local flaps?
   Local flaps of the head and neck require planning and experience. Flaps should be the same size and thickness as the defect; otherwise, problems will develop. The use of local flaps is more difficult in children because of the lack of skin laxity. Preservation of local landmarks, such as the temporal hairline and eyebrows, is vital.

4. In the planning of local flaps, what are the two main vasoelastic biomechanical properties of the skin of which the surgeon must be aware?
   1. **Stress relaxation** occurs when a constant load is applied to the skin, causing it to stretch. With time the load required to maintain the skin in its stretched position decreases.
   2. **Creep** occurs when a sudden load is applied to the skin and is kept constant. The amount of extension increases with the passage of time.

5. Where should incision lines for local flaps and donor areas fall?
   Lines of minimal relaxed tension. The skin tension is at right angles to these lines.

6. In the design of a rotational flap, in what shape should the defect be excised?
   A triangle with the base as the shortest side.

7. In a rotation flap, where is the line of greatest tension?
   The line of greatest tension extends from the pivot point of the flap to the edge of the defect nearest to where the flap previously lay. (See figure at top of next page.)

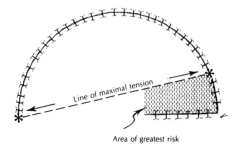

Rotation flap. (From Jackson IT: Local Flaps in Head and Neck Reconstruction. St. Louis, Mosby, 1985, p 10, with permission.)

8. In an advancement flap, what is excessive skin at the base called?
Burow's triangles, which are excised lateral to the flap base.

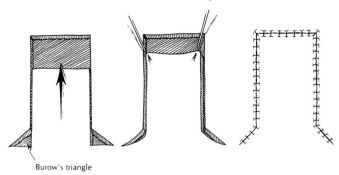

Burow's triangles. (From Jackson IT: Local Flaps in Head and Neck Reconstruction. St. Louis, Mosby, 1985, p 13, with permission.)

9. How many potential flaps can be designed from each Rhomboid defect?
Four.

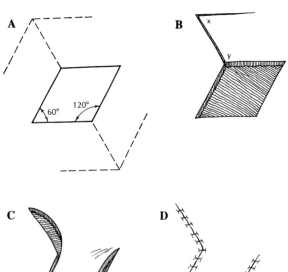

The rhomboid (Limberg) flap. *A,* Four potential flaps can be designed from each rhomboid defect. *B,* As with the Z-plasty, flap elevation should extend slightly beyond the base of the flap. *C* and *D,* The angles of the flap are secured with three-point sutures and the donor site is closed directly. (From Jackson IT: Local Flaps in Head and Neck Reconstruction. St. Louis, Mosby, 1985, p 17, with permission.)

10. What are the common angles of the rhomboid defect created for flap closure?
60° and 120°.

11. Large circular defects can be converted into a hexagon to facilitate closure. How many rhomboid flaps are available for closure of this defect?
Six.

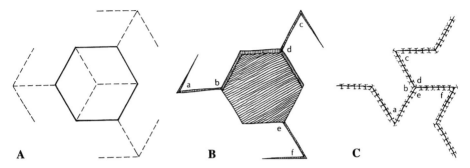

The triple rhomboid. A hexagon can be converted into three rhomboids. Rhomboid flaps can be planned on the 120° angle; thus, six potential flaps are available. Three of these flaps are used for closure of the defect. (From Jackson IT: Local Flaps in Head and Neck Reconstruction. St. Louis, Mosby, 1985, p 19, with permission.)

12. How many rhomboid flaps are most commonly used for closure of a hexagonal defect?
Three.

13. What are the angles used for a Dufourmentel flap?
30° and 150°. This flap adheres to similar principles as the rhomboid flap but is based on 30° and 150° angles instead of 60° and 120° angles.

14. In the design of a Z-plasty, what angles yield what percentage of gain in length?
• 30° → 25%
• 45° → 50%
• 60° → 75%

15. What is the major indication for a W-plasty?
Scar revision.

16. What are the causes of local flap failures in the head and neck?
1. A small flap designed to fill a big hole
2. Hematoma
3. Damaged blood supply (technical error)
4. Making the flap extend outside the blood supply (design fault)
5. Suturing the wound under tension and failing to use a back cut
All of the flaps discussed above can be used for defects in the head and neck.

FOREHEAD

17. Much of the forehead can be anesthetized by infiltration of local agents around which nerves?
The supraorbital nerves, which are located at the junction of the central and medial thirds of the supraorbital rim and arise from cranial nerve (CN) V.

18. The key concept in forehead reconstruction is a firm knowledge of which structures?
Fixed aesthetic structures, such as the eyebrows and hairline.

19. Which area of the forehead has thinner and more pliable skin?
The glabella region.

20. What is the motor supply to the forehead musculature?
The frontal branch of the facial nerve (CN VII), which lies on a line between the ear lobule and a point just lateral to the lateral end of the eyebrow. The frontal branch of the facial nerve lies within the temporoparietal fascia superior to the zygomatic arch. The frontal branch of the facial nerve is located in a deep plane in the facial area and becomes more superficial as it crosses the zygomatic arch into the temporal region. Operative procedures that involve exposure of the zygomatic arch for reconstruction or subperiosteal exposure of the facial skeleton should be performed by dissection deep to the temporoparietal fascia to prevent injury.

21. Where are the lines of minimal tension in the forehead?
Transverse in the forehead and vertical in the glabella region. Scars placed on the diagonal are least satisfactory.

22. To avoid pin cushioning, how should incisions be placed?
Vertically oriented through the skin.

23. What are the four aesthetic units of the forehead?
1. Main forehead   3. Temporal
2. Supra eyebrow   4. Glabella

24. Which technique allows additional length to rotational and other flaps on the forehead?
Galeal scoring with intervals of 0.5–1.0 cm.

25. When scalp mobility and galeal scoring are not sufficient, which technique allows closure of difficult defects?
Bilateral rotational flaps. The defect is triangulated, and bilateral scalp flaps are elevated. The forehead is denervated; however, because bilateral flaps are elevated, symmetry is maintained. Problems may arise if the lateral incisions are carried too posterior to interfere with the blood supply.

26. How is supra eyebrow reconstruction best achieved?
With island flaps based on the superficial temporal artery.

27. Because of the limited amount of forehead skin, epidermolysis can occur. How should it be treated?
Conservatively. Bony exposure may require removal of the outer cortex and permitting the wound to granulate or skin-grafting of the defect. Alternatively, another local flap may be required.

LIPS

28. What are the major functional muscles of the lips and cheeks?
The orbicularis oris is a complex sphincter that functions in conjunction with the muscles of facial expression. Its deep and oblique fibers are positioned in and about the vermilion and function as a sphincter to approximate the lips to the alveolar arch. The superficial elements receive decussating fibers from the buccinator and function to purse and protrude the lips. A major muscle of the cheek is the buccinator, which originates from the alveolar process of the maxilla, mandible, and pterygomandibular raphe and inserts at the corners of the mouth deep to the other muscles of facial expression. The buccinator fibers from above become continuous with the orbicularis of the lower lip and those from below merge with the orbicularis fibers of the upper lip. On the superficial surface of the buccinator are the buccopharyngeal fascia and buccal fat pad. In the region of the third molar, the muscle is pierced by the parotid duct. The action of the buccinator is cheek compression, which serves to assist other muscles in mastication. The principal elevator of the upper lip is the levator labii superiorus. The zygomaticus major draws the lip up and back, whereas the risorius and buccinator clear the gingival sulci. Depression and lip retraction are mainly controlled by the platysma, depressor labii inferiorus, and depressor angulii oris.

29. What are the reconstructive goals of the lip?

1. Complete skin cover
2. Reestablishment of a vermilion
3. Adequate stomal diameter
4. Reestablishment of sensation
5. Competence of the oral sphincter

30. During surgical resection and reconstruction, at what angle should the vermilion-skin junction be crossed?

90°. The vermilion–skin junction should be tattooed with methylene blue using a 25-gauge needle before surgical resection. This approach avoids the loss of the white roll with application of anesthetic combined with epinephrine. Discrepancies in alignment as little as 1 mm may be noticeable.

31. In the staircase or stepladder technique for lip reconstruction, what is the measure of the horizontal component of the step excisions?

The step technique allows closure of defects up to two-thirds of the lower lip. This type of flap retains relatively good sensation and muscle continuity and function and may be adjusted for lateral defects. The horizontal component of the step excisions measure one-half the width of the defect; thus, usually 2–4 steps are required. The vertical dimension of each step is 8–10 mm.

32. What are the indications for an Abbé flap?

The Abbé flap is a highly useful flap that can be used for moderate-sized defects of the upper and lower lip. Indications for the flap include a moderate-sized defect of the lower lip that is off center but spares the commissure, a defect of the philtrum of the upper lip, and the need to restore symmetry to an overly small lower lip as part of a staged reconstruction. The flap should be positioned so that the width of the vermilion of the donor site matches the lip segment being replaced. The flap is designed with the width one-half of the defect so that tissue deficiency will be shared equally between the upper and lower lip. If a discrete aesthetic unit is replaced, the exact corresponding size of the flap should be outlined. Division of the flap occurs at 1–2 weeks.

33. How are defects of the commissure addressed?

The Estlander flap is most useful in medium-sized lateral defects of the upper or lower lip that include the commissure. Its dissection is similar to the Abbé flap, but because it does not have to preserve an intact commissure, it can be performed in one stage. As with the Abbé flap, the Estlander flap is designed to include approximately one-half of the defect. Secondary revisions of the commissure may be required.

34. Which flap restores lip continuity with preservation of motor and sensory function?

The Karapandzic flap, a modification of the Gilles fan flap, maintains the neurovascular pedicle in the soft tissue while rotating and restoring sphincter continuity. For this reason it tends to provide better functional results.

35. The Bernard operation advances full-thickness local flaps with concomitant triangular excisions to allow proper mobilization. What does the Webster modification of the Bernard-Burow cheiloplasty include?

1. Excision of skin and subcutaneous tissue only in Burow's triangles to maintain innervated muscle-bearing flaps.

2. Location of the triangular excisions farther laterally in the nasolabial fold instead of next to the commissure.

3. Paramental Burow's triangles to ease inferior advancement of the cheek tissue.

36. What are the options for the restoration of hair-bearing skin for lip reconstruction?

The nasolabial flap may be used for hair-bearing reconstruction of the upper lip. Full-thickness flaps, however, destroy the innervation to the upper lip. The temporal island scalp flap also may be used for hair restoration.

37. In commissure reconstruction, the restoration of what structure is critical?

The restoration of the orbicularis oris sphincter mechanism is critical for oral competence. This mechanism can be restored by approximation of the muscle with suture.

CHEEK

38. What are the aesthetic units of the cheek?
   The aesthetic units of the face are the topographic zones of the cheek: suborbital, preauricular, and buccomandibular.

39. Small defects of the cheek area are best reconstructed with what type of flaps?
   Defects that are not amenable to primary closure are frequently suited for small local flaps. The laxity and vasculature of the facial skin enables the closure of defects that may not be acceptable in other body locations. The Limberg (rhomboid) local transposition and rotational flaps offer well-vascularized tissue for wound closure. In addition, the use of these flaps over the malar eminence may prevent an ectropion due to skin graft contracture. The nasolabial flap provides well-padded vascularized tissue. The bulky nature of the flap and the requirement of further revisions of the dog-ears may preclude the use of this flap in some cases.

40. Defects approaching 4 × 6 cm are best reconstructed with what type of flap?
   The cervicofacial flap describes a reconstructive method that requires extensive cervical cheek, retroauricular, and chin undermining for flap advancement. The flap can be extended onto the chest if necessary. The rotation of the flap is in a superomedial direction, and a superior dissection lateral to the eye must be performed to prevent possible ectropion as the flap is advanced. In smokers this flap should not be raised in the subcutaneous plane alone. Dissection into the mucosa allows closure of intraoral and through-and-through defects with this flap.

41. Large preauricular defects may require closure with what type of flap?
   Large neck flaps take advantage of the elastic neck tissue. The flap's design may allow a sufficient amount of tissue to be sutured on a plane between the helical attachment and the lateral brow. Lower placement of the flap may lead to an ectropion. The lower level of the flap incision should be above the clavicle. The donor site frequently may require skin grafting, and the use of this flap without delay should be viewed with caution. More stable forms of coverage may include free tissue transfer or alternative flaps.

42. What are the advantages of the cervicopectoral flap?
   The medially based cervicopectoral flap offers many advantages. First, it is vascularized by anterior thoracic perforators off the internal mammary artery. Second, when the flap is delayed it may replace the entire aesthetic unit of the cheek. The flap is elevated deep to the platysma muscle and anterior pectoral fascia.

43. The cheek can be anesthetized by infiltration of local agents around which nerves?
   The infraorbital nerve is located at the junction of the central and medial thirds of the infraorbital rim at a point 0.5–1.0 cm below the rim. The mental nerve exits from the foramen 1–1.5 cm above the inferior border of the mandible (canine premolar teeth). It lies in a vertical plane along with the supraorbital and infraorbital nerves. The mandibular nerve supplies an area extending to the tragus but not incorporating the ear and stopping short of the inferior border of the mandible. The lower cheek and neck are supplied by the anterior cutaneous nerves and the great auricular nerve.

44. What is the motor nerve supply to the muscles of the cheek?
   CN VII to the superficial muscles and CN V to the masseter.

45. Reconstruction over the malar eminence may impinge on what important structures?
   The lower lid and canthal areas. Flap design should be performed to place the minimal amount of tension within this area. Lower lid ectropion can be prevented by securing the advancing flap to the periosteum of the zygoma, thus preventing pull on the lower lid.

HEAD AND NECK

46. What are the optimal characteristics of a technique for head and neck reconstruction?
   Reliability is perhaps the most important factor in any type of oncologic reconstruction. Patients requiring head and neck reconstruction usually have advanced disease, indicating either

limited survival or the need for adjuvant therapy. A failed reconstruction that prolongs hospitalization time and increases cost does not improve the quality of life. Furthermore, prolonged reconstruction is time taken away from family and/or additional adjuvant therapy.

Expediency also must be considered for any reconstructive technique. In most cases a one-stage reconstruction should be employed. Patients seldom benefit from multistaged procedures that take several months to complete, delaying adjuvant therapy and interfering with valuable family time.

In addition to reliability and expediency, reconstruction must provide **function and cosmesis**. Whether restoration of contour is possible depends on the defect size and location and the structures involved. The type and grade of the tumor as well as the psychologic make-up of the patient determine the reconstructive method that will provide the best function and contour.

47. How are defects of the head and neck classified?

Three categories of head and neck defects have been identified by Hanna. The type of defect must be defined before choosing a reconstructive modality.

Class A: defects requiring mandatory cover. Class A defects include exposed brain and/or dura, ocular structures, great vessels of the neck, upper mediastinum and lungs, and/or bone (calvarial or facial bones). Coverage of these structures is critical for wound healing and survival, reinforcing the need for a reliable and expedient method. Flap failures may be life-threatening in such situations.

Class B: defects yielding significant functional deficits. Class B defects include those involving the mucosa and soft tissue of the oral cavity, mandible, lips and cheeks, and/or facial nerve. Reconstruction of these structures is not critical for survival; however, marked functional deficits occur without adequate reconstruction. In particular, oral continence must be maintained.

Class C: defects yielding significant aesthetic deficits. Class C defects involve specialized structures such as the nose, ears, eyes, hair-bearing areas (e.g., mustache, eye brows), and/or external skin contours (without exposed bone). Although loss of these structures may result in a significant loss of cosmesis and quality of life, the timing of reconstruction is less important than with class A and B defects. Immediate reconstruction is often not imperative. Temporized wound coverage with simpler reconstructive methods may be used. Definitive reconstruction may be postponed until adjuvant therapy has been completed.

48. Which flap, based on the superficial temporal vessels, can cover large external or intraoral defects?

The forehead flap can include one-half to two-thirds of the forehead and traditionally was used for intraoral reconstruction with a two-stage procedure. The original flap did not include the contralateral forehead tissue; however, the entire forehead may be included with the dissection. Significant donor site morbidity and microsurgical reconstruction preclude the use of this flap except for a few indications.

49. Although able to supply well-vascularized muscle and fascia from the lateral head, significant donor site deformity may occur from the use of which flap?

The temporal muscle and fascia flap offers viable and well-vascularized tissue for defects around the orbit and upper cheek area. Traditionally the flap also was used for intraoral reconstruction. Significant donor site deformity has encouraged reconstruction by other methods. However, this flap is still useful for orbital and cranial base surgery.

50. What is the vascular supply of the deltopectoral flap?

The deltopectoral flap has three main vascular contributions. Most of the skin from the sternal border to the deltopectoral groove is supplied by the first four perforating branches of the internal mammary artery, primarily the second and third branches. At the upper portion of the deltopectoral groove, branches from the thoracoacromial artery supply the upper midportion of the flap. The area of the flap overlying the deltoid muscle is supplied by perforating vessels. The deltoid portion constitutes a random flap supported on the end of the axially supplied pectoral skin. Delay is frequently necessary to increase viability before transfer. The use of this local flap is currently limited.

51. The deltopectoral flap can be transferred without a delay procedure so long as the skin paddle in the deltoid portion distal to the cephalic groove does not exceed what length/width ratio?

    1:1.

52. The blood supply of the sternocleidomastoid myocutaneous flap is derived from what three sources?

    1. Occipital artery in the proximal one-third
    2. Superior thyroid artery in the middle one-third
    3. A branch from the thyrocervical trunk in the distal one-third.

The main limitation of this flap is its variable blood supply and limited arc of rotation. It has been termed the most tenuous of all the musculocutaneous flaps used for head and neck reconstruction.

53. Which flap is thin with a variable blood supply but may offer both sensation and animation?

The platysma myocutaneous flap has a variable blood supply. Some authors describe the flap as a type II muscle in which the major vascular pedicle is the submental branch of the facial artery and the minor pedicle is the superficial branch of the transverse cervical artery. Other authors disagree, stating that the blood supply is from multiple perforating vessels. Although theoretically advantageous as thin pliable tissue, the flap is generally considered unreliable.

54. Based on the transverse cervical artery, which flap can be elevated in a lateral or descending direction?

The trapezius myocutaneous flap can be designed in several directions. The lateral trapezius flap provides thin, pliable skin over the proximal deltoid area. The origin of the superficial branch of the artery and venous drainage hamper the elevation of this flap. The lower trapezius myocutaneous flap is based on the deep branch of the transverse cervical artery and innervated by the posterior branch of the spinal accessory nerve. The flap is frequently limited by its arc of rotation, and the donor site over the acromioclavicular joint is subject to high operative morbidity.

55. Which versatile flap is based on the pectoral branch of the thoracoacromial artery?

The pectoralis myocutaneous flap is based on the thoracoacromial artery (pectoral branch), which exits the subclavian artery at the midportion of the clavicle and courses medial to the insertion of the pectoralis minor tendon. The flap can be designed with a skin paddle centered over the lower portion of the muscle, which can be placed intraorally if necessary. The flap has been described as raised as high as the orbits; however, in practicality it is difficult to secure the closure without significant downward pull on the muscle. The flap can be modified with an extended random skin component or with two separate skin paddles that can be divided. A rib may be harvested with the flap for bony reconstruction. Higher elevation of the flap can be performed with division of the clavicle.

56. What is the dominant blood supply of the latissimus dorsi muscle?

The dominant blood supply is the thoracodorsal branch of the subscapular artery. The flap is elevated and skeletonized on its vascular pedicle. The muscle is detached from its insertion on the humerus and transferred by tunneling or curving it around to the head and neck defect. The main attributes of the latissimus dorsi are its large size, wide excursion, and little donor site morbidity. The arc of rotation for head and neck defects is difficult and frequently precludes the use of this flap.

BIBLIOGRAPHY

1. Ariyan S: The pectoralis major myocutaneous flap. A versatile flap for reconstruction in the head and neck. Plast Reconstr Surg 63:73–81, 1979.
2. Ariyan S: One-stage reconstruction for defects of the mouth using a sternomastoid myocutaneous flap. Plast Reconstr Surg 63:618–625, 1979.
3. Bakamjian V: Use of tongue flaps in lower lip reconstruction. Br J Plast Surg 17:76, 1964.
4. Bernard C: Cancer de la levre inferieure opere par un procede nouveau. Bull Mem Soc Chir Paris 3:357, 1853.
5. Crow ML, Crow FJ: Resurfacing large cheek defects with rotation flaps form the neck. Plast Reconstr Surg 58:196–200, 1976.

6. Futrell JW: Platysma myocutaneous flap for intraoral reconstruction. Am J Surg 136:504–507, 1978.
7. Goldstein MH: A tissue-expanded vermilion myocutaneous flap for lip repair. Plast Reconstr Surg 73:768–770, 1984.
8. Gonzalez Ulloa M, et al: Preliminary study of the total restoration of the facial skin. Plast Reconstr Surg 13:151, 1954.
9. Hanna DC: Present and future trends in reconstructive surgery for head and neck cancer patients. Laryngoscope 88(Suppl 8):96–100, 1978.
10. Isakksson I, Johanson B: Partial reconstruction of the lower lip. Panminerva Med 9:240, 1967.
11. Jackson I: Local Flaps in Head and Neck Reconstruction. St. Louis, Mosby, 1985.
12. Juri J, Juri C: Cheek reconstruction with advancement-rotation flaps. Clin Plast Surg 8:223–226, 1981.
13. Karapandzic M: Reconstruction of lip defects by local arterial flaps. Br J Plast Surg 27:93–97, 1974.
14. Kolhe PS, Leonard AG: Reconstruction of the vermilion after "lip-shave." Br J Plast Surg 41:68–73, 1988.
15. McGregor IA: The temporal flap in intraoral cancer: Its use in repairing the post-excisional defect. Br J Plast Surg 16:318, 1963.
16. Spira M, Hardy SB: Vermilionectomy. Review of cases with variations in technique. Plast Reconstr Surg 33:39, 1964.
17. Tobin GR, O'Daniel TG: Lip reconstruction with motor and sensory innervated composite flaps. Clin Plast Surg 17:623–632, 1990.
18. Webster RC, Coffey RJ, Kelleher RE: Total and partial reconstruction on the lower lip with innervated muscle-bearing flaps. Plast Reconstr Surg 25:360, 1960.
19. Zide BM: Deformities of the lips and cheeks. In McCarthy JG (ed): Plastic Surgery, vol 3. Philadelphia, W.B. Saunders, 1990, pp 2009–2056.

35. NASAL RECONSTRUCTION

Roy Hong, M.D., and Frederick J. Menick, M.D.

1. What are the nasal subunits? Are they important in reconstruction?

The nose may be divided into nine topographic subunits comprised of the dorsum, tip, columella, and paired sidewalls, alae, and soft triangles. Each subunit has a characteristic skin quality, unit outline, and three-dimensional contour. The normal nose is reestablished only if each of these characteristics is restored. More than obtaining a healed wound, the subunits that describe the nose visually must be restored.

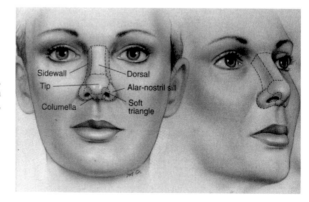

Nasal subunits. (From Burget GC, Menick FJ: Aesthetic Reconstruction of the Nose. St. Louis, Mosby, 1994, with permission.)

2. What are the principles of subunit reconstruction? How are they applied?

If a defect is to be repaired and the nose look normal, the characteristics of each subunit must be reestablished. The surgeon must recreate the unit, not just fill the defect. If a defect encompasses more than 50% of a subunit, it is useful to discard adjacent normal tissue about the defect so that the skin of the entire subunit is replaced, not just the missing skin of the defect. This approach positions border scars in the expected shadows or reflections of subunit borders and ensures a uniform skin quality to the unit. A patch-like effect is avoided. Also, when an entire convex unit is resurfaced with a flap, the inevitable trapdoor contraction that occurs in the underlying scar bed acts to recreate the expected convex contour of the entire subunit. This technique avoids the pincushion effect, which may occur when a small flap is placed within a defect that includes only part of a unit. Missing tissues also must be replaced exactly, bringing neither too much nor too little to the wound. If excessive or too little tissue is placed within a defect, the adjacent landmarks and outline will be distorted outward or inward. Similarly, flaps and grafts should be fashioned with a template designed from the contralateral subunit or the ideal so that the outline and quantity of replaced tissue are exact. Contour is the most important determinant of normal. Judicious subcutaneous sculpturing and the use of primary bone and cartilage grafts to create a nasal framework must be employed primarily to prevent soft tissue collapse and late soft tissue contraction.

3. Is the quality of nasal skin uniform over its surface?

Skin quality (color, texture, and thickness) differs from one region of the nose to the other. The skin of the nasal dorsum and sidewalls is thin, smooth, and pliable. The skin of the tip and alar subunits is thick, stiff, and pitted with sebaceous glands. These regional differences in skin quality suggest different methods of reconstruction based on the location of the defect and method of wound closure. Skin grafts, because of the temporary ischemia associated with revascularization, always appear thin and shiny after transfer. They frequently become hypopigmented or hyperpigmented. Thus, a full-thickness skin graft can be expected to blend well in the smooth-skinned zones of the dorsum or sidewalls. The lax skin of these subunits also lends itself to the use of a local single-lobed flap. In contrast, a thin, shiny skin graft will appear as a patch if placed within the normally thick, pitted skin of the tip or ala. A local or regional flap that will maintain its skin quality is a better choice for tip or alar resurfacing.

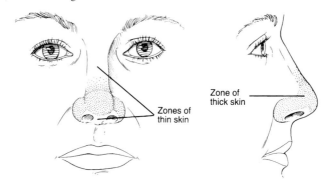

Zones of nasal skin quality. (From Burget GC, Menick FJ: Aesthetic Reconstruction of the Nose. St. Louis, Mosby, 1994, with permission.)

4. How should a nasal defect be analyzed? What are the reconstructive implications?

The nose is covered by skin that matches the face in color and texture, supported by a bone and cartilage framework and lined by thin vascular stratified epithelium and mucosa. The tissue loss from each layer must be identified and replaced with similar material. Lining material must be thin enough to prevent a bulky obstruction of the airway, pliable enough to conform to the desired framework contour, and vascular enough to nourish overlying cartilage or bone grafts. The shape and internal framework of the reconstructed nose must be provided by cartilage or bone grafts. These supporting materials should be placed primarily to prevent soft tissue collapse and late contracture due to scarring associated with wound healing. Finally, covering skin that matches the face in color and texture must be provided.

Just as a surgeon analyzes the anatomic loss, he or she also must examine the aesthetic loss. The wound may be healed but the visual appearance of the nose not restored if the characteristics of the nasal unit and each of its subunits are not reestablished. Each visual subunit must be analyzed and its character restored by using appropriate tissues and lining techniques that recreate the expected visual subunit appearance.

5. What are the advantages and disadvantages of potential donor sites for skin grafting in nasal reconstruction?

For superficial defects with a vascularized bed, full-thickness skin grafts can be used to resurface defects of the upper two-thirds of the nose in the zone of smooth skin but are usually an inappropriate choice for defects within the thicker sebaceous skin of the tip or alae. Preauricular skin provides an ideal match. Grafts of 2–2.5 cm can be harvested from the hairless skin anterior to the ear in both males and females. The donor site is closed primarily. Postauricular skin is also of value but may appear red postoperatively. Supraclavicular skin is available to resurface the entire nose if necessary, although the color match is less satisfactory. Supraclavicular skin usually has a brownish hue once it has healed in place. Split-thickness skin grafts are used only as temporary wound dressings and are infrequently used in nasal reconstruction.

6. What is the role of composite grafts?

The most common donor site for a composite graft is the root of the auricular helix. A skin sandwich containing thin ear cartilage positioned between two layers of skin is available. Adjacent preauricular skin also may be harvested in continuity with the root of the helix and the donor site closed primarily. Composite grafts must be placed on a well-vascularized bed. The size of the graft should be limited to 1.5 cm or less to enhance survival. Postoperative cooling with cold saline compresses may be helpful. Composite grafts are used for full-thickness defects of the alar rim and may provide a relatively simple one-stage reconstruction. In the long term, they usually appear thin and shiny and do not blend perfectly. Nevertheless, composite grafts are a useful option, especially for defects of the alar margin.

7. How are local flaps used in nasal reconstruction?

For small nasal defects, local flaps are an excellent option. Various flaps can be used for defects in the thin, mobile skin of the upper nose. All of them redistribute the relative excess of lax skin within the sidewall and dorsum to cover the defect while allowing primary closure of the donor site. Fortunately, most incisions on the nose heal with good scars. A local flap may be used if the defect is less than 1.5 cm in diameter and if cartilage grafts are not needed. There is not enough excessive nasal skin to redistribute over the nose to cover larger defects, and the tension created by wound closure will collapse a delicate cartilage framework. A forehead or nasolabial flap is required for defects greater than 1.5 cm or those requiring reconstruction of a cartilage framework.

8. What are the advantages of a bilobed flap? Where is it most useful?

The thick sebaceous and adherent skin of the tip and ala does not lend itself to the use of a local flap as easily as the upper nasal two-thirds. The bilobed flap (as modified by Zitelli) is an excellent option for nasal tip and alar defects, however. It redistributes excessive tissue from the upper nose to the tip and alae by transferring skin as a bilobed flap. Limiting the rotation of each lobe to less than 50°, performing a primary excision of the dog-ear, and wide undermining of the submuscular plane just above the perichondrium and periosteum aid in its success. It is difficult to resurface the tip and alae with a classic single-lobed flap. The pedicle blood supply to a single-lobed flap is in jeopardy at the time of dog-ear excision, and the rotation of this stiff tissue through 90° of rotation is difficult.

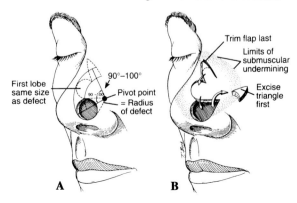

Geometric bilobed flap. (From Burget GC, Menick FJ: Aesthetic Reconstruction of the Nose. St. Louis, Mosby, 1994, with permission.)

9. How is the nasolabial flap used in nasal reconstruction? What is its blood supply?

The use of cheek tissue was popularized by French and German surgeons in the 1800s. The blood supply of a modern flap is based on the perforators from the facial and angular arteries that pass through the underlying levator labii and zygomatic muscles to the skin. The flap design is positioned just lateral to the nasolabial fold; on closure, the scar lies exactly within the nasolabial crease. Its proximal base is positioned over the rich subcutaneous blood supply that enters from its deep aspect. The distal tip of the flap, situated at or just distal to the oral commissure, can be elevated with just a few millimeters of subcutaneous tissue and then rotated on its thick subcutaneous superior pedicle to cover the alar subunit. Three weeks later, the flap pedicle is divided and the alar base inset completed. Nasolabial tissue is an ideal replacement for the alae. However, the amount of available tissue is limited, and attempts at extending the pedicle to reach the tip or dorsum are risky because of an unreliable blood supply.

A nasolabial flap also may be folded on itself to provide both cover and lining for a full-thickness defect. However, the blood supply is put at risk by folding, primary cartilage grafts are difficult to position, and the result usually appears bulky and thick. Excessive skin from the nasolabial fold also may be transferred in one stage as an extension of a random cheek flap. However, a second revision is usually required to recreate the normal alar crease, and it is almost impossible to create a truly aesthetic alar base inset when such a nasolabial flap design is used to rebuild a defect that includes the nasal sill and alar base.

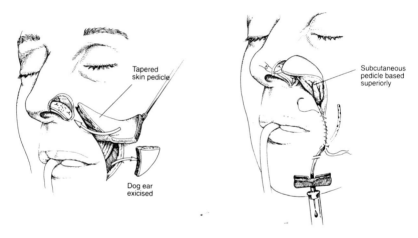

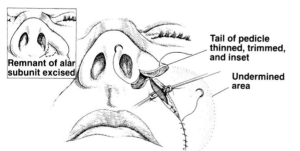

Subunit nasolabial two-stage flap. (From Burget GC, Menick FJ: Aesthetic Reconstruction of the Nose. St. Louis, Mosby, 1994, with permission.)

10. What do you know about the history of nasal reconstruction?

In 600 B.C., Sushruta described the reconstruction of the nose with forehead and cheek flaps in the *Hindu Book of Revelation.* In the late 16th century, Tagliacozzi, an Italian, published a treatise on the use of the pedicle arm flap. The forehead flap was first used in the Western world by Joseph Carpue in England, who had read accounts of the Indian forehead flap in a 1795 issue of *Gentleman's Magazine.* He published two case reports in 1816. In this century, Gillies, Converse, and Millard have pioneered developments.

11. How can forehead tissue be transferred?

Lateral forehead skin can be transferred on the unilateral superficial temporal artery (New's sickle flap) or the contralateral superficial temporal artery (Converse's scalping flap). Both relatively extensive procedures use a hairy scalp pedicle to transfer forehead skin to the nose. The traditional median forehead flap takes central forehead skin based on both right and left supraorbital vascular arcades. However, because of the profuse blood supply to the forehead, midline forehead tissue may be transferred as a paramedian flap based on a unilateral supratrochlear pedicle. Enough skin is available to resurface an entire nose.

12. Describe the blood supply to the paramedian forehead flap.

The blood supply of the central forehead enters vertically from below the supraorbital rim and ascends vertically just above the periosteum. The rich arcade of vessels arising from the supraorbital, supratrochlear, infratrochlear, and dorsal and angular branches of the facial artery pass superiorly from deep to superficial. Above the mid forehead and toward the hairline, the axial vessels lie in the subcutaneous tissue just deep to the dermis. It is safe to elevate the distal 1–2 cm of a paramedian forehead flap with skin and a thin layer of subcutaneous tissue. More inferiorly, the flap should be elevated deep to the frontalis muscle, just above the periosteum, to protect the blood supply. The forehead flap itself should be designed vertically to include the vertical axial blood supply.

13. Is there enough skin to make a nose from the midline forehead? Is the reach too short? How wide should the pedicle be? Should I delay the procedure for safety?

Enough skin to resurface an entire nose can be easily transferred with a paramedian forehead flap. The flap may be designed on either the right or left supratrochlear vessels. Either may be used for midline defects, but the reach of the flap is easier when it is based on the same side as a lateral defect. A template of the required missing forehead skin should be placed at the hairline and designed with a 1.5-cm pedicle above the supratrochlear vessels. The narrow pedicle allows easy rotation without undue tension. If the arc of rotation is short, an additional 1.5 cm can be added by extending the flap tip into hair-bearing scalp. If the patient is a healthy nonsmoker, the distal flap can be thinned to the subcutaneous tissue layer and hair follicles destroyed by excision and light coagulation. An additional 1.5 cm can be obtained by extending the flap pedicle base below the supraorbital rim towards the canthus, snipping fibrous bands under magnification but maintaining vessels intact. The flap should be designed vertically to maintain its axial blood supply. When so designed, the flap does not require delay and has sufficient length to reach all nasal defects, including the columella. Curving the flap eccentrically across the forehead destroys its axial nature and puts the distal flap in jeopardy. There are few indications for flap delay. The resulting scarring and stiffness only make later transfer more difficult.

14. How and why are primary bone and cartilage grafts used in nasal reconstruction?

A nose looks like a nose because of its shape. It is the underlying bone and skeletal framework that provides support, nasal projection, and airway patency and recreates a subtle contour that defines the normalcy of each nasal subunit. Cover and lining alone are inadequate.

15. When and how should bone or cartilage grafts be used?

The soft tissues of cover and lining will collapse without support and be fixed into a shapeless mass by scar. Once scar contraction has occurred, it is difficult to reexpand soft tissues. Thus, bone and cartilage grafts should be placed primarily before wound healing is completed. Cartilage grafts depend on lining for vascularity, and lining and covering skin depend on primary cartilage grafts for support and contour. If missing, a support framework for the dorsum, sidewalls, alae, columella, and tip must be replaced. Although the ala normally contains no cartilage, a cartilage alar batten should be used when the ala is reconstructed to maintain its support and shape and to fight the upward contraction associated with wound healing.

16. What donor tissues are available for nasal support? What are the advantages and disadvantages of each?

If available, septal cartilage is the first choice for most nasal grafts. It can be harvested much as cartilage is removed in a submucous resection, leaving a strong septal L for central midline nasal support. The concha of the ear also provides excellent material for ala and tip support. Rib cartilage or rib osteochondral grafts are used for large support defects of the dorsum. Cranial bone grafts also may be used but have a higher rate of reabsorption. Remember that a nasal framework provides support, braces the soft tissue against myofibroblast contraction, and imparts, when seen through a thin covering skin, a nasal shape. Thus, every nose must have a dorsal buttress, sidewall brace, alar cartilage reconstructions, and a columellar strut support. Although the normal ala contains no cartilage, an alar batten placed along the alar rim provides its shape and support. Although the importance of support has been stressed in this century, only recently has the importance of a precise, complete skeletal framework been emphasized. Limiting nasal support to a cantilever bone graft or rib L-strut does not provide the requirements for long-term success.

17. Practically speaking, what is the most important anatomic layer in nasal reconstruction?

The replacement of missing lining tissue is the most difficult challenge in nasal reconstruction and frequently determines the final outcome. Lining must be vascular enough to nourish primary cartilage grafts, supple enough to conform to the appropriate nasal shape, and thin enough so that the airway is not obstructed. Poor results of nasal reconstruction can often be traced to initial provision of insufficient or poorly vascularized lining tissue.

18. What are the options for nasal lining?

The importance of nasal lining has been emphasized since the work of Gillies in World War I. Traditionally, nasal lining has been supplied with turnover hinge flaps of adjacent intact covering skin, folding of a forehead flap upon itself to supply both cover and lining, or skin grafting the forehead flap at a preliminary operation as it lies in the forehead before transfer. All of these methods have the disadvantage of providing poorly vascularized lining and make the placement of primary cartilage grafts difficult.

In most circumstances, residual intranasal lining is the first choice for reconstruction because of its vascularity, availability, and pliability. Fortunately for surgeons, the septum is perfused by the septal branch of the superior labial artery, which permits elevation and lateral transfer of the septal mucous membrane on a 1.2-cm pedicle based in the soft tissue at the nasal spine. The entire septum, in fact, may be rotated out of the piriform aperture as a sandwich of cartilage between the right and left septal mucosa when based on both superior labial arteries. The facial artery and its angular branches also supply numerous branches to the soft tissues of the lateral nose and alar base.

Frequently, when part of the ala is missing, residual vestibular skin remains intact above the defect. In such circumstances, a bipedicle flap of residual vestibular skin can be incised in the area of the intercartilaginous line and advanced inferiorly to the desired alar rim level. The defect above may be filled with a full-thickness skin graft, raw surface outward, or by an ipsilateral septal mucosal flap based on the ipsilateral superior labial artery. For larger defects, mucoperichondrial flaps based on septal and anterior ethmoid vessels provide significant amounts of highly vascularized thin and supple tissue. The entire septum also may be used as a composite chondromucosal flap to provide both lining and cartilage support. (See figure, top of next page.)

19. Is tissue expansion helpful?

Advocates of tissue expansion have used it prior to nasal reconstruction to increase the available tissue and to assist in primary closure of the forehead. In fact, tissue expansion is rarely necessary. Enough skin can be transferred on an ipsilateral paramedian forehead flap pedicle to resurface the entire nose. Because the pedicle is narrow, closure of the inferior forehead defect is easy. Any defect that remains and cannot be closed primarily is high in the forehead under the hairline. Simply dressed with petrolatum gauze, it will heal by secondary intention and autoexpansion of the forehead. It is unnecessary to skin-graft the forehead defect or to use preliminary tissue expansion. In fact, the capsule that forms around the tissue expander may diminish the pliability of the forehead flap or the quality of the overlying skin. It is also difficult to predict the degree of tissue retraction that follows expansion and the late effects of skin shrinkage. Tissue expansion favors the donor site at the expense of the nose. As a central facial defect, the nose always takes priority. The forehead is a forgiving donor site and is of lesser aesthetic importance. Although rarely required, tissue expansion may be used secondarily after nasal reconstruction to improve the donor site.

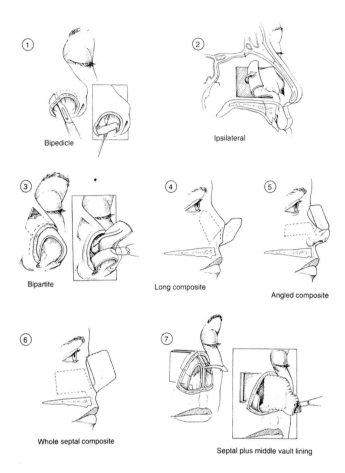

Variations of the septal intranasal lining flaps. (From Burget GC, Menick FJ: Aesthetic Reconstruction of the Nose. St. Louis, Mosby, 1994, with permission.)

20. What are the most frequent mistakes in nasal reconstruction?
- Not visualizing the desired aesthetic result before surgery.
- Not planning each step in three dimensions and imagining the outcome of a reconstruction for the specific location and method of transfer.
- Not taking the time or requisite skill to fabricate your goal.

BIBLIOGRAPHY

1. Barton FE Jr: Aesthetic aspects of nasal reconstruction. Clin Plast Surg 15:155–166, 1988.
2. Burget GC, Menick FJ: Nasal reconstruction: Seeking a fourth dimension. Plast Reconstr Surg 78:145, 1986.
3. Burget GC, Menick FJ: Nasal support and lining: The marriage of beauty and blood supply. Plast Reconstr Surg 84:189, 1989.
4. Burget GC, Menick FJ: Subunit principle in nasal reconstruction. Plast Reconstr Surg 76:239, 1985.
5. Converse JM: Reconstruction of the nose by the scalping flap technique. Surg Clin North Am 39:335, 1959.
6. McCarthy JG, Lorenc PZ, Cutting C, et al: The median forehead flap revisited: The blood supply. Plast Reconstr Surg 76:866–869, 1985.
7. Menick F: Artistry in facial surgery: Aesthetic perceptions and the subunit principle. In Furnas D (ed): Clinics in Plastic Surgery, vol 14. Philadelphia, W.B. Saunders, 1987.
8. Millard DR: Reconstructive rhinoplasty for the lower two-thirds of the nose. Plast Reconstr Surg 57:722, 1976.
9. Zitelli JA: The bilobed flap for nasal reconstruction. Arch Dermatol 125:957, 1989.

36. EYELID RECONSTRUCTION

Daniel J. Azurin, M.D., and Armand D. Versaci, M.D.

1. What are the components of the posterior lamella of the upper lid?

Each eyelid is a bilamellar structure divided by the orbital septum. The anterior lamella of the upper lid is composed of the skin and orbicularis oculi muscle. The posterior lamella of the upper lid is composed of the tarsus, levator aponeurosis, Muller's muscle, and conjunctiva. The levator aponeurosis is unique to the upper lid and is analogous to the capsulopalpebral fascia of the lower lid. The anterior lamella of the lower lid is composed of the skin and orbicularis oculi muscle. The posterior lamella of the lower lid is composed of the tarsus, capsulopalpebral fascia, and conjunctiva. The orbital septum is a fascial membrane of variable thickness that resists the spread of infection, hemorrhage, and inflammation.

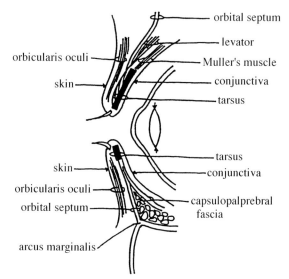

Anterior and posterior lamellae of the eyelids.

2. Describe the anatomy, innervation, and function of the orbicularis oculi muscle.

The orbicularis oculi muscle, which is innervated by the facial nerve, is responsible for lid closure. It is subdivided into the pretarsal, preseptal, and orbital muscles. The orbicularis oculi is continuous with the submuscular aponeurotic system (SMAS) in the upper face as is the platysma in the lower face. The lacrimal pump mechanism is intimately associated with the orbicularis muscle. Contraction of the pretarsal muscle shortens and closes the canaliculi, whereas the preseptal muscle pulls on the lacrimal diaphragm, resulting in a negative pressure within the lacrimal sac. Upon relaxation, tears are driven into the nasolacrimal duct.

3. What is the vertical dimension of the upper and lower tarsus?

The tarsal plates form the structural framework of the eyelids. The vertical height of the upper tarsus is approximately 10 mm. The vertical height of the lower lid ranges from 3.8–4.5 mm.

4. How is levator palpebrae superioris function measured?

The levator muscle, a striated muscle innervated by the third cranial nerve, is responsible for raising the lid. The muscle originates from the superior/posterior orbit (lesser wing of the sphenoid) and broadens into the levator aponeurosis, which in turn inserts onto the tarsus. The levator aponeurosis extends laterally and medially into the horns, each of which attaches to the lateral retinaculum and posterior lacrimal crest, respectively. The lateral horn divides the orbital and palpebral lobes of the lacrimal gland. Levator function is measured by the distance (mm) that the upper lid margin travels from downward gaze to upward gaze with the brow immobilized.

5. What pathologic condition is caused by paralysis or laceration of Muller's muscle?

Muller's muscle is a smooth muscle with sympathetic innervation. It is located in the posterior lamella of the upper lid and has intimate attachments to the levator muscle and the tarsus. It originates from the posterior aspect of the levator muscle and inserts onto the superior border of the tarsus. Muller's muscle provides tone for the upper lid, and injury to this muscle may result in ptosis (2–3 mm).

6. What structures must be transected to explore the orbital floor through a transconjunctival approach?

The transconjunctival approach is an exposure technique through the posterior lamella of the lower lid, beginning with an incision through the conjunctiva. This incision is followed by transection of the capsulopalpebral fascia. At this point, the approach can be either retroseptal or preseptal to reach the orbital floor, which is then explored in a subperiosteal plane. In a standard blepharoplasty, once the capsulopalpebral fascia is transected, the inferior compartments of orbital fat are directly accessible. In exploring the orbital floor, a lateral canthotomy is added for greater exposure. The capsulopalpebral fascia arises from condensations of the investing layers of the inferior rectus and inferior oblique muscles and inserts onto the inferior border of the tarsus. The capsulopalpebral fascia, which is unique to the lower lid, is involved with the coordinated downward movement of the lower lid during downward gaze. It is somewhat analogous to the levator aponeurosis of the upper lid. The orbital septum, orbicularis muscle, and skin are anterior to the capsulopalpebral fascia. Because the anterior lamella is not transgressed, the transconjunctival approach minimizes the problems of lower eyelid retraction, which are significantly more common after the cutaneous approach. The arcus marginalis is the periosteal attachment of the orbital septum to the bony orbital margin.

7. What structures contribute to the lateral retinaculum?

The lateral retinaculum or lateral canthus is a complex integration of a number of structures. It is composed of Lockwood's ligament (inferior suspensory ligament), the lateral extension or horn of the levator aponeurosis, the continuations of the pretarsal and preseptal muscles, and the check ligament of the lateral rectus muscle. This confluence of structures attaches to the lateral orbital wall at Whitnall's tubercle. Whitnall's tubercle is located within the lateral rim of the orbit below the frontozygomatic suture on the frontal process of the zygoma. Therefore, inferiorly displaced zygoma fractures pull the lateral canthus inferiorly, resulting in downward slant of the palpebral fissure. Whitnall's ligament is a check ligament of the levator muscle that limits its excursion and is not a part of the lateral retinaculum.

8. Where does the medial canthus insert?

The medial canthal tendon is a complex structure that attaches onto the medial aspect of the orbit in a tripartite manner. The insertion points include the anterior lacrimal crest and a portion of the nasal bone, the posterior lacrimal crest, and a less well-defined point around the nasofrontal suture. The medial canthal tendon is intimately associated with the lacrimal pump mechanism. The lacrimal sac lies between the anterior and posterior insertions of the medial canthal tendon. Because the anterior attachment extends medially onto the nasal bones, reattachment of this portion to the anterior lacrimal crest may result in an impression of telecanthus.

9. Which extraocular muscle originates from the anterior orbit?

The inferior oblique muscle is the only extraocular muscle that originates from the anterior orbit. It also separates the medial and central fat compartments of the lower lid. The anatomic position of the inferior oblique muscle makes it prone to injury during blepharoplasty. All of the other extraocular muscles originate from the anulus of Zinn near the apex of the orbit.

10. What defines the supratarsal fold?

The supratarsal fold corresponds to dermal attachments of the levator aponeurosis. Above these attachments, the overhanging skin creates a fold. The supratarsal fold is approximately 10 mm above the eyelid margin and is often absent in people of Asian descent. The position of the supratarsal fold is important in the evaluation of patients with eyelid ptosis. A high-positioned supratarsal fold may suggest a levator defect.

11. The fascial framework of the orbit is composed of what structures?
   The fascial framework of the orbit is a connective tissue network that not only provides support to the globe, but also allows coordinated movements among all the orbital contents so that the eye and its associated structures can move in concert. This framework consists of the bulbar fascia or Tenon's capsule, the investing fascial layers of the extraocular muscles, the intermuscular septa, and the check ligaments (condensations of fascia from the medial rectus and lateral rectus, which serve as anchors to the periorbita). Lockwood's ligament is formed by the intermuscular septum between the inferior oblique and the inferior rectus muscle.

12. What are the most common malignant tumors of the eyelids? What is the most common location for a malignant tumor of the eyelids?
   Basal cell carcinoma is by far the most common malignant tumor of the eyelids, followed by squamous cell carcinoma and sebaceous carcinoma. For well-demarcated, nonsclerosing basal cell carcinomas < 2 cm in diameter, a 1–2 mm grossly free margin will be histologically free of tumor in 94–95% of cases. With recurrent or more aggressive tumors, it is necessary to resect larger margins, and it is often wise to delay reconstruction until permanent pathologic specimens are examined. Sebaceous carcinoma of the eyelid is uncommon and difficult to diagnose and carries a poor prognosis. The lower lid is the most common site for occurrence.

13. Which region of the eyelid is most likely to have a recurrent or an advanced tumor?
   Tumors of the medial canthal region are more likely to be advanced and have a higher chance of recurrence. Medial canthal complexity and location make reconstruction difficult. Tumors here are often recognized late and are often inadequately resected.

14. What factors predict postoperative dry eye syndrome?
   Orbital and periorbital morphology along with abnormal ocular histories have been shown to be better predictors of postoperative dry eye complications than Schirmer's test. Morphologic abnormalities include proptosis, exophthalmos, lax lower lids, scleral show, and maxillary hypoplasia. Abnormal histories include such problems as allergic conjunctivitis and corneal ulceration. Schirmer's test is an objective measure of the lacrimal secretory capacity. Schirmer's test I measures both basic and reflex secretion by the amount of wetting that occurs on a 5 × 35-mm filter paper placed on the lower conjunctiva for 5 minutes. Less than 10 mm of wetting is considered abnormal. Schirmer's test II is similar to the first test, except that a local anesthetic is dropped into the eye to block reflex secretions.

15. What are the basic principles of eyelid reconstruction?
   The eyelid is a dynamic, complex, and delicate structure, which carries out indispensable functions related to the eye, serves as a source of beauty, and is not easily duplicated by noneyelid tissues. A clear understanding of the anatomy and functional aspects of the orbital regions is paramount for the success of eyelid reconstruction. The basic principles of eyelid reconstruction include maintenance of the integrity of the upper lid, replacement of deficient tissue with like tissue when possible, maintenance of eye mobility, establishment of an aesthetic balance, and provision of a protective lining, stable skin covering, and internal lid support.

16. A 38-year-old woman with a malignant tumor fixed to the upper tarsus undergoes a full-thickness resection. The resultant defect measures 30% of the horizontal dimension of the lid. What is the most appropriate reconstructive option?
   Once a tumor involves the eyelid margin, a full-thickness excision is required, whereas the same tumor that does not involve the lid margin may only require a partial-thickness excision that can be closed directly or with a skin graft. Numerous methods exist for upper eyelid reconstruction. The horizontal dimension of the defect is an important consideration in selecting a reconstructive method, as are the basic principles outlined in question 15. Generally, for an upper lid defect that is

< 25% of the horizontal length of the lid, the defect can be closed with direct approximation. In elderly patients with lid laxity, defects slightly > 25% can be closed by direct approximation. For defects > 25% of the horizontal dimension that cannot be closed by direct approximation, reconstruction usually consists of a selective lateral cantholysis of the superior crus of the lateral canthal tendon with medial transposition of the lid. The combination of a local skin flap may be necessary. Larger upper lid defects up to 60% of the horizontal dimension require lid switch procedures that borrow like tissues from the lower lid, which are based on the marginal palpebral artery. Lid switch flaps can be designed 25% narrower than the defect width; however, the pedicle should be designed 5–6 mm in vertical dimension to avoid injury to the marginal artery. Defects that are 60–100% of the horizontal dimension are typically reconstructed with either a Cutler-Beard flap or a Mustardé total lid flap. The Cutler-Beard flap is a full-thickness lower lid advancement flap that is advanced under the intact lower lid margin (bridge) and then set into the upper lid defect. The Mustardé total lid flap closes the upper lid defect with a lateral canthotomy and a full-thickness lid switch flap using as much of the lower lid as needed. This procedure is followed by reconstruction of the lower lid donor defect with a composite graft and cheek advancement flap. Both are two-stage procedures. Other local flaps, such as the nasolabial or glabellar flap, combined with mucosal or composite grafts when needed, are sometimes used for lid and periorbital reconstruction.

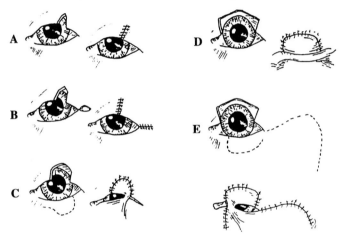

Reconstruction of the upper eyelid. *A,* Direct approximation. *B,* Selective lateral cantholysis and medial transposition of the lid. *C,* Lid switch flap. *D,* Cutler-Beard flap. *E,* Mustardé total lid flap.

17. How much vertical height of upper tarsus is used in the design of a tarsoconjunctival flap for lower lid reconstruction?

As with upper eyelid reconstruction, numerous methods are used to reconstruct the lower lid. Significant differences, however, exist between upper and lower eyelid reconstruction. Because the upper lid is far more dynamic than the lower lid and is also essential for corneal protection, lower lid reconstructions generally do not borrow like tissues from the upper lid; rather, reconstructions usually borrow tissues from other sources, such as the cheek. However, lid-sharing techniques for lower lid reconstruction can be highly successful; the Hugh's tarsoconjunctival flap is a well-accepted example. The Hugh's tarsoconjunctival flap is a staged advancement flap using the posterior lamella of the upper lid to reconstruct a lower lid defect. A horizontal incision is made through the posterior lamella of the upper lid, marking the advancing edge of the flap. The incision is made approximately 5 mm away from the lid margin. Approximately 4–5 mm of inferior upper lid tarsus needs to be preserved to maintain upper lid support and lid margin stability. The flap includes conjunctiva, tarsus, levator aponeurosis, and Muller's muscle. After the flap is advanced and properly inset layer for layer into the defect, a full-thickness skin graft is secured onto the flap for coverage. Flap division is usually performed 6–8 weeks after the first stage.

For lower lid defects that extend up to 25% of the horizontal dimension of the lid, direct approximation, layer for layer, is usually possible. Defects of 25–60% of the horizontal dimension are usually reconstructed with a selective cantholysis and medial transposition of the lid with or without a local skin flap. Defects of 75–100% of the horizontal dimension require either a Hugh's tarsoconjunctival flap (two stages) or a Mustardé cheek flap (one stage) with composite grafting for lid support and lining. The tarsoconjunctival flap is best suited for defects that have a vertical dimension of 4–5 mm. Marginal defects of either the upper or lower lid can be reconstructed with a bipedicle skin/muscle Tripier flap in conjunction with a composite graft, such as a septal chondromucosal graft.

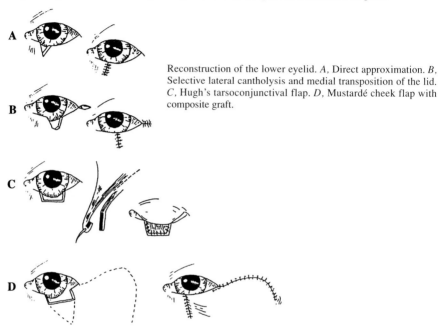

Reconstruction of the lower eyelid. *A*, Direct approximation. *B*, Selective lateral cantholysis and medial transposition of the lid. *C*, Hugh's tarsoconjunctival flap. *D*, Mustardé cheek flap with composite graft.

18. Is lower lid ectropion a common complication after a Cutler-Beard flap reconstruction?
    No. Upper lid retraction may occur after the division of a Hugh's tarsoconjunctival flap secondary to scar formation and foreshortened Muller's muscle fibers in the donor bed. During the design and execution of the Cutler-Beard flap, care must be taken to avoid injury to the marginal artery of the lower lid. The marginal artery courses parallel to the lid margin approximately 3–4 mm from the edge. The inset-advanced Cutler-Beard flap is usually left in place for 6–8 weeks. Any unused portion is returned to the lower lid after division. Because of significant elongation in the flap, lower lid ectropion is not a typical complication. The Mustardé cheek advancement flap may cause lower lid ectropion secondary to flap retraction and gravitational forces. Notching at the area of marginal reapproximation is a common problem.

19. Is the contralateral eyelid a preferred site for skin graft harvest?
    An optimal area for skin graft harvest in terms of color and texture is the contralateral eyelid; however, the amount of skin is limited. The following sites are preferred areas for skin graft harvest: retroauricular, preauricular, and supraclavicular. The infraclavicular region yields a graft with poor color match.

20. Describe the evaluation of lid ptosis.
    Ptosis of the upper lid may be classified as congenital, neurogenic, myogenic, aponeurotic, or mechanical. The underlying cause, degree of ptosis, amount of levator function, position of the globe, presence of a Bell's phenomenon, and position and contour of the upper lid fold are important in the evaluation of the ptotic lid. The degree of lid laxity, or the result of a "snap back" test, is not a critical factor; however, lid tone is important. The Tensilon test is useful in the diagnosis of ocular myasthenia. Topical phenylephrine is useful in evaluating Horner's syndrome, a neurologic form of ptosis.

21. For most patients with lid ptosis, what is the most important factor in determining which operation to perform?

The most important factor in selecting the optimal surgical approach for patients with lid ptosis is the measure of levator function. The normal lid covers 1–2 mm of the upper limbus of the cornea. Levator function (excursion) is measured by the distance (mm) that the upper lid margin travels from downward gaze to upward gaze with the brow immobilized. Although many ptosis repair techniques exist, four are most frequently used: the Fasanella-Servat operation, aponeurosis surgery, levator resection, and brow suspension.

22. What is the underlying cause of congenital ptosis?

Congenital ptosis is present at birth and involves an isolated dystrophy of the levator muscle.

23. A patient who has lid ptosis secondary to an attenuated levator aponeurosis, 4 mm of ptosis, and a levator function of 8 mm is best treated by which ptosis procedure?

Levator function is classified as good (> 10 mm), fair (4–10 mm), or poor (< 4 mm). The degree of ptosis is classified as mild (1–2 mm), moderate (3–4 mm), or severe (> 4 mm). In general, the Fasanella-Servat operation is optimal in patients with good levator function and mild ptosis. Aponeurosis surgery is most appropriate for patients with good levator function and moderate ptosis. Levator resection is used when the levator function is fair and the degree of ptosis is moderate. Brow or frontalis suspension techniques are used in patients with poor levator function and severe ptosis. Suspension procedures are mostly applied to treat severe congenital ptosis. The Fasanella-Servat operation involves a conjunctival, tarsal, and Muller's muscle resection. Aponeurosis surgery involves direct repair or advancement of the levator aponeurosis. Levator resection surgery involves resection of the levator aponeurosis. Brow or frontalis suspension entails suspending the lid margin to the frontalis muscle. The neosynephrine test helps to determine if the Fasanella-Servat operation will yield a satisfactory result. If 10% neosynephrine drops do not elevate the lid significantly, the Fasanella-Servat operation will probably result in undercorrection.

24. Match the following:

1. Ectropion	A. An abnormal skin fold that may cause inversion of the eyelid
2. Epicanthus	B. Frequently caused by chemical burns
3. Blepharophimosis	C. Associated with ptosis of the upper lids
4. Entropion	D. A fold of skin overhanging the medial canthus
5. Epiblepharon	E. Ocular irritation secondary to turned-in lashes
6. Trichiasis	F. May involve significant lid retraction leading to exposure keratinization
7. Symblepharon	G. May be caused by horizontal laxity

Ectropion is an eversion of the eyelid margin, often first producing scleral show. It may lead to serious oculopathies, such as exposure keratinization

Epicanthus is an overhanging skin fold that partially hides the medial canthus. Congenital epicanthus most frequently occurs in Asians.

Blepharophimosis is a congenital malformation associated with ptosis and epicanthal folds, telecanthus, and shortening of the horizontal fissure of the lids

Entropion is the inversion of the eyelid. Horizontal lid laxity may lead to involutional entropion. This malposition of the lid often causes corneal irritation from friction elicited by turned-in lashes.

Epiblepharon is an abnormal skin fold that folds over the skin margin, usually resulting in the inversion of the eyelid margin

Trichiasis refers specifically to eyelashes that are turned against the globe with the lid remaining in its normal position.

Symblepharon is a cicatricial fusion between the globe and the inner surface of the eyelid. It usually occurs as a complication of a chemical burn.

Answers: 1 F, 2 D, 3 C, 4 G, 5 A, 6 E, 7 B.

25. What factors contribute to entropion?

Congenital entropion may result from an abnormal tarsal plate. Involutional entropion is usually the result of horizontal lid laxity or an overriding preseptal muscle. Cicatricial entropion occurs secondary to the shortening of the posterior lamella. Facial paralysis, particularly of the orbicularis oculi muscle, results in a paralytic ectropion.

26. What factors contribute to ectropion?
Congenital ectropion is usually caused by a deficiency of eyelid skin. Involutional or senile ectropion is most often a result of laxity of the tarsus, canthal structures, and lid retractors. Cicatricial ectropion is a relative deficiency of skin and muscle from various causes, ranging from retraction and contraction (of the anterior lamella) to the excessive removal of skin during blepharoplasty. Paralytic ectropion is a complication of facial nerve palsy. Repair of ectropion depends on the underlying pathology. Enophthalmos from periorbital fat atrophy decreases posterior lid support and leads to involutional entropion.

27. How does the Asian eyelid differ from the Occidental eyelid?
The Asian eyelid differs from the Occidental eyelid by the common presence of epicanthal folds and lack of a supratarsal fold. The supratarsal fold is defined by dermal attachments of the levator aponeurosis, which is lacking in the Asian eyelid. Often retroorbicularis fat is also increased. Furthermore, the preaponeurotic fat may extend lower in the Asian eyelid secondary to a lower insertion of the orbital septum to the levator aponeurosis.

28. Describe tear secretion and the composition of tear film.
Tear secretion is either basic or reflexive. The precorneal tear film is composed of three layers. The innermost layer is the mucin layer, composed mainly of polysaccharides secreted by the conjunctival goblet cells. This layer stabilizes the tear film, provides lubrication, and prevents desiccation. The intermediate layer is the aqueous layer, which accounts for 90% of the tear film and is composed of an aqueous (98% water) solution secreted by the accessory and main lacrimal glands. The most superficial layer is mainly composed of lipids secreted by the meibomian, Zeis, and Moll glands. This layer also stabilizes the tear film and minimizes evaporation. The tear film break-up test measures the amount of time required for discontinuities or "holes" to form in the tear film when the eye is not allowed to blink. A time of < 10 seconds is considered abnormal.

29. What are the indications for performing dacryocystorhinostomy?
Dacryocystorhinostomy (DCR) is a surgical technique that opens the lacrimal sac directly into the nasal cavity. DCR is most commonly performed on patients with lacrimal obstruction distal to the common canaliculus, including patients with paralysis of the pump mechanism. DCR may be used to treat chronic dacryocystitis. For obstruction of the common canaliculus a canaliculodacryocystorhinostomy is performed. If both upper and lower canaliculi are obliterated, a conjunctivodacryocystorhinostomy is performed.

30. During the reduction of an avulsed medial canthal tendon, injury to the nasolacrimal duct is suspected. What is the appropriate course of action?
The initial management of traumatic telecanthus and nasoethmoidal fractures does not include exploration of the nasolacrimal duct. In this situation, delayed obstruction is not common and would be treated by DCR. Unnecessary initial exploration may cause trauma to the lacrimal drainage system.

31. After selective cantholysis and medial transposition of the lid for reconstruction of a moderate upper lid defect a patient complains of severe pain, photophobia, blurred vision, epiphora, and a foreign body sensation on the eye. Extraocular movements are intact and fundoscopic exam appears normal. Does the initial appropriate management include releasing all the incisions and administering mannitol?
Retrobulbar hematoma is a serious complication after eyelid surgery and may lead to blindness. Sudden-onset pain, proptosis, and conjunctival edema indicate the likelihood of a retrobulbar hemorrhage. The patient also may have limited extraocular movements, periorbital ecchymosis, and firmness to the eye. Immediate intervention is necessary, including opening all wounds and pharmacologically decompressing the orbit, such as by the administration of mannitol. An emergent ophthalmologic consultation should be obtained. The patient's complaints, however, are consistent with a corneal injury. After the application of a topical anesthetic, the eye should be irrigated and examined.

Fluorescein dye, which is dropped onto the corneal surface and then illuminated with a Wood's lamp, readily confirms the diagnosis of corneal abrasion. The patient is then treated with a topical antibiotic. A topical short-acting cycloplegic may be applied if ciliary spasm is significant; however, local anesthetics should not be continued (or ever prescribed for the patient) because they delay reepithelialization, mask complications, and decrease the protective sensibility of the eye. Although the vast majority of corneal abrasions heal rapidly within 1–3 days without complication, the possibility of superinfection and recurrent epithelial erosions must be kept in mind.

BIBLIOGRAPHY

1. Carraway JH: Levator advancement technique for eyelid ptosis. Plast Reconstr Surg 77:395, 1986.
2. Carraway JH: Reconstruction of the eyelids and correction of ptosis of the eyelid. In Aston SJ, Beasley RW, Thorne CHN (eds): Grabb and Smith's Plastic Surgery, 5th ed. Philadelphia, Lippincott-Raven, 1997, pp 529–544, 1997.
3. Jelks GW, Jelks EB: Reconstruction of the eyelids. In Cohen M (ed): Mastery of Plastic and Reconstructive Surgery. Boston, Little, Brown, 1994, pp 864–882.
4. Jelks GW, Smith BC: Reconstruction of the eyelids and associated structures. In McCarthy JG (ed): Plastic Surgery. Philadelphia, W.B. Saunders, 1990, pp 1671–1784.
5. McKinney P: The value of tear breakup and Schirmer's test in preoperative blepharoplasty evaluation. Plast Reconstr Surg 84:572–576, 1989.
6. Peist K: Malignant lesions of the eyelids. J Dermatol Surg Oncol 18:1056–1059, 1992.
7. Siegel R: Involutional entropion: A simple and stable repair. Plast Reconstr Surg 82:42–46, 1988.
8. Siegel R: Essential anatomy for contemporary upper lid blepharoplasty. Clin Plast Surg 20:209–212, 1993.
9. Weinstein G: Lower eyelid reconstruction with tarsal flaps and grafts. Plast Reconstr Surg 18:991–992, 1988.
10. Zarem B: Minimizing deformity in lower blepharoplasty. The transconjunctival approach. Clin Plast Surg 20:317–321, 1993.
11. Zide B: Surgical anatomy of the orbit. New York, Raven Press, 1985, pp 47–50.

37. EAR RECONSTRUCTION

Bruce S. Bauer, M.D., and Paul Fortes, M.D.

1. What are the normal size, position, protrusion, and axis of the ear?

The normal adult ear height is between 5.5–6.5 cm. The width varies from 66% of the height in children to 55% of the height in adults. Eighty-five percent of ear development occurs by age 3 years, and full development between ages 6–15 years. For children 4 years of age, a subnormal ear height (i.e., < 2 SD) is below 4.5 cm. General guidelines are as follows:
• The ear should lie one ear length posterior to the lateral orbital rim.
• The lateral protrusion of the helix from the scalp is between 1.5–2.0 cm.
• The mean inclination of the ear from the vertical is 20° posteriorly.

2. Using the diagram below, name the landmarks of the external ear.

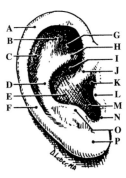

Answers listed on following page. (From Leber DC: Ear reconstruction. In Georgiade GS, Georgiade NG, Riefkol R, Barwick WJ (eds): Textbook of Plastic, Maxillofacial and Reconstructive Surgery, 2nd ed. Baltimore, Williams & Wilkins, 1992, p 494, with permission.)

A. Helical rim	E. Concha	I. Cymbum concha	M. Cavum concha
B. Superior crus	F. Tail of helix	J. Root of helix	N. Intertragal notch
C. Scapha	G. Triangular fossa	K. External auditory meatus	O. Antitragus
D. Antihelix	H. Inferior crus	L. Tragus	P. Lobule

3. What is the vascular supply of the ear?
Arterial supply:
1. Superficial temporal artery: supplies lateral surface of auricle
2. Posterior auricular artery: branch of external carotid artery. Dominant blood supply to posterior surface of ear, lobule, and retroauricular skin in 93% of cases.
3. Occipital artery: minor contribution. Dominant blood supply to posterior ear in only 7% of cases.

Venous outflow:
1. Posterior auricular veins: drain into external jugular vein.
2. Superficial temporal and retromandibular veins: drain anterior auricle.

4. Can an amputated ear be replanted?
Yes. An amputated ear may be replanted by microanastomosis of the posterior auricular artery (diameter 0.6–2.0 mm) and a posterior auricular vein (diameter 0.8–2.5 mm) to donor vessels, provided that these vessels can be identified.

5. Describe the nerve supply of the auricle. Why can a patient with an oropharyngeal carcinoma present with ear pain?
Great auricular nerve (C2, C3): Sensation to lower half of lateral surface of the ear and lower portion of the cranial surface of the ear.
Auriculotemporal nerve (branch of V_3): Sensation to superolateral surface of ear and anterior and superior surface of external auditory canal.
Lesser occipital nerve: Sensation to superior cranial surface of ear.
Arnold's nerve (auricular branch of vagus): Sensation to concha and posterior auditory canal.
Patients with cancers of the oropharynx (tonsil, base of tongue, soft palate) may complain of ear pain referred via the branches of the vagus nerve that innervate both the oropharynx and concha.

6. What is the embryologic origin of the external ear? Why is this knowledge significant in treating malignant tumors of the external ear?
During embryologic development, the auricle arises from the first (mandibular) and second (hyoid) branchial arches. Three anterior hillocks of the first branchial arch form the tragus, helical crus, and superior helix. Three posterior hillocks of the second branchial arch form the antihelix, antitragus, and lobule. The first branchial groove forms the external auditory meatus.

Cutaneous carcinomas of the external ear may spread via lymphatic channels that follow embryologic development. Cancers of the tragus, helical crus, and superior helix drain into the parotid nodes. Cancers of the antihelix, antitragus, and lobule drain into the mastoid nodes. Cancers of the concha and meatus may drain into the parotid and mastoid nodes. Clinicians must be alert to these drainage patterns making diagnoses and prescribing treatment.

7. What is the incidence and etiology of microtia?
Microtia (hypoplastic deformity of the auricle), occurs once in 6000–8000 births. Male to female ratios are 2:1, and right to left to bilateral ratios are 5:3:1.

Microtia is thought to be a component of first and second branchial arch syndrome (hemifacial microsomia) with varying degrees of hypoplasia of the bony and soft tissues of the involved half of the face. The proposed mechanism is thought to be obliteration of the stapedial artery during early embryonic life. Agents implicated have included viruses (rubella), drugs (thalidomide), and multifactorial inheritance.

8. What factors enter into the timing of microtia reconstruction?
Body image concept begins to form around 4–5 years of age. Therefore, reconstruction usually is timed at or before school age. Rib growth is also sufficient for cartilage framework construction

by age 5 years. By this age the normal ear has grown to within 6–7 mm of full vertical height. Even if microtia reconstruction is done as early as age 2 years, studies show that the reconstructed ear "keeps up" with the normal ear in growth.

9. In what cases and at what time is middle ear surgery indicated?

Complete deafness is very rare in microtia because the inner ear, or neurosensory apparatus, is normal. Children have normal speech and adapt well without middle ear surgery. Middle ear surgery is generally reserved for bilateral microtia patients and is done **after** auricular reconstruction. In selected cases middle ear reconstruction can be performed in patients with unilateral microtia, but should be planned following completion of the external reconstruction to avoid further complicating these procedures.

10. What are the basic steps in microtia reconstruction?

(1) Cartilage framework construction, (2) dissection of auricular vestige and placement of framework, (3) lobule transposition, (4) tragal construction and conchal excavation, and (5) helical rim elevation. The sequence of procedures and what is accomplished in each stage varies depending on the technique chosen by the operating surgeon, but it is agreed that the cartilage framework be placed in the first stage to make maximal use of the unscarred bed of the vestige. Opinions also vary on whether the lobule should be rotated in the first or second stage; current techniques demonstrate a significant benefit of lobule rotation at the time of cartilage graft placement. Nagata has demonstrated that the tragus can be reconstructed as part of the initial framework rather than a separate stage. Following other techniques, the lobule rotation, tragal construction, and elevation of the helical rim are performed in either the second or third stage of reconstruction.

11. Which costal cartilages are harvested for the construction of the framework in microtia reconstruction?

A cartilage framework is constructed from varying portions of the 6th–9th costal cartilages depending on the technique selected. Authors vary on whether to use ipsilateral or contralateral cartilages, basing their decision on how the cartilage segments are most easily spliced. Opinions also differ on whether to retain perichondrium on the graft or to leave it behind in the donor area. While maintaining some perichondrium on the graft helps to maintain long-term graft integrity, some feel that maintaining at least the visceral perichondrium in the donor site may minimize the risk of subsequent donor site deformity.

12. What options are available if the skin envelope is insufficient?

On some occasions there is insufficient skin available to cover the cartilage framework. These circumstances arise either as a result of associated facial deformity (hemifacial microsomia, Goldenhar's and Treacher Collins syndromes) in which the auricular vestige is malpositioned and the hairline is low-lying, or in cases of excessive scarring surrounding the vestige (from either trauma or prior unsuccessful surgery).

While tissue expansion has been used in selected ear reconstruction cases, the associated risk of expander complications, such as exposure, are significantly higher in this region than in other areas, and expansion is generally not recommended. This is particularly the case in the treatment of significant facial scarring around the vestige or in the remaining ear segment following trauma.

The most readily available tissue for reconstruction in these cases is the temporoparietal fascial flap (TPFF), or on occasion its extension into the postauricular area. This flap is usually based on the superficial temporal artery, but is best raised on both superficial temporal and postauricular vessels for total auricular reconstruction. In cases of severe tissue loss and deep scarring it may be necessary to use the contralateral TPFF by microvascular transfer. In most cases of fascial coverage of the framework the fascia is covered with a split thickness skin graft. The authors prefer a 0.016 inch thick graft from the upper inner arm. This is a well concealed donor site with excellent color match in the majority of cases.

13. Discuss some of the complications of ear reconstruction. How would you remedy them?

• **Rib donor site problems:** Pneumothorax; atelectasis. When recognized intraoperatively, aspirate the pneumothorax with a red rubber catheter and repair the pleural rent during positive pressure ventilation. Incentive spirometry and pulmonary toilet are indicated for atelectasis.

• **Ischemia or necrosis of the skin envelope with graft exposure:** Graft exposure mandates aggressive care, either antibiotic ointment for very small areas of exposure or coverage with well vascularized tissue. Failure to gain coverage may result in either partial or complete framework loss. Primary closure may be attempted after trimming the edge of the exposed cartilage, but rarely is the adjacent skin healthy enough to allow advancement and closure. Coverage with a narrow temporoparietal fascial flap or postauricular fascial flap and skin graft is often safer and provides better vascularization of the underlying cartilage.

• **Ischemia of transposed earlobe:** If performed during the first stage, lobule transposition requires leaving an adequate subdermal pedicle attached to the lobule in the location of the intertragal notch. Leaving the transposition for a second stage may be safer in experienced hands.

• **Hematoma and seroma:** Ensure complete hemostasis, and always place a suction drain in the pocket.

• **Resorption of framework/failed reconstruction:** Avoid cartilage exposure, but if it occurs treat it aggressively. Leave the perichondrium on the graft that is in contact with the skin. Failed reconstruction usually requires starting anew.

• **Flaws in planning:** Poor ear position, poorly designed framework.

CONTROVERSIES

14. Faced with a patient with a traumatic avulsion of the ear, you are unable to identify an uninjured vessel to perform an anastomosis; what should be done with the avulsed part?

In cases where replantation with anastomosis of a healthy vessel is not possible, there is still some controversy as to the optimal treatment. While anecdotal cases have described salvage of an entire ear by replantation without microvascular anastomosis, this approach cannot be relied on and typically results in total or near total loss of the avulsed segment. In the past it was suggested that the skin be carefully dissected from the amputated part and the cartilage be buried beneath the skin in the abdominal area or retroauricular area to be later retrieved and used as the framework for subsequent reconstruction. Unfortunately, in almost all cases, this approach results in deformation and loss of the cartilage substance with a nonuseable graft of cartilage being retrieved from the banking site. Selected single cases have been reported in which the denuded cartilage was covered with either a regional fascial flap or distant flap with subsequent microvascular transfer. In the majority of these cases the final result of the reconstruction has poor definition.

Brent and others, including the authors, agree that a far superior result can be obtained in experienced hands with debridement and preservation of the remaining ear segment with subsequent formal staged reconstruction with cartilage framework, TPFF, and skin graft coverage. Unless the operating surgeon has experience with more complex alternative fascial flap coverage techniques, the use of the fascia acutely for coverage of the replanted cartilage will significantly complicate further reconstruction when an unacceptable outcome results.

15. What principles of treatment are observed for a burned ear? How are segmental defects reconstructed?

1. Reconstruction begins with preservation of viable tissue, not with early surgical intervention.

2. Exposed, nonviable cartilage will not heal, and surgical debridement and reconstruction need to be performed.

3. Excision of dry, nonsuppurative eschar should be condemned. Sulfamylon cream is the most effective topical antibacterial because of its eschar penetration.

4. Segmental cartilage resection of tragus, antitragus, inferior crus, and midportion of the antihelix does not alter the overall appearance of the ear. Local skin flap advancement or skin graft may be all that is needed.

5. Segmental loss of helix can be reconstructed with a local chondrocutaneous advancement (Antia) flap, wedge excision and closure, contralateral conchal cartilage graft with local skin flap, or composite grafts (if defect < 1 cm).

6. Sulfamylon is the preferable topical antibiotic for treatment vs. Silvadene because of its superior cartilage penetration.

7. Major loss of ear cartilage and soft tissue requires reconstruction with costal cartilage framework, temporoparietal fascial flap, and split-thickness skin graft.

16. What are the three most common cancers of the auricle?

Squamous cell carcinoma (50–60%), basal cell carcinoma (30–40%), and melanoma (2–6%). About 12% of head and neck squamous cell carcinoma and basal cell carcinoma occur on the periauricular areas. Invasion of the perichondrium necessitates excision of the underlying cartilage.

BIBLIOGRAPHY

1. Allison GR: Anatomy of the auricle. Clin Plast Surg 17:209–212, 1990.
2. Bauer BS: The role of tissue expansion in reconstruction of the ear. Clin Plast Surg 17:319–325, 1990.
3. Brent B: Reconstruction of the auricle. In McCarthy JG (ed): Plastic Surgery. Philadelphia, W.B. Saunders, 1990, pp 2094–2152.
4. Brent B, Byrd HS: Secondary ear reconstruction with cartilage grafts covered by axial, random, and free flaps of temporoparietal fascia. Plast Reconstr Surg 72:141–151, 1983.
5. Eriksson E, Vogt PM: Ear reconstruction. Clin Plast Surg 19:637–643, 1992.
6. Furnas DW: Complications of surgery of the external ear. Clin Plast Surg 17:305–318, 1990.
7. Menick FJ: Reconstruction of the ear after tumor excision. Clin Plast Surg 17:405–415, 1990.
8. Rosenthal JS: The thermally injured ear: A systemic approach to reconstruction. Clin Plast Surg 19:645–661, 1992.
9. Thomson HG, Winslow J: Microtia reconstruction: Does the cartilage framework grow? Plast Reconstr Surg 84:908–915, 1989.
10. Tolleth H: A hierarchy of values in the design and construction of the ear. Clin Plast Surg 17:193–207, 1990.
11. Bauer BS: Aesthetic ear surgery. In Marchac D, Granek MS, Solomon MP, et al (eds): Male Aesthetic Surgery. Boston, Butterworth-Heinemann, 1996, pp 255–286.

38. LIP RECONSTRUCTION

John T. Seki, M.D., and Christine Haugen, M.D.

1. What are the key anatomic features of the lip?

The key landmarks include the vermilion border, commissure, tubercle, philtral columns, and Cupid's bow.

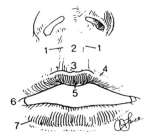

Topographic anatomy of the lips. *1*, Philtral columns. *2*, Philtral groove or dimple. *3*, Cupid's bow. *4*, White roll upper lip. *5*, Tubercle. *6*, Commissure. *7*, Vermilion. (From Zide BM: Deformities of the lips and cheeks. In McCarthy JG (ed): Plastic Surgery. Philadelphia, W.B. Saunders, 1990, p 2009, with permission.)

2. What is the significance of the vermilion border?

The vermilion border, also known as the white roll or the mucocutaneous line, is the transition zone between the mucosa of the lip and the skin. In the surgical repair of this mucocutaneous junction, anatomic alignment is critical as even a 1-mm discrepancy is noticeable at a conversational distance. In addition, even after anatomic alignment, the subsequent scar may droop secondary to gravity and require further revision.

3. What is Cupid's bow?

Cupid's bow is the central portion of the upper mucocutaneous line at the base of the philtral columns. Defects of Cupid's bow may be covered by a mustache in males. In females, however, absence of this landmark leads to a flattened appearance of the upper lip.

4. What is the primary function of the lips?

The main function of the lips is to provide oral competence. This function is controlled by the orbicularis oris muscle. Its muscle fibers originate at an area of mingling of various muscle bundles lateral to the commissure (known as the modiolus), cross the lip at the midline, and insert at the opposite philtral column.

5. What are the muscles of the upper and lower lip?

The orbicularis oris produces an oral sphincter integral to facial expression and oral competence; the levator labii superioris, zygomaticus major, and levator anguli oris elevate the upper lip; the depressor labii inferioris (quadratus) and depressor anguli oris (triangularis) are depressors of the lower lip and angle of the mouth; the mentalis muscle elevates the central portion of the lower lip.

6. What is the motor and sensory innervation of the upper and lower lip?

The buccal and zygomatic branches of the facial nerve supply motor innervation to the upper lip. The marginal mandibular branch of the facial nerve supplies motor innervation to the lower lip. Sensory innervation of the upper lip is provided by the infraorbital branch of the trigeminal nerve, whereas the mental nerve supplies the lower lip.

7. Discuss the vascular anatomy and the lymphatic drainage of the lips.

The facial artery emerges bilaterally between the mandible and anterior border of the masseter muscle and divides at the commissure to form the superior labial artery, which supplies the upper lip, and the inferior labial artery, which supplies the lower lip. Venous drainage occurs mainly via branches of the facial vein. Lymphatic drainage is facilitated by the submandibular nodes, which drain the upper lip and lateral lower lip, and the submental nodes, which drain the central lower lip.

8. How is an infraorbital nerve block performed?

The infraorbital foramen is 4–7 mm distal to the infraorbital rim. Transcutaneous injection with local anesthetic is performed lateral to the nasal ala and medial to the nasolabial fold. Intraoral or transmucosal techniques require infiltration superior to the canine eminence.

9. How is a mental nerve block performed?

Avoid injection of anesthesia into the mental foramen. To locate the mental nerve, roll the lower lip outward and stretch the mucosa; the mental nerve should be visible at the canine root, lateral to the canine sulcus.

10. Is the mental nerve block sufficient for anesthesia of the chin?

No. To block the region below the labiomental fold, an inferior alveolar nerve block should be performed at the medial border of the mandibular ramus.

11. Can the lip be locally infiltrated with an anesthetic agent?

Yes. The advantage to local anesthesia with the addition of epinephrine is hemostasis. However, the increased volume can distort the anatomy, especially at the vermilion border. It is imperative to mark the edges of the mucocutaneous junction with methylene blue dye before infiltration of local anesthetic.

12. How should lesions near the vermilion border be managed?

Lesions near the vermilion border should be excised in a vertical ellipse. If the lesion is oriented horizontally, excision may be performed transversely. The mucocutaneous line should be avoided if possible. If the lesion crosses the vermilion, the incision must cross the mucocutaneous line at a 90° angle. In all planned excisions that cross the vermilion, dye should be used to mark the junction before infiltration of local anesthetic.

13. Should sutures be placed directly on the mucocutaneous junction to align the vermilion border?

No. Erythema may develop at the suture line secondary to inflammation and distort the mucocutaneous line. Sutures may be placed immediately above and below the vermilion border for proper alignment.

14. How much tissue loss still permits a satisfactory primary closure?
Up to 25% of the lip may be excised without subsequent functional or aesthetic defect. In elderly patients, this percent may be increased to one-third because of tissue laxity.

15. How should full-thickness lip lacerations be repaired? What suture materials should be used?
The buccal mucosa may be repaired with 4-0 or 5-0 chromic suture, either interrupted or running. The muscles must be well aligned and reapproximated to preserve proper sphincter function; 4-0 vicryl or monocryl may be used. The dermal layer may be closed with 5-0 monocryl or vicryl and the skin with either running or interrupted 6-0 nylon.

16. Why is the lower lip more often a site for tumors than the upper lip?
The lower lip receives more direct actinic radiation (i.e., sun exposure), making it the site for 95% of all lip cancers.

17. What are the key considerations in lip reconstruction?
The size of the oral aperture is important to provide adequate access for dental repair and denture insertion or removal. Sensation should be carefully preserved because a decrease may lead to impaired ability to retain liquids in the oral cavity. Preservation of neurovascular supply during flap mobilization, proper anatomic alignment, and restoration of function and cosmesis are critical. Revisions after initial flap reconstruction may be necessary.

18. What is the major complication of flap reconstruction?
Reduction of the size of the oral stoma is the major complication.

19. Why is the lower lip a more suitable donor for reconstruction than the upper lip?
The lower lip has no distinguishing features such as the Cupid's bow, philtrum, or tubercle. It may sustain greater tissue loss and can donate tissue for upper lip reconstruction.

20. Do V wedge resections provide adequate margins for squamous cell cancer of the lower lip?
No. V excisions are suboptimal because tumor tends to spread downward or laterally. Furthermore, the apex of the excision crosses the labiomental fold and may promote hypertrophic scars. The W excision or the modified flared W-plasty allows a wider excision; the modified W-plasty avoids crossing the labiomental fold.

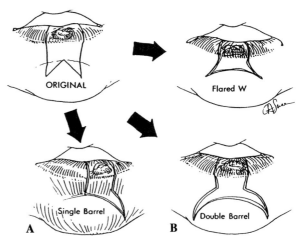

The W-plasty results in a scar that crosses the labiomental fold, often providing a hypertrophic band. Modifications such as the flared W (*upper right*) or the barrel incisions (*A, B*) yield a more favorable scar. (From Zide BM: Deformities of the lips and cheeks. In McCarthy JG (ed): Plastic Surgery. Philadelphia, W.B. Saunders, 1990, p 2016, with permission.)

21. What options are available for repair of localized mucosal and vermilion defects?
Notch or saddle deformities of the lower lip involving the vermilion may be managed by excision and Z-plasty. Other options include the V-Y mucomuscular advancement flap and the lateral mucomuscular advancement flap. (See figure at top of next page.)

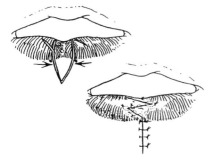

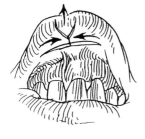

Significant notch deformities may require excision and Z-plasty to prevent further retraction. (From Zide BM: Deformities of the lips and cheeks. In McCarthy JG (ed): Plastic Surgery. Philadelphia, W.B. Saunders, 1990, p 2015, with permission.)

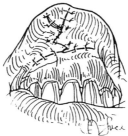

V-Y mucomuscular advancement flap may be used for a midline whistle deformity or deficiency of the tubercle. (From Zide BM: Deformities of the lips and cheeks. In McCarthy JG (ed): Plastic Surgery. Philadelphia, W.B. Saunders, 1990, p 2028, with permission.)

22. Describe the flaps commonly used for lip reconstruction.

The following are full-thickness, musculomucocutaneous flaps:

Abbé flap: V-shaped lower lip flap based on the inferior labial artery and designed opposite the area of defect for the central upper lip region. The flap is raised, transposed 180°, and inset. The donor site is closed directly. Second-stage division of the pedicle and final inset take place 14 days later.

Estlander flap: triangular flap based on the superior labial artery and designed for reconstruction of lateral lower lip defects involving the commissure. The flap is transposed 180° from the upper lip to the lower lip. This procedure results in a smaller oral stoma and indistinct commissure, which may require further revision.

Gillies fan flap: fan-shaped rotational advancement flap based on the superior labial artery and designed for large defects involving greater than 50% of the lower lip. The flap is made lateral to the defect around the nasolabial fold with a 1-cm back-cut. This procedure also may reduce the oral aperture.

McGregor flap: rectangular-shaped flap modified from the Gillies fan flap and based on the superior labial artery. This flap is rotated around the commissure without altering the size of the oral stoma. The width of the flap equals the vertical height of the defect, whereas the length of the flap equals the width of the defect plus the width of the flap. A mucosal advancement flap is required to reconstruct the lip mucosa.

Karapandzic flap: rotational neurovascular advancement flap designed for upper or lower lip defects or both simultaneously. Semicircular incisions are performed from the edge of the skin defect toward the nasal ala bilaterally. The facial nerve branches and the branches of the superior and inferior labial arteries must be preserved. *(Figure continued on following page.)*

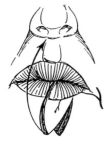

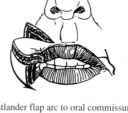

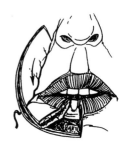

Abbé flap arc to central upper lip

Estlander flap arc to oral commissure and lower lip

Gillies fan flap to central upper lip

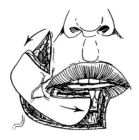
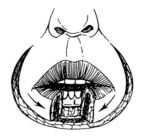

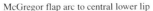

| McGregor flap arc to central lower lip | Karapandzic flap arc to central lower lip |

Full-thickness musculocutaneous flaps for lip reconstruction. These flaps may be based on the right or left superior or inferior labial arteries and are useful for lip and oral sphincter reconstruction. (From Mathes SJ, Nahai F (eds): Orbicularis oris flap. In Mathes SJ, Nahai F (eds): Reconstructive Surgery: Principles, Anatomy, and Technique. New York, Churchill Livingstone, 1997, with permission.)

BIBLIOGRAPHY

1. Fonseca RJ, Walker RV (eds): Oral and Maxillofacial Trauma. Philadelphia, W.B. Saunders, 1991.
2. Hollinshead WH, Rosse C (eds): Textbook of Anatomy, 4th ed. New York, Harper & Row, 1985.
3. Mathes SJ, Nahai F (eds): Orbicularis oris flap. In Mathes SJ, Nahai F (eds): Reconstructive Surgery: Principles, Anatomy, and Technique. New York, Churchill Livingstone, 1997, pp 301–320.
4. Netter FH: Atlas of Human Anatomy. Summit, NJ, Ciba-Geigy Corporation, 1989.
5. O'Daniel TG: Lip reconstruction. In Marsh JL (ed): Decision Making in Plastic Surgery. St. Louis, Mosby, 1993, pp 134–135.
6. Zide BM: Deformities of the lips and cheeks. In McCarthy JG (ed): Plastic Surgery. Philadelphia, W.B. Saunders, 1990, pp 2009–2037.

39. RECONSTRUCTION OF THE ORAL CAVITY

Eser Yuksel, M.D., Adam Weinfeld, B.A., and Saleh M. Shenaq, M.D.

1. What are the borders and contents of the oral cavity?

The oral cavity extends from the vermilion of the lips to the junction of the hard and soft palates superiorly and to the line of the circumvallate papillae of the tongue inferiorly. It contains the lips, buccal mucosa, alveolar ridges, retromolar triangle, floor of the mouth, hard palate, and anterior two thirds of the tongue.

2. Which risk factors are associated with oral cancer?

Tobacco products are the most significant risk factor; alcohol consumption is second. Noncessation of smoking after diagnosis of a primary tumor increases the risk of developing a second primary tumor, increases the rate of recurrence, and decreases the response to radiotherapy. Poor oral hygiene, mechanical irritation by dental appliances, use of mouthwash, smokeless tobacco, syphilis, Plummer-Wilson syndrome, chronic candidiasis, and chronic exposure to toxic irritants are additional risk factors for intra-oral cancer.

3. What are the benign and premalignant lesions of the oral cavity?

Mucocele formation due to the obstruction of minor salivary glands, sialolithiasis, pleomorphic adenoma, necrotizing sialometaplasia of the hard palate, dermoid cysts of the floor of the mouth, granular cell myoblastoma, hemangioma and lymphangioma, mucosal polyps, fibroma, median rhomboid glossitis, aphthous ulcers, tuberculous granulomas, and lichen planus are benign lesions of the oral cavity. Leukoplakia and erythroplakia are premalignant lesions; they are bright white or bright red in color, respectively. Histologic examination of these premalignant lesions reveals existing dysplasia or consequent malignant transformation.

4. What is the distribution of oral cavity cancers by location and histologic types?

Malignant tumors of the oral cavity account for approximately 30% of all head and neck cancers. The tongue is the most common site for oral cavity cancers, accounting for 22–30% of all cases. The floor of the mouth follows the tongue as a common site of malignancy. Squamous cell carcinoma represents more than 90% of oral cancers. Adenocarcinomas are second in frequency. Subtypes of squamous cell carcinomas are differentiated, undifferentiated (transitional, spindle cell), adenoid squamous, and verrucous carcinoma. Verrucous carcinoma has a tendency to grow more radially than vertically.

5. How can you predict the outcome and formulate a treatment for intraoral carcinoma?

Tumor size and thickness and presence of cervical nodal involvement are major determinants of outcome; however, immunohistologic quantification of tumor angiogenesis may help to predict the aggressiveness of the tumor. Tumor-node-metastasis (TNM) classification is still the basis for formulating treatment. Surgery remains the main treatment modality, although extended procedures cause functional problems with swallowing and speech. Reconstructive procedures are designed to minimize functional and aesthetic problems. Despite its acute morbidity (mucositis, odynophagia, swelling) and long-term morbidity (loss of taste perception, dry mouth, tissue necrosis), radiotherapy often is used as an adjuvant therapy in advanced cases.

6. What are the objectives of oropharyngeal reconstruction?

The objectives are to maintain oral continuity, to facilitate swallowing, to prevent aspiration, to preserve satisfactory speech, and to provide primary wound healing in one stage. These functional restorations require adequate tongue mobility and oral sealing.

7. Squamous cell carcinoma of the tongue is most frequently located at the base. True or false?

False. Three-quarters of all tongue cancers are located in the anterior mobile portion. Forty percent of all tongue cancers have nodal involvement, and 20% of all cases demonstrate bilateral nodal involvement. Elective node dissection is recommended for tumors thicker than 10 mm. Tumors of the posterior third of the tongue are less well differentiated, and 75% of cases have nodal involvement at the time of diagnosis.

8. Describe the goals and methods for reconstruction of tongue defects.

Restoration of tongue mobility and sensation are primary goals of reconstruction. T1 lesions treated with wedge excision of tumor and 1–2-cm margins generally can be reconstructed with primary closure or local lingual flaps. After partial or hemiglossectomies, local flaps or innervated free flaps are the choices for reconstruction. Muscle flaps may be used for reconstruction of subtotal to total glossectomy cases.

9. How are palatal defects reconstructed?

Palatal island flaps, temporalis muscle flaps, lingual flaps, or fasciocutaneous free flaps serve well for the reconstruction of palatal defects. Extensive composite defects caused by maxillectomy may require free muscle and/or bone composite flap transfers.

10. What is the reconstructive strategy for floor of the mouth (FOM) defects?

The selection of a proper method is based on the quantity of tissue removed, tongue mobility, and radiotherapy. Primary closure or skin grafting is adequate for defects of limited size. Skin grafts also can reconstruct larger FOM defects without restricting tongue mobility. Removal of the mylohyoid complex necessitates regional or free flap reconstruction. Reconstruction of the lingual nerve may be accomplished with innervated free flap transfers. Muscle flaps are used in greater volume defects to prevent the pooling of saliva and food in this region. Composite defects that include bone require vascularized bone transfers in addition to volume and surface reconstruction.

11. Buccal mucosa defects should not be left to heal by secondary intention. True or false?

False. Small defects may be closed primarily or allowed to heal by secondary intention. Reconstruction of larger defects with skin or mucosal grafts is rapid and reliable. Temporalis muscle or fascia flaps, with or without skin grafts, can be used for thicker or less vascularized defects. Other regional flaps may be utilized for volume and surface reconstruction. For through-and-through cheek defects, cervical rotation advancement flaps (prior radiotherapy or neck dissection should be ruled out) or free fasciocutaneous flaps can be used.

12. Periosteum is always a physiologic barrier for bone involvement in alveolar ridge malignancies. True or false?

False. In cases of previous radiotherapy, the periosteum loses its ability to serve as a barrier for local invasion because irradiation alters the structural integrity of periosteum. This factor should be considered during surgical planning. Stage I and II malignancies can be treated with resection of the primary tumor with a marginal mandibulectomy and local flap coverage. Advanced cases require en bloc resection of full-thickness mandibular segment and treatment of the affected neck. Mandibular reconstruction modalities are applied for the reconstruction in such cases (osteocutaneous free flaps).

13. List the reconstructive options for oral malignancies.

Alternatives for Surface and Volume Reconstruction of Intraoral Defects

Basic approaches	Regional flaps *(cont.)*
Secondary healing	Cervical rotation-advancement flaps
Primary closure	Sternocleidomastoid muscle flaps
Grafts	Trapezius muscle flaps
Split-thickness skin grafting	Latissimus dorsi muscle flaps
Full-thickness skin grafting	Pectoralis major muscle flaps
Local flaps	Free flaps
Mucosal flaps	Jejunum flaps
Lingual flaps	Gastro-omental flaps
Palatal flaps	Radial forearm flaps
Regional flaps	Lateral arm flaps
Platysma flaps	Ulnar flaps
Nasolabial flaps	Scapular flaps
Temporalis muscle and fascia flaps	Groin flaps
Forehead flaps	Rectus abdominis muscle flaps
Posterior auricular flaps	Dorsalis pedis flaps

14. Free flap transfers are the method of choice in most cases. True or false?

False. The reconstructive technique depends on the size and composition of the defect. The reconstructive approach must follow the sequence of priority from primary closure to skin grafting, local flaps, regional flaps, and distant flaps. The specific functional requirements may alter the treatment choices in individual cases.

15. What are the advantages and disadvantages of free flap applications in oral reconstruction?

Advantages	Disadvantages
Superior wound healing	Require microsurgical skill
Better functional and aesthetic outcome	Longer operation time (risk of anesthesia
Higher quality of life	in debilitated and older patients)
Shorter hospitalization	
Use of neurotized flaps	
One-stage, immediate reconstruction	
Suitable for simultaneous two-team approach	
Ability to restore composite defects	
Fewer complications in irradiated patients	

16. Which arteries and veins in the head and neck region are preferred as recipient vessels for microvascular anastomoses?

Branches of the ipsilateral external carotid system are suitable for arterial anastomoses, including the superior thyroid artery, lingual artery, facial artery, and superficial temporal artery. In irradiated or operated cases, contralateral neck vessels or the ipsilateral common carotid artery may be selected. For veins, tributaries of the superficial and deep jugular system are convenient.

17. Describe the elevation of the platysma flap and outline the indications for intraoral reconstruction.

This flap is based on the submental branch of the facial artery and raised on a subcutaneous superior muscle pedicle. The skin island is designed on a transverse axis distally. The pedicle area is supported by anastomoses with both labial arteries, the superior thyroid artery and superior labial artery. Because a motor branch of the facial nerve and sensory branches innervate the musculocutaneous unit, this flap may be used to give motor function to the lip and to provide sensation to the reconstructed area. It can be transposed 180° to reconstruct defects of the tongue and FOM. Previous irradiation to the neck area is the main contraindication for use of this flap.

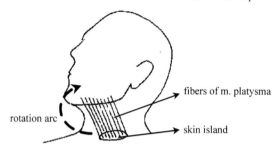

fibers of m. platysma

rotation arc

skin island

Platysma flap.

18. What are the limitations of the temporalis muscle and fascia flaps for oral reconstruction?

The temporal muscle flap (TMF) is based on the deep temporal vessels, whereas the temporal fascial flap (TFF) is based on the superficial temporal vessels. Either may easily be transposed to the buccal region, palate, and lateral portions of FOM. The length of the pedicle precludes its use for the tongue and central portion of FOM. Flaps can be lined with skin grafts; however, adaptation and epithelialization of the flaps' raw surface are satisfactory even with secondary healing. Muscle is included in the flap when bulk is needed. The main problems after flap transfer are temporal depression (in TMF cases) and limitations of the oral aperture.

19. Can the posterior auricular flap (PAF) be used for tongue reconstruction?

Yes. The PAF may be transferred as an island or free flap based on the posterior auricular vessels for oral cavity reconstruction. Dissection of this flap is a difficult and time-consuming procedure, and the area of the skin island is limited. Complications due to the extensive dissection and close proximity to the facial nerve have been reported. However, a less visible donor site scar and the pliability of the transferred skin places this flap among the alternatives for intraoral reconstruction when simultaneous neck dissection is carried out.

20. Explain the extension arc of nasolabial musculocutaneous flaps.

Inferiorly based nasolabial flaps may be transferred transbuccally to reconstruct buccal defects and FOM defects of 2.5 cm by 7.0 cm. It is essential not to include hair-bearing skin in the flap. Unlike the subcutaneous pedicle flaps, the muscle-incorporated flaps (nasalis, levator superioris, zygomaticus muscles) may be transposed for distances greater than 2 cm and undergo minimal contraction.

21. Classify the lingual flaps.

Dorsal lingual flaps must not cross the median raphe. They are elevated at 8-mm thickness to include mucosa, submucosa, and superficial musculature. Posteriorly based dorsal tongue flaps may be used to reconstruct moderate defects of the retromolar triangle. Anteriorly based dorsal tongue flaps offer greater mobility and may be used to repair anterior cheek and commissure defects. Transverse dorsal tongue flaps may be used in bipedicle fashion to reconstruct FOM defects when the tongue is extra long.

Flaps from the lingual tip. Perimeter flaps and dorsoventrally based flaps may be raised.

Ventral surface flaps. These flaps may be used for FOM defects; however, the donor area must be skin-grafted to avoid limitation in tongue mobility.

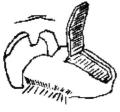

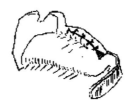

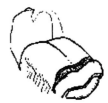

A. Posteriorly based dorsal tongue flap

B. Anteriorly based dorsal tongue flap

C. Transverse dorsal tongue flap

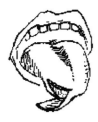

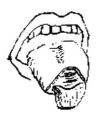

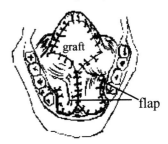

D. Perimeter flap of tip

E. Dorsoventrally based tip flap

F. Ventral surface flap

Lingual flaps.

22. What is the role of palatal flaps in oral reconstruction?

Total palatal mucoperiosteal tissue (up to 24 cm^2) can be raised on a single greater palatine artery. This flap can be transposed to cover neighboring defects of the buccal mucosa, retromolar triangle, tonsillar region, and soft palate. The donor area is left to granulate. The palatal mucosa is not pliable, and caution must be taken to avoid pedicle torsion. As with other local flaps, previous irradiation to the oral cavity precludes the use of palatal flaps.

23. What are the drawbacks of the forehead flap?

(1) Poor aesthetic results of the donor site, (2) need for staged operations, and (3) extensive dissection area.

24. When should the latissimus dorsi (LD) muscle and musculocutaneous flaps be used?

The LD muscle or musculocutaneous flaps may be used to cover extensive defects of the oral cavity, especially when volume reconstruction is needed and/or recipient bed conditions are poor. When both internal and external linings are required, this flap may be used with one side grafted or with separate skin islands.

25. What are the limitations of the pectoralis major (PM) muscle and musculocutaneous flaps?

- Donor site scar is not aesthetic (unacceptable in female patients).
- Pedicle produces bulk in the subcutaneous tunnel.
- Hair-bearing skin is a disadvantage for intraoral reconstruction.
- Too much bulk may cause problems in tongue and FOM reconstruction.
- Dissection is carried out over a large area.
- The close proximity to the recipient site prevents a simultaneous two-team approach.

26. Can the sternocleidomastoid (SCM) musculocutaneous flap be raised over an inferior pedicle?

Yes. The skin island may be outlined over the inframastoid area and the flap may be based on an inferior blood supply; however, it usually requires sacrifice of the eleventh nerve. The SCM has three blood supplies (superior, middle, and inferior); the flap is more frequently raised on the superior pedicle with a distally placed skin island over the supraclavicular area. In functional neck dissection cases, this flap may be used for intraoral reconstruction.

27. Describe the variants of the trapezius muscle and musculocutaneous flaps for intraoral reconstruction.

The trapezius musculocutaneous flap may be elevated along the descending portion of the transverse cervical artery with a vertical skin island or in a transverse direction, mobilizing the upper portion of the muscle on the transverse cervical artery. The flap is elevated only with the portion of the muscle necessary to incorporate the pedicle area and provide a base with the skin paddle.

28. What is the first-line choice in free flap reconstruction for tongue and FOM defects?

The radial forearm fasciocutaneous flap.

29. What are the advantages of the radial forearm flap for intraoral reconstruction?
- Thin pliable skin is suitable for intraoral lining.
- Distant donor area enables a simultaneous two-team approach.
- Reliable and constant pedicle and internal vascular architecture provide satisfactory flap circulation.
- Incorporation of cutaneous nerves serves to restore sensation to the reconstructed area.
- Lack of bulkiness avoids limitation of tongue mobility for tongue and FOM reconstruction.
- Consistency of the fasciocutaneous unit allows osteointegration of the alveolar ridge.
- Versatility of the skin island-pedicle alignment facilitates comfortable anastomoses.
- Brachioradialis muscle may be included with the flap when additional bulk is needed.
- A partial-thickness segment of radius may be harvested within the flap for bone and soft tissue reconstruction.

30. What are the advantages and disadvantages of the jejunum free flap for intraoral reconstruction?

Advantages: It is best for correction or prevention of xerostomia in irradiated patients and retains secretory ability. Use of bowel components to provide coverage and bulk as well as lining is possible. Jejunal reconstruction of tongue and FOM defects allows full range of tongue motion. The vascular pedicle is reliable and suitable for microsurgical anastomoses. The flap can be harvested endoscopically. Reconstruction is a one-stage procedure.

Disadvantages: The intraabdominal procedure carries the associated donor site risks. Hypersecretion and extreme mobility of the flap lining are additional drawbacks.

31. Describe the vascular anatomy and harvest of the jejunum flap.

An arcade formed by branches of the superior mesenteric artery supplies the jejunum. Each branch (usually larger than 1.5 mm in diameter) can support a segment of jejunum up to 24 cm long. Usually a segment of proximal jejunum (within the first two feet) is used for reconstruction.

After the identification of the ligament of Treitz through a left upper quadrant transverse incision, a suitable proximal segment is located. The vascular pedicle is dissected toward its superior mesenteric origin. All other anastomosing vessels are tied off, leaving the pedicle as the only blood supply to the flap. Next, the proximal and distal ends of the jejunal segment are divided, usually with a stapling device. Once the viability of the flap is assessed, the vascular pedicle is divided close to its origin and the flap is transferred. The tubular flap can be converted to a flat flap by opening it through its antimesenteric border longitudinally. Bowel continuity in the donor site is reestablished.

32. Evaluate the lateral arm flap for tongue reconstruction.

The lateral arm flap provides soft, supple, mobile, innervated tissue of 12 cm $\times$ 18 cm for tongue and FOM reconstruction. It receives its blood supply from the radial collateral artery (1.2 mm in diameter). The lateral brachial cutaneous nerve can be transferred within the flap to reconstruct the lingual nerve. This flap possesses similar advantages to the radial forearm flap; however, the course of the vascular pedicle may vary.

33. What is the role of the laser in oral cavity cancer?

Transoral laser resection of oral cavity carcinomas is widely used in the absence of nodal involvement. The surface is left to granulate and satisfactory epithelialization is observed. Low morbidity and successful control of the disease have supported the use of laser resection in combination with staged neck dissection in advanced cases when mandibular or deep visceral involvement is ruled out.

BIBLIOGRAPHY

1. Ariyan S: Cancer of the upper aerodigestive system. In McCarthy JG (ed): Plastic Surgery. Philadelphia, W.B. Saunders, 1990.
2. Bakamjian VY: Lingual flaps in reconstructive surgery for oral and perioral cancer. In McCarthy JG (ed): Plastic Surgery. Philadelphia, W.B. Saunders, 1990.
3. Eckel HE, Volling P, Zorowka P, Thumfart W: Transoral laser resection with staged discontinuous neck dissection for oral cavity and oropharynx squamous cell carcinoma. Laryngoscope 105:53–60, 1995.
4. Hagan WE: Nasolabial musculocutaneous flap in reconstruction of oral defects. Laryngoscope 96:840–845, 1986.
5. Leonard AG, Kolhe PS: The posterior auricular flap: Intra-oral reconstruction. Br J Plast Surg 40:570–581, 1987.
6. Panje WR: Immediate reconstruction of the oral cavity. In Thawley SE, Panje WR (eds): Comprehensive Management of Head and Neck Tumors. Philadelphia, W.B. Saunders, 1987.
7. Panje WR: Oral cavity and oropharyngeal reconstruction. In Cummings CW (ed): Otolaryngology—Head and Neck Surgery. St. Louis, Mosby, 1992.
8. Papadopoulos ON, Gamatsi IE: Platysma myocutaneous flap for intraoral and surface reconstruction. Ann Plast Surg 31:15–18, 1993.
9. Wells MD, Edwards AL, Luce EA: Intraoral reconstructive techniques. Clin Plast Surg 22:91–108, 1995.

40. MANDIBLE RECONSTRUCTION

Norman Weinzweig, M.D.

1. Who was Andy Gump?

Caricaturized in the 1930s, Andy Gump was a real-life person with head and neck cancer who had an unreconstructed resection of the anterior mandible. A statue in his memory stands in Lake Geneva, Wisconsin.

2. Describe the functional deficits associated with the Andy Gump deformity.

The Andy Gump deformity results from loss of height, width, and projection of the lower third of the face due to resection of the anterior mandibular arch with anterior and medial deviation of the lateral mandibular segments by the residual mylohyoid muscles and superior displacement by the medial pterygoid, masseter, and temporalis muscles. Loss of the anterior mandible results in impairment of oral competence, speech, deglutition (swallowing), and mastication. Loss of support for the hypomandibular complex contributes to aspiration, dysphagia, oral incompetence, and difficulty with mastication.

3. What functional deficits are associated with lateral mandibulectomy?

Loss of continuity in the lateral and posterior segments is far less severe than with central defects. Lateral mandibulectomy defects result in cheek contour deformity with deviation of the symphysis from the midline when the mouth is open. Upward and lateral displacement of the mandibular remnants results from uninhibited pull of the opposite intact muscles of mastication and scar contracture on the resected side. This displacement creates difficulty with bimaxillary relationships and occlusion.

4. What are the main goals and considerations in mandibular reconstruction?

- Primary wound healing
- Early functional oral rehabilitation
- Restoration of aesthetics
- Restoration of the patient's body image

5. What are the advantages of immediate mandibular reconstruction?

Immediate reconstruction provides the best opportunity to achieve optimal aesthetic and function outcome after loss of the mandible. Delayed reconstruction, on the other hand, is associated with deformity and functional deficits as the resected ends of the mandible become tethered by soft tissue scarring, fibrosis, and contracture and often cannot be fully corrected.

6. How do you manage a patient with a shotgun wound to the face?
- Airway, breathing, circulation (ABCs) of resuscitation
- Tracheostomy—often necessary to secure an airway
- Serial debridements of devitalized soft tissue and bone
- Temporary stabilization of the mandibular fragments with rigid plate(s) or external fixation
- Definitive composite reconstruction when the patient's overall status permits

7. What are conventional techniques for mandibular reconstruction?
- Free bone grafts
- Alloplastic materials (metallic implants, metal or Dacron trays packed with cancellous bone)
- Freeze-dried, autoclaved, or irradiated bone allografts
- Pedicled flaps

These techniques have poor or, at best, unpredictable results due to variability of the traumatized, irradiated, or avascular recipient beds. Reconstructions often require multiple-staged procedures with long hospitalizations; patients often succumb before completion of the reconstruction.

8. What are the indications for a no-bone reconstruction?
- Poor surgical candidates
- Short life expectancy
- Edentulous patients with only small posterior mandibulectomy defects

9. What is the role of nonvascularized bone grafts?
- Limited to small lateral defects (< 5 cm) in patients with excellent soft tissue coverage who have not received and will not receive radiation
- Condylar reconstruction in children

10. What are the advantages of reconstruction plates, with or without soft tissue reconstruction?
- Ease of application
- Rigid fixation
- Lack of donor site morbidity
- Reduced operative time
- Condylar replacement
- Reconstruction of extensive bony defects in elderly and infirm patients

Best indicated in patients with poor prognosis, lateral defects, and good soft tissue coverage who have not received and will not receive radiation.

11. What are the disadvantages of reconstruction plates, with or without soft tissue reconstruction?
- Lack of long-term reliability
- Stress on mandibular fragments may cause screw loosening, plate fatigue, and fracture
- Inadequate soft tissue coverage or radiated tissues result in plate extrusion in many anterior reconstructions
- No bone stock for osseointegrated dental implants

12. What are the advantages of the radial forearm osteocutaneous flap?
- Up to 14 cm of straight unicortical bone
- Multiple osteotomies may create an anterior mandible or hemimandible
- Thin, pliable, abundant, relatively hairless skin
- Excellent intraoral lining; conforms well to sulci and prevents tethering of tongue
- Can be split into separate skin paddles for intraoral mucosal lining and external skin coverage
- Flexibility in three-dimensional orientation of bone and skin paddle(s)
- Possible reinnervation by coaptation of lateral or medial antebrachial cutaneous nerves with lingual, mental, or great auricular nerves may facilitate oral rehabilitation
- Long pedicle; large caliber vessels; dual venous drainage

13. What are the disadvantages of the radial forearm osteocutaneous flap?
- Donor radius fracture
- Skin graft loss with tendon exposure
- Displeasing appearance of donor site
- Prolonged extremity immobilization
- Osseointegration *not* possible

14. What are the major reasons for donor radius fracture?
- Harvesting an excessive amount of bone
- Perpendicular osteotomies with cross-cutting of the radius, which further weakens it
- Inadequate length of postoperative immobilization of arm
- Failure to prevent pronation and supination by application of a long-arm cast

15. How can donor radius fracture be prevented?
The radial forearm osteocutaneous flap has received a bad reputation because of donor radius fracture. This complication can be prevented by avoiding the problems cited above as well as by a modification of the standard technique in which the radius is harvested as a keel-shaped segment of bone. Early series reported incidences of fracture ranging from 10–67%. However, two recent series by Weinzweig et al. and Swanson et al. demonstrated a combined fracture incidence of only 2.9% (1 of 34). The solitary fracture was perhaps preventable.

16. What are the advantages of the iliac crest osteocutaneous flap?
- Up to 14 cm of thick corticocancellous bone
- Natural bone curvature (its unique shape resembles a hemimandible)
- Best bone stock for osseointegration

17. What are the disadvantages of the iliac crest osteocutaneous flap?
- Soft tissue too bulky for intraoral lining unless glossectomy is performed
- Poor tissue for intraoral, chin, and submental contour
- Least degree of three-dimensional flexibility of skin and bone
- Skin reliability is unpredictable
- Delayed ambulation and gait disturbances
- Contour deformity at donor site, especially when a large amount of bone is harvested
- Abdominal wall weakness or herniation
- Injury to lateral femoral cutaneous nerve

Modifications include use of the internal oblique muscle and skin graft for intraoral lining and split inner cortex bone harvest.

18. What are the advantages of the scapular osteocutaneous flap?
- Up to 14 cm of straight lateral scapular bone
- Independently vascularized bone and skin paddle(s)
- Greatest three-dimensional flexibility
- Good external skin coverage
- Osseointegration possible
- Minimal donor site morbidity

19. What are the disadvantages of the scapular osteocutaneous flap?
- Bulky soft tissue for intraoral lining
- Osteotomies can devascularize bone segments
- Two-team approach not facilitated
- Seroma formation

20. What are the advantages of the fibular osteocutaneous flap?
- Up to 25 cm of straight bicortical bone— by far the largest amount of bone
- Multiple osteotomies
- Osseointegration possible
- Minimal donor site morbidity

21. What are the disadvantages of the fibular osteocutaneous flap?
- Unreliability of skin paddle (no longer a problem)
- Limited amount of skin available
- Objectionable appearance of skin-grafted donor site
- Delayed ambulation
- Neurapraxia

22. Compare the common vascularized composite tissue transfers and donor sites for oromandibular reconstruction.

*Comparison of Common Vascularized Composite Tissue Transfers
for Oromandibular Reconstruction*

DONOR SITE	BONE LENGTH (cm)	QUALITY	SOFT TISSUE QUALITY	RELIABILITY	HARVEST	MORBID-ITY	PEDICLE
Fibula	25	Excellent	Skin/muscle, excellent, potentially sensate	Good	A, B	Minimal	Peroneal artery, up to 15 cm
Scapula	14	Good	Skin/muscle, good, not sensate	Excellent	D	Moderate	Subscapular artery, up to 10 cm
Iliac crest	14	Excellent	Skin/muscle, fair, not sensate	Good	A, C	Moderate to severe	Deep circumflex iliac artery, 5–6 cm
Radial forearm	10	Poor	Skin, excellent, potentially sensate	Excellent	A,B	Moderate to severe	Radial artery, up to 15 cm

A, two-team approach; B, easy; C, intermediate; D, more difficult.

Comparison of Free Flap Donor Sites for Mandible Reconstruction

	TISSUE CHARACTERISTICS			DONOR SITE CHARACTERISTICS	
DONOR SITE	BONE	SKIN	PEDICLE	LOCATION	MORBIDITY
Fibula	A	C	B	A	A
Ilium	B	D	D	B	C
Scapula	C	B	C	D	B
Radius	D	A	A	C	D

A, excellent; B, good; C, fair; D, poor.

23. Provide algorithms for microvascular mandibular reconstruction.

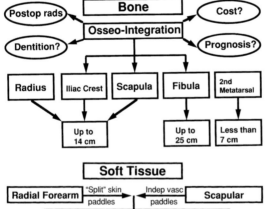

Algorithm for mandibular reconstruction: bone component.

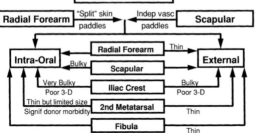

Algorithm for mandibular reconstruction: soft tissue component.

24. Is there a role for sequential free flaps?

Sequential or simultaneous free flaps combine the best qualities of bone and soft tissue of the individual flaps; however, they prolong operative time, add complexity to the case, and increase donor morbidity. Their role, if any, is limited to extensive bone and soft tissue defects not satisfactorily reconstructed by a single flap.

25. What is the role of dental rehabilitation by osseointegration?

Dental rehabilitation by osseointegration achieves the ideal end-goal in mandibular reconstruction, maximizing aesthetic and functional outcome. Unfortunately, few patients are candidates for osseointegration and even fewer actually have it performed. It is difficult to justify this approach, which requires several stages over 6–9 months, in patients with advanced intraoral malignancies who have poor prognoses (approximately 50% of such patients die within 1.5–2 years). Moreover, many patients were edentulous or had poor dentition before tumor ablation. In addition, the significant cost associated with this procedure may not be covered by many insurance companies. Lastly, the fate of osseointegrated implants in the face of postoperative radiation is uncertain.

26. What are important considerations in reconstruction (or construction) of the pediatric mandible?

The pediatric mandible is dynamic, constantly changing with growth and development. Reconstructive options are based on the higher osteogenic potential, the tremendous capacity of the temporomandibular joint (TMJ) for remodeling, and the implicit requirement for growth. The mandibular body and parasymphysis are filled with developing tooth buds. One must consider not only the three-dimensional problems of aesthetics and occlusion but also the fourth dimension of time. Techniques include conventional bone and cartilage grafting, orthognathic surgery, distraction osteogenesis, and microvascular free tissue transfer, alone or in combination. Because of the above factors, the diversity of reconstructive options in pediatric cases is greater than in adult cases.

27. Name three primary indications for mandibular reconstruction in the child.

1. Posttraumatic—management of significant fractures with bone loss and treatment of their sequelae of growth disturbances and TMJ ankylosis.

2. Congenital—hypoplasia associated with oculoauricular vertebral (OAV) syndrome, including hemifacial microsomia and craniofacial microsomia.

3. After resection of facial tumors or radiation therapy for orbitofacial tumors.

BIBLIOGRAPHY

1. Coleman JJ III: Mandible reconstruction. Oper Tech Plast Reconstr Surg 3(4):213–302, 1996.
2. Hidalgo DA: Aesthetic improvements in free-flap mandible reconstruction. Plast Reconstr Surg 88:574, 1991.
3. Hidalgo DA: Fibula free flap: A new method of mandibular reconstruction. Plast Reconstr Surg 84:71, 1989.
4. Millard DR, Maisels DO, Batstone JHF: Immediate repair of radical resection of the anterior arch of the lower jaw. Plast Reconstr Surg 37:15, 1969.
5. Shenaq SM, Klebuc MJA: The iliac crest microsurgical free flap in mandibular reconstruction. Clin Plast Surg 21:37, 1994.
6. Shusterman MA, Reece GP, Kroll SS, et al: Use of the AO plate for immediate mandibular reconstruction in cancer patients. Plast Reconstr Surg 88:588, 1991.
7. Shusterman MA, Reece GP, Miller MJ, et al: The osteocutaneous free fibula flap: Is the skin paddle reliable? Plast Reconstr Surg 90:787, 1992.
8. Soutar DS, Widdowson WP: Immediate reconstruction of the mandible using a vascularized segment of radius. Head Neck Surg 8:232, 1986.
9. Steckler RM, Edgerton MT, Gogol W: Andy Gump. Am J Surg 138:545, 1974.
10. Swanson E, Boyd JB, Manktelow RT: The radial forearm flap: Reconstructive applications and donor-site defects in 35 consecutive patients. Plast Reconstr Surg 85:258, 1990.
11. Swartz MM, Banis JC, Newton E: The osteocutaneous scapular flap for mandibular and maxillary reconstruction. Plast Reconstr Surg 77:550, 1986.
12. Taylor GI: Reconstruction of the mandible with free iliac bone grafts. Ann Plast Surg 9:361, 1986.
13. Weinzweig N, Weinzweig J: Current concepts in mandibular reconstruction by microsurgical free flaps. Surg Technol Int VI:338–346, 1997.

14. Weinzweig N, Jones NF, Shestak KC, et al: Oromandibular reconstruction using a keel-shaped modification of the radial forearm osteocutaneous flap. Ann Plast Surg 33:359, 1994.
15. Wells MD, Luce EA, Edwards AL, et al: Sequentially linked free flaps in head and neck reconstruction. Clin Plast Surg 21:59, 1994.

41. SCALP RECONSTRUCTION

Sai S. Ramasastry, M.D., F.R.C.S., and Ahmed Makki, M.D., F.R.C.S.

1. What are the common causes of scalp defects?

Scalp defects may result from trauma, tumor excision, and tissue necrosis due to burns or radiation therapy.

2. What are the five anatomic layers of the scalp?

S = **S**kin. Scalp skin is considered the thickest skin in the body and may be used as a donor site for split-thickness skin grafts.

C = Sub**c**utaneous tissue, which contains hair follicles and sweat and sebaceous glands, blood vessels, lymphatics, and nerves.

A = **A**poneurosis (galea aponeurotica) that connects the frontalis muscle with the occipitalis muscle.

L = **L**oose connective tissue, which allows the scalp to be mobile on the cranium.

P = **P**ericranium, which invests the skull bone.

Scalp avulsion injuries occur at the level of the loose areolar tissue.

3. What is the arterial supply of the scalp?

The scalp is endowed with an extensive circulatory network. Anteriorly, it is supplied by the supraorbital and supratrochlear arteries, which are end vessels of the ophthalmic artery arising from the internal carotid. Laterally, it is supplied by the superficial temporal artery, a branch of the external carotid, supplying the temporal, parietal, and frontal regions. Posteriorly, it is supplied by two lateral and two medial branches of the occipital artery, a branch of the external carotid. The postauricular artery, also a branch of the external carotid, supplies the posterolateral scalp.

4. What factors affect the selection of a scalp reconstruction method?

1. Replace like tissue with like tissue. The scalp should be reconstructed with hair-bearing skin whenever possible.

2. Wound repair depends on location, size, and depth of the wound.

3. Careful preoperative and intraoperative planning.

4. Wounds without tissue loss, no matter how long after injury, may be closed by direct approximation.

5. Overzealous debridement is unnecessary because the robust circulation often allows salvage of the tissues.

6. In large defects, skin grafting, scalp flaps, and non-scalp flap transfer from a regional or distant site come into play.

5. What are the principles of the management of acute scalp wounds?

1. The goal is to obtain a healed wound while preventing desiccation, infection, and bone necrosis.

2. Wounds with vascularized tissue covering the bone, such as the pericranium, may be covered by skin grafts.

3. Keep the tissues moist in every acute situation.

4. If all layers are absent and the calvarial bone is exposed, immediate coverage must be provided by either local flaps or distant flaps.

5. If the tissue defect also involves the bone, vascularized soft tissue coverage must be provided. Bone may be replaced at the same time or at a later date.

6. What are the indications and advantages of using a skin graft for coverage of scalp wounds?

A skin graft is an option for partial-thickness wounds. The recipient bed must be well vascularized and free of infection. Split-thickness skin grafts provide a simple, fast, and economic way to obtain reliable wound healing. In some situations, the calvarial bone can be drilled on the outer cortex of the bone and decorticated to allow granulated tissue growth to facilitate skin graft take.

7. Can a skin graft be used to cover decorticated outer table skull?

Yes. Two to three days after decortication of the outer table of the skull, a skin graft remains an option in special circumstances. This method provides an epithelial cover for the skull. The procedure is most useful as a temporary measure before definitive scalp reconstruction—for example, by tissue expansion.

8. How do you manage scalp wounds after radiation therapy or tumor resection?

The presence of multiple scalp incisions makes the use of scalp tissues somewhat problematic. Previous radiation therapy complicates the situation because of its deleterious effect on local tissue blood supply. When it is important to protect the bone or underlying brain tissue, one must provide soft tissue coverage with an independent and robust blood supply. This task often requires transfer of a regional flap or the microvascular transfer of a free flap.

9. Do periosteal flaps have any role in scalp reconstruction?

When bone is exposed, skin graft coverage may not be possible. Local pericranial flaps may be used in such cases for bone coverage, thus providing the vascularized bed necessary for skin graft take.

10. What is the major indication for use of regional or distant flaps for scalp reconstruction?

Large defects involving greater than 30% of the scalp that must be closed acutely and cannot be reconstructed with a skin graft or local flap. This situation is seen most commonly after full-thickness excision of a scalp tumor.

11. What are the indications for the use of free flaps for scalp reconstruction?

Free tissue transfer should be reserved for patients for whom reconstruction by conventional pedicle flap is not feasible. Free flaps are becoming increasingly used in the acute coverage of large defects after burns, radiation, and, occasionally, full-thickness excision of large tumors. In most cases, however, a carefully planned local transposition or rotation flap may be equally effective.

12. What are the advantages of free flaps?

Microvascular free tissue transfer allows one-stage coverage of large defects with exposed bone or underlying brain tissue.

13. What are the most commonly used free flaps for scalp reconstruction?

1. Omental flaps
2. Latissimus dorsi muscle flaps followed by split-thickness skin grafts
3. Radial forearm flaps

14. What makes a radial forearm flap an ideal free flap for the scalp?

The radial forearm flap is a versatile flap for the reconstructive surgeon because of its thinness, durable skin quality, aesthetic match, and relative ease of dissection. It provides a reliable single-stage method to cover difficult scalp defects when other local methods are unsuitable. One of the drawbacks is its relatively small size. Preexpansion of the radial forearm flap may be used to cover a large scalp defect. In addition, the radial forearm flap is relatively non–hair-bearing.

15. What are the disadvantages of free flaps for scalp reconstruction?

The flaps are often bulky and do not provide hair-bearing tissue for reconstruction. Technical difficulties and donor site problems associated with microsurgical tissue transfer are additional drawbacks.

16. What are the available options for reconstruction of scalp bony defects?
1. Cranial bone graft, which is available in the same operative field
2. Split rib graft
3. Cancellous bone graft from a distant bone site
4. Alloplastic materials, such as methyl methacrylate

17. What is the role of tissue expansion in scalp reconstruction?
Tissue expansion has become the preferred method of secondary scalp reconstruction. It offers the reconstructive surgeon a better option than the conventional methods of skin grafts or transfer of non–hair-bearing, regional, or microvascular flaps for reconstruction of large defects that cannot be repaired with adjacent hair-bearing flaps. Reconstruction of large scalp defects depends on the ability to cover them with hair-bearing tissue. When the area of alopecia is large, the normal scalp is not sufficient to cover the defect resulting from excision of alopecia. Using tissue expansion techniques, large wounds can be totally resurfaced while normal hair growth is maintained.

18. What is the major drawback of tissue expanders?
The main disadvantage of tissue expansion is the long duration of treatment.

19. What is the main concern in the use of scalp tissue expansion in children?
There is a risk of skull deformation after a prolonged period of expansion. Little is known about the long-term effects on the skull and the ability of the skull to remodel after removal of the expander.

20. What are the potential complications of scalp tissue expansion?
Infection, exposure of the expander, extrusion, and device failure.

21. What are the advantages of an expanded free scalp flap?
Expansion of a large free scalp flap before transfer allows direct closure of the flap donor site, thereby avoiding the need for a skin graft or local flap to close the donor site.

BIBLIOGRAPHY

1. Alpert BS, Buncke HJ, Mathes SJ: Surgical treatment of the total avulsed scalp. Clin Plast Surg 9:145, 1982.
2. Argenta LC, Watanabe MJ, Grabb WC: The use of tissue expansion in head and neck reconstruction. Ann Plast Surg 11:31, 1983.
3. Arnold PG, Rangarathnam CS: Multiple-flap scalp reconstruction: Orticoshea revisited. Plast Reconstr Surg 69:605, 1982.
4. Hallock GG: Cutaneous coverage for the difficult scalp wound. Contemp Surg 38:22, 1991.
5. Jackson IT, et al: Use of external reservoirs in tissue expansion. Plast Reconstr Surg 80:266, 1987.
6. Orticochea M: Four-flap scalp reconstruction technique. Br J Plast Surg 20:159, 1967.
7. Orticochea M: New three-flap reconstruction technique. Br J Plast Surg 24:184, 1971.
8. Shestak KC, Ramasastry SS: Reconstruction of defects of the scalp and skull. In Cohen M (ed): Mastery of Plastic and Reconstructive Surgery. Boston, Little, Brown, 1994, pp 830–841.
9. Tolhurst MB, et al: The surgical anatomy of the scalp. Plast Reconstr Surg 87:603, 1991.

42. SURGICAL ANATOMY OF THE FACIAL NERVE

Soheil Younai, M.D., and Brooke R. Seckel, M.D.

1. From which foramen does the main trunk of the facial nerve exit the skull, and what type of fibers does it contain?
The main trunk of the facial nerve leaves the skull from the stylomastoid foramen, and at this point it only contains motor and sensory fibers, because its parasympathetic fibers leave the cranial fossa along with other cranial nerves.

2. How do you locate the main trunk of the facial nerve during a parotidectomy?

As the facial nerve trunk travels from the stylomastoid foramen to the parotid body, it passes anterior to the posterior belly of the digastric muscle, lateral to styloid process and the external carotid artery, and posterior to the facial vein. At the beginning of a parotidectomy start by mobilizing the tail of the parotid superiorly and retracting the anterior border of the sternocleidomastoid laterally in order to identify the posterior belly of the digastric muscle. Follow this muscle superiorly toward its insertion at the mastoid tip. After bluntly separating the parotid from its attachment to the cartilage of the external auditory canal, the tragal pointer comes into view. The facial nerve trunk lies approximately 1 cm deep and slightly anteroinferior to the tragal pointer.

3. "Great nerves travel together." How does this apply to the relationship of the facial nerve to other cranial nerves?

   a. Facial nerve accompanies the acoustic nerve (CN VIII) as they leave the cranial fossa via the internal acoustic meatus.

   b. Facial nerve's parasympathetic fibers travel with the trigeminal nerve (CN V).

      i. V_1-lacrimal nerve to the lacrimal gland.

      ii. V_2-pterygopalatine nerve to the nasal and palatal glands.

      iii. V_3-lingual nerve via chorda tympani to the taste buds of the anterior two thirds of the tongue, and submandibular and sublingual glands.

   c. Facial nerve's sensory fibers travel with the auricular branch of the vagus nerve (CN X) to provide sensation to the external auditory meatus.

4. Does the facial nerve innervate the posterior or the anterior belly of the digastric muscle?

The facial nerve innervates the posterior belly of the digastric muscle, while the trigeminal nerve innervates its anterior belly.

5. What muscle does the facial nerve innervate in the middle ear and what does it do?

The facial nerve innervates the stapedius muscle which dampens loud noise.

6. Which brachial cleft arch does the facial nerve arise from? Which brachial cleft arch does the trigeminal nerve arise from?

The first brachial cleft arch gives rise to the trigeminal nerve, while the second arch gives rise to the facial nerve.

7. What are the major branches of the facial nerve before and after it enters the parotid?

The facial nerve trunk has six major branches which are the temporal, zygomatic, buccal, mandibular, cervical, and auricular. The auricular branch comes off before the facial nerve turns into the parotid body, and innervates the superior auricular, posterior auricular, and occipitalis muscles, as well as providing sensation to the area behind the ear lobe. Within the parotid, the facial nerve divides into two main divisions, the temporofacial and the cervicofacial, which further divide into the temporal, zygomatic, buccal, mandibular, and cervical branches.

8. What is the relationship of the facial nerve to the SMAS?

As the facial nerve branches leave the parotid body they are covered by a very thin layer of parotidomasiteric fascia. The SMAS is located superficial to this layer.

9. What is Bell's palsy?

Bell's palsy is paralysis of the facial nerve. It was first described by Charles Bell in 1814 after he noted the features of facial paralysis in a laboratory monkey with a transected facial nerve. There have been over 75 different etiologic factors identified for Bell's palsy, including (1) Congenital (Möbius syndrome), (2) Traumatic (iatrogenic laceration, fractures, gunshot wound), (3) Neoplastic (tumors of parotid, central nervous system, head, and neck), (4) Neurologic (cerebral vascular accident, degenerative), (5) Infections (bacterial, viral), (6) Metabolic, and (7) Idiopathic. The specific findings in facial paralysis depend on the level of the lesion, which are summarized in the following table:

Level of Injury	Paralysis	Signs/Symptoms	Test
Extracranial	Muscles of facial expression	Inability to close eyes Lower lid laxity/ectropion Eyebrow ptosis Asymmetric facial animation Oral sphincter incompetence/drooling	Facial movement Electrodiagnostic tests
Tympanomastoid	Chorda tympani: a) Taste fibers	a) Loss of taste in anterior two thirds of tongue	Bitter taste test
	b) Parasympathetic innervation to sublingual and submandibular glands	b) Dry mouth	Salivary test
	Stapedius muscle	Hyperacoustic sounds	Stapedial reflex
Geniculate ganglion/greater petrosal nerve	Lacrimal nerve	Dry eye	Schirmer's test
	Parasympathetic to nasal and palatal secretory glands	Dry nose	
Internal Auditory canal	CN VII + VIII	+ Loss of hearing + Loss of balance	Audiology Electronystagmogram
CNS	Supranuclear Nuclear Infranuclear/cerebellopontine angle	All of the above (unilateral upper motor neuron lesion does not affect muscle function of forehead or eyes)	Central neurologic examination

10. Do the facial muscles of expression receive their innervation along their superficial or deep surface?

It depends. Facial muscles such as the mentalis, levator angularis superioris, and the buccinator are located deep within the facial soft tissue. Because these muscles lie deep to the plane of the facial nerve, they receive their innervation along their superficial surfaces and may be damaged during rhytidectomy if the dissection is carried out superficially. On the other hand, all other facial muscles of expression are located superficial to the plane of the facial nerve and thus receive their innervation along their deep or posterior surfaces. For example, the platysma, orbicularis oculi, zygomaticus major and minor are situated superficial to the level of the facial nerve; therefore, during rhytidectomy the dissection should be performed superficial to the surface of these muscles in order to avoid their denervation.

11. What is the course of the frontal branch of the facial nerve?

The frontal branch of the facial nerve travels approximately along a line from 0.5 cm below the tragus to 1.5 cm above the lateral end of the eyebrow.

12. What is the relationship of the frontal branch of the facial nerve to the SMAS and temporoparietal fascia?

Temporoparietal fascia is the extension of the SMAS superior to the zygomatic arch. Inferior to the zygomatic arch the frontal branch of the facial nerve travels deep to the SMAS. As it crosses over the zygomatic arch it becomes very superficial. At this point it is sandwiched between the periosteum (extension of the deep temporal fascia) and the temporoparietal fascia (extension of the SMAS). Superior to the zygomatic arch, the frontal branch of the facial nerve travels within or on the undersurface of the temporoparietal fascia, and superficial to the superficial layer of the deep temporal fascia.

13. What are the "facial danger zones"?

They are defined areas in the face and neck that correspond to the location of the important nerves. A surgeon must know their exact locations to avoid injuring them during rhytidectomy.

Facial Danger Zones	Midpoint Location	Nerve	Relationship to SMAS	Sign of Injury
1	6.5 cm below the external auditory canal	Great auricular nerve	Beneath	Numbness inferior two-thirds of ear
2	Below a line drawn from 0.5 cm below tragus to 2.0 cm above lateral eyebrow	Temporal branch of facial nerve	Within	Paralysis of fore-head
3	Midmandible 2.0 cm posterior to oral commissure	Marginal mandibular branch of facial nerve	Beneath	Paralysis of lower lip
4	Anterior to parotid gland and posterior to zygomaticus major muscle	Zygomatic and buccal branch of facial nerve	Beneath	Paralysis of upper lip
5	Superior orbital rim above midpupil	Supraorbital and supra-trochlear nerves	Beneath	Numbness of fore-head, upper eye-lid, nasal dorsum
6	1.0 cm below inferior orbital rim below midpupil	Infraorbital nerve	Beneath	Numbness of side of upper nose, cheek, upper lip
7	Midmandible below second premolar	Mental nerve	Beneath	Numbness of half of the lower lip

14. What is the incidence of facial nerve injury during a standard rhytidectomy? Which nerve is damaged most often? What are the chances for recovery?

The incidence of facial nerve paralysis after rhytidectomy in a series of over 6,500 reported cases is approximately 0.7%. Of all of these only 0.1% were permanent. The most frequently injured branches were the temporal and the marginal mandibular. Most patients recovered within 6 months.

CONTROVERSY

15. Does the marginal mandibular branch of the facial nerve really run at the margin of the mandible?

Cadaver dissections reveal that posterior to the facial artery the marginal mandibular nerve runs above the inferior border of the mandible in 81% of specimens. In the other 19%, it runs in an arc, the lowest point of which is 1 cm or less below the inferior border of the mandible. Anterior to the facial artery, all of the branches of mandibular rami are above the inferior border of the mandible.

On the contrary, clinical observations made during hundreds of parotidectomies and rhytidectomies have shown that the mandibular branch **always** runs between 1–2 cm below the lower border of the mandible. It has also been noted that in some individuals with lax and atrophic tissues, the branches were even 3–4 cm below the inferior border of the mandible.

BIBLIOGRAPHY

1. Anderson JE (ed): Grant's Atlas of Anatomy. Baltimore, Williams & Wilkins, 1983, pp 7:16–18.
2. Baker DC, Conley J: Avoiding facial nerve injuries in rhytidectomy: Anatomical variations and pitfalls. Plast Reconstr Surg 64:781–795, 1979.
3. Baker DC: Facial paralysis. In McCarthy JG (ed): Plastic Surgery. Philadelphia, W.B. Saunders, 1990, pp 2237–2255.
4. May M: Facial paralysis: Differential diagnosis and indications for surgical therapy. Clin Plast Surg 6:277–282, 1979.
5. Miehlke A: Surgery of the salivary glands and the extratemporal portion of the facial nerve. In Naumann HH (ed): Head and Neck Surgery: Indications, Techniques, Pitfalls. Philadelphia, W.B. Saunders, 1980, pp 421–440.
6. Pansky B: The facial (VII) nerve. In Review of Gross Anatomy. New York, Macmillan, 1984, pp 32–35.
7. Seckel BR: Facial Danger Zones: Avoiding Nerve Injury in Facial Plastic Surgery. St. Louis, Quality Medical Publishers Inc., 1993.
8. Stuzin JM, Wagstrom L, Kawamoto HK, Wolfe SA: Anatomy of the frontal branch of the facial nerve: The significance of temporal fat pad. Plast Reconstr Surg 83:265–271, 1989.

43. REANIMATION OF THE PARALYZED FACE

Julia K. Terzis, M.D., and Jeffrey Caplan, M.D.

1. What are the key questions in obtaining the history of a patient with facial paralysis?

Onset is the most important aspect of the history in determining the cause of a patient's facial paralysis. Acute onset is most likely associated with infection, trauma, medication, or vascular causes. Slow onset is most indicative of a tumor. Other important questions are the presence of hyperacuity, dizziness, and changes in tearing, taste, and hearing.

2. What should you look for on physical exam?

The patient should be observed at rest, while talking, laughing, smiling, and drinking. Special attention should be focused on whether the patient has a blink reflex, whether the blink reflex is symmetrical, or whether the patient stares at the observer and blinks only from one eye. Movements of the commissure of the mouth, nasolabial fold, and forehead and the ability to depress or elevate the lips are important for assessing symmetry. The patient should be asked to close the eyes tightly, puff the cheeks, and smile both broadly and lightly. Downward movement of the lips demonstrates depressor and platysma function.

3. How does an upper motor neuron lesion present? Why?

Upper motor neuron lesions present with an ipsilateral lower face paralysis. Upper face function is usually preserved because of bilateral innervation of the upper face from the cerebral cortex.

4. How does an intratemporal lesion of the facial nerve present compared with an extratemporal lesion?

The intratemporal portion of the facial nerve contains both sensory and motor fibers:
1. The superficial petrosal branch innervates the lacrimal glands.
2. The nerve to the stapedius helps to dampen loud noises.
3. The chorda tympani provides sensory fibers to the anterior two-thirds of the tongue.

Because the extratemporal facial nerve has only motor fibers, extratemporal lesions involve no sensory deficits; the stapedius and lacrimal glands are not affected.

5. What tests can differentiate between an intratemporal and extratemporal lesion of the facial nerve?

1. Schirmer's test looks at lacrimation of the normal and paralyzed sides. A 25% decrease in tear production is abnormal.
2. The stapedius reflex test measures the ability of the stapedius to dampen loud sounds.
3. The electrogustometry test measures the sensation of the anterior two-thirds of the tongue by using a galvanic current.

6. Which branch of the facial nerve is most commonly injured during a routine face lift?

The mandibular branch is the most commonly injured because it courses inferior to the parotid just beneath the superficial masseter fascia superiorly and along the lower border of the mandible. It is usually injured during removal of fat from the submental and submandibular areas.

7. How long after injury to the facial nerve can some function be restored with microsurgery?

The timing of surgery is critical. If immediate repair of the damaged facial nerve is possible, it should be done. Immediate repair prevents scar and neuroma formation and permits easier identification of the injured nerve ends; it also allows better fascicle alignment, leading to improved results.

If reconstruction is delayed because of the patient's condition, a period up to 3 weeks will still allow optimal results. After this time, the quality of the results deteriorates because of contraction of the severed ends, thickening of the muscle membrane, proximal neuroma formation, and proliferation of fibrous tissue. In general, for a complete lesion, the optimal time for repair is within 3 months. If the lesion is partial, however, good results may be obtained even after 2 years.

8. **Once the diagnosis is made, how does one establish a strategy of reconstruction?**

The strategy of reconstruction is determined by the extent and level of the injury. If both proximal and distal stumps are available, direct repair is recommended. If only the proximal stump is available, attempts should be made to neurotize the facial muscles directly with nerve grafts. If only the distal nerve stump of a facial nerve branch is available, ipsilateral nerve transfers or cross-facial nerve grafting (CFNG) should be considered. If the main facial nerve is extensively damaged, other available ipsilateral donors may have to be used, such as the hypoglossal nerve, spinal accessory nerve, or trigeminal nerve, usually in combination with CFNG.

9. **What preoperative tests are mandatory in facial paralysis work? Why?**

Plain radiographs of the skull usually demonstrate lesions such as menigiomas and outline any bony invasion that may be present. Bilateral temporal bone polytomography helps to visualize the right and left facial nerve canals and is an important test in differentiating developmental absence of the facial nerve from acquired lesions. Coronal-cut CT scan helps to demonstrate transverse skull fractures, and longitudinal views demonstrate temporal bone damage. Electromyography (EMG) helps to assess which muscles are partially or totally innervated and to define which targets need to be reinnervated.

10. **What are the advantages and disadvantages of ipsilateral nerve grafting?**

Ipsilateral nerve grafting is the treatment of choice for lesions of isolated branches of the facial nerve. It gives faster, stronger regeneration in a shorter time. However, ipsilateral nerve grafting to the main trunk of the facial nerve is invariably followed by severe mass action and synkinesis.

11. **What is cross-facial nerve grafting (CFNG)?**

CFNG is a technique that borrows motor axons from the normal facial nerve and delivers them via interposition nerve grafts to the contralateral paralyzed side. CFNG allows the possibility of synchronized, coordinated movements as well as the possibility of self-expression. Although it can be done as a one-stage or two-stage procedure, most surgeons prefer the two-stage approach. The advantage of the two-stage approach is that the distal stump of the cross-facial nerve grafts can be assessed histologically at the second stage before coaptation with the branches of the facial nerve on the injured side.

12. **What are the advantages and disadvantages of CFNG?**

CFNG is a physiologic approach that, if done properly, gives satisfactory reinnervation to the damaged contralateral facial nerve. Disadvantages include invasion of the normal facial nerve, donor deficits from the harvesting of the nerve grafts, need for interposition nerve grafts with two coaptation sites, and a long interval for target reinnervation. CFNG is considered a relatively weak motor donor and thus provides best results if used in the first 3 months after the onset of facial paralysis.

13. **In the CFNG procedure, how does one determine when the regenerating facial nerve motor fibers have crossed the face?**

Clinical exam is used to assess the nerve grafts postoperatively. After consulting the intraoperative drawings, Tinel's sign is elicited. Tinel's sign is observed when the paralyzed side is percussed and the patient feels tingling in the appropriate site on the normal face. The degree of tingling sensation usually corresponds to the effectiveness of regeneration of the particular nerve graft. In addition, conduction velocities can be obtained noninvasively and are a useful and objective means to evaluate each CFNG individually.

14. **Describe the postoperative management after a completed CFNG procedure.**

The most important factor in postoperative care is protection of the coaptation sites of the CFNG. A splint is placed around the patient's head, limiting the patient's ability to open the mouth. Manipulation of the area in which the repairs are located should be limited. Antiemetics are given because a sudden episode of projectile vomiting will invariably disconnect the repair. Talking also should be limited. In 6 weeks, massage should be instituted in the cheek to soften the area and decrease scar formation around the nerve repairs. Intensive slow-pulse stimulation of the denervated muscles prevents atrophy while the facial motor fibers are regenerating. After the second stage, a certain degree of facial muscle reinnervation takes place. The same postoperative precautions are taken, and slow-pulse stimulation again is recommended at 6 weeks along with intensive physical therapy and facial exercises. Physical therapy includes training the patient to use both sides of the face in a symmetric, coordinated fashion and each side of the face independently. Furthermore, biofeedback is a useful tool that facilitates the reeducation process.

15. What are the indications for free muscle transfer in facial paralysis?

If the denervation time (time after injury) is excessively long, the facial muscles invariably atrophy. In such cases, free muscle transfers are required. EMG demonstrates the degree of denervation of the facial musculature. If there is no hope of adequate reinnervation by ipsilateral or contralateral nerve grafts alone, foreign muscle in the form of a free vascularized muscle transplant is indicated.

16. What criteria determine the choice of foreign donor muscles?

The choice of muscle depends on the dynamic requirements of the nonparalyzed side. The selected muscle should provide a range of excursion that corresponds to the opposite normal side. The origin and insertion must appropriately fit the line of excursion intended to be restored. Muscle transplantation can be done to correct mild asymmetry or complete paralysis of the nasolabial fold and angle of the mouth. The free muscle must have a reliable neurovascular pedicle and be dispensable, easily contoured, and capable of generating sufficient force to provide the needed symmetry to the face. The most commonly used muscles in facial reanimation are the gracilis and pectoralis minor.

17. What are the advantages and disadvantages of the gracilis free muscle transfer?

Advantages

• A predictable, long, and constant neurovascular pedicle makes the gracilis a very dependable transfer.

• Harvesting of the gracilis is relatively easy because of easy reach; thus, trimming, debulking, and contouring are facilitated.

• After transfer and upon reinnervation, the muscle can generate sufficient force to obtain the desired excursion.

Disadvantages

• The gracilis is bulky and too long for facial reanimation purposes and always requires sculpturing to fit the face.

• The debulking process, if extensive, may cause injury to the end plates and result in a successful transfer that cannot generate adequate force.

• The gracilis has only one direction of pull; thus, it is best used for restoring certain types of smile, especially retraction and modest elevation of the modiolus.

18. What are the advantages and disadvantages of the pectoralis minor muscle transfer?

The best indication for the use of the pectoralis minor flap is developmental facial paralysis in young children (see figure, top of next page). In 4–5-year-old children the dimensions of the muscle are ideal. It also may be used in nonathletic adults who have not built up the muscles of the upper torso.

Advantages

• Donor site morbidity is minimal.

• The muscle has ideal form and shape for the face.

• The muscle can yield adequate excursion in the needed direction of pull.

• If the hilus of the muscle is placed over the zygomatic arch, its slips of origin can be separated and fashioned to substitute not only for the zygomaticus major muscle but also for the elevators of the upper lip as well as the retractors of the commissure. Thus one can obtain a multidirectional pull. Dual innervation is the most important advantage. The upper third is innervated by a branch of the lateral pectoral nerve, whereas the lower two-thirds are innervated from the medial pectoral nerve. Dual innervation allows independent movements of the upper and lower parts of the muscle. This advantage can be used to address the separate needs of animation of the eye and the mouth or of animation of the commissure vs. the upper lip.

Disadvantages

• The position of the muscle is deep; thus, harvesting is difficult for the inexperienced.

• Debulking the muscle is difficult; thus, it has to be debulked during ischemia time, which may have functional repercussions.

• Because the neurovascular pedicle is short, one needs to carry the recipient vessels on the posterior surface of the muscle to accomplish the anastomoses.

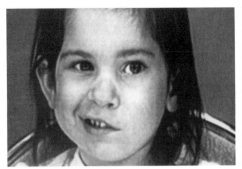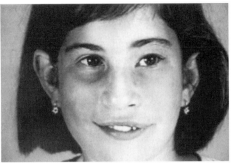

Exemplary outcome from microsurgical reconstruction. *Left,* The patient with developmental facial paralysis pre-operatively. *Right,* The patient 3 years after cross-facial nerve grafts and pectoralis minor transplantation.

• The pectoralis muscle has a variable dominant vascular supply. The lateral thoracic artery is the main artery in most cases, but a contributing branch from the thoracoacromial trunk occasionally shares codominance, making the muscle nontransferable because of the small size of both vessels.
• The muscle cannot be used in adults with highly developed upper torsos.

19. When does one consider crossover procedures? Why?

In irreversible damage to the facial nerve, other ipsilateral motor nerves are considered as donors of motor fibers, including the hypoglossal, spinal accessory, and trigeminal nerves. The downside to these donors is that resulting facial movement is not coordinated with the normal side.

20. What is the "baby sitter" principle?

The baby sitter principle uses ipsilateral cranial nerves to send strong motor fibers quickly to the denervated facial muscles. This technique can stop the denervation clock and maintain the bulk of the facial muscle while at the same time the first stage of cross-facial nerve grafting is done. Donors include the hypoglossal, trigeminal, or spinal accessory nerve. Only 30–40% of the donor nerve is used. Thus, morbidity associated with these transfers is minimal. At the second stage, the distal ends of the CFNG are coapted to the peripheral branches of the involved facial nerve. The babysitter is not severed at this time; instead, it is kept to give additional motor fibers to the affected facial musculature. The babysitter serves only to preserve bulk to the facial muscles; the CFNG functions as the pacemaker that enables coordinated animation.

21. What are the advantages and disadvantages of local muscle transfers?

The masseter and temporalis muscles are the most often used local muscle transfers. They offer more expedient return of function (within weeks) and are easier to perform than free muscle transfers. The main disadvantage: their function is not synchronized with the function of the contralateral face.

22. What are the prerequisite criteria for the diagnosis of Möbius syndrome?

Möbius syndrome is a developmental disorder characterized by bilateral facial paralysis. This condition usually involves the sixth and seventh cranial nerves. It also may involve the third, fifth, ninth, and twelfth cranial nerves. Limb abnormalities occur in 25% of cases, and the pectoral muscles are abnormal in 15% of cases. Occasionally, the paralysis is unilateral, but such patients still have contralateral involvement of the cranial nerves.

23. What are the reconstructive goals in a child with Möbius syndrome?

The reconstructive goals are to provide symmetric and functioning nasolabial folds that may mimic a smile. Reconstruction is done in multiple stages. The first stage focuses on bringing motor donors to one side of the face by using the ipsilateral partial spinal accessory nerve and/or branches of the trigeminal nerve with or without interposition nerve grafts. The second stage involves provision of muscle targets in the form of a free muscle transplant. These procedures are repeated for the contralateral face with the goal of producing symmetric results. The contralateral facial nerve and ipsilateral hypoglossal nerve usually cannot be used because they are often absent or abnormal.

24. Discuss current microsurgical approaches for the paralyzed eye sphincter.

When reconstructing the eye, the surgeon should determine if the upper lid, lower lid, or both need to be corrected. If a lower lid ectropion exists, the lower lid needs support. Support can be provided through a minitendon transfer to the lower lid. The usual donor is the palmaris longus tendon. To restore animation to the upper lid, a gold weight may be considered. The weight allows gravity to close the eye when the levator is relaxed. The gold weight is indicated in older patients or patients who are not amenable to frequent visits for adjustments. If the patient is young and cooperative and has residual but not normal blink reflex, an eyespring is the treatment of choice. Eyesprings can be tedious to place and invariably need adjustment. The results are superior to gold weights both aesthetically and functionally. Local and free muscle transplantation in combination with CFNG can replace the missing eye sphincter and provide coordinated and dynamic eye closure, but the procedure should be left in the hands of an experienced surgeon.

25. What are the surgical options for correction of unilateral lower lip palsy?

Unilateral lower lip paralysis is a challenging problem. If direct coaptation of the damaged mandibular nerve is not an option, other donors must be found. A small segment of the hypoglossal nerve can be coapted directly to the damaged distal mandibular nerve. If neural microsurgery is not indicated because of the longevity of the palsy, a muscle transfer may be necessary. The most commonly used muscles are the platysma and the digastric, which are transferred to help with depression of the lower lip.

26. What are the indications for use of digastric vs. platysma muscle in lower lip reanimation?

Because the platysma is innervated by the facial nerve, it gives coordinated depressor function when used for reanimation of the lower lip. When the ipsilateral platysma is absent or paralyzed, the digastric muscle may be used in combination with a CFNG.

27. What outcomes can be obtained with free muscle transfers for long-lasting facial paralysis?

According to a review by the senior author of 100 cases of free muscle transplants for facial paralysis, 94% of patients had improved results postoperatively. Eighty percent were rated moderate or better by an independent panel of four judges that included one doctor, one medical student, one photographer, and one journalist.

Other results showed:

1. Women received higher scores and had a slightly earlier onset of muscle function than men.
2. Younger patients had earlier onset of muscle function than older patients.
3. Patients with developmental facial paralysis did better than patients with posttraumatic or infectious causes.
4. Pectoralis minor transplants recovered function more quickly than gracilis transplants.
5. Intraoperative ischemia time did not correlate with onset of muscle function as long as the ischemia time was kept below 3 hours.

BIBLIOGRAPHY

1. Baker DC: Facial paralysis. In McCarthy JG (ed): Plastic Surgery. Philadelphia, W.B. Saunders, 1990, pp 2237–2319.
2. Hamilton SGL, Terzis JK, Carraway JT: Surgical anatomy of the facial musculature and muscle transplantation. In Terzis JK (ed): Microreconstruction of Nerve Injuries. Philadelphia, W.B. Saunders, 1987, pp 571–586.
3. Lee KK, Terzis JK: Management of acute extratemporal facial nerve palsy. In Terzis J (ed): Microreconstruction of Nerve Injuries. Philadelphia, W.B. Saunders, 1987, pp 587–600.
4. Liberson WT, Terzis JK: Some novel techniques of clinical electrophysiology applied to the management of brachial plexus palsy. Electromyogr Clin Neurophysiol 67:371, 1987.
5. Manktelow RT: Free muscle transplantation for facial paralysis. In Terzis JK (ed): Microreconstruction of Nerve Injuries. Philadelphia, W.B. Saunders, 1987, pp 607–615.
6. Terzis JK: The "babysitter" principle: A dynamic concept in facial reanimation. In Castro D (ed): Proceedings of the Sixth International Symposium on the Facial Nerve, Rio de Janeiro, 1988.
7. Terzis JK: Pectoralis minor: A unique muscle for correction of facial palsy. Plast Reconstr Surg 5:767, 1989.
8. Terzis JK, Noah ME: Analysis of 100 cases of free-muscle transplantation for facial paralysis. Plast Reconstr Surg 99:1905, 1997.
9. Zucker RM, Manktelow RT: A smile for the moebius syndrome patient. Ann Plast Surg 22:188, 1989.

VI. Breast Surgery

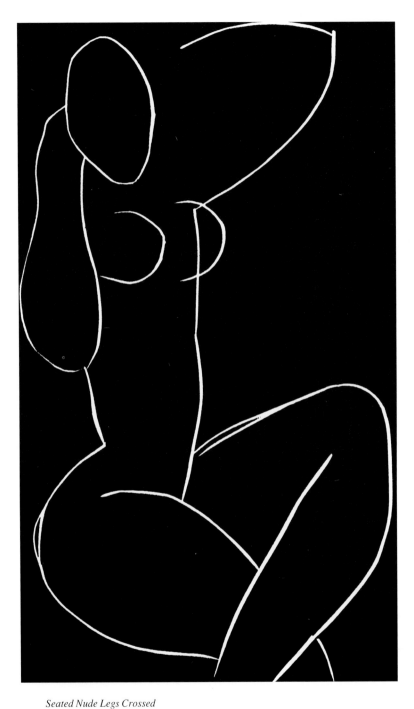

Seated Nude Legs Crossed
Henri Matisse
1941–1942
Linogravure
Editions Hazan, Paris
© 1998 Succession H. Matisse, Paris/Artists' Rights Society (ARS), New York

44. AUGMENTATION MAMMAPLASTY

Scott L. Spear, M.D., and James Ben Burke, M.D.

1. When was the first augmentation mammaplasty performed?

In 1895 Czerny successfully transplanted a lipoma from the back to a submammary position. A number of materials, including paraffin, glass beads, free fat grafts, free dermal grafts, polytetrafluoroethylene, free silicone oil, and polyvinyl alcohol sponges, have been tried with poor success. The modern age of augmentation mammaplasty began with the implant of a silicone gel-filled prosthesis in 1962 by Cronin and Gerow.

2. What are the indications for augmentation mammaplasty?

The primary indication for augmentation mammaplasty is inadequate volume of the breast, which may be either developmental or involutional. Augmentation also may be performed for psychological reasons, including feelings of inadequacy, low self-esteem, lack of self-confidence, and sexual inhibition.

3. Does the preoperative shape of the breast affect the results obtained by augmentation mammaplasty?

The width, cleavage, projection, and size of the breast can be manipulated by the dimensions of the pocket and the shape of the implant. Ptosis of up to 2–3 cm can be corrected with a subglandular or subpectoral placement of the implant or by lowering the inframammary fold with submuscular placement of the implant. Deformities of the breast may require use of implants of different sizes with or without the addition of mastopexy.

4. What incisions are used in augmentation mammaplasty? Describe their benefits and drawbacks.

Three incisions are most often used for augmentation mammaplasty. The **periareolar incision** is a semicircular incision at the border of the nipple-areolar complex. The **inframammary incision** is located at the inframammary fold; it does not extend medially beyond the medial border of the nipple-areolar complex. The **axillary incision** is located in the hair-bearing region of the axilla. Recently the endoscope has been used via the axillary or umbilical incisions, but this technique is not universally performed. Each of these approaches has benefits and drawbacks. With the periareolar incision, scarring is usually minimal, but there may be an increased incidence of nipple paresthesia. The inframammary incision offers excellent exposure but may result in a more noticeable scar. The axillary incision leaves no scar on the breast but may provide decreased exposure of the operative field.

5. Which breast implants are currently available?

Before April 1992, silicone gel-filled implants were the most common implants used for augmentation. Subsequently the Food and Drug Administration (FDA) has ruled that silicone gel-filled implants can be used only for breast reconstruction after cancer ablation surgery and replacement of silicone gel-filled implants in previously augmented patients. At present, saline-filled implants in a smooth or textured envelope are available. The shape is either round or contoured; the round implant is more commonly used.

6. Where is the implant placed in augmentation mammaplasty?

The implant may be subglandular, submuscular, or subpectoral. The subglandular placement is below the breast tissue and above the muscular fascia. The submuscular placement is above the chest wall and below portions of the pectoralis major and minor, serratus anterior, rectus abdominis, and external oblique muscles. The subpectoral placement is above the chest wall and below the pectoralis major muscle superiorly and in the subglandular, subfascial, or subcutaneous plane inferiorly.

7. Should the same technique be used for all patients undergoing augmentation mammaplasty?

Every surgeon believes that his or her technique is the best, and to some extent this is true. Still, a few caveats should be remembered. Ptosis may be better addressed with either a subglandular or subpectoral placement. The implant is generally more camouflaged with submuscular or subpectoral placement. Regardless of the technique, the surgeon should listen to what the patient desires; in turn, the patient deserves to be well informed about the possible limitations of the procedure.

8. What type of anesthesia is used?

Either general or local anesthesia is acceptable. The choice depends on the comfort and expertise of the surgeon and, most importantly, the desires and expectations of the patient.

9. Should prophylactic antibiotics be used?

The incidence of infection in augmentation mammaplasty is 2.2%. Because the implant is a foreign body, infection can be a catastrophic event requiring its removal. The most commonly isolated organism is *Staphylococcus epidermidis*. Thus, in addition to an adequate skin preparation, cephalothin, 1 gm intravenously, should be administered prior to the skin incision. Postoperatively the patient should be given 5–7 days of cephalexin, 500 mg 4 times/day.

10. What are the operative risks?

All surgical procedures have inherent risks, including bleeding and infection. Hematoma in augementation mammaplasty occurs in 0.5–3.0%; large hematomas require drainage. The reported incidence of infection is 2.2%. Nerve injury occurs in approximately 15%. Malposition of the implant has been reported and is related to improper positioning of the pocket, improper placement of the inframammary fold, and scarring. Unsightly scars are reported with both the periareolar and inframammary incisions.

11. What is the routine postoperative care after augmentation mammaplasty?

Postoperative care can be as basic as a simple dressing to the wounds. Wearing of a bra is advocated for comfort and support. Molding of the breast also may be accomplished with a bra, especially for an inferiorly displaced inframammary fold. An elastic wrap on the superior pole of the breast may be used to keep the implant low in the pocket or to maintain the proper orientation of contoured implants. Restriction of activities is dictated by the patient's tolerance of discomfort.

12. Does augmentation mammaplasty interfere with subsequent breastfeeding?

No studies have specifically addressed this question. Nonetheless, augmentation should involve little if any injury to native breast tissue. Breastfeeding is patient-dependent and should not be contraindicated in augmented women.

13. Is there a change in sensation of the nipple after augmentation mammaplasty?

The anterior branch of the fourth lateral intercostal nerve provides the main sensory component to the nipple-areolar complex. The nerve enters the breast at the chest wall 1.5–2.0 cm from the lateral edge of the gland. The reported incidence of nerve injury in subglandular placement is 15%. The major cause of nerve injury is aggressive lateral dissection. With submuscular and subpectoral placement, nerve injury is reported to be less frequent.

14. What is the classification of capsular contracture?

Baker presented his classification of capsular contracture in 1975.

Grade I	Soft
Grade II	Minimal contracture; implant palpable but not visible
Grade III	Moderate contracture; implant palpable and discernible
Grade IV	Severe contracture; hard symptomatic breast, sometimes with distortion

The incidence of encapsulation with silicone gel-filled implants is approximately 30%; for saline-filled implants it is much lower (less than 5% of patients).

15. What is the average increase in size after augmentation mammaplasty?

The increase in size of the breast depends on many factors, including the state of the skin of the breast. Small-breasted patients have less available skin, and patients with involutional atrophy have more skin, allowing use of a larger implant. Augmentation can be staged with a smaller implant acting as a tissue expander and larger implant placed later. Other factors include body habitus, breast shape and size, and shape of the implant.

16. Is there a risk of rupture of the breast implant?

All manufactured devices have a finite life expectancy. Patients should be counseled that the risk of failure of the implant depends on the physical properties of the device and the time elapsed since implantation. The risk is cumulative and spectulated to be approximately 2% per year. Rupture of saline-filled implants has negligible risks other than replacement of the implant.

17. Is an increased risk of autoimmune disease associated with augmentation mammaplasty?

In the late 1980s and early 1990s there were anecdotal reports of autoimmune disease associated with silicone gel-filled implants in augmented patients. However, recent large controlled cohort studies have shown no correlation between silicone gel-filled implants and an increased risk of autoimmune diseases. The FDA has mandated that all patients undergoing augmentation mammaplasty be followed for potential adverse consequences attributable to the implants.

18. Is the incidence of cancer increased in patients who have undergone augmentation mammaplasty?

In the general population, the risk of breast cancer is approximately 1 in 9 women. Approximately 2 million women are estimated to have undergone augmentation with silicone gel-filled implants. Of this subpopulation, it is anticipated that 200,000 will develop breast cancer. Multiple studies have failed to show any increased induction or increased incidence of breast cancer in augmented patients.

19. Is mammography adversely affected by augmentation mammaplasty?

The effectiveness of mammography in the augmented breast has been debated for years. However, Eklund concluded that compression mammography allows greater visualization of the breast tissue. Effective visualization of the maximal amount of breast tissue with mammography may be influenced by various factors, including the radiographic technique, degree of encapsulation, and placement of the implant. Within these limits, mammography should be used as indicated and supplemented by physical examination.

BIBLIOGRAPHY

1. Biggs TM, Humphreys DH: Augmentation mammaplasty. In Smith JW, Aston SJ (eds): Grabb and Smith's Plastic Surgery, 4th ed. Boston, Little, Brown, 1991, pp 1145–1156.
2. LaTrenta GS: Breast augmentation. In Rees TD, LaTrenta GS (ed): Aesthetic Plastic Surgery, 2nd ed. Philadelphia, W.B. Saunders, 1994, pp 1003–1049.
3. Spear SL, Dawson KL: Augmentation mammaplasty. In Cohen M (ed): Mastery of Plastic and Reconstructive Surgery. Boston, Little, Brown, 1994, pp 2099–2113.

45. REDUCTION MAMMAPLASTY

Deborah J. White, M.D., and G. Patrick Maxwell, M.D.

1. What is the blood supply to the breast?

The primary blood supply to the breast comes from (1) perforating branches of the internal mammary artery (60%); (2) branches from the axillary artery (mostly the lateral thoracic artery but also pectoral branches and the highest thoracic artery); and (3) lateral branches from the third, fourth, and fifth posterior intercostal arteries. Rich anastomoses between these arteries allow survival of the breast with varying breast reduction techniques as long as sufficient vessels remain.

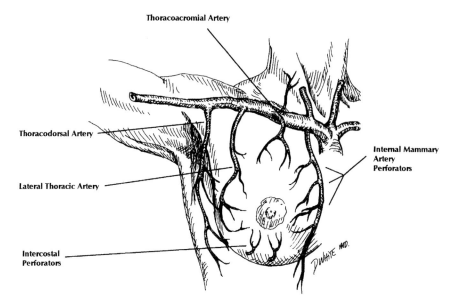

Blood supply to the breast.

2. What is the nerve supply to the breast? Nipple?

Sensory innervation to the breast is from (1) the supraclavicular nerves from the third and fourth branches of the cervical plexus; (2) the anterior cutaneous branches from intercostal nerves 2–6; and (3) the anterior branches of the lateral cutaneous nerves 3–6. The lateral cutaneous branch of T4 is believed to be the primary innervation to the nipple.

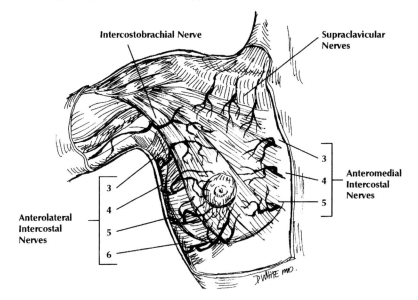

Nerve supply to the breast.

3. What are the most popular techniques in the United States for breast reduction?

The inferior pedicle and central pedicle techniques enjoy great popularity. However, other methods are still in use, and new ones are gaining favor.

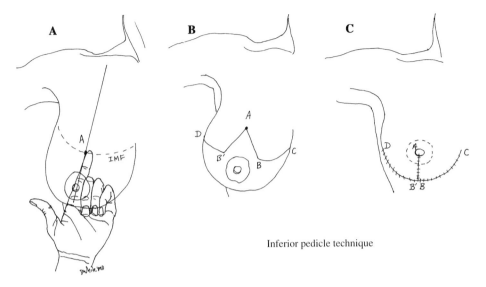

Inferior pedicle technique

4. What are the advantages and disadvantages of the above techniques?

Both of the above approaches can be used with prefabricated templates or measurements, or with more freehand "cut-as-you-go" techniques for shaping the skin envelopes. Both are relatively easy to learn and produce consistent results. They have good safety records and can be used for a large range of reductions from small to over 2 kg/side, even in breasts with extremely long pedicles. Although they may appear somewhat boxy initially, this problem resolves with time; the shape is usually acceptable. Nipple sensation and lactation potential are usually well preserved.

Disadvantages include large scars that not uncommonly become hypertrophic, a tendency to have a wide shape with medial and lateral fullness, and a tendency to "bottom out" with time, leaving superior pole hollowness and nipples that point up.

5. Can bottoming out be prevented?

Possibly. Pennington of Australia described a technique in which the inferior pedicle is sutured at a fixed distance from the inframammary fold. So far this technique has shown good shape maintenance without the all-too-common lengthening of the areola to the inframammary fold. However, long-term results are not yet available, and historically techniques that rely on sutures to hold tissue under tension tend to fail.

6. What are common indications for breast reduction?

Physical complaints: shoulder grooving; neck, back, and shoulder pain; mastodynia; maceration and infection of the inframammary regions; neurologic sequelae secondary to neck problems (e.g., ulnar nerve impingement); and difficulty in finding clothing that fits and is attractive. Respiratory complaints are not associated with mammary hypertrophy.

Psychological complaints: embarrassment, feelings of physical unattractiveness, self-consciousness, unwillingness to exercise, loss of sexual appeal and femininity.

7. How are macromastia and virginal hypertrophy different?

Virginal (or juvenile) hypertrophy is a relatively rare condition seen in prepubertal and pubertal females. Pathology is limited to the breast and leads to bilateral or unilateral gigantomastia. Treatment is surgical, although recurrence is common, and tamoxifen citrate therapy reportedly has been successful. Local hypersensitivity to estrogen has been proposed as a cause.

8. At what age should breast reduction be performed?

Ideally, one should wait for the patient to achieve full breast maturation, generally several years after the onset of menstruation. However, if the oversized breasts interfere with the patient's activities and self-esteem, the procedure may be performed earlier. The patient and her family must understand that the procedure may need to be repeated if the breasts continue to grow. They also must understand the extent of the scarring and the potential for loss of sensation and loss of the ability to lactate.

9. What are some of the recent innovations in breast reduction methods? What are their advantages and disadvantages?

1. **Reduction by liposuction alone (controversial).** In patients with minimal-to-moderate breast hypertrophy, satisfactory breast shape and nipple location, good skin tone, and fatty breasts, this alternative can be appealing. Only small scars are produced, and the skin can retract, resulting in a decrease of the sternal notch to nipple distances. It is almost impossible to predict preoperatively what percentage of the breast is fat, but older patients tend to have more fat than younger patients. Many plastic surgeons believe that fat should not be suctioned from or added to breast tissue because of oncologic concerns. Lejour published a study examining the material removed from breasts with traditional suction; no glandular tissue was found on pathologic exam. Postoperative mammograms have not been shown to have changes that can be confused with malignancy.

2. **Reduction using ultrasound-assisted liposuction (UAL) (even more controversial).** UAL can remove fat from even the most dense breast tissue, but studies have not yet been done with the aspirate. Studies from the gynecologic and neurologic literature have shown that tumor histology can be performed on ultrasonic aspirate with great accuracy.

3. **Short scar techniques.** Marchac and Chiari have shown excellent results with much smaller scars in the inframammary fold along with attractive breast shapes.

4. **Vertical technique.** Popularized by Lejour, this technique has gained popularity because of the reduced number of scars and the attractive and long-lasting breast shape. The biggest drawbacks are a steep learning curve and an unappealing immediate postoperative appearance that may take over 1 month to resolve.

5. **Periareolar techniques.** These techniques accomplish breast reduction and reshaping via an incision around the areola alone. Common problems with periareolar surgery include flattening of the breast shape with loss of nipple/areolar projection and widening of the scars and areolae. Benelli's "round block" technique, in which a permanent pursestring suture is placed, may prevent the scar and areolar spread. Góes of Brazil obtained good projection and shape with the use of a Vicryl/polyester mesh between the gland and skin; however, use of this material would be difficult for medicolegal reasons in the United States.

10. Is lactation possible after breast reduction?

Yes, depending on the technique. Obviously, procedures that leave the underlying gland attached to the nipple (such as the inferior and central pedicle techniques) are much more likely to be successful at preserving the ability to breastfeed. In one study, 100% of the women who became pregnant after inferior pedicle reductions lactated, although 65% did not breastfeed for various personal reasons.

11. How has the postoperative hospital stay changed over the past 10 years?

Hospital stay has changed from over 1 week with the patient's arms secured to prevent movement a few decades ago to overnight or outpatient status. The patient is allowed to use her arms cautiously.

12. Is autologous blood donation recommended?

No. The use of electrocautery, careful hemostasis, and epinephrine-containing solutions has made the loss of large amounts of blood a rare event.

13. Are drains necessary?

Many surgeons use them for several days (until the drainage reaches a certain level), whereas others remove them the next morning and some do not use them at all. No studies have been done.

14. Are patients satisfied with the results?

This procedure has excellent long-term patient satisfaction, despite the scars. In most series, over 95% of patients would have the surgery again and would recommend it to others. Patients are more comfortable buying clothes and exercising and feel better about their self-image. The majority of patients report a postoperative decrease in physical symptoms.

15. When are free nipple grafts recommended?

Less and less often. Surgeons have reported success with other reduction techniques with even massive gigantomastias. The procedure tends to produce poor nipple projection and sensation and destroys lactation potential but is very quick. Elderly patients (with no need for lactation) and patients with medical problems or poor health have traditionally been candidates. Patients with gigantomastia have a greater risk of nipple/areolar necrosis (and necrosis of the distal pedicle), especially with long pedicles, and are also believed to be candidates. Many believe that a better breast shape can be obtained with the free nipple graft technique. Poor nipple or areolar perfusion intraoperatively that is unresponsive to other measures is also an indication for conversion to a free nipple graft.

16. What is the incidence of occult breast cancer in reduction specimens?

A large retrospective study of 5008 reductions showed an overall incidence of breast malignancies to be approximately 0.4%. One-fourth were detected by physical examination before surgery, one-fourth were discovered on frozen section of a suspicious area during surgery, and just over one-half were found in routine pathology specimens. It is extremely important to record carefully the site from which breast tissue is removed. It is a disaster to receive a report of an occult malignancy and not to know from which breast it came.

17. What are the most common complications from reduction mammaplasty?

- Asymmetry
- Not enough tissue removed
- Too much tissue removed
- Poor shape
- Poor scarring
- Delayed healing at base of T incision
- Change in nipple/areolar sensation
- Infection
- Partial or total loss of nipple
- Skin loss or necrosis
- Fat necrosis

18. Do nipple grafts regain sensation? Erectile capacity?

Yes, to varying degrees. Erectile capacity also may be regained, particularly if the graft is fairly thick and smooth muscle tissue is left behind.

19. How can nipple viability be determined intraoperatively?

Pale-skinned women with light nipple color usually can be evaluated by looking for a healthy pink color and by assessment of capillary refill. White or dark nipple color indicates poor blood supply or venous congestion, respectively. Observing whether the cut edges bleed or poking a large-gauge needle into the tissue and looking for bright red blood also may help. **Dark-skinned women** may present more of a challenge. Visual inspection can be supplemented with fluorescein and/or laser Doppler evaluation. Laser Doppler perfusion values that are consistently 1.0–2.0 ml/min/100 gm indicate marginal perfusion and should be followed closely; values less than 1.0 ml/min/100 gm are considered to have low perfusion, which needs to be addressed.

20. What do you do if the nipples look compromised?

Try releasing some incisions and checking whether the pedicle is kinked. If the pedicle is not twisted and releasing some incisions revives the nipples, the closure may be too tight. This problem can be remedied in some cases by removal of more breast tissue either by an open technique or by liposuction. If no maneuvers improve the dire condition of the nipple or if the Doppler readings remain below 1.0ml/min/100 gm, consider conversion to free nipple grafts. There are reports of successful leech use in the postoperative period.

21. What do you do with lateral dog ears?

The inverted T incision often leaves large lateral dog ears, especially on heavy women with large breasts that may appear to continue back to the scapula. Large incisions in this area can be disappointing, especially for the young patient who wishes to wear a bikini. Standard methods of eliminating dog ears at wound ends may be used, along with attempts to work the excess skin medially. Often liposuction of the dog ear is beneficial, although it may be difficult because of the fibrous nature of the lateral chest. In such cases UAL may be extremely efficacious (controversial). Direct excision of the fat may also be used.

22. What about medial dog ears?

The inverted T incision often leaves medial dog ears on large, wide, breasts. One generally tries to work the excess tissue medially, but if this is impossible, it is acceptable in certain cases to extend the incisions across the midline and connect them. Again, liposuction (SAL or UAL) or direct fat excision may be useful, bearing in mind the increased propensity for sternal wounds to become hypertrophic.

23. What would be the ideal breast reduction?

Attractive shape, preservation of sensation, preservation of ability to breastfeed, long-lasting shape, reliable tissue survival, and minimal scars (the order of importance depends on patient preference).

CONTROVERSY

24. Are the patient's chances of developing breast cancer affected by breast reduction?

Perhaps. Recent studies suggest that patients with large breasts are at an increased risk for breast cancer and that breast reduction may decrease this risk (relative risk = 0.6–0.7 compared with controls). The decreased risk may be due to the removal of potential foci of breast cancer. Another study showed no increased risk of breast cancer with larger breasts unless the patient also had a positive family history or proliferative disease. In patients with these risk factors, larger breasts were associated with increasing relative risk; 1.2, 1.4, and 2.1 for small, medium, and large breasts with proliferative disease and 1.6, 2.0, and 2.7 for small, medium, and large breasts and a positive family history.

BIBLIOGRAPHY

1. Benelli L: A new periareolar mammaplasty: The "round block" technique. Aesth Plast Surg 14:93–100, 1990.
2. Brinton LA, Malone KE, Coates RJ, et al: Breast enlargement and reduction: Results from a breast cancer case-control study. Plast Reconstr Surg 97:269–275, 1996.
3. Chiari A Jr: The L short-scar mammaplasty: A new approach. Plast Reconstr Surg 90:233–246, 1992.
4. Dupont WD, Page DL: Breast cancer risk associated with proliferative disease, age at first birth, and a family history of breast cancer. Am J Epidemiol 125:769–779, 1987.
5. Góes JCS: Periareolar mammaplasty: Double skin technique. Rev Soc Bras Cir Plast 4:55–63, 1989.
6. Goldwyn RM: Pulmonary function and bilateral reduction mammaplasty. Plast Reconstr Surg 53:84, 1974.
7. Gross MP, Apesos J: The use of leeches for treatment of venous congestion of the nipple following breast surgery. Aesth Plast Surg 16:343–348, 1992.
8. Harris L, Morris SF, Freiberg A: Is breast feeding possible after reduction mammaplasty? Plast Reconstr Surg 89:836–839, 1992.
9. Kupfer D, Dingman D, Broadbent R: Juvenile breast hypertrophy: Report of a familial pattern and review of the literature. Plast Reconstr Surg 90:303–309, 1992.
10. Lejour M: Vertical Mammaplasty and Liposuction. St. Louis, Quality Medical Publishing, 1994.
11. Marchac D, de Olarte G: Reduction mammaplasty and correction of ptosis with a short inframammary scar. Plast Reconstr Surg 69:45–55, 1982.
12. Maxwell GP, White DJ: Breast reduction with ultrasound-assisted liposuction. Oper Techn Plast Reconstr Surg 3:207–212, 1996.
13. Morimoto T, Komaki K, Mori T, et al: Juvenile gigantomastia: Report of a case. Surg Today 23:260–264, 1993.
14. Pennington D: Pedicle plication/suspension in the Robbins reduction mammaplasty. Presented at the Australasian Society of Aesthetic Plastic Surgery Annual Conference. Queenstown, New Zealand. July 6–10, 1997.
15. Roth AC, Zook EG, Brown R, et al: Nipple-areolar perfusion and reduction mammaplasty: Correlation of laser Doppler readings with surgical complications. Plast Reconstr Surg 97:381–386, 1996.
16. Snyderman RK, Lizardo JG: Statistical study of malignancies found before, during, or after routine breast plastic operations. Plast Reconstr Surg 25:253–256, 1960.
17. Toledo LS, Matsudo PKR: Mammoplasty using liposuction and the periareolar incision. Aesth Plast Surg 13:9–13, 1989.

46. MASTOPEXY

Daniel J. Azurin, M.D., Jack Fisher, M.D., and G. Patrick Maxwell, M.D.

1. What defines an aesthetically pleasing breast?

Opinions about what defines the ideal breast vary greatly among different societies and subcultures. The average or normal breast may not coincide with an aesthetically pleasing breast. Furthermore, patients occasionally request that you surgically alter their breast into a form that may be both unnatural and aesthetically unpleasing. However, certain criteria define the aesthetically pleasing breast. Variables of particular importance are position, contour, symmetry, size, and proportion of both the breast mound and nipple-areolar complex. Tactile aspects are as significant as visual ones, including softness, mobility, and sensibility.

2. Describe the form and dimensions of the normal breast.

The breast is best situated on the anterolateral chest wall with the majority of its mass or fullness located in the inferior hemisphere. The lines of contour should converge smoothly on the nipple-areolar complex, which serves as the focal point of the breast. The inferior hemisphere should have a full convexity spanning from the areola to the inframammary fold (a distance of approximately 5–6 cm from the inferior areolar edge to the inframammary fold), whereas the superior hemisphere should possess less volume and have only a subtle, sloping convexity on the lateral view (spanning a distance of approximately 19–21 cm from the sternal notch to the nipple). A small amount of ptosis is natural and pleasing. The nipple-areolar complex projects slightly from the underlying breast mound on an inclined plane. It represents the point of maximal projection of the breast and is located slightly inferior and lateral (to the midclavicular line) on the breast mound. As breast volume increases, the nipple-areolar complex moves more inferiorly and laterally. The diameter of the areola should be approximately 35–45 mm, depending on the overall size of the breast. The size of the breast should be in proportion to the patient's chest, torso, hips, and buttocks. Full cleavage, which is desired by many patients, in reality results only from external forces, such as a brassiere. Attempts to create such full cleavage require unacceptable compromise to other aesthetic factors of the breast. Despite the fact that true symmetry between both breasts is rare, symmetry is extremely important for a good aesthetic outcome. Preoperative asymmetries must be studied and made known to the patient, because often symmetry can be only approached at best; in some cases, preexisting asymmetries are even more evident after surgery.

3. Describe the developmental phases of the breast.

The breast originates from the ectoderm. The milk line and subsequently the milk ridge are formed at approximately the fifth week of intrauterine life. Prior to involution, the milk ridge gives rise to the ectodermal milk hill. Incomplete involution of the milk ridge results in supernumerary nipples and accessory breast tissue. The milk hill vascularizes and forms the mammary structures. After birth, with the withdrawal of maternal steroids and the decline of fetal prolactin, the mammary tissues are not altered again until adolescence. Under multiple hormonal influences, the breast begins to grow and differentiate. During adolescent development there is usually no breast ptosis. Development continues until the woman's maximal height is attained, typically at the age of 16. From this point the breast matures as the parenchyma and nipple-areolar complex gravitate inferiorly and laterally, with continued superior hemipshere (upper pole) flattening and settling of the breast fullness into the inferior hemisphere. At menopause, the breast undergoes significant glandular involution and a decrease in vascularity. Glandular tissue is reduced and fat content is increased. Thus the youthful appearing breast is full and uplifted, whereas the aging breast is flattened and ptotic. Breast ptosis, a relentless process, is a sign of aging.

4. What are the supporting structures of the breast?

The skin envelope and fascial attachments (Cooper's ligaments) are the major supporting structures of the breast. The thickness and quality of the skin brassiere greatly contribute to the support of the breast and, thus, to breast shape. The quality of skin is affected by aging, hormonal influences (cyclic engorgement), and physical forces, such as gravity and expansible factors (weight gain, pregnancy, prosthetic expansion). Thin skin with loss of elasticity will not support the weight of the breast, resulting in ptosis. Striae, found typically in the supraareolar and periareolar areas, are the result of tears in the dermis and represent thin, inelastic skin. Skin of poor quality may lead to less than optimal aesthetic results and earlier recurrence of ptosis. Suspensory ligaments of Cooper are connective tissue attachments that run from the deep fascia underlying the breast through the parenchyma and attach to the overlying dermis. Cooper's ligaments provide parenchymal support. As with skin, loss of elasticity or attenuation of these ligaments results in ptosis.

5. What are the characteristics of a ptotic or sagging breast?

The ptotic breast is characterized by the inferior-lateral descent of both the glandular breast and the nipple-areolar complex. In the early stages of ptosis, the nipple areolar complex and gland descend at the same rate. More advanced stages of breast ptosis, however, are marked by a nipple-areolar complex descent out of proportion to the glandular descent. Thus the nipple-areolar complex assumes a dependent position on the lower pole convexity of the breast rather than the youthful position at the point of maximal projection higher on the breast mound. As the breast parenchyma moves downward, the upper hemisphere or pole of the breast becomes flatter with loss of significant breast volume. Attentuation of both the skin and Cooper's ligaments results in redundant, loose, and inelastic skin with striae; in addition, the breast has a considerable increase of mobility on the chest wall. Furthermore, the tendency toward increased fat content after lactational or menopausal glandular involution results in a breast that is less firm.

6. What factors contribute to breast ptosis?

Although hypertrophic breasts certainly exhibit ptosis, breast ptosis is usually associated with the combination of volume loss and compromise of the skin brassiere. Loss of breast volume commonly results from significant weight loss, postpartum atrophy, or postmenopausal involution. Gravity exerts a continual ptotic pull on the breast, elongating Cooper's ligaments and stretching the skin. Heavy mammary prostheses contribute to ptosis. The quality of the skin is influenced by a number of factors, such as aging. Simple cyclic or lactational engorgement, weight gain, and expandable prosthetic devices may stretch the skin detrimentally. Thin, inelastic skin creates an ineffective natural brassiere.

7. Describe the classification system for grading breast ptosis.

The classification system set forth by Regnault is perhaps the most useful. This system and similar modifications focus on the position of the nipple-areolar complex relative to the inframammary fold and breast mound. The patient should be in an upright standing position. **First-degree or minor ptosis** is defined as location of the nipple-areolar complex at or slightly above the inframammary fold and above the lower hemispheric convexity of the breast. **Second-degree or moderate ptosis** is defined by descent of the nipple-areolar complex to a position below the inframammary fold, but it is situated on the anterior projection of the breast mound. **Third-degree or major ptosis** is defined by a nipple-areolar complex that is not only below the inframammary fold but also on the dependent position of the inferior convexity of the breast mound. In severe forms of third-degree ptosis, the nipple points directly downward. In **pseudoptosis**, the nipple-areolar complex remains above the inframammary fold, the breast mound descends below the inframammary fold, and other characteristics of breast ptosis are present, such as glandular hypoplasia. **Glandular ptosis** refers to an otherwise normal breast (with the nipple-areolar complex at or above the inframammary fold) except that the breast mound or glandular portion has descended below the inframammary fold. The degree of breast ptosis is an extremely important consideration in choosing an operative technique for correction.

8. What are the goals of mastopexy?

Mastopexy is a surgical procedure that attempts to reverse the normal progression of breast ptosis, thus restoring the breast to a more youthful form. Indeed, some breasts never enjoy a full, nonptotic appearance, even in youth. Important in the management of breast ptosis are not only the particular abnormalities of the patient's breast but also her desires and expectations. The goals of mastopexy are to reposition the nipple-areolar complex, to reposition the breast mound and optimize its contour and volume, to remove redundant skin and tighten the skin brassiere, and to provide support for the breast in a lasting manner. Mastopexy techniques, which have paralleled the evolution of breast reduction techniques, are also used to treat congenital deformities (such as tubular breasts), correct asymmetries (congenital or acquired), and optimize the aesthetic outcome after explantation of augmented breasts.

9. Are the effects of mastopexy permanent?

No. As soon as the mastopexy procedure is completed, ptotic forces, such as aging and gravity, resume their relentless attack on the breast.

10. What are the major drawbacks to mastopexy?

Compared with other aesthetic breast procedures, mastopexy is particularly challenging and full of compromise:

1. Mastopexy requires that incisions be made directly on the breast. Depending on the degree of ptosis and mastopexy technique, the scars may be quite extensive. The patient must be willing to accept the extent of scars as a trade-off for a more youthful and aesthetically pleasing breast.

2. The effects of surgery are only temporary (even though the scars are permanent).

3. The medium for surgical manipulation most often includes thin, inelastic skin of poor quality and involuted breast parenchyma with attenuated internal support and frequently decreased vascularity.

4. The inherent upper pole flatness of the ptotic breast cannot be addressed by simple mastopexy alone; correction typically requires an implant.

5. Although mastopexy delivers a more uplifted breast, the necessary repositioning and redraping of the breast makes the breast appear smaller.

6. In addition to nonspecific problems such as tissue loss, hematoma, seroma, and infection, loss or alteration of sensibility is always a possibility.

11. What are the advantages and disadvantages of implants after mastopexy?

The addition of an implant can enhance size and contour. Of interest, an implant also increases the longevity of the uplifting effects of mastopexy and often reduces the length of incisions needed to perform an adequate mastopexy. However, the skin envelope of a ptotic breast may not able to handle adequately the weight and possible expansibility of an implant. Furthermore, the addition of an implant brings with it the associated complications and risks of breast prostheses. A tightened breast without an implant also loses some projection.

12. How are scars tolerated on the breast?

Because scars are probably the greatest drawback to aesthetic breast surgery, there is a constant effort to minimize the length of incisions and to place incisions in hidden areas. Decreasing incision length, however, may limit the ability to achieve the optimal aesthetic result. Although periareolar and intraareolar incisions are located on the most prominent and focused position of the breast, the resultant scars are the most predictable and best tolerated. Areolar scars are less likely to become hypertrophic than inframammary scars. Areolar scars may still be subject to significant widening if placed on tension. In addition, intraareolar scars are unpigmented; therefore, they may be readily apparent on a darkly pigmented areola. A median inferior longitudinal (vertical) scar is also generally well tolerated on the breast compared with the inframammary horizontal scar. Scars on the thorax are typically unpredictable and often unsightly, especially scars that approach or encompass the sternal region, such as an overextended medial limb of an inframammary incision. All attempts should be made to keep incisions off the superior hemisphere of the breast and the medial lower quadrant, because these areas are often not covered by clothing.

13. What are the blood supply and innervation to the breast?

Familiarity with breast anatomy is paramount to achieving optimal results, preserving sensibility, and avoiding complications, especially in reoperative surgery. The three main routes of arterial blood supply to the breast are the internal mammary artery, lateral thoracic artery, and intercostal arteries. The dominant supply originates from the internal mammary artery (approximately 60%), a branch of the subclavian artery. The internal mammary artery gives off perforating vessels that enter the breast approximately 2 cm lateral to the sternal edge. The nipple-areolar complex depends on the underlying breast parenchyma and an enhanced subdermal plexus for its blood supply. This dermal blood supply is fed chiefly by the lateral thoracic artery with significant contributions from anastomosing internal mammary vessels. Postmenopausal (often ptotic) breasts have decreased blood flow. Smoking, diabetes, and atherosclerosis also contribute to decreases in blood flow. In reoperative surgery, every attempt must be made to establish the precise nature of previous operations. Cutting across a previous flap carries the risk of vascular compromise. The innervation to the nipple-areolar complex is primarily from the fourth anterolateral intercostal nerve, which travels lateral-to-medial beneath to deep fascia before coursing upward through the breast parenchyma to innervate the nipple and areola. The third and fifth anterolateral intercostals (along with their medial counterparts) also contribute to the overlapping innervation of the nipple-areolar complex. In evaluating the breast parenchyma from the pectoralis, care must be taken not to dissect too far laterally because of the risk of nipple denervation.

14. What are the pertinent anatomic features in planning a mastopexy procedure?
All of the following anatomic features must be examined before undertaking a mastopexy: degree of ptosis and nipple-areolar position; breast volume; distribution of breast volume; breast contour; length, position, and definition of the inframammary fold; lower pole constriction; quality of the skin; fascial attachments (breast mobility); lateral breast/chest folds; and symmetry. Of these features, the degree of breast ptosis predominantly dictates which form of mastopexy is best suited to achieve the optimal aesthetic goals.

15. What are the various surgical options available for treatment of breast ptosis?
The many techniques for correction of breast ptosis represent the broad spectrum in degrees of ptosis and underscore the fact that no ideal technique currently exists. Treatment must be individualized. In general, the surgical options of mastopexy are categorized by the manner or pattern in which redundant skin is removed or tightened. More accurately, the lax skin is usually deepithelialized and invaginated rather than actually excised to preserve the subdermal plexus supplying the nipple-areolar complex. The nipple-areolar complex can be moved and the breast tightened by partial or full circumareolar skin excisions. For greater degrees of breast ptosis with more skin redundancy, in which the nipple-areolar complex must move a further distance, a vertical excisional component is added. As the degree of ptosis increases, a horizontal excisional component (placed at the inferiormost point of the vertical excision) must be added, ultimately resulting in a full inverted T incision. Augmentation or various parenchymal flaps, foldovers, and "pexies" are occasionally added to the mastopexy procedure. The typical surgical options for ptosis correction are augmentation only, circumareolar mastopexy, circumareolar excision with a vertical or oblique excisional component, circumareolar excision with a vertical excisional component and a short horizontal extension, and circumareolar excision with a full inverted T excisional component.

Glandular and minor degrees of ptosis may be treated with an implant only or a circumareolar skin excision (donut mastopexy). Implants should be used to fill the skin envelope volume rather than to expand it. Attempting to correct greater degrees of ptosis with an implant requires the use of large-volume implants that may be aesthetically unpleasing. In addition, the poor-quality skin envelope may not be able to tolerate such expansion. Without the necessary skin tightening, the native ptotic breast may hang over the less mobile and higher positioned underlying implant. This postoperative contour deformity, termed a "double bubble," is not easily corrected. Donut mastopexies tighten the breast envelope but do not raise the position of the nipple-areolar complex. In addition, this procedure tends to flatten the central breast. If undue tension is placed on the suture line, the scar and/or the areola may widen. The addition of a vertical excision below the nipple-areolar complex allows more tightening and greater ability to raise the nipple-areolar complex. For major ptosis, an additional horizontal excisional component is often required. If an implant is used, the breast should be augmented before defining the final nipple-areolar complex position because augmentation decreases the amount of ptosis and thus changes the optimal position for the nipple-areolar complex. (See figures at top of next page.)

16. What is a Benelli mastopexy?
A donut mastopexy refers merely to a concentric skin excision around the areola; the outer dermal circumference is reapproximated to the areola. A Benelli mastopexy refers to a method of pursestringing the outer dermal circumference with a strong nonresorbable suture. This maneuver eliminates the tension placed on the areola by a donut mastopexy. The addition of the pursestring or "round block" overcomes many of the inherent problems of previous forms of concentric mastopexies, thus expanding their indications and optimizing their results. A Benelli mastopexy, in the strictest sense, also includes a remodeling of the breast parenchyma by pexying the retroglandular surface to underlying periosteum at the aponeurotic prepectoral level in a crisscross fashion.

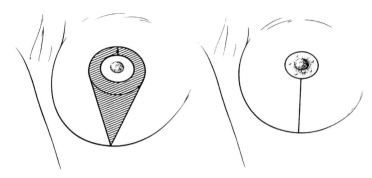

For minor ptosis, the circumareolar excision with a vertical ellipse tightens the skin and lifts the nipple without the need for an inframammary incision. This incision can be shortened because the vertical component is used primarily to close the defect from the transposed nipple-areola. It also tends to shorten with postoperative scar contraction. (From Bostwick J: Aesthetic and Reconstructive Breast Surgery. St. Louis, Mosby, 1983, p 234, with permission.)

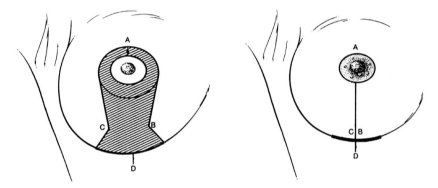

For moderate ptosis, the circumareolar excision with a vertical and short horizontal ellipse produces a short in-framammary scar and tightens the breast while shortening the inframammary distance. (Modified from Bostwick J: Aesthetic and Reconstructive Breast Surgery. St. Louis, Mosby, 1983, p 235.)

17. What is tailor-tacking?

Tailor-tacking allows the surgeon to view the result before making any incisions. Proposed areas of resection or deepithelialization are simply invaginated and the outer edges are tacked together, usually with staples, to simulate a resection with edge-to-edge closure. When the desired result is achieved, the outer edges are marked, the tacks are released, and all areas within the marks are identified for removal. This method is particularly useful for determining the correct position for the nipple-areolar complex.

18. What is meant by a constricted breast or inferior-pole hyperplasia?

In a constricted breast the inframammary fold is tight and elevated. Because of a deficiency of lower pole skin and breast tissue, the distance between the lower edge of the areola and the infra-mammary fold is short. As a result, the upper pole rotates over the high, tight inframammary fold. The appearance suggests constriction and ptosis. The ptosis is not related to an inferiorly descended nipple-areolar complex, but rather to a higher inframammary fold and inferior breast hypoplasia. Correction includes releasing and lowering the fold, along with radial releases inferiorly and expansion inferiorly. Severe constriction is represented by the tubular breast.

19. What are the common complications of mastopexy?

Complications common to mastopexy are recurrent ptosis, nipple-areolar complex asymmetry, breast asymmetries, upper pole flattening, poor scarring, and nipple-areolar necrosis. Most complications are the result of poor planning. Nipple-areolar complexes that are malpositioned superiorly are particularly troublesome, because it is usually necessary to place scars on the superior hemisphere to lower the nipple-areolar complex.

BIBLIOGRAPHY

1. Benelli L: A new periareolar mammaplasty: The "round block" technique. Aesth Plast Surg 14:93–100, 1990.
2. Bostwick J: Aesthetic and Reconstructive Breast Surgery. St. Louis, Quality Medical Publishing, 1990.
3. Brink RR: Evaluating breast parenchymal maldistribution with regard to mastopexy and augmentation mammaplasty. Plast Reconstr Surg 86:715–721, 1990.
4. Dinner M, Artz J, Fogelietti M: Application and modification of the circular skin excision and pursestring procedures. Aesth Plast Surg 17:301–309, 1993.
5. Erol OO, Spira M: A mastopexy technique for mild to moderate ptosis. Plast Reconstr Surg 65:603–609, 1980.
6. Gasperoni C, Salgarello M, Gargani G: Experience and technical refinements in the "donut" mastopexy with augmentation mammaplasty. Aesth Plast Surg 12:111–114, 1988.
7. Georgiade N, Georgiade G, Riefkohl R: Aesthetic Surgery of the Breast. Philadelphia, W.B. Saunders, 1990.
8. Georgiade G, Riefkohl R, Levin LS: Plastic, Maxillofacial, and Reconstructive Sugery, 3rd ed. Baltimore, Williams & Wilkins, 1997.
9. Grotting J: Reoperative Aesthetic and Reconstructive Surgery. St. Louis, Quality Medical Publishing, 1995.
10. Gruber R, Jones H: The "donut" mastopexy: Indications and complications. Plast Reconstr Surg 65:34–38, 1980.
11. Lejour M: Vertical mammoplasty and liposuction of the breast. Plast Reconstr Surg 94:100–114, 1994.
12. Netscher D, et al: Aesthetic outcome of breast implant removal in 85 consecutive patients. Plast Reconstr Surg 100:206–219, 1997.
13. Puckett C, Meyer V, Reinisch J: Crescent mastopexy and augmentation. Plast Reconstr Surg 75:533–539, 1985.
14. Regnault P, Daniel R: Aesthetic Plastic Surgery. Boston, Little, Brown, 1984.
15. Regnault P, Daniel R, Tirkantis B: The minus-plus mastopexy. Clin Plast Surg 15:595–599, 1988.
16. Ship A, Weiss P, Engler A: Dual-pedicle dermoparenchymal mastopexy. Plast Reconstr Surg 83:282–289, 1989.
17. Westreich M: Anthropomorphic breast measurement: Protocol and results in 50 women with aesthetically perfect breasts. Plast Reconstr Surg 100:468–479, 1997.
18. Whidden P: The tailor-tack mastopexy. Plast Reconstr Surg 62:347–354, 1978.

47. DISEASES OF THE BREAST

Kirby I. Bland, M.D., F.A.C.S., and Daniel S. Kim, M.D.

1. What is the incidence, risk probability, and mortality for breast cancer?

The 1997 estimated incidence for female breast cancer is 180,200 with a 1 in 8 lifetime probability of developing invasive cancer. It is the most common cancer in women. The estimated mortality for 1997 is 43,900, which is second only to lung cancer.

2. Which factors increase the risk of breast cancer?

Major risk factors include advanced age, family history, personal history, ductal carcinoma in situ (DCIS) or lobular carcinoma in situ (LCIS), benign atypical proliferation, and first pregnancy at ≥ 40 years of age. Minor risk factors include early menarche, late menopause, obesity, and nulliparity.

3. Can breast cancer be inherited? What is the risk of developing breast cancer with a BRCA1/BRCA2 mutation?

Breast cancer is believed to be hereditary in 4–9% of all cases. One in 200–400 women are carriers of the BRCA1 mutation. Estimated lifetime risk of breast cancer is 85% for mutations on BRCA1 and 2.

4. What is DCIS? Is it a precancerous state? What is the risk of invasive cancer? What is the treatment? What about LCIS?

DCIS is ductal carcinoma in situ and is a precursor of invasive cancer. The risk for developing invasive cancer is considered to be in the range of 30–50% over 10 years. The gold standard treatment is total mastectomy. Because of the success in using conservation therapy for invasive cancer, this treatment is being applied to DCIS. National Surgical Adjuvant Breast and Bowel Project–17 (NSABP–17) is examining lumpectomy versus lumpectomy and radiation therapy. Early data reveal a significant decrease in event-free survival and invasive cancer with radiation therapy. However, there is no change in overall survival and distant disease.

LCIS is lobular carcinoma in situ and is a marker rather than a precursor for invasive cancer. It carries a 10–37% risk of breast cancer, most incidences occurring more than 15 years later. Fifty to sixty-five percent of the invasive cancers are not lobular but ductal in origin and can occur in either or both breasts. If operative intervention is chosen, anything less than total mastectomy is inappropriate because the disease process is multicentric and often bilateral.

5. When should a woman begin mammographic screening? Has mammography made a difference?

The American Cancer Society recommends annual mammography for women beginning at age 40. The Hospital Insurance Project (HIP) study demonstrated a 33% mortality reduction with mammographic screening. Screening in the group aged 40–49 years has been controversial. A meta-analysis of eight randomized clinical trials of mammography screening reveals an 18% mortality reduction in women aged 40–49 years. Seven of the trials were population-based and a meta-analysis of these showed a 26% reduction in this age group. Swedish trials have yielded even higher mortality reductions of up to 44%.

6. What features make a mammographic lesion suspicious for malignancy? Do all lesions require biopsy?

Suspicious lesions consist of fine microcalcifications and/or density lesions such as masses, architectural distortions, and asymmetries. Microcalcifications that are fine, branching, clustered, pleomorphic, and numerous are most suspicious. Masses that are stellate and irregular are also most suspicious. The combination of such masses with microcalcifications gives the highest yield for malignancy. Any suspicious lesions should be biopsied with needle localization or stereotactic core needle biopsy if available. Lesions deemed less suspicious by the surgeon and radiologist may be followed closely by mammography.

7. Is there a role for fine-needle (FNA) aspiration for palpable breast masses? Is there a role for mammography?

Yes. FNA is an inexpensive, quick, and easy technique to differentiate solid from cystic masses with low morbidity. If nonbloody fluid is obtained and the mass disappears, the patient may be followed closely by physical exam and mammography. If the fluid is bloody or the mass persists or recurs after two aspirations, the patient should undergo open biopsy. The fluid should also be sent for cytologic evaluation. If no fluid is found, the mass is assumed to be solid and the patient should undergo outpatient open biopsy. If the cytology is positive, the patient may undergo a one-step procedure including open biopsy and frozen section confirmation prior to conservation therapy or mastectomy. However, a two-step approach is preferred.

Mammography should be obtained in all women over 30 years of age with a palpable breast mass. The combination of physical examination, mammography, and FNA yields a diagnostic accuracy approaching 100%.

8. What is conservation therapy?

Conservation therapy includes lumpectomy, axillary lymph node dissection (ALND), and ipsilateral breast irradiation. The lumpectomy should have free margins, often requiring re-excision. If the disease is multicentric, total mastectomy is appropriate. ALND should include at least 10 lymph nodes for adequate sampling. Usually only level I and II nodes are excised.

9. Name the borders of the axilla.

• Anterior wall: pectoralis major, subclavius, and pectoralis minor muscles and clavipectoral fascia
• Posterior wall: subscapularis, latissimus dorsi, and teres major muscles
• Medial wall: upper 4 or 5 ribs and the intercostal spaces covered by the serratus anterior muscle
• Lateral wall: coracobrachialis and biceps muscles

10. Which nerves can be identified during an ALND? What is their role?

The **intercostobrachial nerve** supplies sensory innervation to the upper medial aspect of the arm and is preserved if possible.

The **long thoracic nerve**, respiratory nerve of Beu, originates from roots C5, C6, and C7 of the brachial plexus and provides motor stimulation to the serratus anterior muscle. It usually can be found adjacent to the lateral thoracic artery's origin and runs along the serratus anterior. Transection results in a "winged scapula."

The **thoracodorsal nerve** originates from the posterior cord of the brachial plexus and can usually be found posterior to the origin of the subscapular vessels. It provides motor innervation to the latissimus dorsi muscle and should be preserved unless it is encased in tumor. There is minimal morbidity associated with its transection as compared with the long thoracic nerve. However, for myocutaneous flaps that utilize the latissimus dorsi muscle, the thoracodorsal neurovascular bundle must be spared to ensure flap function, form, and viability.

The **medial pectoral nerve** supplies motor innervation to the pectoralis major muscle and 40% of the time it wraps around the lateral border of the pectoralis minor muscle. This nerve should be spared.

11. What are the dissection boundaries of a mastectomy?

The skin flaps are raised superiorly to the clavicle, medially to the sternum, inferiorly to the rectus sheath, and laterally to the latissimus dorsi muscle.

12. How does tamoxifen work? Who may benefit from tamoxifen?

Tamoxifen's mechanisms of action have not been fully elucidated; however, its primary action is mediated through its antiestrogen effect. Tamoxifen provides significant prolongation of both recurrence-free and overall survival in both node-negative and node-positive patients. The benefit is greater for women aged 50 and older. It is also more beneficial when the tumor is estrogen receptor-positive.

13. Does chemotherapy have a beneficial effect?

Chemotherapy has a beneficial effect both on disease-free survival and overall survival. Both node positive and negative patients and women under 50 receive a greater benefit. Combination chemotherapy is superior to single agents and CMF (cyclophosphamide, methotrexate, and 5-fluorouracil) is probably the combination of choice. Newer combinations, particularly for more advanced disease, include doxorubicin.

14. What are the most common areas of recurrence?

Locally, breast cancer recurs in the breast and regional lymph nodes. Distant metastases can affect almost any site. The most common are lung, liver, and bone and, less commonly, the gastrointestinal tract, adrenals, brain, and soft tissues.

15. What is the 5-year survival rate according to AJCC (American Joint Committee on Cancer) staging?

Stage I, 85%; stage II, 66%; stage III, 41%; and stage IV, 10%.

16. What is the most common solid breast mass in women under 30? Does this lesion have malignant potential?

The most common solid breast mass in this age group is a fibroadenoma, a benign tumor composed of both stromal and epithelial elements. Women may be managed with FNA and observation or excisional biopsy, depending on the patient's age.

17. What are the most common organisms cultured from nipple discharge in a woman with a breast abscess? What is the treatment?

Staphylococcus aureus and streptococci. Most abscesses are subareolar and occur within the first few days of breast-feeding. Treatment is conservative and combines broad-spectrum antibiotics, warm soaks, and a mechanical breast pump. More serious infections may require intravenous antibiotics and incision and drainage. The incisions should be small and circumareolar for optimal cosmesis.

18. A woman presents with diffuse, bilateral breast pain associated with her menstrual cycle. Palpation reveals multiple nodular irregularities. What is the disorder? Is it premalignant?

Fibrocystic disorder. It is not a premalignant state unless it is associated with atypia. Thirty percent of fibrocystic change is proliferative with cellular atypia. If there is a dominant mass, it should be aspirated and treated like any other suspicious cyst or mass.

BIBLIOGRAPHY

1. Bassett LW: Mammographic analysis of calcifications. Radiol Clin North Am 30:93–105, 1992.
2. Biesecker BB, Boehnke M, Calzone K: Genetic counseling for families with inherited susceptibility to breast and ovarian cancer. JAMA 269:1970–1974, 1993.

3. Bland KI, Vezeridis MP, Copeland EM: Breast. In Schwartz SI, Daly JM, Galloway AC, Fischer JE (eds): Principles of Surgery, 7th ed. New York, McGraw-Hill, 1998.
4. Bland KI, Copeland EM (eds): The Breast: Comprehensive Management of Benign and Malignant Diseases, 2nd ed. Philadelphia, W.B. Saunders, 1998.
5. Chung M, Chang HR, Bland KI, Wanebo HJ: Younger women with breast carcinoma have a poorer prognosis than older women. Cancer 77:97–103, 1996.
6. Early Breast Cancer Trialists' Collaborative Group: Systemic treatment of early breast cancer by hormonal, cytotoxic, or immune therapy. Lancet 339:1–15, 71–85, 1992.
7. Gloeckler LA, Henson DE, Harras A: Survival from breast cancer according to tumor size and nodal status. Surg Oncol Clin North Am 3:35–53, 1994.
8. Iglehart DJ: The Breast. In Sabiston DC (ed): Textbook of Surgery, 15th ed. Philadelphia, W.B. Saunders, 1997.
9. Leitch MA, Dodd GD, Costanza M, et al: American Cancer Society guidelines for the early detection of breast cancer: Update 1997. CA Cancer J Clin 47:150–153, 1997.
10. Lynch HT, Lynch J, Conway T, et al: Hereditary breast cancer and family cancer syndromes. World J Surg 18:21–31, 1994.
11. McKenna RJ: The abnormal mammogram radiographic findings, diagnostic options, pathology, and stage of cancer diagnosis. Cancer 74:244–255, 1994.
12. Parker SL, Tong T, Bolden S, Wingo PA: Cancer statistics, 1997. CA Cancer J Clin 47:5–27, 1997.

48. BREAST RECONSTRUCTION

Kenneth C. Shestak, M.D., F.A.C.S., Jeffrey W. Szem, M.D., David D. Zabel, M.D., and Chet L. Nastala, M.D.

1. Is there evidence that breast reconstruction adversely affects disease-free survival?

Current studies have repeatedly demonstrated that the risks of local recurrence and development of a second breast cancer are similar in patients undergoing breast reconstruction and patients undergoing mastectomy alone. In fact, a trend toward a decrease in the death rate and rate of distant metastasis is seen in the breast reconstruction group in some studies.

2. Is skin-sparing mastectomy oncologically sound?

When performed properly, skin-sparing mastectomy does not increase the risk of local or distant recurrence. In one study involving over 100 patients with T1 and T2 breast cancer, no difference in recurrence rates was seen in the group undergoing skin-sparing mastectomy.

3. Are there significant differences in immediate and delayed breast reconstruction?

Immediate reconstruction offers many advantages compared with delayed reconstruction. A superior cosmetic result can generally be achieved while reducing the cost and anesthetic risk for a two-stage procedure. The previously perceived need to live with a postmastectomy defect before reconstruction has been challenged by the current belief that a more positive body image can be maintained with a breast mound that is reconstructed immediately. Delayed procedures involve recreation of the previous defect, often associated with significant scar tissue. In addition, previously dissected pedicles make such surgery more challenging. Difficulties with native skin loss of the mastectomy flaps can be overcome by careful dissection, clinical examination, and use of fluorescein to assess skin viability. Simultaneous ablation and breast reconstruction have made immediate reconstruction safer and improved the overall aesthetic outcome.

4. Is the goal of symmetry more easily achieved with implants or autogenous reconstruction?

In reconstructing one breast after mastectomy, the goal of symmetry may be quite challenging. Submuscular implant reconstruction may be ideal for a patient with small to moderate-sized breasts. Implant sizes in this instance typically range from 200–400 cc. In unilateral reconstruction with larger breasts, particularly with increasing ptosis, symmetry can be better achieved with autogenous tissue. When autogenous tissue reconstruction is contraindicated, better symmetry may be achieved with implant reconstruction and simultaneous reduction mammaplasty, mastopexy, or even augmentation of the contralateral breast.

5. What is the best method to create a breast mound with ptosis?

Preserving superior and medial fullness by correct inset of the TRAM flap into the mastectomy defect creates a more aesthetic breast mound. Accurate determination of the weight and skin dimensions of the mastectomy specimen is critical to reconstructing the aesthetic contour. Recreating the inframammary fold with sutures and preserving the majority of the fold when a pedicled TRAM is used are maneuvers to recreate ptosis.

6. What is the major complication of implant reconstruction without previous tissue expanders?

The incidence of capsular contracture with poor aesthetic result is high. Loss of implant may result from breakdown of the incision, loss of native tissue flaps, or infection when an implant is used for immediate reconstruction. Increased tension on native skin flaps and decreased perfusion to the wound margin may occur in an effort to maximize implant volume. A safer approach is tissue expander placement at low volume followed by expansion. Of particular concern is the use of implant reconstruction in the previously irradiated breast. The incidence of capsular contracture, exposure, and loss of implant is increased.

7. What are the major indications for tissue expansion?

Postmastectomy defects leading to loss of breast volume and reduction of the skin envelope may be adequately corrected by insertion and inflation of tissue expanders. Although autogenous tissue reconstruction may provide better symmetry, in some circumstances tissue expansion with subsequent implant placement is a better alternative. Examples include patients who do not wish to undergo a flap reconstruction, thin patients without excessive tissue readily available for transfer, patients in whom flap reconstruction is not possible for technical reasons, and patients who are elderly and have comorbid medical illness.

8. What are the major advantages of tissue expansion?

Tissue expansion breast reconstruction uses local tissue that has the advantage of providing superior texture and color match comparable to that of the contralateral breast. The sensation in the native breast skin flaps is also preserved. Significant donor site scars, often seen with autogenous reconstruction, may be avoided with this technique.

9. What are the most common complications of tissue expansion? Is there a difference between immediate and delayed tissue-expanded breast reconstruction?

Complications of tissue expansion reconstruction are a function of the wound, the device, the process of expansion and the quality of tissue cover at the site of the mastectomy. Wound complications of hematoma, seroma, and infection may occur. Skin necrosis and wound breakdown are appreciated more frequently after mastectomy secondary to pressure applied to the skin flaps. They also may result more often in immediate reconstruction, whereas in delayed reconstruction the flaps have more time to mature. Complications from the device are usually due to failure from leakage, which may occur secondary to structural failure or damage of the implant from needle punctures at the time of suturing or periodic refilling. Increasingly recognized is the effect of the expansion process in producing subcutaneous adipose tissue and muscle atrophy. Complications during the process of expansion are related to skin necrosis and breakdown with exposure of the device from too rapid filling. This may represent one of the critical complications of tissue expansion requiring secondary operations to cover the device with local flaps and/or to remove it.

10. What are the differences between smooth wall tissue expanders and textured dimensional based devices?

Smooth surface expanders have a tendency to move and usually create a spherical periprosthetic space. Dimensional devices, which are textured, are shaped to approximate breast form and are designed to create a breast that dimensionally simulates the remaining breast. All implantable materials elicit a host cell response leading to a fibrous scar or capsule. Textured expanders allow ingrowth of collagen from the periprosthetic capsule, which assists in fixing an implant's position. These textured devices theoretically divert the linear deposition of scar along its surface in attempts at limiting scar contraction around the device. Implant and expander fixation may provide improved definition of the inframammary fold and better breast shape in the upright position.

11. What is the cause of skin wrinkling or rippling after implant reconstruction?

Superior pole wrinkling is seen more commonly with saline implants than with silicone gel prostheses. These defects may represent underfilling of the device with saline volume and result from the ubiquitous gravitational forces that pull the implant inferiorly, leaving waves or folds in the upper pole of the implant that can be transmitted through the overlying tissues at the mastectomy site. Rippling is also related to the textured surface, which produces a thinner capsule and also may produce traction on the overlying tissues, resulting in so-called traction rippling.

12. What is the frequency of implant rupture?

Current studies indicate that the rate of rupture for silicone gel implants approximates 50% with follow-up of more than 10 years after insertion. Although similar studies for saline devices have only a 5-year follow-up and show a 1% per year cumulative rupture rate, deflation of saline implants from studies during the early 1990s has shown such rates to be 5–15%. Mechanical failure and deflation have been attributed to "fold-flaw" cracking. It is possible that subpectoral positioning of the implant may decrease the rate of this fatigue phenomenon; muscle pressure prevents creasing of the implant and failure at the seams.

13. Can tissue expansion be accomplished in an irradiated tissue bed?

Radiation to the postmastectomy area should be considered a relatively strong contraindication to tissue expansion. Expansion results in application of force to the overlying tissue as the expander is inflated, subjecting the skin flaps to periods of relative ischemia that may lead to necrosis and exposure of the implant. Tissue expansion in this setting is characteristically much slower and has a high incidence of capsular contracture after completion of the breast reconstruction process.

14. What is a TRAM flap? What are the main variations for breast reconstruction after mastectomy?

TRAM stands for **t**ransverse **r**ectus **a**bdominis **m**yocutaneous flap. It is a technique of autogenous tissue reconstruction of the breast mound using the rectus abdominis muscle and overlying skin and fat. As originally described, the rectus muscle is dissected carefully with maintenance of the continuity between the anterior rectus fascia and the overlying subcutaneous fat and skin. The myocutaneous composite is then tunneled through the epigastric subcutaneous tissue to the location of the mastectomy defect. The procedure may be performed as a unipedicled flap with the blood supply based on the superior epigastric artery and vein or as a bipedicled flap using both rectus muscles to support a larger amount of skin and fat for creation of a larger breast mound with a more vigorous blood supply. The TRAM flap also may be performed as a microvascular free flap using the inferior epigastric vessels to provide vascular supply.

15. What comorbid conditions should be considered in patient selection for TRAM flap reconstruction?

The patients at highest risk for complications include severely obese patients, chronic smokers, patients with abdominal wall scars from antecedent procedures, and patients who have undergone previous radiation therapy. Autoimmune disease, diabetes mellitus, chronic obstructive pulmonary disease, and heart disease also increase the chance of perioperative surgical complications. These factors are not contraindications per se, but must be carefully considered in the decision to perform a TRAM flap reconstruction and may alter the technique selected for flap transfer (pedicled vs. free flap).

16. What measures can be undertaken to increase the blood supply of a pedicled TRAM flap?

1. **Delay.** Two weeks before the performance of the muscle transposition, the deep inferior epigastric artery and vein may be ligated in an effort to bolster the blood supply to the more inferior aspects of the muscle and the overlying skin and subcutaneous fat.

2. **Supercharging.** The inferior epigastric vessels are anastamosed to the thoracodorsal vessels. Such a maneuver provides a second blood supply to the inferior aspect of the flap, the area in which the perforators to the skin and subcutaneous fat are located.

17. What are the main recipient vessels for a free TRAM flap?

The thoracodorsal vessels are the recipient vessels of choice. This is important for the general surgeon to understand so that these vessels are not injured during mastectomy and axillary dissection. The preferred position of the anastamosis is the point just proximal to the take-off of the serratus branch. If the thoracodorsal vessels are not available, the internal mammary vessels are a good second choice.

18. What common complications are specific to TRAM flaps?

Fat necrosis is the most common complication. Its incidence has been reduced by performance of free TRAM reconstructions. Partial flap loss occurs more commonly than total flap loss. Skin envelope complications also may occur. In the setting of immediate reconstruction, the use of intravenous fluorescein and a Wood's lamp may help to avoid leaving behind a compromised mastectomy flap, thereby reducing the chance of native breast flap necrosis. Abdominal hernias occur at varying rates, depending on methods of closure and patient selection. Wound complications such as infection and dehiscence occur with an incidence similar to other plastic surgical operations. Of course, size mismatch, poor aesthetic result, and need for revision surgery are also considered complications.

19. Are there any absolute contraindications to TRAM flap reconstruction?

Prior abdominoplasty divides the perforator vessels to the central abdominal skin and is a contraindication, although case reports have demonstrated the success of the TRAM flap if the skin and adipose tissue are revascularized by using the omentum as an angioneogenic substrate. Previous subcostal incisions dividing the superior epigastric pedicle or laparoscopic ports through the muscle should raise suspicion that blood supply may be inadequate. In this instance, preparation for supercharging or free microvascular tissue transfer may be required.

20. What are the most common alternatives to breast reconstruction if the TRAM flap is not available?

Alternative sites for autogenous reconstruction include the gluteal flap, latissimus flap, lateral thigh flap, and Rubens flap. Donor site deformity, availability of donor tissue, difficulty of the technique, the surgeon's experience, and the ability to create a new breast mound are important factors that influence choice.

21. Describe the vascular anatomy of the Rubens flap.

This periiliac fat pad is commonly seen in subjects of the famous Renaissance painter. Based on the deep circumflex iliac artery and vein, this flap may be an appropriate alternative to TRAM reconstruction.

22. Can breast reconstruction be performed using the latissimus dorsi muscle without an implant?

Entirely autogenous breast reconstruction can be performed by enlarging the skin paddle overlying the latissimus muscle in a fleur-de-lis pattern or by including greater amounts of fat and fascia with a standard elliptical skin paddle. In larger women with redundant tissue in the flank, more adipose tissue may be available. Matching a large breast is difficult, and the donor site may present a significant cosmetic deformity. The volume of the transferred tissue can be increased by including the parascapular dorsal thoracic fascia supplied by perforators anterior to the latissimus muscle. Small to moderate-sized breasts may be appropriately matched without an implant.

23. How do you determine whether the thoracodorsal pedicle is likely to be intact in the setting of a previous modified radical mastectomy?

Have the patient stand with her hands on her iliac crests and elbows forward. The latissimus dorsi contraction can be palpated along the axillary line. Paralysis, significant weakness of the muscle, or scapular winging is an indication that the pedicle has most likely been previously divided.

24. Can the latissimus dorsi flap be used if the thoracodorsal pedicle has been divided?

Often the thoracodorsal pedicle is divided proximal to the serratus branch. A reversal of flow in the serratus branch allows the latissimus dorsi to remain vascularized. In this setting, however, a decrease in the length of the pedicle will decrease the arc of rotation of the latissimus flap.

25. Are there significant differences in the cost of implant-based reconstruction vs. autogenous tissue breast reconstruction?

Surprisingly, the initial cost advantage of implant-based reconstruction is lost when corrected for unsuccessful reconstruction and the costs of subsequent surgery are included. Autogenous breast reconstruction is more cost-effective, when all resources are considered, than reconstruction with prosthetic implants.

BIBLIOGRAPHY

1. Birdsell DC, Jenkins H, Berkel H: Breast cancer diagnosis and survival in women with and without breast implants. Plast Reconstr Surg 92:795, 1993.
2. Elliot LF: Option for donor sites for autologous tissue breast reconstruction. Clin Plast Surg 21:177, 1994.
3. Evans GR, Shusterman MA, Kroll SS, et al: Reconstruction and the radiated breast: Is there a role for implants? Plast Reconstr Surg 96:1111, 1994.
4. Germann G, Steinau HU: Breast reconstruciton with the extended latissimus dorsi flap. Plast Reconstr Surg 97:519, 1996.
5. Hartrampf CR, Noel RT, Drazan L et a: Rubens' fat pad for breast reconstruction—A peri-iliac soft tissue free flap. Plast Reconst Surg 95:217, 1995.
6. Kroll SS, Evans GR, Reece GP, et al: Comparison of resource costs between implant based and TRAM flap breast reconstruction. Plast Reconstr Surg 97:364, 1996.
7. Maxwell GP, Falcone PA: Eighty-four consecutive breast reconstructions using a textured silicone tissue expander. Plast Reconstr Surg 89:1022, 1992.
8. Moon HK, Taylor GI: The vascular anatomy of the rectus abdominis myocutaneous flap. Plast Reconstr Surg 82:815, 1988.
9. Petit JV, Lee MG, Mouriesse H, et al: Can breast reconstruction with gel-filled silicone implants increase the risk of death in secondary primary cancer in patients treated by mastectomy for breast cancer? Plast Reconstr Surg 94:115, 1994.
10. Slavin SA, Colen S: Sixty consecutive breast reconstructions with inflatable expanders: A critical appraisal. Plast Reconstr Surg 86:910, 1990.
11. Sozer SO, Cronin ED, Biggs TM, Gallegos ML: The use of the transverse rectus abdominis musculocutaneous flap after abdominoplasty. Ann Plast Surg 35:409, 1995.
12. Watterson PA, Bostwick J III, Hester TR, et al: TRAM flap anatomy correlated with a 10 year clinical experience with 556 patients. Plast Reconst Surg 95:1185, 1995.

49. NIPPLE-AREOLA RECONSTRUCTION

John William Little, M.D., F.A.C.S.

1. Should nipple-areola reconstruciton be an integral part of breast reconstruction or an added option for certain patients?

It should be an integral part of the overall surgical plan for every breast reconstruction. Until a realistic nipple-areola has been added, a breast has not been reconstructed—only a breast mound. One of the key psychological benefits of breast reconstruction is relief from the daily reminder of mastectomy and its mortal implications. The more realistic the reconstruction, the more likely the relief. Nipple-areola reconstruction contributes greatly to such realism. In truth, if the majority of a surgeon's patients do not elect nipple-areola reconstruction, the results of the breast-mound reconstruction are probably not very good. A previous study confirms a high correlation between the presence of a nipple-areola and the patient's overall satisfaction with breast reconstruction to a level that is statistically highly significant. In addition, the morbidity for the procedure is negligible.

2. Should nipple-areola reconstruction be performed at a second stage after primary reconstruction of the mound?

Generally, yes, if there is reasonable symmetry between the breasts at the second stage. If significant additional work will be required on the breast mound or the contralateral breast to improve symmetry at the second stage, the nipple-areola reconstruction should be postponed to a third stage, when proper position can be more precisely determined. In such circumstances the nipple-areola is typically added in an office setting with local anesthesia alone and no additional medication. There is little justification for nipple reconstruction at the time of the initial breast mound reconstruction because exact positioning becomes very difficult. Furthermore, single-stage breast reconstruction creates an unrealistic expectation on the part of the patient and a difficult burden for any surgeon who is critical of the final result.

3. Is banking of the nipple-areola in the groin area an appropriate alternative to reconstruction if the primary cancer is located away from the nipple-areola?

No. Such banking cannot be justified on an oncologic basis in the presence of an invasive cancer. Studies in the Scandinavian literature have revealed breast cancer cells in the areola, not to mention nipple, of specimens in which the primary cancer was at a significant distance from the nipple-areola. Furthermore, the cosmetic outcome of such twice-transferred composite grafts is inferior to what can be produced de novo.

4. Do options for nipple reconstruction include composite grafts from the toe or earlobe?

No. Such grafts are woefully inadequate for the purpose of nipple reconstruction. The only grafting source that is effective remains a composite graft from the opposite nipple. Although this technique continues to be used by many surgeons, the overall price is a reduced and scarred opposite nipple in a woman who has already suffered the sensory and psychological assault of mastectomy. Assuming that the sharing technique results in two nipples of equal size, the final projection of the nipple pair will be less than one-half of what could have been achieved if the remaining nipple had been respected and matched by existing techniques.

5. What is the treatment of choice for nipple reconstruction?

Local flap. Virtually any opposite nipple can be matched by a local flap technique with a minimum of morbidity and distortion at the donor site if the proper technique is selected.

6. Is the best way to determine nipple-areola position by measurement from the other side?

Only in part. Such measurements should be made, but they are only the initial step in determining the proper final position. Measurements should be taken of the transverse midsternal line-to-nipple distance as well as the sternal notch-to-nipple distance. Then the appropriate-sized areola should be sketched around the intersection site. The surgeon-scientist must then become surgeon-artist and stand back to observe the overall impact of symmetry. Because of inherent asymmetries in nearly all final results in breast mound reconstruction, the best final position may well fall somewhat off the precise mathematic determination. The final position is an artistic compromise among various factors.

7. Are flap techniques for nipple reconstruction interchangeable and merely a matter of the surgeon's preference?

No. Some are inherently unsound in design and are not sufficiently reliable to be recommended. Others present a strict limitation to the amount of final projection.

8. What type of nipple reconstruction is inherently unreliable?

Reconstruction based on a central subcutaneous pedicle without dermal continuity, such as the quadrapod design. Although such techniques may give impressive results in the operating room and immediate postoperative period, long-term projection is unreliable; far too many results suffer late loss of projection.

9. Do the best designs in nipple reconstruction allow closure of the donor site, avoiding the need for grafting?

No. Such designs, which include the double opposing flap and the star flap, may be excellent for matching small or moderate-sized nipples but prove generally inadequate for larger nipples. Donor-site closure limits the amount of possible projection in designs that attempt to match opposite large nipples.

10. Is the skate flap the best design to use for matching an opposite large nipple?

Yes. The technique can be executed both with or without a skin graft; when large dimensions are required, however, a skin graft invariably is required. An opposite nipple of virtually any size can be matched with this technique with proper preoperative planning (see figure on next page).

11. Is there a disadvantage to the use of a skin graft in the final outcome of the nipple-areola?

No, as long as the area of graft falls within the pattern of the final areola. Full-thickness skin grafts placed on an appropriate deep dermal bed are far preferable in the overall outcome of nipple-areola reconstruction than spread scars that follow primary closure under tension.

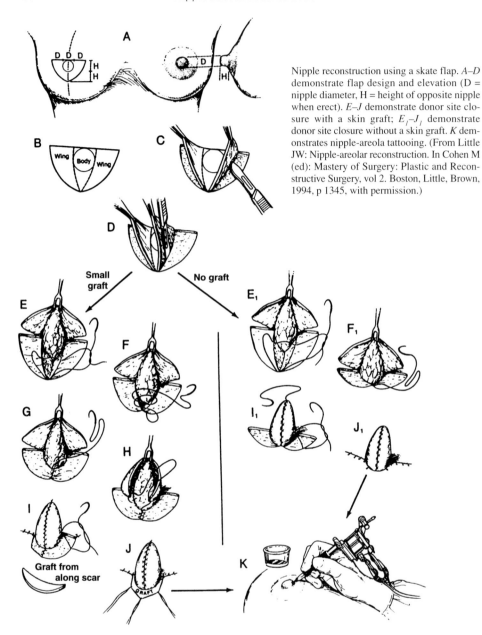

Nipple reconstruction using a skate flap. *A–D* demonstrate flap design and elevation (D = nipple diameter, H = height of opposite nipple when erect). *E–J* demonstrate donor site closure with a skin graft; E_1–J_1 demonstrate donor site closure without a skin graft. *K* demonstrates nipple-areola tattooing. (From Little JW: Nipple-areolar reconstruction. In Cohen M (ed): Mastery of Surgery: Plastic and Reconstructive Surgery, vol 2. Boston, Little, Brown, 1994, p 1345, with permission.)

12. Can subsequent intradermal tattoo hide spread donor-site scars after nipple reconstruction?

No. Spread scars present poor beds for the receipt of intradermal tattoo pigments and mar the final result. Well-healed full-thickness skin grafts, on the other hand, accept such pigments as well as surrounding native tissues and are not discernible within the pattern of the final areola.

13. What are the other disadvantages to spread scars after primary closure of nipple donor sites?

Final increased surface tension at the site of nipple reconstruction favors late loss of nipple projection for reasons not yet elucidated. Furthermore, tension at the site of nipple reconstruction flattens the aspect of the breast silhouette where maximal convexity is desired. Donor-site closure under tension is wrong-minded. Three strikes—you're out!

14. In using a local flap to reconstruct the missing nipple, should the dimensions of the planned nipple match those of the opposite nipple?

No. The dimensions of the reconstructed nipple should match only the diameter of the opposite nipple. Nipple height should be at least twice that of the opposite stimulated nipple. Partial loss of projection is inherent in any design for nipple reconstruction and must be factored into the final result.

15. Are some nipples too large to match by nipple reconstruction?

No. The skate technique with skin graft can match virtually any nipple size if the appropriate dimensions are used in the preoperative plan. Early in his experience with the skate technique, the author documented many late results exceeding 2 and 3 cm of final projection. All of these cases required drastic reduction. A final result in nipple reconstruction that does not match the other side in projection typically represents an error in planning, with an inadequate initial design. Errors in execution or inherent local ischemia at the donor site are far less common causes.

16. Does raising the skate flap with full-thickness wings produce a better overall result?

No, not when a large nipple is being matched and a skin graft is required. Even a small amount of reticular dermis covering the donor site allows closure of the composite defect because of the suture-holding ability of the fibers. Furthermore, the final exposed bed is far more receptive for grafting than is fat.

17. Do the best results in areola reconstruction follow the grafting of skin that later becomes pigmented spontaneously?

No. Although grafting from an opposite areola undergoing reduction remains appropriate as reconstruction in kind, only occasionally is enough skin available to replace the missing areola completely. Furthermore, with the sophisticated techniques currently available in breast mound reconstruction, alteration of the opposite breast is much less necessary or desirable than in the past. The transfer of skin that will become pigmented after grafting, such as from the upper inner thigh, allows no control over final coloration and matches the opposite areolar color only by chance. Furthermore, such darkened grafts invariably lose color over time, typically becoming indiscernible from surrounding breast skin within 5–10 years after transfer. Finally, the high morbidity rates of donor sites from such grafts cannot be justified.

18. What is the treatment of choice for areola reconstruction?

Tattoo. The only justification for grafting during areola reconstruction is to close the nipple donor site when matching a large opposite nipple. Otherwise, tattoo alone gives the best result in areola reconstruction because it allows accurate matching of both shape and surface area of the opposite areola as well as the best available color match.

19. Are coloration or tattoo techniques at the time of nipple reconstruction helpful?

No. Techniques that tattoo the nipple at the time of nipple reconstruction increase the likelihood of flap failure. Techniques that tattoo before nipple reconstruction miss the point and waste an extra stage. Location for the tattoo remains imprecise, and the opportunity for fine tuning of the ultimate result is forfeited. Finally, techniques that paint pigments beneath grafts, although imaginative, are impractical, both in terms of their unpredictability in final coloration and their reliance on otherwise unnecessary areolar grafting.

20. When is the ideal time for nipple-areola tattoo?

Generally 4 months after nipple reconstruction, when the majority of nipple shrinkage has occurred and final resolution has come to the second-stage balancing procedure. At this point final adjustments to both breast mound and nipple-areola may be carried out with minor surgery, liposuction, and tattoo.

21. Is one of the most important attributes of nipple reconstruction a centric position within the areola?

No. A far more important attribute of nipple-areola reconstruction is symmetry of the areolar color patch compared with the opposite side. If at the time of final tattoo it becomes necessary to shift the areolar pattern from a position that is concentric to the nipple, an eccentric nipple within a symmetric areola is a far better compromise than the alternative.

22. Is the best equipment for nipple-areola tattoo the delicate machinery supplied by manufacturers specializing in medical equipment?

Not necessarily. The most important attribute of tattoo equipment for nipple-areola reconstruction is sufficient torque to imbed pigments in skins of various thicknesses, such as that overlying the latissimus dorsi muscle, as well as sites that may be inherently scarred. These requirements are often very different from the characteristics of machines that imbed pigments in the delicate skin of an eyelid, for example.

23. Does nipple-areola reconstruction require a long learning curve until acceptable results can be achieved?

Not really. In truth, the earliest experiences with intradermal tattoo produce results that are superior to those available by any other means, including the transfer of grafts that later darken at random. On the other hand, matching the hue, tint, and depth of color of an opposite areola is an artistic challenge for even the experienced surgeon-tattooist; quite naturally, the accumulation of experience aids in achieving such matched results.

24. Should the final color immediately after tattoo match the opposite nipple-areola?

No. It must be significantly darker. Hemosiderin is invariably imbedded with the tattoo earth pigments, producing a dark appearance to the proper immediate result. This initial darkness fades within the first few weeks after tattoo. The final tattoo, in turn, continues to fade slowly over the months and years ahead. Secondary tattoo, however, is especially rapid and straightforward, because areolar borders are already determined. The particular patient may require a secondary boost of color, and this possibility should be discussed before the initial tattoo.

BIBLIOGRAPHY

1. Little JW: Nipple-areolar reconstruction. Adv Plast Reconstr Surg. 3:43, 1986.
2. Little JW, Spear SL: Nipple-areolar reconstruction. Perspect Plast Surg 2:1, 1988.
3. Little JW: Nipple-areolar reconstruction. In Marsh JL (ed): Current Therapy in Plastic Surgery. Philadelphia, B.C. Decker, 1989.
4. Little JW, Spear SL: Nipple-areolar reconstruction and tattoo. In Russell RC (ed): Instructional Courses, vol. 2. St. Louis, Mosby, 1989.
5. Little JW: Nipple-areolar reconstruction and correction of inverted nipple. In Noone RB (ed): Plastic and Reconstructive Surgery of the Breast. Philadelphia, B.D. Decker, 1991.
6. Little JW: Nipple-areolar reconstruction. In Cohen M (ed): Mastery of Surgery: Plastic and Reconstructive Surgery. Boston, Little, Brown, 1994.
7. Little JW: Nipple-areola reconstruction. In Spear SL, Little JW, Lippman ME, Wood WC (eds): Surgery of the Breast: Principles and Art. Philadelphia, Lippincott-Raven, 1998.
8. Spear SL, Convit R., Little JW: Intradermal tattoo as an adjunct to nipple-areolar reconstruction. Plast Reconstr Surg 83:907, 1989.
9. Wellisch DK, Schain WS, Noone RB, Little JW: The psychological contribution of nipple addition in breast reconstruction. Plast Reconstr Surg 80:699, 1987.

50. GYNECOMASTIA

Nicholas J. Speziale, M.D., and Mary H. McGrath, M.D., M.P.H.

1. What is gynecomastia?

Gynecomastia is excessive development of the male breasts.

2. In what age groups does gynecomastia occur?

Physiologic or idiopathic gynecomastia with no pathologic basis commonly develops in the newborn, during puberty, and in old age.

3. How common is gynecomastia in each age group?

Palpable breast tissue transiently develops in over 60% of all newborns because of transplacental passage of estrogens. Pubertal gynecomastia has been reported in 64% of adolescent boys with a peak incidence at 14–14.5 years and an average duration of 1–2 years. During middle age, about 30% of men develop gynecomastia. The prevalence gradually increases to > 60% in the seventh decade.

4. How does pubertal gynecomastia present?
Bilateral enlargement of the breasts to a mean diameter of 2–2.5 cm. Gynecomastia also may present unilaterally or bilaterally with asymmetry.

5. Are patients with gynecomastia symptomatic?
Most patients are asymptomatic. If symptoms occur, they generally include breast tenderness or soreness or occasional troublesome nipples.

6. What questions are pertinent in taking the history?
1. What is the duration of the breast enlargement?
2. Is there any breast pain or tenderness?
3. Is the patient taking any medication?
4. Is there any history of weight gain or loss?
5. Is there any history of hepatic disease or hyperthyroidism?

7. What physical findings should be sought?
1. **Breast:** if gynecomastia exists, thickened breast tissue should be palpable under the nipple. If there is a small, hard, eccentrically located mass or if skin dimpling is found, suspect carcinoma.
2. **Testes:** if testes appear small, consider a chromosome study. If asymmetric, evaluate for testicular tumor with ultrasound.
3. **Liver:** assess for hepatomegaly or ascites.
4. **Thyroid:** assess for enlargement and nodularity.
5. **Assess nutritional status.**

8. Classify the etiologies of gynecomastia.
Physiologic, pathologic, and pharmacologic.

9. What are the most common causes of pathologic gynecomastia?
Cirrhosis, malnutrition, hypogonadism, Klinefelter's syndrome, neoplasms, renal disease, hyperthyroidism, or hypothyroidism.

10. What tumors may lead to gynecomastia?
Testicular tumors (i.e., Leydig cell and Sertoli cell tumors, choriocarcinomas), adrenal tumors, pituitary adenomas, and lung carcinomas.

11. What drugs may cause gynecomastia?

Estrogens	Cimetidine	Marijauna	Diazepam
Spironolactone	Digoxin	Reserpine	Theophylline

Mnemonic: **S**ome (**s**pironolactone) **m**en (**m**arijuana) **c**an (**c**imetidine) **d**evelop (**d**iazepam) **r**ather (**r**eserpine) **e**xcessive (**e**strogens) **t**horacic (**t**heophylline) **d**iameters (**d**igoxin).

12. Does gynecomastia ever resolve?
• During puberty, gynecomastia often regresses spontaneously within 2 years.
• In drug-related gynecomastia, withdrawal of the medication leads to regression.
• If gynecomastia is of long duration, it is unlikely to regress spontaneously.

13. What is in the differential diagnosis?
Gynecomastia, pseudogynecomastia, and breast carcinoma.

14. What is pseudogynecomastia?
Pseudogynecomastia is an increase in male breast size that results from fat deposition. There is no hyperplasia of breast tissue, and involvement is bilateral.

15. Is there any relationship between gynecomastia and breast cancer in adult males?
No. Numerous clinical studies have failed to show an increased incidence of breast cancer in men with gynecomastia. There is no evidence of an increased incidence in patients on long-term estrogen therapy or with drug-induced gynecomastia. No histologic evidence supports a relationship.

16. What laboratory values should be obtained?

Prepubertal Males	Pubertal Males	Adult Males	
Estradiol*	Estradiol*	Estradiol*	Thyroid function tests
LH/FSH	LH/FSH	LH/FSH	Liver function tests
HCG†	HCG†	HCG†	Renal function tests
Adrenal CT scan	Testosterone‡	Testosterone‡	Chest radiograph

LH = luteinizing hormone, FSH = follicle-stimulating hormone, HCG = human chorionic gonadotropin.
* If estradiol is increased, check adrenal CT scan to rule out feminizing tumor.
† If HCG is increased, check an ultrasound of the testes to rule out tumor.
‡ If testosterone is low and LH/FSH are elevated, check karyotype to rule out Klinefelter's syndrome.

17. What is the role of medical therapy?
    Testosterone can be effective in the treatment of gynecomastia secondary to testicular failure. **Tamoxifen** has been shown to reduce gynecomastia in middle-aged men. **Danazol** acts as a gonadotropin inhibitor, reducing both the pain and extent of gynecomastia.

18. What are the indications for surgery in patients with gynecomastia?
 • Adolescent males with enlargement persisting for 18–24 months
 • Symptomatic patients
 • Gynecomastia of long duration leading to fibrosis
 • Patients at risk for carcinoma (e.g., patients with Klinefelter's syndrome)

19. Describe the surgical classification of gynecomastia.
    Grade 1: small visible breast enlargement without skin redundancy
    Grade 2A: moderate breast enlargement without skin redundancy
    Grade 2B: moderate breast enlargement with skin redundancy
    Grade 3: marked breast enlargement and marked skin redundancy

20. Discuss surgical techniques for gynecomastia (see figures on following pages).
    1. **Mild-to-moderate gynecomastia.** Excision of breast tissue through either a semicircular incision along the inferior aspect of the areola or a transverse incision in the apex of the axilla.
    2. **Moderate-to-large gynecomastia.** With more severe cases, skin resection and nipple transposition techniques become necessary. After resecting skin, the nipple-areola complex is rotated superiorly and medially based on a single dermal pedicle.
    3. **Massive gynecomastia.** In the most severe cases, en bloc resection of excessive skin and breast tissue and free nipple grafting can be performed. The final scar is placed within the inframammary crease using a cresenteric transverse incision. The nipple-areola graft is then placed on the dermis overlying the fifth rib.

21. What is the role of liposuction in the treatment of gynecomastia?
    Liposuction is most helpful as an adjunct to excision by smoothing the edges of the resection. The ideal candidate is the patient with fatty breasts responsive to fat aspirations. Although cannulas have been designed to break up fibrous septa, it is usually necessary to excise a small button of breast tissue.

22. What is the most common complication after surgery?
    Hematoma or seroma formation is very common secondary to extensive soft tissue dissection through a small incision with a substantial dead space. Good hemostasis and placement of a drain may be helpful. Evacuate any hematomas that may occur. Other less common complications include nipple slough and infection.

23. What techniques may prevent unwanted results?
    1. Be sure to leave an adequate layer of subcutaneous fat over the pectoralis fascia to prevent a concave breast.
    2. Perform liposuction to produce a smooth contour peripherally.
    3. Leave a 1-cm thick layer of adipose or glandular tissue beneath the areola to avoid nipple inversion.

A and *B,* Mastectomy for gynecomastia through a semicircular
intraareolar incision. *C* and *D,*
Resection of cone-shaped mass
of breast tissue tapering away at
periphery with sufficient fat left on
pectoral fascia. (From McGrath
MH: Gynecomastia. In Jurkiewicz
MJ, Krizek TJ, Mathes SJ, Ariyan
S (eds): Plastic Surgery: Principles
and Practice. St. Louis, Mosby,
1990, p 1128, with permission.)

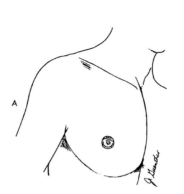

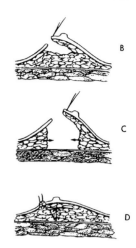

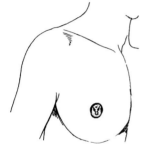

Operations for reduction of moderate-to-large breasts with
nipple transposition or reduction and transposition of periareolar skin around stationary nipple. *A,* Superior periareolar incision with skin excision. *B,* Nipple transposition on
single dermal pedicle with oblique breast scar. *C,* Nipple
transposition on vertical dermal bipedicle with transverse
breast scar. (From McGrath MH: Gynecomastia. In
Jurkiewicz MJ, Krizek TJ, Mathes SJ, Ariyan S (eds):
Plastic Surgery: Principles and Practice. St. Louis, Mosby,
1990, p 1130, with permission.)

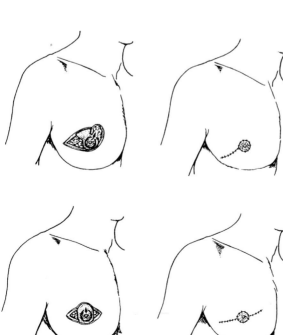

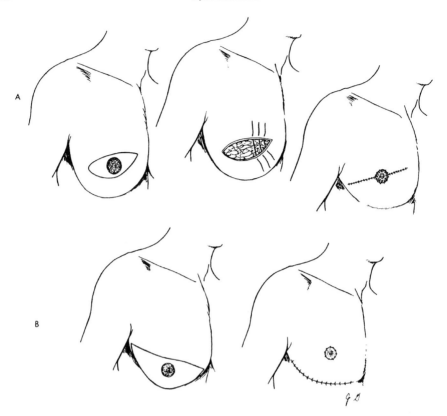

Operation for excessively large breasts with radical excision and free transplantation of nipple. *A,* Grafting of nipple onto dermal bed prepared in center of breast scar. *B,* En bloc excision with nipple grafting and inframammary crease scar. (From McGrath MH: Gynecomastia. In Jurkiewicz MJ, Krizek TJ, Mathes SJ, Ariyan S (eds): Plastic Surgery: Principles and Practice. St. Louis, Mosby, 1990, p 1132, with permission.)

BIBLIOGRAPHY

1. Braunstein GD: Gynecomastia. N Engl J Med 328:490–495, 1995.
2. Eaves FF III, et al: Endoscopic techniques in aesthetic breast surgery. Clin Plast Surg 22:683–695, 1995.
3. Glass AR: Gynecomastia. Endocrinol Metab Clin North Am 23:825–837, 1994.
4. Hands LJ, Greenall MJ: Gynecomastia. Br J Surg 78:907–911, 1991.
5. Mladick RA: Gynecomastia: Liposuction and excision. Clin Plast Surg 18:815–822, 1991.
6. McGrath MH: Gynecomastia. In Jurkiewicz MJ, Krizek T, Mathes SJ, Ariyan S (eds): Plastic Surgery: Principles and Practice. St. Louis, Mosby, 1990, pp 1119–1136.
7. Ruberg RL, Smith DJ: Plastic Surgery: A Core Curriculum. St. Louis, Mosby, 1994.

VII. Aesthetic Surgery

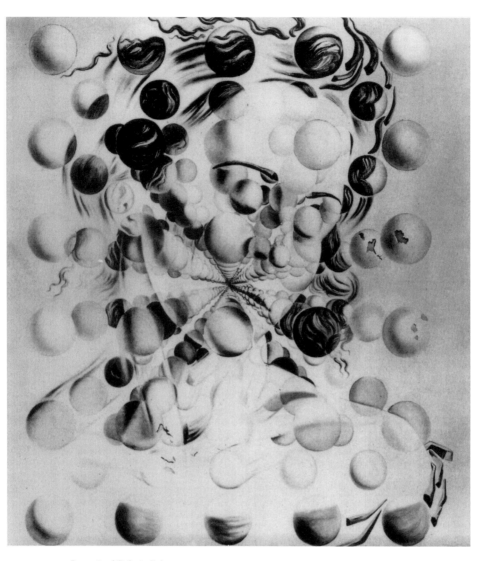

Portrait of Gala in Spheres
Salvador Dali
1952
Oil on canvas
Private Collection, New York
© 1998 Demart Pro Arte B.V.®, Geneva/Artists' Rights Society (ARS), New York

51. EVALUATION OF THE AGING FACE

Jack A. Friedland, M.D., and John W. Smith, M.D.

1. Give examples of trigger events that may cause a person to seek consultation for aesthetic facial rejuvenation.
1. Observation of a friend who has undergone facial rejuvenative surgery with good results
2. Self-criticism and realization of signs of aging in the face, eyes, and neck
3. Realization of a need for self-enhancement that may pave the way for career advancement
4. Realization of the need for self-enhancement to keep competitive in the work environment
5. Realization that a social relationship with a younger person would be enhanced by a more youthful appearance

2. What elements comprise the initial aesthetic facial surgery consultation?
1. Evaluation and discussion of the patient's desires as well as current and past medical history
2. Thorough physical examination, which is best done with the patient comfortably seated in front of a large mirror with appropriate lighting. In addition, a reversing mirror may be used to demonstrate to the patient their actual appearance rather than the image that they see in a standard mirror.
3. Consideration of appropriate laboratory and radiographic tests to determine general health status. If a specific medical problem becomes apparent, consultation with the patient's physician should be done.
4. Visual examination, including acuity, Schirmer test (if indicated), and visual fields (if indicated)
5. Photographic documentation of preoperative status
6. Patient education
   • Videotapes
   • Instructional brochures
   • Discussion of arrangements for surgery with office staff (patient coordinator, nurse, secretary)

3. What factors contribute to the aged appearance of the face?
1. Atrophy and loss of skin tone due to sun damage
2. Genetic inheritance
3. Morphologic changes of the facial bones
4. Health-related problems
5. Emotional stress
6. Large gains or losses in weight
7. Chronic abuse of alcohol
8. Chronic smoking of cigarettes
9. History of trauma
10. Chronic facial muscular contractions
11. Environmental damage due to excessive sun exposure and pollution

4. What intrinsic changes of the skin may be seen in the aging face?
1. Loss of elasticity
2. Keratoses, epitheliomata, and other hyperpigmented lesions
3. Fine lines and wrinkles
4. Decreased amount of subcutaneous adipose tissue due to atrophy
5. Abnormal pigmentation
6. Environmental damage

5. Outline the chronologic appearance of signs of aging in the face and neck.
Decade of the 30s: the upper eyelid skin becomes redundant and crow's feet form lateral to the canthi.
Decade of the 40s: the nasolabial folds become more prominent; transverse forehead furrows and vertical glabellar frown lines develop.
Decade of the 50s: rhytids develop in the neck; the jaw line becomes less distinct. Jowls form; the tip of the nose droops.

Decades of the 60s, 70s, and 80s: cutaneous and subcutaneous tissues atrophy, contributing to the formation of increased wrinkles and sagging of the skin.

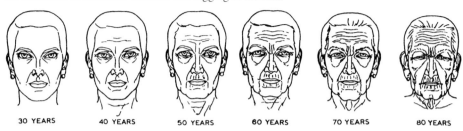

| 30 YEARS | 40 YEARS | 50 YEARS | 60 YEARS | 70 YEARS | 80 YEARS |

Changes observed in the external appearance of the aging face. (From Gonzalez-Ulloa M, Flores ES: Senility of the face—basic study to understand its causes and effects. Plast Reconstr Surg 36:239, 1965, with permission.)

6. What changes in the facial skeleton occur with aging?

1. Decreased height of mid and lower portions of face
2. Slight increase in facial width
3. Increased prominence of chin
4. Increased prominence of frontal sinus
5. Increased prominence of zygomatic arch
6. Increased facial depth

7. Which retaining ligaments provide support to the soft tissues and skin of the face over the bony skeleton?

1. Zygomatic osteocutaneous ligaments
2. Mandibular osteocutaneous ligaments
3. Platysma-auricular ligaments
4. Anterior platysma-cutaneous ligaments

The most important of these are the zygomatic and mandibular ligaments.

Retaining ligaments of the cheek that must be divided for proper skin drapage. Zygomatic ligament (Mc-Gregor's patch) and mandibular ligaments tether the skin to the facial skeleton. The platysma-auricular ligament and the anterior cutaneous ligaments are condensations of platysma fascia that extend to the dermis. (From Furnas DW: The retaining ligaments of the cheek. Plast Reconstr Surg 83:11, 1989, with permission.)

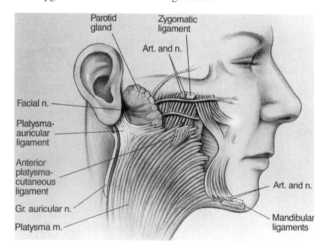

8. What signs of facial aging are correctable by aesthetic rejuvenative surgery?

1. Sag and laxity of the skin of the cheeks and neck
2. Prominence of the nasolabial folds
3. Deepening of the nasolabial and perioral commissural creases
4. Formation of jowls with laxity and sag of the facial skin over the border of the mandible, causing the jaw line to become less distinct
5. Formation of rhytids in various areas of the face
6. Atrophy of the skin and subcutaneous adipose tissues
7. Ptosis of the soft tissues of the anterior aspect of the chin

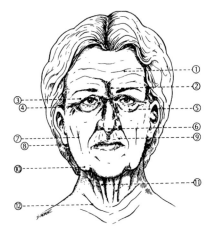

Stigmata of the aging face. Common findings include (1) ptotic and wrinkled brow, (2) glabellar laxity and frown lines, (3) ptotic eyebrows, (4) periorbital folds and lids, (5) redundant lower eyelid skin, (6) droopy nasal tip, (7) laxity of cheeks, (8) ptotic earlobes, (9) perioral wrinkling, (10) jowls, (11) platysmal bands, and (12) laxity of cervical skin. The possible combinations are infinite, and each patient must be carefully analyzed to formulate a treatment plan. (From Baker TJ, et al: Surgical Rejuvenation of the Face. St. Louis, Mosby, 1995, with permission.)

9. What signs noted on physical examination of the forehead can be corrected by aesthetic facial rejuvenative surgery?

1. Transverse furrows
2. Vertical glabellar frown lines
3. Ptosis of the brows
4. Fullness and hooding of the upper eyelids
5. Fullness in the glabellar region
6. Transverse creases over the dorsum of the nose in the area of the radix
7. Crow's feet

10. What is the normal or ideal position for the female eyebrow?

1. The brow is located approximately 1 cm above the superior orbital rim (whereas it lies approximately at the level of the rim in men).

2. The medial aspect of the brow is delineated by a vertical line drawn superiorly and perpendicular through the alar base.

3. The lateral aspect of the eyebrow is delineated by an oblique line drawn from the lateral aspect of the alar base through the lateral canthus.

4. The medial and lateral ends of the brow are approximately at the same horizontal level. The highest portion or apex of the brow is delineated by a vertical line extending superiorly from the lateral aspect of the corneal limbus.

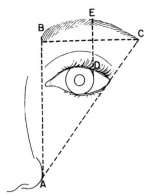

Spatial relationships of the ideal female eyebrow. (From Ellenbogen R: Transcoronal eyebrow lift with concomitant upper blepharoplasty. Plast Reconstr Surg 71:490, 1983, with permission.)

11. What signs of aging in eyelids are correctable by aesthetic rejuvenative surgery?

1. Increased amount and laxity of skin of the lids
2. Increased protrusion of periorbital fat
3. Ptosis of the brows, which, along with upper eyelid skin redundancy, causes hooding
4. Crow's feet, or rhytids, in the lateral canthal region
5. Ptosis of the lacrimal glands

6. Formation of xanthelasma
7. Hypotonicity and horizontal laxity of the lower lids

12. Is an ophthalmologic consultation required for all patients before undergoing aesthetic rejuvenation of the eyelids?

No—unless the patient is found to have a previously unknown defect in visual acuity or tear production or an anatomic deformity is discovered on physical examination that may require further ophthalmologic testing or treatment.

13. What signs of aging in external ears can be corrected by aesthetic rejuvenation?

1. Increased prominence due to an increase in the conchoscaphoid angle and/or unfurling of the antihelix
2. Increased size of the earlobes
3. Increased size of pierced earlobe holes due to chronic wearing of heavy earrings

14. What signs of aging of the nose are correctable by aesthetic rejuvenative surgery?

1. Drooping nasal tip or decrease in the nasolabial angle
2. Thickening of the skin of the nose
3. Enlargement and thickening of alar cartilages
4. Elongation of the nose
5. Widening of the nostrils

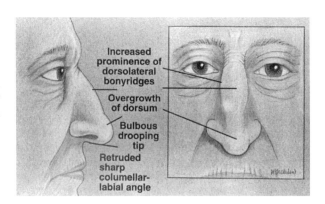

Signs of the aging nose. (From Gruber RP, Peck GC: Rhinoplasty: State of the Art. St. Louis, Mosby, 1993, with permission).

15. What signs of aging in the perioral region can be corrected by surgical rejuvenation?

1. Vertical rhytids extending from the vermilion borders of the upper and lower lips
2. Increased vertical height of the white portion of the upper lip
3. Flattening of the contour of the upper lip
4. Thinning and decreased fullness of the vermilion of the upper and lower lips
5. Downturning of the lateral oral commissures
6. Appearance and deepening of "marionette" lines

16. What signs of aging in the neck can be corrected by aesthetic rejuvenation?

1. Wrinkling of the skin
2. Formation of vertical bands in the platysma muscle
3. Formation of a less acute and more obtuse cervicomental angle (due to laxity of the platysma and/or excessive deposition of subcutaneous and subplatysmal adipose tissue)
4. Laxity and sag of the submental and anterior and lateral cervical skin
5. Ptosis of the submandibular glands

17. Why are preoperative photographs necessary?

1. They assist in preoperative planning and patient discussion.
2. They are invaluable for reference during surgery.
3. They are useful for postoperative counseling and review.
4. They provide necessary medicolegal documentation.

18. What visual records are used to document preoperative appearance?
Most surgeons prefer **preoperative photographs** that become part of the patient's permanent office records. Photographs may be taken with a 35-mm camera, high-grade portrait lens (105 mm preferred), and appropriate lighting. The images are recorded in black and white or color and can be printed in $3'' \times 5''$, $4'' \times 6''$, or even $5'' \times 7''$ sizes. Some surgeons use life-size $11'' \times 14''$ prints and mark on a clear acetate film placed over them to demonstrate goals and hoped-for changes in appearance. Others prefer to record images on 35-mm color film. **Computer imaging** allows innumerable poses and computer modifications that enable patients and surgeons to visualize preoperative defects as well as hoped-for postoperative improvements. Electronic images are easily made into permanent slides or prints.

19. What standard views of the face and neck are taken for photographic documentation?
Anteroposterior, right lateral, right oblique, left lateral, and left oblique.

20. What additional views may be taken to demonstrate deformities?
1. Close-up of the eyes to demonstrate fine lines and asymmetry of the lids
2. Close-up of the eyes looking up to demonstrate bulging of the periorbital fat in the lower lids
3. Smiling profile to demonstrate change in position of the nasal tip
4. "Worm's eye" view to demonstrate the basilar orientation of the inferior aspect of the nose and its relationship to the cheeks and lip
5. Flexed lateral view to demonstrate laxity and sag of the skin of the lower face and neck
6. Posteroanterior view to demonstrate protrusion of the ears from the side of the head (concha-scaphoid angle)
7. Close-up of the mouth at rest, smiling, and puckering to demonstrate muscular function, asymmetry, and rhytids

21. Does the consultation for aesthetic facial rejuvenative surgery differ for men and women?
No. However, physical characteristics and psychological considerations may be greatly different and must be explored and adequately discussed.

22. What differences are noted between men and women in evaluating patients for aesthetic facial surgical rejuvenation?
1. The position of the eyebrows is different. In women, the brow is usually located above the superior orbital rim, whereas in men it is located at or slightly below the rim.
2. Different patterns of hair growth in the scalp. Men tend to have recession of the frontal forehead hairline with loss and thinning of hair much earlier in life than women.
3. The presence of a beard in men, which causes an increase not only in the thickness of the skin but also in the blood supply due to a richer subdermal plexus.
4. Psychologic differences. Active men like to be in control of all aspects of their situation and are less likely to follow postoperative instructions such as restriction of activity and taking medication. Men seem to be less demanding about the results of surgery and usually have more realistic goals.

23. What is the best age at which to undergo aesthetic facial rejuvenative surgery?
There is no one best age. The timing of surgery depends on (1) the patient's desires, (2) the patient's general health status, (3) the patient's mental health status, (4) the presence of signs of aging that the plastic surgeon believes can be surgically corrected, and (5) history of sun exposure and presence of environmental damage to the skin.

24. Is there an age at which the patient is "too old" to undergo facial rejuvenative surgery?
No—as long as the patient's general mental and physical health status are deemed satisfactory.

25. How long do the results of facial rejuvenative surgery last?
The answer depends not only on the general health status of the patient but also on the age at which the procedure is performed. Usually foreheadplasties and eyelidplasties do not need to be repeated, but facialplasties are considered to last for 8–10 years.

26. Where can facial rejuvenative surgery be performed?
Facial rejuvenative surgery may be performed in a hospital, a free-standing ambulatory outpatient surgical facility, or a physician's office. Any of these options is acceptable as long as the appropriate

equipment for performance of the surgery and resuscitation is available. In addition, the necessary trained and certified medical personnel must be available.

27. What type of anesthesia is most appropriate for facial rejuvenative surgery?
The type of anesthesias depends on the procedure, the patient's general health status, and the surgeon's preference. For some procedures, local anesthetics may be sufficient. However, for the great majority of procedures, local anesthetics must be combined with intravenous sedation and analgesics. General anesthesia is used for procedures requiring complete relaxation (such as complete relaxation of the abdominal muscles during abdominoplasty).

28. Who may *not* be considered candidates for facial rejuvenative surgery?
1. Patients who have difficulty with describing or delineating the changes they desire
2. Patients who feel that their deformities are greater than they actually are
3. Patients with unrealistic expectations
4. Patients with severe mental or physical health problems who are poor surgical risks
5. Patients who are addicted to cigarettes, alcohol and/or drugs
6. Patients with nonsupportive family members

29. Who else may not be considered good candidates for aesthetic facial rejuvenative surgery?
1. Patients who are overly concerned about minimal defects
2. Patients who are too demanding or direct the physician about what to do and how to do it
3. Patients who constantly interrupt when explanations are given by the physician
4. Patients who have previously undergone surgery by another physician with less than desirable results and are antagonistic and defensive

30. What five rare skin conditions may present as premature aging with or without skin laxity? Is facial aesthetic surgical rejuvenation indicated?
1. **Ehlers-Danlos syndrome:** a rare, genetically transmitted disease of connective tissue characterized by thin, friable, and hyperextensible skin, hypermobile joints, and subcutaneous hemorrhages. It may be associated with posttraumatic bleeding and poor wound healing. It is caused by a genetic defect with inadequate production of the enzyme lysyl oxidase. Rhytidectomy is not indicated.
2. **Cutis laxa:** a degeneration of the elastic fibers in the dermis, associated with chronic obstructive pulmonary disease, pulmonary infections, cor pulmonale, GI and GU diverticuli, and hernias. The genetic defect is a deficiency of lysyl oxidase. Aesthetic facial rejuvenation is indicated and beneficial as long as the patient's general health status is satisfactory.
3. **Progeria:** a rare disorder of unknown etiology, transmitted in an autosomal recessive manner and characterized by growth retardation, craniofacial disproportion, baldness, protruding ears, pinched nose, micrognathia, atherosclerotic heart disease, and shortened life span. Plastic surgery is not indicated.
4. **Werner's syndrome (adult progeria):** a rare autosomal recessive disorder that consists of scleroderma-like skin changes, including patchy induration associated with baldness, aged facies, hypo/hyperpigmentation, short stature, high-pitched voice, cataracts, diabetes, muscle atrophy, osteoporosis, various neoplasms, and premature atherosclerosis. Plastic surgery is not indicated because of the presence of diabetic microangiopathy.
5. **Pseudoxanthoma elasticum:** a degenerative disorder of the elastic fibers with premature skin laxity. Aesthetic facial rejuvenative surgery is beneficial.

BIBLIOGRAPHY

1. Baker TJ, Gordon HL, Stuzin JM: Surgical Rejuvenation of the Face. St. Louis, Mosby, 1995.
2. Cohen M (ed): Mastery of Plastic and Reconstructive Surgery. Boston, Little, Brown, 1994.
3. Georgiade GS, Georgiade NG, Riefkohl R, Barwick WJ: Textbook of Plastic, Maxillofacial and Reconstructive Surgery. Baltimore, Williams & Wilkins, 1992.
4. Gruber RP, Peck GC: Rhinoplasty: State of the Art. St. Louis, Mosby, 1993.
5. Lewis JR (ed): The Art of Aesthetic Plastic Surgery. Boston, Little, Brown, 1989.
6. Rees TD, LaTrenta GS: Aesthetic Plastic Surgery. Philadelphia, W.B. Saunders, 1994.
7. Smith JW, Aston SJ: Grabb and Smith's Plastic Surgery. Boston, Little, Brown, 1991.

52. FOREHEAD AND BROW LIFT

Paul L. Schnur, M.D., and Scott A. Don, M.D.

1. Describe the arterial and nerve supply to the forehead.

It is necessary to understand the anatomy in the dissection of a forehead flap or endoscopic dissection of the brow. The forehead receives blood from both the internal and external carotid arteries. The frontal branches of the superficial temporal artery arise from the external carotid artery. The supratrochlear and supraorbital arteries arise from the internal carotid artery via the ophthalmic artery. The supraorbital and supratrochlear cutaneous nerves are derived from the ophthalmic division of the trigeminal nerve (cranial nerve V_1). The supraorbital nerve exits through the supraorbital foramen to innervate the lateral part of the forehead and the front of the scalp. The supratrochlear nerve exits medial to the supraorbital nerve and supplies the middle portion of the forehead.

2. Describe the anatomy of the frontal nerve.

The frontal nerve is a branch of the facial nerve. It emerges from beneath the parotid gland on a line extending from a point 0.5 cm below the tragus to a point 1.5 cm superior to the lateral position of the eyebrow. The nerve enters the frontalis muscle on its deep surface at a point where the orbicularis oculi intersects the lateral aspect of the frontalis muscle (approximately 1.5 cm above the lateral aspect of the eyebrow).

3. What is the function of the musculi frontalis?

Eyebrow elevation. The musculi frontalis are vertically oriented, paired muscles that blend in the midline. The muscles originate from the epicranial aponeurosis (galea) at the level of the anterior hairline and extend inferiorly to cover most of the forehead and insert into the dermis of the forehead skin.

4. What three facial muscles oppose the brow-lifting activity of the musculi frontalis?

Corrugator supercilii, procerus, and orbicularis oculi muscles.

5. Which muscles of the face are responsible for the deep transverse forehead lines, vertical glabellar creases, and transverse wrinkles at the root of the nose?

Frontalis, corrugator, and procerus muscles, respectively.

6. Describe Ellenbogen's criteria for the ideal eyebrow position and contour.

1. The brow begins medially at a vertical line extending from the ipsilateral alar base and ipsilateral medial canthus.
2. The brow ends laterally at an oblique line extending through the ipsilateral alar base and lateral canthus.
3. The medial and lateral ends of the eyebrow lie at approximately the same horizontal level.
4. The apex of the brow lies directly above the lateral limbus of the eye.
5. The brow arches above the supraorbital rim in women and lies approximately at the level of the rim in men.

7. What systematic approach should be used to evaluate the contour of the eyebrow?

The contour of the brow is evaluated in thirds: medial, central, and lateral. If the medial eyebrow is lower than the lateral, the patient looks angry or distressed. In contrast, a lower lateral eyebrow gives the patient a concerned or sad appearance. An excessive medial elevated eyebrow gives the patient a surprised look.

8. What are the indications for a forehead and brow lift?

Primary indications include ptosis of the forehead and eyebrows and fullness of the lateral upper lids. The forehead and brow lift also helps to correct transverse forehead lines, glabellar creases, and transverse folds at the root of the nose.

9. Where is the plane of dissection for the development of the forehead flap?

The flap for a coronal brow lift is elevated in the areolar plane between the galea and the pericranium. The other potential planes of dissection are subcutaneous or subperiosteal.

10. What is a supraciliary eyebrow lift?

It is a procedure that elevates the eyebrow by excision of skin directly above the eyebrow. This relatively simple excision produces dramatic eyebrow elevation but leaves a permanent visible scar, thus limiting its popularity. The procedure is best limited to men with thick eyebrows or women willing to accept a scar that may or may not be covered by makeup.

11. What is a midforehead lift?

This procedure helps to correct deep forehead creases and brow and glabellar ptosis. The incision is placed centrally in a prominent horizontal forehead crease to allow direct interruption of the frontalis muscle and elevation of the eyebrows (with optional excision of the medial muscles). The procedure leaves a visible scar and thus is limited to men with deep forehead creases.

12. What is a bitemporal lift?

This procedure has the advantage of elevating the lateral brow while concealing the paired incisions in the temporal hair. There is no muscle resection. It is primarily indicated for younger patients with lateral orbital hooding.

13. Before the development of the endoscope, what were the most popular techniques for forehead and brow lift?

The bicoronal and modified anterior hairline forehead lift. In the standard bicoronal lift, the incision in the frontal and temporal regions is placed far enough posteriorly so that after resection of the redundant scalp it remains approximately 5 cm behind the hairline. In the modified anterior hairline lift, the incision follows the hairline in the frontal region and then turns posteriorly in the temporal region for 7–9 cm before curving caudally toward the top of the ear.

14. What factors determine the preference for a standard bicoronal or a modified anterior hairline incision?

Patient choice, height of the hairline, and thickness of the hair determine which incision should be used. For patients with a normal anterior hairline and without excessive thinning of the hair, a standard coronal incision is preferred. When the anterior hairline is high, the modified incision is used.

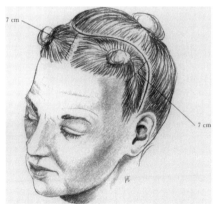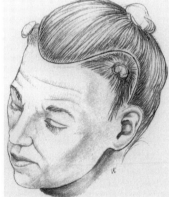

Left, Standard coronal incision for normal hairline. *Right,* Modified coronal incision for high hairline. (From Aston S, Thorne CH: The forehead and brow. In Rees TD, Latrenta GS (eds): Aesthetic Plastic Surgery, 2nd ed. Philadelphia, W.B. Saunders, 1994, p 733, with permission.)

15. What are the potential complications of a forehead and brow lift?

The incidence and severity of complications from a forehead and brow lift are quite low, and virtually all complications are apparent in the early postoperative period. The complications include hematoma, transient loss of sensation (< 5% permanent loss), tightness, chronic pain, hair loss, unacceptable scars, irregularities, and skin necrosis.

16. What are the major operative principles of an endoscopic forehead lift?
1. Several small incisions are made within the hairline.
2. An extensive subperiosteal dissection is performed to include the orbital rim and the root of the nose.
3. Release and resection of the corrugator and procerus muscles.
4. Preservation of the supratrochlear and supraorbital neurovascular elements.
5. Forehead elevation and fixation with percutaneous microscrews or other techniques allow reattachment to bone at a higher position.

17. What are the advantages of an endoscopic forehead lift?
No scalp resection, less scarring, decreased and less permanent numbness, and less bleeding. This procedure is beneficial for patients with alopecia and permits a comfortable, fast recovery.

18. What are the disadvantages of an endoscopic forehead lift?
New training and instruments are necessary, careful patient selection is essential, deep wrinkles of the forehead and glabellar area are not completely eradicated, and correction of severe eyebrow ptosis is limited.

BIBLIOGRAPHY

1. Chajchir A: Endoscopic subperiosteal forehead lift. Aesth Plast Surg 18:269–274, 1994.
2. Cohen M: Mastery of Plastic and Reconstructive Surgery. Boston, Little, Brown, 1994.
3. McCarthy JG: Plastic Surgery, 9th ed. Philadelphia, W.B. Saunders, 1990.
4. Regnault P: Aesthetic Plastic Surgery. Boston, Little, Brown, 1984.
5. Smith JW: Plastic Surgery, 4th ed. Boston, Little, Brown, 1991.
6. Toronto R: The subperiosteal forehead lift. Clin Plast Surg 19:477–485, 1992.

53. BLEPHAROPLASTY

Robert S. Flowers, M.D., and Eugene M. Smith, Jr., M.D.

1. What is blepharoplasty?
Blepharoplasty comes from two Greek words—*blepharon*, meaning eyelid, and *plastikos*, meaning fit for molding. Blepharoplasty is any procedure that is performed to shape or modify the appearance of the eyelids. It may be performed purely to remove bagginess, fatty protrusions, and lax hanging skin around the eyes or to correct a "lazy" or blepharoptotic eyelid. This last procedure is more often referred to as blepharoptosis repair. Blepharoplasty also refers to the creation of lid creases on eyelids that have no visible infolding and a similar operation on eyelids with ill-defined or asymmetric folds.

Traditionally, blepharoplasty denotes the removal of skin and perhaps a sliver of muscle from the upper lids, together with protruding or excessive orbital fat. On the lower lid, blepharoplasty suggests an elevation of skin or skin-muscle flaps and removal of skin, muscle, and/or fat.

2. What is the difference between blepharochalasis and blepharodermatochalasis (dermatochalasis)? Between steatoblepharon and blepharoptosis?
True **blepharochalasis**, a rare inherited disorder that appears in childhood, is characterized by repetitive episodes of eyelid edema that eventually lead to attenuation and/or dehiscence of the levator aponeurosis with resultant ptosis. The periorbital tissues stretch out, and dehiscence of the canthal tendons sometimes occurs. More often blepharochalasis refers to the stretching of the skin of the eyelids associated with aging. A more accurate term for involutional loosening of the eyelid skin is **dermatochalasis**. The puffiness of fat that is either excessive or protruding through a lax septum is

steatoblepharon. **Blepharoptosis** is drooping of the upper eyelid. When the eyebrow is ptotic, fat, together with the eyelid skin, hangs over the margin and may cause the illusion of ptosis when the eyelid occupies a normal position. The proper term for this condition is **pseudoblepharoptosis**.

3. Is blepharoplasty the procedure of choice for brightening and refreshing the eye region?

Since its inception, traditional blepharoplasty has been touted as the procedure to brighten and refresh the eye region. Commonly it fails miserably in this quest. Failure comes from two sources: (1) poor design of the blepharoplasty surgical procedure, which was conceived for a static model rather than the dynamic tissues of the human face, and (2) poor patient selection.

4. What is compensated brow ptosis?

In considering the upper portion of the orbit, it is absolutely essential to understand the concept of compensated brow ptosis. Most people presenting for blepharoplasty have a resting position of the eyebrow that is far too low for effective and/or comfortable forward and lateral vision. It is also too low for optimal aesthetics. This situation is remedied by constant contraction of the frontalis muscle when the eyes are open. Removal and/or invagination of overhanging tissues from the upper eyelids partially or totally relaxes the brow-elevating musculature. Frontalis muscle contraction checks the descent of the eyebrow and lid skin at a point just short of visual interference or weighty discomfort for the lids. Upper blepharoplasty procedures in people with compensated brow ptosis allow the eyebrow to position itself lower in the resting eye-open posture after surgery compared with the preoperative position. The usual result is a lid with precisely the same amount of overhang as before surgery, leading to a second or even a third redo with yet more upper lid tissue excision.

Only in people with an adequately high resting position of the brow and little-to-no compensated brow ptosis is upper blepharoplasty a procedure of choice for brightening and refreshing the eye region, and only in unusual adults with superb lid tonicity does lower lid blepharoplasty satisfy these conditions. In all others the effect of lower blepharoplasty is to drop lid posture, increase scleral show, and markedly sadden the patient's appearance. Unfortunately, patients requesting blepharoplasty who satisfy these criteria are few and far between.

5. If blepharoplasty is not the procedure of choice, what is?

Coronocanthopexy is the basic foundation for aesthetic repair around the orbital region without deforming the lids, periorbital aesthetics, or aperture shape. It maintains normal healthy eyelids without sacrificing any of the precious and irreplaceable eyelid tissue. Dropped posture of the lower lids, due to attenuation of the canthal tendon and reduced lid tonicity, is commonly responsible for what appears to be excessive skin. Canthopexy restores position, tone, and the normal upward tilt to the eye, whereas blepharoplasty (including transconjunctival fat removal) adds downward cicatricial traction on an already weakened eyelid, lowers the lid posture, and imparts a saddened appearance along with a decreased aperture width. When a secure canthopexy accompanies blepharoplasty, whatever tissue is truly excessive may be removed without adversely altering the shape of the eye. Elevation of the lid tightens the orbital septum and adds restraint to bulging fat.

The key effect of a frontal lift is to check the brow against precipitous descent after blepharoplasty. When the eyebrow is properly positioned, the lid appearance often suggests a youthful version of the patient. Coronocanthopexy often totally eliminates the need to resect skin. If redundant or excessive skin remains when the brow is examined postoperatively (positioning it at its estimated postoperative posture), a simple excision of skin (and/or a tiny sliver of orbicularis) just above the supratarsal crease will suffice to create the desired correction. With the lateral brow properly positioned, it is rarely necessary to extend the lid excisions beyond the edge of the orbital rim.

6. What is the youngest age at which a patient should consider blepharoplasty?

A functional blepharoplasty is indicated sometimes within the first few weeks of life if the upper eyelids block the infant's vision, as in severe cases of congenital blepharoptosis. If one or both eyelids block the child's vision, normal visual pathways may not develop, leading to irreversible visual loss in one or both eyes. This phenomenon is called amblyopia. In epiblepharon, an anomaly common in young Asian children, the lower lid eyelashes are in contact with the cornea. Surgery may be required to correct this deformity. Cosmetic blepharoplasty also may be considered in children and young teenagers, especially those of Asian ancestry, with heavily pseudoblepharoptotic lids. In general, it is preferable to wait until a person is old enough to cooperate under IV-assisted local anesthesia.

7. Is the preaponeurotic fat continuous with the deeper orbital fat?

Yes. The preaponeurotic fat is an important landmark during blepharoplasty and blepharoptosis surgery. It is usually the first fat encountered in making an incision through the orbicularis muscle and orbital septum, and portions of preaponeurotic fat are commonly removed during blepharoplasty. The lateral fat is contained anteriorly within a sling made by the fusion of the orbital septum and levator aponeurosis in the upper lid. Because the aponeurosis of the levator muscle is immediately posterior to this orbital fat, it is called preaponeurotic fat. All of it is in continuity with the deeper orbital fat.

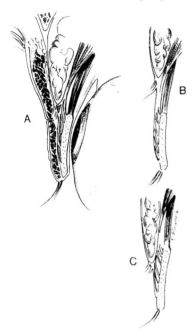

Upper eyelid anatomy. *A*, Note fusion of the levator aponeurosis and orbital septum to form the septoaponeurotic vehicle that serves as a ball-bearing mechanism for eyelid opening and closure. Sympathetically innervated Mueller's muscle inserts into the superior tarsus. *B* and *C*, The septum and aponeurosis may fuse at variable levels in the eyelid. In Caucasians the attachment is usually higher, whereas in Asians it is usually more inferior.

8. Is it important to remove most of the fat from the lateral or central-lateral upper eyelid during blepharoplasty?

No. The contrary is true. The central-lateral fat, together with its sheath, provides a "ball-bearing" mechanism for the septoaponeurotic vehicle, which serves an important function during eyelid opening and closure. Excessive or aggressive removal of central fat may produce scarring capable of interfering with lid opening and result in blepharoptosis or lagophthalmos. Most people have a deep, hollowed-out area between the medial and lateral (central-lateral) compartments in the upper orbit. Loss of fat worsens this deformity and creates excessively deep-set upper lids or a superior sulcus deformity.

9. What structure is often mistaken for fat in the upper eyelid?

The lacrimal gland. Beware of color and texture differences, and be careful when removing fat from the lateral portion of the upper lid. Injury to the lacrimal gland may result in dryness of the eyes and the possible need for permanent use of artificial tears and lubricating ointments. If the gland is abnormally large, it is far better to tuck the gland beneath the orbital rim with one or more sutures, anchoring its capsule to the deep periosteum, than to resect the gland itself.

10. Does removal of the palpebral lobe of the lacrimal gland have any deleterious consequences? What about the orbital lobe?

Removal of either the palpebral or orbital lobe of the lacrimal gland may adversely affect tear secretion. The lacrimal gland is divided into the palpebral and orbital portions by the lateral horn of the levator aponeurosis. The ducts for secretion of tears travel from the orbital lobe through portions of the palpebral lobe to reach the superior lateral fornix. Thus, cuts in or removal of the palpebral lobe may decrease tearing by severing ducts and interrupting the passage of tears. Injury or removal of the orbital lobe of the lacrimal gland may adversely affect the secretion of tears by eliminating the secretomotor innervation to both the orbital and palpebral lobes.

11. What is a retrobulbar hemorrhage? What are the common causes and possible consequences?
A retrobulbar hemorrhage is bleeding that occurs posterior to the orbital septum or globe in sufficient quantity to exert pressure on the globe. It may result from trauma, orbital surgery (including fat removal during blepharoplasty), injection of anesthetic in the retroseptal space, and frontal or brow lifting with violation of the orbital septum during dissection. It is much more common in hypertensive patients or normotensive patients with intraoperative elevation of blood pressure and patients who use aspirin or other medications with anticoagulant properties. The risk of retrobulbar hemorrhage can be minimized by controlling pain and blood pressure preoperatively and intraoperatively, by precisely cauterizing all fat and vessels before transecting them, and by using blunt-tipped needles for deep orbital anesthesia. Except in severe exophthalmos, all significant retrobulbar hemorrhage usually causes visible protrusion of the globe.

Too much pressure on the globe may lead to irreversible loss of vision. The intraocular pressure at first remains within normal range but may increase rapidly if the cause goes untreated. Normal intraocular pressure is 10–22 mmHg. Pressures of 30–40 mmHg should sound an alarm and motivate the surgical team to control contributing factors immediately. Intraocular pressure above 40 mmHg represents real risk of visual compromise and demands immediate treatment. Intraocular pressures approaching diastolic levels put the eye in imminent danger of vein occlusion or retina or nerve infarction, causing severe or total loss of vision.

12. How is a retrobulbar hemorrhage treated?
Treatment requires prompt recognition followed by measures to decrease pressure on the globe. Prompt control of pain and blood pressure elevation are often the most pressing needs, with application of light intermittent pressure on the orbit until these factors are controlled. A blunt instrument placed into the orbit through an existing incision may allow some blood to drain. Maximal exposure and illumination are essential in attempting to identify and cauterize the offending vessel, which is rarely found. Lateral cantholysis may be necessary to allow the orbital tissues and eyelids to bulge forward to decrease the orbital pressure transmitted to the globe. Some physicians recommend the immediate use of mannitol or acetazolamide (Diamox) to lower the intraocular pressure.

Immediately after recognizing the condition, during or after a blepharoplasty or blepharoptosis surgery, reopen the incision and orbital septum, and drain the orbit with a blunt instrument. Another technique involves using a hemostat to create an opening in the orbital floor to decompress the orbit emergently. This technique is rarely indicated unless all other maneuvers fail. Anterior chamber decompression is not indicated.

13. What are the advantages and disadvantages of a transconjunctival blepharoplasty?
Transconjunctival incisions are useful lower eyelid surgical approaches when only fat (steatoblepharon) removal or orbital septum tightening with little or no removal of skin (minimal dermatochalasis) is required. Resultant scarring still exerts downward traction on the lower lid, although typically less than with skin or skin-muscle flap approaches. The incisions are within the lower conjunctival sac, going through the lower lid retractors to acquire access to the lower eyelid fat. One clear advantage is the absence of visible external incisions, but conjunctival hemorrhage is often greater and hinders cosmetic concealment. Disadvantages include occasional difficulty in locating the proper tissue planes to identify the fat in respective compartments; inability to remove lower eyelid skin; inability to tighten lower eyelid laxity, which is usually present; increased risk of injury to the inferior oblique muscle by inexperienced probing; and postoperative downward lid traction that can be both profound and surprising.

14. What effect does blepharoplasty or tissue removal from the upper eyelid have on the position of the eyebrows?
Most people requesting upper eyelid surgery have significant compensated eyebrow ptosis; that is, they must contract the frontalis muscle to effect comfortable, unobstructed forward and lateral vision. A clue to this condition may be transverse forehead creasing or corrugation, but young people

and others with lots of subcutaneous padding may telescope the skin when the frontalis muscle contracts and show no transverse wrinkling. In all people with compensated brow ptosis, the brow posture drops after upper blepharoplasty. Therefore, all patients require a careful preoperative evaluation that compares the eye-closed resting (uncompensated) and elevated (compensated) brow positions with the corresponding eyes-open positions. Full relaxation of the brow is often best achieved with the eyes closed. The position of the eyebrows with the eyes closed and the forehead relaxed is the position toward which the eyebrows will drop after an upper lid blepharoplasty without a concurrent procedure to secure proper eyebrow position.

15. Does lower lid skin or skin-muscle resection change the shape of the eye? If so, how?

Resection of even a small or conservative amount of lower eyelid skin in the presence of a lax lower lid will result in aesthetically unpleasing results. Skin resection, in the setting of lower eyelid laxity, results in a rounded lower eyelid with increased scleral show, directly mirroring the triangular section of skin typically removed. This altered shape of the lower eyelid gives the patient a sadder and more tired appearance. A significant amount of corneal and conjunctival exposure with characteristic symptoms typically accompanies lower eyelid retraction, and ectropion may occur if laxity of the lower eyelids is not addressed before or during lower eyelid blepharoplasty with a canthopexy procedure.

16. What are the most common causes of postoperative eyelid ptosis?

The most common cause of postoperative ptosis is undiagnosed preoperative ptosis. Ptosis (blepharoptosis) describes a drooping of the upper eyelid. In a patient undergoing cosmetic or functional blepharoplasty, the type of ptosis most commonly encountered is due to dehiscence of the levator aponeurosis. Blepharoptosis also accompanies asymmetric brow ptosis. The more blepharoptotic upper eyelid is usually on the same side as the lower eyebrow. After traditional blepharoplasty the preexisting ptosis is usually exaggerated during the first 4–8 weeks postoperatively because lid edema adds weight to the lid, thereby exaggerating the ptosis. Another common cause is accidental resection of the levator aponeurosis when the orbicularis is lifted and resected. Other common causes include cicatricial restriction of lid opening and closing, usually as a result of excessive tissue removal (especially fat), hemorrhage within the surgical field, and inflammation.

17. How is blepharoptosis categorized?

Congenital ptosis is present at the time of birth, whereas **acquired ptosis** occurs after birth. These broad categories can be divided into additional types based on the specific etiology. Various terms describing both congenital and acquired varieties include dysmyogenic, myogenic, neurogenic, involutional (or senile), aponeurotic, traumatic, cicatricial, mechanical, and structural. Many of these descriptive classifications overlap; a disease process may fit under more than one category.

Myogenic (dysmyogenic) blepharoptosis, the most common congenital type, results from dysgenesis or faulty development of the levator muscle. Much of the striated muscle is replaced with fibrous tissue and sometimes fat, resulting in limited contractile ability and capacity to relax. A child with congenital myogenic ptosis may have unilateral or bilateral involvement with decreased ability to open and close the eyes. Examples of acquired myogenic ptosis include muscular diseases, such as muscular dystrophy, oculopharyngeal dystrophy, or chronic progressive external ophthalmoplegia (CPEO), and orbital trauma with muscle injury.

Neurogenic blepharoptosis results from faulty innervation of the upper lid retractors. Ptosis is profound with complete interruption of innervation to the levator muscle (through the superior division of the oculomotor nerve) and subtle with interruption of the sympathetic innervation to the superior tarsal (Mueller's) muscle. One example of congenital or acquired neurogenic ptosis is Horner's syndrome with sympathetic disruption, resulting in miosis, anhydrosis of the skin, and mild blepharoptosis.

Mechanical or traumatic blepharoptosis may result from any condition that interferes with the levator muscle or its innervation.

18. What is the treatment of postsurgical lagophthalmos?

Postsurgical lagophthalmos (inability to close the eyelids completely or to cover the globe adequately on caudal gaze) is common. It is often temporary but may be permanent. If too much skin has been resected, the patient may have skin deficiency with a temporary or permanent lagophthalmos. Usually inherent mechanisms protect against it by dropping the brow dramatically. Local anesthesia contributes to its appearance in the immediate postoperative period by blocking the orbicularis oculi more than the levator muscle. Postoperative edema of the upper lids during the first weeks after surgery commonly interferes with normal eyelid blinking and may aggravate drying of the eye. We prefer to give all patients artificial tears and/or lubricating eye ointment for routine surgical aftercare. In general, 30 mm of skin is required for a normally functioning lid with a normally positioned brow; less than this often requires life-long use of artificial tears, lubricants, and other measures to prevent drying.

19. What forms the supratarsal fold?
The upper eyelid supratarsal fold is also referred to as the upper eyelid or supratarsal crease. *Supratarsal* implies that the fold or crease is above the superior border of the tarsus, but such is not always the case, particularly in Asians. The crease is formed by insertions of fibrous extensions of the levator aponeurosis into the skin. It is important to reestablish these connections during blepharoplasty so that the incision is appropriately hidden within the lid crease. Of interest, the lid always enfolds at the point at which the sling created by the aponeurosis and septum descends into the lid. Indeed, even with no fibrous connections into the skin, a lid fold would be created by the rotary motion of this sling, which surrounds the ball-bearing-like orbital fat.

20. What is the double eyelid operation often requested by Asians or people of Asian ancestry?
Most people of East Asian ancestry, including those from China, Japan, Korea, and Southeast Asia, have a visible crease on the eyelid—at least during the first two or three decades of life. In many people they are quite well formed. In others the lid folds begin to be visible only on the central to lateral part of the eyelid. Because this fold (or crease) divides the lid into two sections (i.e., the part above and the part below the crease), the eyelids are referred to as *double*. An eyelid with no visible crease is referred to as *single*. These terms are uniformly used by most persons of East Asian ancestry. Often one eyelid is double and the other is single, or one lid fold is simply much more clearly defined than the other. Most people have an understandable desire for symmetry. The many different methods of lid fold creation fall into two groups: the closed or suture technique and the open technique. The senior author (Flowers) has often used a combination of the two when a conservative lid fold was desired with minimal postoperative swelling and morbidity.

In the **closed technique**, three or four tiny incisions are made at the desired level of fold creation on the external lid to allow the knot of suture to disappear into the substance of the lid, with a suture closing the skin overlying it.

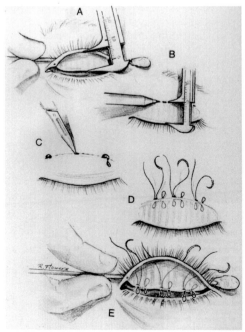

Upper eyelid crease fixation using the closed or suture technique. *A*, The vertical height of the tarsus is measured. *B*, The superior edge of the tarsus is marked on the skin. *C*, Several small incisions are made along the marked line. *D* and *E*, Full-thickness nonabsorbable sutures are passed through the eyelid to create eyelid crease fixation at the superior edge of the tarsus. (From Flowers RS: Upper blepharoplasty by eyelid invagination: Anchor blepharoplasty. Clin Plast Surg 20: 193–207, 1993, with permission.)

In the **open technique**, an incision is made across the lid. Skin and/or muscle is excised, after which the pretarsal skin flap is attached to the tarsus, aponeurosis, or both. If the fold is made small, it can be attached to the conjoint tendon or the pretarsal extension of the aponeurosis.

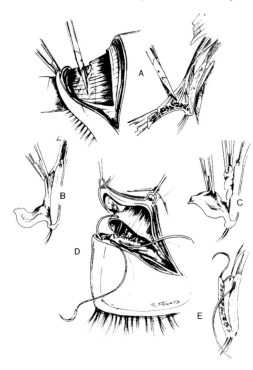

Open technique of upper eyelid crease fixation. *A,* The orbital septum is opened, and the pretarsal extension of the aponeurosis is dissected free from the pretarsal orbicularis. *B* and *C,* Pretarsal portions of the eyelid are debulked if needed. *D* and *E,* The inferior cut edge of the aponeurosis is secured to the edge of the pretarsal skin and the superior anterior tarsus using absorbable buried sutures. (From Flowers RS: Upper blepharoplasty by eyelid invagination: Anchor blepharoplasty. Clin Plast Surg 20: 193–207, 1993, with permission.)

In the **combination technique**, skin, with or without a sliver of muscle, is removed just above the level of suture creation of the lid fold. The lid sutures are placed through the open portion of the lid, and no additional small incisions are necessary on the lid.

A conservative **medial epicanthoplasty** is helpful in achieving a long aperture and avoiding the appearance of esotropia and/or telecanthus. It also assists in creating a lid crease that originates outside or just above the remaining small epicanthus and looks maximally normal.

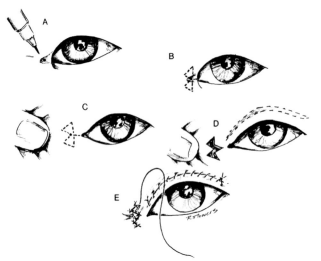

Flowers' modification of the Uchida medial epicanthoplasty. *A,* Mark the center point of the W 0.5–1.0 mm lateral to the desired medial endpoint of the canthus. *B* and *C,* The size of the W is varied with the size of the epicanthal fold. The V is made toward the medial canthus. *D,* The W incisions should not connect with the blepharoplasty incision. *E,* The W incision is typically closed with seven interrupted sutures. (From Flowers RS: Upper blepharoplasty by eyelid invagination: Anchor blepharoplasty. Clin Plast Surg 20:193–207, 1993, with permission.)

21. Where is the peripheral arterial arcade of the eyelid located?

The peripheral arterial arcade is located superior to the tarsus between the levator aponeurosis and Mueller's muscle. Many of these little arteries are within the substance of Mueller's muscle where it inserts into the tarsus. Great care must be taken in placing sutures into the cephalad margins of the tarsus to avoid these vessels. Puncture leads to hemorrhage into Mueller's muscle, which occasionally causes lid ptosis that may persist for 2 or 3 months after surgery.

An arcade is also located in the lower eyelid between the inferior tarsal muscle and lower eyelid retractors. These peripheral arcades anastomose with the marginal arcades that are located near the lid margins of both upper and lower eyelids. The marginal and peripheral arterial arcades serve as points of anastomosis between the internal and external carotid systems. These arcades receive contributions from the angular artery, which is a branch of the facial artery from the external carotid system, and from the terminal portions of the orbital artery, which arises from the internal carotid system.

22. When is a coronal lift contraindicated?

1. When one or more previous blepharoplasties have excised too much skin from the upper eyelids. Further brow elevation will result in lagophthalmos.

2. When manual elevation of the brows preoperatively reveals lid retraction with exposure of the upper limbus. In such cases a frontal lift should be performed only with a levator-lengthening procedure.

3. When a deep and unattractive hollowed-out upper lid is exposed or made worse by manual brow elevation, simulating the results of a surgical frontal lift.

4. When small eyelid apertures (measured horizontally, medial to lateral) are present. This is particularly relevant in men.

23. When is it appropriate to resect frontalis muscle?

Rarely, if ever. Sometimes a combination of blepharoplasty and frontal lift is required to eliminate transverse forehead wrinkling, especially when brow ptosis is profound and dermatochalasis or pseudoblepharoptosis of the eyelid is advanced.

24. Why does the medial brow commonly drop after blepharoplasty and/or elevation of the lateral brow?

The frontalis muscle inserts more effectively into the medial brow than into the lateral brow. When most people raise their eyebrows, the medial end elevates more than the lateral brow. The thin residual lateral overhang drives the frontalis contraction, causing an overcorrection of the medial brow to clear adequately the lateral upper lid overhang. When the lateral overhang is cleared through either blepharoplasty or lateral brow elevation (via direct excision or frontal lift), the medial brow will always drop. The cause is frontalis muscle relaxation.

25. How does one plan a medial epicanthoplasty?

Prominent epicanthal folds are common in many people, particularly Asians. These little canopies covering the medial apertures are best corrected with a small W-shaped incision, with the wide part of the W facing laterally and the small part facing medially. The middle portion of the W should be level with and point directly to the medial canthus. After completion of the design, excision of small skin triangles from the wings of the W follows—often joined centrally by a 1–2-mm bridge. Closure is done with interrupted 6-0 sutures. This is an excellent technique for removing small or large epicanthal folds common to all races. We believe that the most effective approach to epicanthal folds is this Flowers modification of the Uchida "split V-W" epicanthoplasty. (See figure at bottom of previous page.)

26. How does one avoid lash or lid eversion and areas of lid retraction associated with invagination blepharoplasty?

In performing an invagination blepharoplasty, the surgeon must take care not to attach the pretarsal skin segment under excessive tension when anchoring it to the tarsus and/or aponeurosis. Tension on the pretarsal skin causes the eyelashes to evert or turn upward, giving an abnormal "surprised" appearance, whether the procedure is done in Asians or Caucasians. Tension on the pre-tarsal skin can be adjusted by changing the level at which the skin is anchored on the tarsus. Careful measurements of the height of the tarsus and the amount of skin for resection during blepharoplasty should be part of the preoperative assessment. In most normal adults a minimum of 30 mm of skin be-tween the eyebrow and eyelashes should remain to allow attractive lid contour and normal function. The amount of excessive skin overhang obscuring the pretarsal lid multiplied by two gives an ap-proximation of how much skin needs to be removed. One-and-a-half to 2 mm should be added to the pretarsal measurement to allow for the tightly stretched skin and invagination "turn-in" and another millimeter to accommodate the distal end of the overhang.

27. Are wedge resections and tarsal strip canthopexies recommended procedures for tightening the lower lid?

Various techniques are available for tightening the lower lid. Traditional wedge resections usu-ally shorten the aperture and sometimes result in notching of the lid margin. Thus, they should be re-served for gaping ectropions. The tarsal strip procedure, if done properly on carefully selected patients, may prove extremely helpful. Our preferred technique for tightening the lower lid in the vast majority of patients is a canthopexy anchoring the lateral retinaculum of the lower eyelid into the bone just inside the lateral orbital rim. Anchoring the retinaculum into bone results in a tighten-ing and/or lateral canthal lift and provides permanent and secure lateral canthopexy with long-term excellent results. Wedge resections fail to correct the commonly dropped tilt of the intercanthal axis lid while shortening the lid aperture.

28. What are the pros and cons of the endoscopic forehead lift?

The main advantage of the endoscopic forehead lift is less total scar length on the scalp, which may be of particular benefit for men or even women with various balding patterns. Another advantage is a potential for less bleeding because fewer scalp vessels are cut in the process. Usually only 3–5 incisions measuring 1.5–2.0 cm are made within the hairline for endoscopic techniques.

The disadvantages of the endoscopic forehead lift are numerous. Complete removal of the cor-rugator muscles, which is one of the most important aspects of forehead lifting, is difficult. It is also more difficult to identify tissue planes accurately, which increases the risk of injury to important motor branches of the facial nerve. It is far more difficult to perform periosteal anchoring flaps for extra help in positioning the eyebrows—especially with asymmetrically ptotic brows. Another major problem is that canthopexies into the bone are far more difficult through an endoscopic approach. Lastly, the blind subperiosteal dissection leads to common transection of aberrant or anomalous courses of the supraorbital and supratrochlear nerves.

An open technique allows thorough visualization of the corrugator, depressor supercilii, and procerus muscles; access to the periosteum above the orbital rim for periosteal flap anchoring proce-dures; good access to the orbital rim for canthopexies and contouring; and full and comprehensive visualization of the tissue planes.

29. Are transblepharoplasty methods of corrugator muscle resection and brow elevation ef-fective for eliminating deformity? How do they compare with other techniques?

Transblepharoplasty approaches may improve the deformity but do not compare with the effec-tiveness of a direct maximal excision. When removal of the corrugator muscle is incomplete, there are other methods to decrease the corrugator frown, such as repeated injections with botulinum toxin, collagen injections, cutting the motor nerve to the corrugator, or placement of alloplasts. But these are ways of compensating for an operation that failed to achieve its goal. The route to the cor-rugator muscles through a blepharoplasty incision is lengthy and somewhat tedious, making precise corrugator removal without injury extremely difficult. Precise identification of the supratrochlear nerve and its isolation from the corrugator muscle before muscle excision become quite difficult. Transblepharoplasty approaches, in our opinion, are typically inadequate for complete removal of the corrugator muscle.

30. When is a direct excision of lower eyelid skin indicated?

Direct excision of varying amounts of lower eyelid skin is often indicated for patients who have true excess rather than merely a dropped lid posture or pseudoexcess. Extreme care must be taken so that skin removal does not result in a pulling down or rounding of the lower eyelids. This problem always occurs unless some type of lid support procedure or canthopexy is also performed. Counsel all patients about the impossibility of completely removing the wrinkles of the lower eyelid—especially during smiling. Often some type of resurfacing, either with laser modalities or chemical peel, may be the preferred treatment, but consideration should be given to canthopexy support. Skin may, of course, be removed independently or as a portion of a skin-muscle flap, depending on the surgical procedure. Our preference is a short skin flap combined with a muscle procedure near the base of the skin flap, which gives access to the deeper tissues of the lid. It is unusual to need more than several millimeters of lower eyelid skin removal.

31. What is the best method to rid a patient of the deep grooves commonly present near the junction of the eyelid and cheek skin?

Deep grooves near the junction of the eyelid and cheek are either tear trough deformities or nasojugal grooves. With the tear trough deformity, the problem is primarily a bone defect. The nasojugal groove represents the muscular deficiency between the orbicularis oculi muscle and the angular head of the levator labii superioris (levator labii superioris alaque nasi).

Different techniques have been used through the years. Loeb, Flowers, Hamra, and others have described techniques in which pedicles of orbital fat are mobilized into these areas. Free fat can be injected or transplanted as another method. The Flowers tear trough implant is the best option when a palpating finger clearly discerns and defines a suborbital malar bony defect. In such instances, an eyelet cut within the implant accommodates passage of the infraorbital nerve. The implant fits nicely into the defect, allowing attachment to the inferior orbital rim periosteum. Small holes made throughout the implant allow tissue ingrowth and fixation. Implants may be inserted through subciliary, transconjunctival, intraoral, or direct incisions, but the transconjunctival incision is best reserved for patients without prominent supraorbital ridges. Free grafts commonly leave irregularities, and fat injections leave palpable and often visible ridges, which are unacceptable to patients.

32. How does one permanently secure the brow into its desired (elevated) position?

Many techniques have been used. Surgeons involved in endoscopic brow-lifting sometimes use screws, plates, or permanent sutures to anchor the brow until adequate healing and fibrosis are able to secure the brow in its new position. Similar techniques can be used with open large flap procedures, but fixation hardware is less frequently required. With the open procedures, markedly improved fixation is available by removal of the superficial temporal fascia or subgaleal tissue in the parietotemporal area. This method allows good fibrosis of the forehead flap to the skull. It is easy to overcorrect the medial brow and difficult to adequately correct the lateral brow. For these reasons, periosteal flaps are often used in developmentally low brows as a method for securing them into an elevated location. Superiorly based periosteal flaps are inserted into an incision made within the eyebrow hairs at the junction of the medial and lateral thirds of the eyebrows. The flap is taken just at the border of the temporalis fascia. This technique limits the caudal descent of the brow, but the brow can still be raised by frontalis animation. It is far better than methods that fix the brow in place without allowing movement.

33. What is Whitnall's ligament?

It is a condensation of the sheath overlying the anterior superior part of the levator muscle. Medially, it arises from connective tissue of the frontal bone posterior to the trochlea. Laterally, it attaches to the capsule of the orbital lobe of the lacrimal gland and to the frontal bone portion of the lateral orbital wall approximately 10 mm above the lateral orbital tubercle. This structure is the point at which the direction of pull of the levator muscle changes from a horizontal to a vertical direction, and it serves to limit the elevation of the eyelid with check ligaments. During blepharoptosis procedures it is important not to suture Whitnall's ligament to the tarsus or other eyelid structures because this may result in a permanent lagophthalmos or inability to close the eyes. The superior transverse ligament was first described by Whitnall in 1910.

34. What is Lockwood's ligament?

It is a hammocklike system with contributions from the inner muscular septae, Tenon's capsule, and the lower eyelid retractors. Posteriorly, Lockwood's ligament arises from fibrous attachments from the inferior side of the inferior rectus muscle and continues anteriorly as the capsular palpebral fascia and lower eyelid retractors. This suspensory system has medial and lateral horns that extend into the retinacula. The medial retinaculum, in turn, attaches to the posterior lacrimal crest, and the lateral retinaculum attaches to the lateral orbital tubercle of Whitnall. The suspensory system of the globe was initially described by Lockwood in 1886.

35. In patients with eyelid liner tattoos, where should the lower eyelid blepharoplasty incisions be placed?

If a person wants the tattoos removed, a subciliary incision superior to the tattoos usually allows its eradication, provided that sufficient lower lid skin is present. Do not forget the supporting maneuver. If the patient wants to preserve the tattoos, make the lid incision just at the caudal margin of the tattooed eyeliner. This method helps to prevent the eventual "bleed" of the tattoo pigment into eyelid skin. Tattoos on the gray line cannot be removed.

36. Which cranial nerve innervates the lacrimal pump that drains the tears?

The seventh cranial nerve innervates the orbicularis oculi. The deep heads of the medial pretarsal and preseptal orbicularis oculi contract and exert traction on the fascia immediately lateral to the lacrimal sac, known as the lacrimal diaphragm. This traction during contraction of the orbicularis creates a relatively negative pressure within the lacrimal sac that draws tears through the puncta and cannaliculi into the lacrimal sac. Relaxation of the orbicularis oculi allows the lacrimal sac to collapse, and the tears traverse the nasolacrimal duct to the nose.

37. During blepharoplasty, where is the "white" fat?

The medial or nasal upper eyelid fat typically has a color that is paler—white or yellow-white—than other fat of the eyelids and orbit. The lateral fat of the upper eyelid has a deeper yellow color. The medial fat pad of the upper lid may move anteriorly more prominently than the other fat pads, resulting in a large bulge of the upper medial eyelid just inferior to the trochlea of the upper medial orbit. Often there is a hollowed-out defect in the area between the white medial fat compartment and the lateral "yellow" fat compartment, where the nasal portion of the aponeurotic sling housing the fat migrates superiorly.

DISCLOSURE

The tear trough implants discussed in this text were designed by Robert S. Flowers, M.D., and manufactured by Implantech. Currently they are marketed by Mentor Corporation. Dr. Flowers receives a small royalty for each pair of implants purchased.

BIBLIOGRAPHY

1. Flowers RS: Upper blepharoplasty by eyelid invagination: Anchor blepharoplasty. Clin Plast Surg 20:193–207, 1993.
2. Flowers RS: Optimal procedure in secondary blepharoplasty. Clin Plast Surg 20:225–237, 1993.
3. Flowers RS: Canthopexy as a routine blepharoplasty component. Clin Plast Surg 20:351–365, 1993.
4. Flowers RS: Tear trough implants for correction of tear trough deformity. Clin Plast Surg 20:403–415, 1993.
5. Flowers RS: The biomechanics of brow and frontalis function and its effect on blepharoplasty. Clin Plast Surg 20:225–268, 1993.
6. Flowers RS: Cosmetic blepharoplasty—state of the art. Adv Plast Reconstr Surg 8:31–67, 1992.
7. Flowers RS: Periorbital aesthetic surgery for men. Clin Plast Surg 18:689–729, 1991.
8. Smith EM, Dryden RM: Eyelids: Anatomy, ectropion, entropion, blepharoptosis, blepharoplasty and abnormalities. In Chern KC, Wright KW (eds): Review of Ophthalmology: A Question and Answer Book. Baltimore, Williams & Wilkins, 1997.

54. THE NASOLABIAL FOLD

Marcello Pantaloni, M.D., and Jeffrey Weinzweig, M.D.

1. What are the nasolabial crease (NLC), nasolabial fold (NLF), and malar fat pad?

The NLC, or sulcus, is the facial line between the upper lip and cheek, extending from the alae nasi to the lip commissure. The crease may extend superiorly to the side of the nose and inferiorly below the commissure. The NLF is the bulging fat pad and skin lateral to the NLC. The malar fat pad is the triangular fat pad with its base along the NLC and, in young people, its apex along the body of the zygoma. It lies over the zygomaticus major muscle, levator labii superioris muscle, and orbital portion of the orbicularis oculi muscle.

2. What are marionette lines?

Bilateral inferior extensions of the NLC below the commissure resemble the vertical lines on the lower face of a ventriloquist's dummy and are thus referred to as marionette lines.

3. What is one of the more noticeable aesthetic changes between a young adult and the same person 30 years later?

Deepening of the NLC and accentuation of the fold with concomitant inferior, lateral, and anterior displacement of the check mass and the tissue lateral to the fold occur with aging. The inferior migration of the cheek mass leaves a noticeable hollow in the infraorbital area.

4. What is the anatomy of the NLF area?

In the superficial layer the subcutaneous tissue from the adjacent cheek area crosses the NLF in the upper lip, where it changes to a dense, thin fascial-fatty layer closely attached to the skin and to the superficial portion of the orbicularis oris muscle. Beneath the subcutaneous tissue the submuscular aponeurotic system (SMAS) extends across the NLF and merges with the superficial portion of the orbicularis oris muscle of the upper lip. The deep layer of the orbicularis oris muscle merges with the superficial layer at the NLF, together with the SMAS.

5. What are mimetic muscles? What is the relationship between the SMAS and the mimetic musculature near the NLF?

The mimetic musculature is composed of individual muscles that receive their innervation from the facial nerve and are responsible for facial movement. The mimetic muscles and superficial facial fascia (SMAS) function as a single anatomic unit in producing movement of the facial skin. The SMAS is intimately associated with the mimetic muscles; muscle contracture is translated into movement of overlying facial skin through the vertical fibrous septa extending from the SMAS into the dermis. Anatomically the SMAS divides into superficial and deep fascial leaves and invests or surrounds the superficially lying mimetic muscles (platysma, orbicularis oculi, zygomaticus major and minor, and risorius). The investiture of the mimetic muscles by the SMAS forms a single functional anatomic layer with muscle and fascia working in continuity to produce movement of facial skin.

6. What is the anatomic and clinical difference between the tissue medial and lateral to the NLC?

The tissue medial to the crease has subcutaneous muscle attachments that protect against the effect of gravity. Lateral to the crease the muscle does not insert into the skin and thus remains without deep support. For this reason, the lateral tissue descends at a quicker rate than the medial tissue.

7. What are the retaining ligaments of the face?

Facial skin is supported in normal anatomic position by retaining ligaments that run from deep, fixed facial structures to the overlying dermis. The two types of retaining ligaments are (1) true osteocutaneous ligaments, which are a series of fibrous bands that run from periosteum to dermis (e.g., zygomatic and mandibular ligaments), and (2) supporting ligaments formed by a coalescence between the superficial and deep facial fascias in certain regions of the face (e.g., parotidocutaneous and masseteric cutaneous ligaments). (See figure at top of next page.)

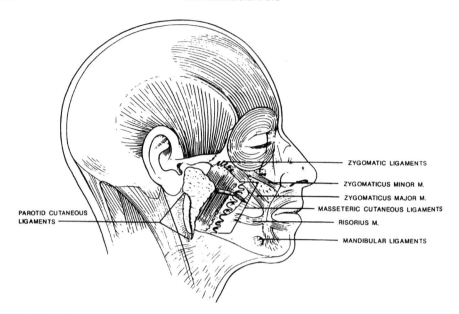

Facial soft tissue is supported in normal anatomic location by a series of retaining ligaments. The zygomatic and mandibular ligaments are examples of osteocutaneous ligaments that originate from periosteum and insert directly into dermis. The masseteric and parotid cutaneous ligaments are formed as condensations between the superficial and deep facial fascias. Rather than originating from periosteum, these ligaments originate from relatively fixed facial structures such as the parotid gland and the anterior border of the masseter muscle. Attenuation of support from these ret aining ligaments is responsible for many of the stigmata seen in the aging face, including deepening of the NLC and increased prominence of the NLF. (From Stuzin JM, Baker TJ, Gordon HL: The relationship of the superficial and deep facial fascia: Relevance to rhytidectomy and aging. Plast Reconstr Surg 89:441, 1992, with permission.)

8. Which of the retaining ligaments suspend the malar fat pad?

The zygomatic ligaments, which are a series of fibrous septa that originate from the periosteum of the malar region. They begin where the zygomatic arch joins the body of the zygoma and continue over the malar eminence. A particularly stout ligament originates along the most medial portion of the zygoma near the zygomaticomaxillary suture. The fibers composing the zygomatic ligament extend through the malar fat pad (McGregor's patch) and attach to the dermis of the malar skin to suspend the fat pad over the underlying zygomatic eminence.

9. Does any other anatomic structure contribute to supporting the malar fat pad?

The maxillary eminence. Patients with a greater anterior slope of the maxilla have increased support of the cheek tissue and less prominent NLF.

10. What is the cause of a prominent NLF?

Aging is associated with attenuation of the zygomatic retaining ligaments. Because of ligamentous laxity, the malar soft tissue migrates downward along the direction of the zygomaticus major muscle, bulging against the NLC. The skin lateral to the crease stretches and becomes redundant, forming a prominent NLF.

11. What are the sequential migration vectors of the cheek mass?

Initially, the migration vectors are inferior and parallel to the contraction of the mimetic muscles and perpendicular to the NLC. When inferior movement is restrained by the dermal-fascial attachments of the NLC, the tissue slides laterally and anteriorly over the crease with accentuation of the NLF.

12. What is the role of midface muscle in a prominent NLF?

The mimetic muscle contraction transmits a shearing force on the fascial attachments between the SMAS and overlying subcutaneous tissue and skin. The malar fat pad migrates downward and forward, producing a prominent NLF. Accentuated contraction of the levator muscle, as seen with smiling, pulls cephalically and deepens the NLC with further bulging of the ptotic fat pad.

13. What is the effect of facial nerve paralysis on NLF appearance?

Facial nerve paralysis results in less prominence of the fold because the tissue medial to the crease no longer has underlying support and descends in a similar fashion to the lateral tissue.

14. What can you inject or insert in the NLC to improve its appearance?

Both autologous tissue and implants may be used. Fat and collagen can be injected in the NLC. In addition, fat, dermis and dermal-fat grafts as well as silicone and Gore-Tex implants are often inserted beneath the NLC.

15. When should fat injection of the NLC be considered?

Fat injection of the NLC is used rarely. This technique is considered in patients who wish to avoid more aggressive and definitive procedures. The best candidate for fat injection is the patient with thick skin and slight prominence of the fold.

16. Who is the best candidate for direct crease excision?

The patient with a deep crease, thin skin (a rare combination), and a fold that is not very prominent is the best candidate for crease excision.

17. What can we offer a patient with thick skin and slight fold prominence who prefers a minimally invasive procedure?

Fat injection or a dermal-fat graft may be used. The fat is obtained from the deep plane of the lower abdomen and injected beneath the crease after releasing the fibrous bands between dermis and muscle. With this technique it is important to overcorrect; the result is unpredictable because of the variable survival of the injected fat cells.

The dermal-fat graft may be harvested from the suprapubic area or groin and inserted beneath the crease after releasing the bands and undermining the NLF. The thickness of the graft must be directly proportional to the thickness of the skin. The graft thickens the soft tissue and prevents reattachment of fibrous bands to the dermis. Some surgeons use a SMAS graft. For both techniques the principal advantage is the minimal scar; the disadvantage is the unpredictable and modest improvement achieved.

18. How can the malar fat pad be repositioned?

Elevation and tightening of the skin-subcutaneous flap or the SMAS flap can reposition the malar fat pad.

19. How extensive need the SMAS dissection be to elevate the malar fat pad to its original position and decrease NLF prominence?

The SMAS dissection must reach the malar region, continuing medially beyond the area of subcutaneous undermining over the inferolateral orbicularis oculi muscle. The zygomatic and masseteric ligaments must then be released as well as the ligaments medial to the zygomaticus minor muscle. The division of these restraints allows greater mobility of the malar portion of the SMAS and the NLF. The malar fat pad, along with the SMAS, is repositioned over the zygomatic eminence, perpendicular to the NLC and parallel to the zygomaticus major muscle. The amount of undermining varies for each patient; for severe midface laxity and migration of the fat pad, undermining should reach the NLC level.

20. With the extended SMAS dissection, what step should be performed at the level of the zygomaticus major muscle to maximize resuspension of the malar fat pad?

Because of the tethering effect of the mimetic muscles, to which the SMAS is closely attached, traction exerted on the cheek flap is not transmitted to the NLF. This tethering effect is maximal at the bony origin of the zygomaticus major muscle. To maximize the traction on the NLF prominence, the SMAS is transected at the level of the zygomaticus major muscle and the dissection is continued above the superficial leaf of the SMAS. This maneuver frees the SMAS from the attached mimetic muscles and allows the force pulling on the skin and fat superior and lateral to the NLC to be transmitted to the NLC.

21. What change do you expect in the NLF with superior and lateral SMAS pulling without releasing the SMAS from the zygomaticus major muscle?

The pulling of the SMAS shortens the mimetic muscles between the modiolus and their bony origin. The overlying soft tissue moves for a smaller distance than the muscle. The pull is transmitted from the SMAS to the orbicularis oris muscle medial to the crease. The medial tissue moves superiorly and laterally for a greater extent than the lateral tissue, which is attached less strongly to the underlying structures. The consequences of these dynamic changes are deepening of the NLC and accentuation of the NLF. A similar situation can be seen during smiling. The actions of the zygomaticus major muscle and deep orbicularis oris muscle transmit a similar pulling to the medial tissue via the joining structure, the SMAS.

22. In the malar fat pad suspension technique, the fat pad vector is the skin flap. Describe this approach.

The skin-subcutaneous flap incorporates the malar fat pad, which needs to be completely dissected from the underlying retaining ligaments. The platysma-SMAS flap is elevated as needed. A fixation suture is sewn from the apex of the fat pad to the superficial fascia of the malar eminence or deep temporal fascia. The suture is placed along a line perpendicular to the NLC about 2 cm above and 1 cm in front of the ear until the pad is maximally elevated.

23. When the malar fat pad is based within a skin flap vector, what is the direction and the amount of fat pad lifting needed to correct the NLF?

The direction of the lifting is superolateral and roughly perpendicular to the crease. With mild laxity the fat pad can be repositioned and adequately supported by the cheek flap alone. With more severe laxity a wider and stronger repositioning is needed, necessitating a suspension technique.

24. What is the role of suction-assisted lipectomy in corrective surgery of the NLF?

After raising the SMAS for the extent required to obtain repositioning of the ptotic malar pad, any residual fullness of the NLF area can be sculpted under direct vision using a 3 or 4 mm liposuction cannula. Alternatively, direct excision of fat in this region can be performed, but the risk of bleeding is higher with this technique.

25. What is the role of the subperiosteal approach in corrective surgery of the NLF?

The subperiosteal approach allows detachment of the central third of the face at the subperiosteal level. After SMAS and subcutaneous dissection, superior and lateral pulling allows transmission of the forces to the full thickness of the NLC and NLF areas that are completely freed from the underlying bone. Movement of the tissue to a higher and more lateral position results in flattening of the NLF.

26. What is the recommended amount of undermining below the fat pad to correct the NLF?

The amount of undermining varies for each patient but should be extensive. For mild midface laxity and mildly prominent NLF, the undermining should extend beyond the malar eminence over the inferolateral orbicularis oculi muscle to the origin of the zygomaticus major muscle. For more severe midface laxity and migration of the fat pad, the entire fat pad should be undermined to the level of the NLC.

BIBLIOGRAPHY

1. Barton FE Jr: Rhytidectomy and the nasolabial fold. Plast Reconstr Surg 90:601, 1992.
2. Barton FE Jr: The SMAS and the nasolabial fold. Plast Reconstr Surg 89:1054, 1992.
3. Barton FE Jr, Gyimesi IM: Anatomy of the nasolabial fold. Plast Reconstr Surg 100:1276, 1997.
4. Furnas DW: The retaining ligaments of the cheek. Plast Reconstr Surg 83:11, 1989.
5. Furnas DW: Strategies for nasolabial levitation. Clin Plast Surg 22:265, 1995.
6. Guyuron B: The armamentarium to battle the recalcitrant nasolabial fold. Clin Plast Surg 22:253, 1995.
7. Owsley JQ: Elevation of the malar fat pad superficial to the orbicularis oculi muscle for correction of prominent nasolabial folds. Clin Plast Surg 22:279, 1995.
8. Rubin LR, Mishriki Y, Lee G: Anatomy of the nasolabial fold: The keystone of the smiling mechanism. Plast Reconstr Surg 83:1, 1989.
9. Stuzin JM, Baker TJ, Gordon HL: The relationship of the superficial and deep facial fascias: Relevance to rhytidectomy and aging. Plast Reconstr Surg 89:441, 1992.
10. Yousif NJ, Mendelson BC: Anatomy of the midface. Clin Plast Surg 22:227, 1995.
11. Zufferey J: Anatomic variations of the nasolabial fold. Plast Reconstr Surg 89:225, 1992.

55. RHYTIDECTOMY

*Rexford A. Peterson, M.D., F.A.C.S., Tia Peterson,
and Daniel C. Mills, II, M.D., F.A.C.S.*

1. What is a face lift?

A face lift is a multiprocedure surgical operation for the purpose of rejuvenation of the facial contours, including all regions of the face and the anterior and lateral cervical areas.

2. What is the most important first step in face lift surgery?

Diagnosis. When a physician arrives at a diagnosis, the appropriate treatment is usually clear. In face-lift surgery, the detailed structure-by-structure observation, examination, and evaluation of the cervicofacial regions form a valuable diagnostic record that points to the appropriate surgical approach. Recommendations for aesthetic facial corrections may be custom-designed for each person, while envisioning future needs for the maintenance and preservation of the improvement to be gained. If your patients have similar vision and the will and ability to pursue the same goals, a continuing, more youthful appearance may be preserved for as long as 15 years.

3. To determine the proper facial rejuvenation procedure(s) for any patient, what else must you know?

In order to achieve patient satisfaction, it is essential to ascertain the patient's goal(s). Many patients present themselves having already "diagnosed" their situation and "prescribed" their treatment. (They have already decided they would like a face lift before an appointment with a plastic surgeon is scheduled.) For instance, patients may come to you saying they want "liposuction" of the anterior neck, thinking it will "lift" the neck and cheeks, whereas a SMAS (superficial musculoaponeurotic system) face lift or "composite" face lift would be required to achieve that goal.

In order to give the best advice to aesthetic plastic surgery patients, it is necessary to understand *their* goals in rejuvenation surgery. Understanding comes from *listening* to the patient. It is also necessary to evaluate objectively all the features of the head, face, and neck regions. Preoperative Evaluation and Recommendation forms[6] provide excellent medicolegal data, which reveal the scope of your exam and observations. The evaluation should be a careful, thorough record of all areas of the face and neck.

After listening to the patient's goals and recording a complete facial evaluation, the surgeon writes a menu of recommended face-lift and ancillary procedures considered ideal for the patient's facial conditions.

4. What are the different types of face-lift procedures?

There are four basic types of face-lift surgeries:
1. Skin only
2. Skin and submuscular aponeurotic system (SMAS)-platysma
3. Skin and SMAS-platysma and mid-face suspension
4. Deep plane and/or a combination of 1, 2, and 3

5. Which do you recommend for a patient who has never had a face lift?

The recommendation depends on the results of the evaluation. A skin-only face lift is recommended if the primary face-lift patient has early laxity and rhytids of the face and neck skin but *does not have* platysmal cords, SMAS laxity, jowls, marionette down lines, submalar concavity, or any other feature of deep facial tissue relaxation due to aging. The presence, degree, and extent of SMAS-platysmal laxity *and* contour abnormalities determine the type of face lift to be recommended, and the choice of additional concomitant procedures such as areas of liposuction, chin or malar augmentation, mid-face suspension, lip augmentation, chin contouring, forehead-brow lifting, and perhaps others.

If the SMAS-platysma and nasolabial tissues are ptotic, the skin is also ptotic, for these musculofascial tissues are *of the skin.* Hence, one recommends a skin and deep-layer (SMAS-platysma) face lift, at the least. Early, before skin redundancy and rhytids have become pronounced, skin-only lifting may suffice but also may be combined with endoscopic lifts. If the deep tissues need lifting in all regions, it is our opinion to rely on double-layer, skin, and deep-tissue lifting techniques.

6. What are the indications for plication of the medial margins of the platysma in a primary face lift?

Ptosis of the platysma in the anterior cervical region, with the presence of redundant, lax medial platysmal bands or cords.

7. Would you do another SMAS-platysma deep-tissue lift on a person who had one several years before?

A previous complete SMAS lift may well contraindicate a secondary extensive deep-layer lift, because the SMAS may be thinner and more difficult to dissect, thus risking injury to the facial nerve. An alternate option would be a plication of the cheek and mandibular area SMAS (as recommended by Skoog[11]) and a secondary lift-imbrication of the platysma.

8. What would you recommend for a patient who has had an extensive SMAS lift and desires further lifting?

You cannot answer this question without a thorough re-evaluation to establish a new diagnosis and surgical treatment plan. However, these and *all* face-lift patients will be significantly improved by skin-only lifts, with small to moderate dissection-undermining. These cheek-and-neck tucks may be combined with pertinent corrections of the deep tissues, such as plication of the cheek SMAS, lifting and imbrication of the platysma, mid-face suspension, medial platysmal plication, etc., as may be indicated by the patient's diagnosis.

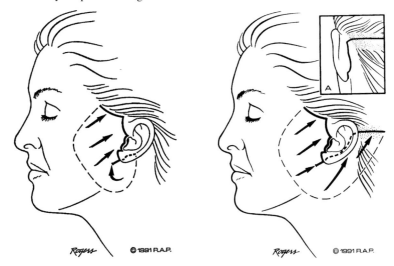

Left, Skin-only mini-lift. Incision schematic for a mini-tuck or secondary cheek tuck, showing placement of a temporal hairline incision to avoid obliteration of the temporal sideburns as well as the skin undermining dissection and lift vectors. The incision into the facial flap at the ear lobe is directed toward the mentum. *Right,* Skin-only midi-lift. Incision, skin undermining, and left vectors for a "midi-tuck" procedure. (Copyright © 1991, R.A. Peterson, M.D., F.A.C.S., with permission.)

9. What are the indications for a secondary skin-only face lift?

Recurrent minor skin laxity of the face and neck after a previous face lift of any type.

10. Do repeated tucks cause a drawn or "face-lifted" appearance?

No. The minimal skin undermining dissection prevents a drawn appearance. The facial contours, expressions, and skin continue to look good and natural. Such patients usually have a better appearance 15–20 years after a primary face lift than they had before their first operation. However, an excessively "lifted" appearance will result if secondary operations remove additional temporal and/or postauricular hair-bearing skin. A high hairline thus created is disfiguring and a stigma of a poorly planned operation.[7]

11. What is the best secret in face-lift surgery?

First lift, then . . . tuck . . . tuck . . . tuck.

12. When does a patient need a deep-plane lift of the mid-face?

When there is ptosis of the mid-face (the region medial from the lateral canthi of the lids to the corners of the mouth). Ptosis may include significant nasolabial and nasojugal creases, marionette down lines, and sagging of the malar tissues below the infraorbital rim.

13. What contours are rejuvenated by a mid-face lift?

The contours of the infraorbital, malar, and submalar areas become more youthful in appearance. The downward marionette lines from the oral commissures and the adjacent cheek contours are improved and may even be eradicated.

14. What is the vector of lift in a mid-face suspension?

In a line that is perpendicular to the nasolabial fold, from the lateral nasal ala to the lateral canthus of the eyelids.

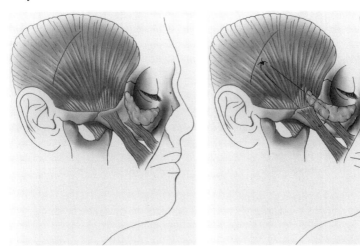

Left, Mid-face suspension incisions. Through a lower blepharoplasty incision a pocket is dissected down to the deep plane to mobilize the tissues of the mid-face. This pocket is packed, and an incision is made in the temporal scalp to the plane between the superficial portion of the deep temporal fascia and the superficial temporal fascia. The plane is dissected down to and along the zygomatic arch and connects with the dissection of the mid-face. *Right,* Mid-face suspension. A suspension suture is placed via the blepharoplasty approach in the SOOF as well as in the the periosteum. The suture ends are drawn up through the temporal incision area and anchored on the superficial portion of the deep temporal fascia. The vector of lift is 90° from the nasolabial line. (Copyright © 1996, D.C. Mills, M.D., F.A.C.S., with permission.)

15. How are the lifted tissues of the mid-face anchored?

To maintain the lift of the mid-face, it is necessary to anchor the tissues to something unyielding, such as through the periosteum at the suborbicularis oculi fat (SOOF) into the superficial portion of the deep temporal fascia. Suspension to nonstable tissues, such as other fat or SMAS, does not give as good a result.

16. What are the indications for an endoscopic face lift?

An endoscopic face lift is a valid procedure for young patients having mid-face ptosis without significant skin laxity of the face or neck. However, it is *not* indicated for every face-lift patient and is not a substitute for the open face lift requiring correction of laxity of the skin, SMAS, platysma, and mentum.

Small temporal and preauricular incisions provide endoscopic access for lifting and suspension of the deep tissues, including the malar region periosteum. The mid-face endoscopic lift may be combined with an endoscopic forehead-brow lift and upper/lower blepharoplasties. These procedures are less invasive than larger, open-technique lifts.

If using an open face-lift technique, there is no need to extend the dissection endoscopically, as a fiberoptic retractor provides direct vision for the mid-face suspension procedures. The methods of face-lift techniques you may choose will have evolved in continuum from the works of Skoog, Millard, Peterson, Owsley, Connell, Tessier, Ortiz-Monaterio, Hamra, Ramirez, Stuzin, Heinrichs, and subsequent face-lift authors.

17. What are the common tell-tale signs of face-lift surgery?
- Visible scars (from poorly planned incisions and lift dynamics)
- Overlifting of the temporal hairline
- Stepped occipital hairline
- Distorted traguses and distorted auditory meatuses, no longer shielded by appropriate tragal positions (caused by excessive cheek flap tension and a retrotragal incision)
- Distorted earlobes (from an error in skin flap vector dynamics and incision placement)
- "Drapery swag" of the cheek and neck skin due to incorrect lift vectors
- Lack of balance in the lift of the face and neck (e.g., a patient with tightened smooth cheeks, but deformities such as a ptotic, wrinkled brow/forehead region, a senile chin ("witch's chin") deformity, or persistent platysmal cords)
- Inadequate lifting in any facial region

18. What are the acceptable incisions for the preauricular incision and the indications for each?
The **contoured pretragal incision** is a good choice (1) if the tragus is protruding and there is a preauricular rhytid, (2) in older patients, (3) in male patients, and (4) for smokers or other patients with the possibility of impaired cutaneous circulation. After lifting the cheek flap and avoiding undue skin tension, repair should be done with fine, inverted dermal sutures and carefully placed fine surface sutures. Incisions following the contours of the helix, tragus, and lobule normally result in invisible scars.

Indications for a **tragal edge incision** are (1) small, flat, nonprotruding traguses, (2) youthful female patients *without* a pronounced pretragal rhytid, and (3) nonsmokers. The tragal edge incision provides an invisible incisional scarline without having to wrap the lifted cheek skin inside the tragus, thereby avoiding the distortion of the normal tragal contours that may occur with a retrotragal incision.

Indications for a **retrotragal incision** are similar to the those for the tragal edge incision. However, this incision may cause deformity or obliteration of the tragal contour and may distort the tragal shielding of the auditory meatus, causing the appearance of an enlarged cavernous meatus. These deformities are overt signs of face-lift surgery.

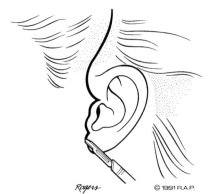

Contoured pretragal incision pattern. The contoured pretragal incision is the best incision placement for patients who match the discussed indications. The scar is essentially invisible and does not distort the tragus or auditory meatus. (Copyright © 1991, R.A. Peterson, M.D., F.A.C.S., with permission.)

19. How does a surgeon obtain an invisible scar in the postauricular skin?
First, by logical thought about the effect of tissue tensions as dynamic forces that can cause migration of incisional scars to conspicuous areas.

Second, by placing vertical incisions behind the ear precisely in the sulcus between the ear and mastoid area and repairing these carefully, as follows:

1. The vertical postauricular incision should be made in the exact junction of the postauricular skin and the posterior ear skin by placing it deep in the postauricular sulcus.

2. The incision should be turned horizontally across the scalp at a point at least two-thirds of the distance from the lobular sulcus to the superior extremity of the concha. The angle should be almost 90° and the horizontal incision into the scalp along the occipital ridge about 7.5 cm in length.

3. Tension is placed on the cervicofacial flap at the temporal incision and mastoid incision edges in a supero-oblique direction.

4. The cervicofacial skin flap is repaired to the lobule with a dermis-conchal fascia-lobular dermis inverted suture.

5. The postauricular and occipital flap is placed under tension with three Allis clamps spaced about 2 cm apart on the superior horizontal edge of the flap, taking care to spread out the upward tension away from the ear.

6. A *very narrow* strip of postauricular skin is excised adjacent to the the vertical (or sulcus) edge to avoid convergent draping of cervical rhytids toward the ear.

7. The postauricular skin flap is aligned for a perfect match with the posterior conchal skin. The dermis of the postauricular flap is repaired deep into the sulcus (which may, if desired, be made deeper by electrosurgical incision) and to the dermis of the postauricular skin with one or two inverted 5-0 sutures.

8. The skin edges are repaired with a continuous 5-0 suture from the lobular to the superior incisional angle.

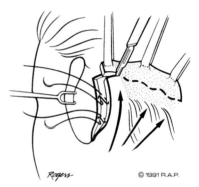

Postauricular resection. Very little skin (4 mm or less) is excised along the anterior edge from lobule to scalp. Note the vectors of the lift dynamics. (Copyright © 1991, R.A. Peterson, M.D., F.A.C.S., with permission.)

20. How does a surgeon avoid creating a "step" or surgical distortion of the occipital hairline?

Again, it is a matter of analyzing the tension dynamics of the postauricular skin flap and scar lines and placing the incisions so that excised skin will alter the hairline only minimally, if at all. Do not ever assume that male or female patients desire to lose hair-bearing skin behind the ears; therefore, strive to accomplish goals of concealing the scars without too much hair loss.

1. The appropriate amounts of scalp and postauricular flap skin are removed by excising the superior flap edge in a wavy, undulating line or sweeping curve within the scalp from the posterior apex of the incision to the hairline. Matching a longer, curved flap incision to the shorter, straight superior skin edge incision makes it possible to restore the natural alignment of the hair in the primary face lift.

2. The wavy scalp excision is repaired to the straight incision in the scalp with half-buried 4-0 interrupted sutures and a continuous 5-0 suture.

3. Care is taken to spread out the tension posteriorly, as well as superiorly, to prevent the previously mentioned "draping" effect. A pre-planned inferior Burrow's triangle incision can be placed in the posterior edge of the flap to assist in this goal.

21. What are causes of pulled, distorted ear lobules after rhytidectomy?

Improper incision placement, faulty lift dynamics, excessive excision of skin adjacent and inferior to the ear lobule, and failure to repair the cheek flap to the nonyielding conchal fascia under the lobule.

22. What are vector dynamics in face lift?

The direction and magnitude of the tension forces of the integumentary lift, which should be in balance throughout the contours of the face, mandible, and neck.

23. What are the major consequences of faulty lift vector dynamics in face-lift surgery?

- Wide, conspicuous scars, distorted by tension contractures
- Unnatural temporal and occipital hairlines
- Ear protrusion
- Earlobe stretching
- Tragal protrusion and exposure of the auditory meatuses
- Inadequate posterior ear skin
- Flattened postauricular sulcus
- Unnatural draping of the skin and tissues of the cheek, jaw area, and neck, conspicuous when the head tilts forward ("the drapery effect")

If skin vectors and excisions are correctly planned, these distortions are preventable in primary lifts. In secondary face lifts, the surgeon is somewhat at the mercy of the first surgical result and may not be able to correct prior distortions completely, although the "drapery swag" and lobular pulling defect can be improved by balancing the vector forces of the cheek and neck lift and orienting them more horizontally anterior and posterior to the ear.

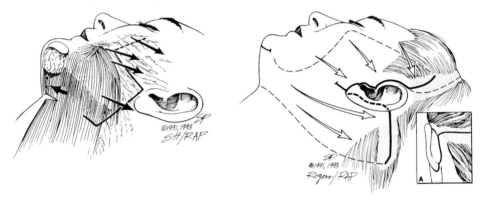

Left, Lift vectors of SMAS. (Note: This is a *see-through* graphic and does not depict skin incisions. The chin has been illustrated as surgically contoured.) This view illustrates the vector lift of the deep tissues, i.e., platysma, pattern of the SMAS flap, and premalar and premaxillary fat. *Right,* Lift vectors of skin, showing the proper skin face-lift vectors as well as the area of undermining (dotted lines on the cheeks and neck) and the temporal, preauricular, postauricular, and occipital incisions with possible coronoplasty (also a dotted line) incision placement. (Copyright © 1991, R.A. Peterson, M.D., F.A.C.S., with permission.)

24. In what order should you accomplish the following procedures during major face-lift surgery: (a) coronoplasty, (b) blepharoplasties, (c) face and neck lifts, and (d) chin and submental platysmal plication?

1. Upper and/or lower blepharoplasties. Your best skills should be focused first on the most precise and delicate procedure.

2. The chin and submental platysmal plication. The medial platysmal plication establishes a midline anchor from which to lift the facial and neck tissues bilaterally.

3. Face and neck lifts, which are individually completed to gain the new contours of the face, mandible, and neck.

4. The forehead and brow lifts. If the forehead and brow are lifted after the blepharoplasties, there is no increased risk of opening the upper lids too widely if excision of the eyelid skin and muscles has been correctly planned so as not to be excessive. The benefits of a forehead-brow lift are gained by excision of corrugator supercilii muscles and chosen segments of galea (deep frontalis fascia), and excision of skin or scalp as may be indicated.

25. Should you completely transect the cervical platysma to obtain a better cervicomandibular contour?

No—for the following reasons:

1. Complete platysmal transection may cause paralysis of the platysma superior to the severance, and the tissues may become flaccid and atrophic.

2. The submaxillary glands, which are located in an aperture in the deep cervical fascia, may prolapse into the weakened platysma and become an unsightly bulge, which is especially noticeable if the glands are large.

3. Complete platysmal transection creates unnatural anatomic relationships that are not an improvement when repaired and may cause distortion of the cervical contours.

26. In which patients should you recommend a chin-contouring procedure?

Even minor ptosis of the chin (mentum) should be corrected, or it will be accentuated after a SMAS lift and lipocontouring of the submental and submandibular areas. The SMAS lift should begin with improvement of the chin and submental contours and advancement-repair of the submental platysma bilaterally to the midline.

27. What is a "witch's chin" deformity?

A witch's chin deformity results from ptosis of the integumentary and muscular tissues of the mentum, a consequence of aging. However, it also may occur for other reasons, such as chin implant surgery or sliding genioplasty surgery by the intraoral approach, wherein the mandibular attachments of the lip and chin musculature are cut across or stripped away from the mandible by periosteal elevation. Subsequently, the chin sags below the mental protuberance, and the platysma and subcutaneous fat may become lax and ptotic. Jowls may appear and a genio-mandibular sulcus or concavity occurs below and lateral to the sagging chin.

28. Can the senile chin be corrected by chin augmentation implants?

Not by chin implant alone. Excellent correction is possible, however, by a combination of procedures, including a chin implant to lift the mentum and contouring procedures with inferior advancement and repair of a superiorly based, horizontally elliptical dermafat flap of the ptotic mentum into the submental area onto the superficial platysma. When a witch's chin deformity exists, chin contouring procedures are an essential part of the SMAS face lift.[5]

29. What are jowls?

Ovoid masses of fibrofatty subcutaneous tissue immediately adjacent and lateral to the inferior extremity of the nasolabial creases.

30. How can jowls be corrected?

After the SMAS flap lift and/or mid-face deep-plane lift is completed, it is convenient to liposuction the ovoid mass of subcutaneous tissue, mostly fat, that may overhang the mandibular margin. A small suction cannula (1.5–3.0 mm diameter) may be inserted through the incision just under the earlobe into the jowl. The ovoid mass is suctioned away, taking care to confine the suction first to the jowl, and, as necessary, very carefully, to the submandibular area to define the mandibular margin and contour the regions adjacent to the previous lipectomy of the submental area.

31. What happens if this jowl reduction lipectomy is even slightly excessive?

Concave contour defects may result. If recognized during surgery, these contour concavities should be corrected immediately by implantation of excised platysma-fascia-fat.

32. What complications are associated with face-lift surgery?

- Bleeding, hematoma
- Infection
- Poor tissue healing: ischemia, objectionable scarring
- Nerve injuries
- Device problems
- Anesthesia problems
- Medication reactions

33. What causes hematoma after face-lift surgery?

- Postoperative pain, which causes anxiety and hypertension with subsequent bleeding. After general anesthesia, this sequence may begin *in the operating room.*

- Nausea and vomiting, through the physical motion of the act of vomiting and also from sudden blood pressure fluctuations
- Ingestion of aspirin or other anticoagulant medications before or immediately after surgery

34. Can the frequency of postoperative hematoma be minimized?

Yes—by good hemostasis, effective pressure dressings, prevention of postoperative anxiety, pain, hypertension, and vomiting.

35. Can hematoma be avoided entirely?

Not likely—but one should strive for a frequency of 1–3%. (The senior author once had 200 consecutive patients without hematoma, then 5 in a brief period.) The time to be watchful for the earliest signs of bleeding is immediately after surgery in the recovery room and up to 12 hours after surgery. Within minutes of extubation after general anesthesia, the patient's waking awareness of pain and other postanesthetic factors may cause hypertension, which, untreated, causes hematoma formation. One should anticipate this postoperative hypertension and ask the anesthetist to treat the hypertension prophylactically before extubation and during recovery. The *surgeon, anesthesiologist,* and *recovery nursing staff* all must involve themselves in the process of hematoma prevention.

36. Is the incidence of face-lift hematoma more frequent in male or female patients?

In males. They are more subject to labile hypertension, are inwardly nervous, anxious, and afraid of pain, and wish to stay in command. Unless counseled beforehand, they may react to pain by tearing off a dressing. They are, with infrequent exception, not candidates for intravenous sedation and local anesthesia. Male patients should be pre-advised that they have to abdicate executive authority and release command to the surgeon throughout the surgical experience.

37. What is the treatment for expanding hematoma?

If recognized early, the treatment is suction-aspiration (using liposuction cannulas) under IV sedation (and local infiltration anesthesia, if necessary). Manual pressure is applied for several minutes after removing the hematoma. A new compression dressing is wrapped in place, and the patient is observed for recurrence for at least one-half hour. If a large expanding hematoma has formed, suction-aspiration should be tried first, but one may need to take out the sutures, remove the clots, and locate and control bleeding points by electrocautery. The incisions are again repaired and a new compression dressing is applied for 48 hours.

38. What is the most dreaded face-lift complication?

Ischemia of face-lift skin flaps with major tissue loss. Cervicofacial skin flaps are relatively thin and, therefore, potentially at risk for impairment of circulation in any face lift, but more so in the *at-risk* group. Occasionally, unexpected skin ischemia in front of, under, or behind the ears is seen in other patients. These ischemic areas are at the farthest points from the sources of the blood supply— the boundary of skin undermining—and may require immediate relief by removal of adjacent incisional sutures to assist in regaining viable circulation.

39. Which patients are more at risk for flap ischemia?

Smokers, "second-hand smokers," diabetics, hypertensives, and any other patients who may have narrowing of small blood vessels, including the arteriolar network in the dermis and subcutaneous tissue.

40. What do you recommend for the prevention of face-lift flap ischemia?

1. Smokers should *entirely* discontinue smoking 3 weeks before surgery or longer if possible and should be off all nicotine substitution medication programs during this period. They should not smoke for approximately 10 days after surgery.

2. Slow-acting niacin may be helpful in counteracting the effects of smoking on the small vessels. If tolerated, 250 mg of slow-acting niacin is prescribed 3 times/day for 3 weeks before surgery.

3. If smoking cannot be discontinued, the skin undermining and lift tension certainly should be reduced. Most of the lift should be taken on the musculofascial level, and the skin flaps should be draped with lighter tension than is usual for a nonsmoking patient.

4. Skin undermining and skin flap tension should be minimized in all patients with thin skin or potentially diminished circulation.

5. Hypertension should be controlled before, during, and after surgery.

6. At surgery, one should apply smooth dressings and avoid excessive tightness.

7. The patient should sleep with the head and chest elevated for approximately 7 days after surgery.

8. The patient should not sleep on either cheek for approximately 7 days.

9. The patient should be instructed never to use a heat pack, heating pad, or hot water bottle on either cheek until sensory perception returns to these areas. If the patient disregards this instruction, third- and even fourth-degree burns may result.

41. What course of action should a surgeon follow upon seeing a dusky, plum-colored flap a day or two after surgery?

Press on the dusky area with a digit for a second or two. If the area blanches, the surgeon should consider putting the patient on time-release niacin therapy or perhaps oxygen inhalation therapy. One may even consider treatment in a hyperbaric chamber to increase tissue oxygenation. The involved area of the flap should be coated with an antibiotic ointment, Vaseline gauze, and a light dressing. It is essential that the patient is examined the next day for evaluation, and daily until the trend has subsided.

If the pressed area does *not* blanch, the surgeon should release both the skin surface sutures and the deep dermal sutures adjacent to the involved area sufficiently to provide relaxation of the flap and free *all* tension from the ischemic skin. This approach may seem radical, but, in fact, it is the *most conservative* treatment one can do and offers the only real viable (and viability) alternative. Thus, circulation is often restored partially or totally to the relaxed ischemic skin flap.

If this maneuver is to succeed, it must be *timely*—that is, at the earliest moment one can diagnose ischemia, even on the first day after surgery. Examination of the face-lift flaps is a valid reason for removing the head wrap dressing on the first postoperative day.

In addition, the patient should receive niacin therapy, oxygen inhalation therapy, protective lubrication of the skin, and a protective light dressing that should be removed daily for progress evaluation.

If ischemia progresses, one can expect necrosis and demarcation of the vascularly impaired cheek or neck flap to be complete in 10–14 days. If ischemia is reversed, the flap can be revised in a month or two. If the viable flap contracts into perfect position, the scar may be revised *ad lib* with a mini- or midi-tuck, which will improve the cheek contours.

42. How should you treat the granulating area of the sloughed face lift?

There are two treatment methods.

1. Allow the granulating wound to epithelialize and gradually contract. This approach, however, may require months of wound care by the patient and surgeon, an interval that is psychologically debilitating to both.

2. In the office, frequent wound care dressing, first daily, then two times weekly, and finally once every week or two. When the edges of the granulating wound exhibit epithelialization from the adjacent skin, a very thin split skin graft may be taken from the patient's lateral thoracic area as an outpatient office procedure to gain closure. This can usually be accomplished approximately 4–6 weeks after the ischemic complication. In a few months, one may begin serial, staged excisions and mini- or midi-lifts until the skin graft has been removed or reduced by the maximum amount.

43. What is the most likely cause of nerve injuries in face-lift surgery?

In first-time face lifts, cautery hemostasis may be the most frequent cause of nerve injuries, but direct division by scissors seems more probable in the deep-plane lifts. The facial nerve branches (N VII) are potentially more susceptible to injury in SMAS deep-plane lifts. The small terminal branches from the buccal and zygomaticus major and minor muscles may be most vulnerable. Sutures advancing the SMAS may impinge on nerves, particularly the great auricular nerve (GAN).

44. In face-lift surgery, which nerve is most susceptible to injury?

The GAN can be harmed by dissection of the skin flap from the fibrofatty tissue over the sternocleidomastoid (SCM) muscle.

45. Where is the GAN?

In a large series of patients, the senior author located the GAN at 6.0–6.5 cm from the tragus of the ear at the anterior margin of the SCM and 9.0–9.5 cm as it emerged from the posterior margin of the SCM. The variability and sometimes delicate nature of the GAN make it vulnerable between these two points.

46. If you recognize injury to the GAN at surgery, what should you do?

Repair it with fine sutures and cover the repair with the platysmal portion of the deep tissue flap.

47. What symptoms may occur after surgery if the GAN is injured?

• Numbness in the inferior portions of the ear and ear lobule
• Painful, neuralgic sensations in the SCM and ear areas
• Painful neuroma at the site of injury and sometimes symptoms of causalgia

48. What should you recommend if the symptoms persist for several weeks or months?

Secondary neurolysis and repair, but sometimes discomfort persists.

49. What is the easiest way to identify the branches of the facial nerve during a face lift?

• It is quite easy to locate the buccal branches in the buccal pocket, under the SMAS, 5.5–6.0 cm horizontally anterior from the ear lobe sulcus.
• The mandibular branch is located about 1.0 cm inferior to the mandibular margin, deep to the cervical fascia, and 4.0–4.5 cm from the ear lobe sulcus.
• The zygomatic branch may be found under the fascia of the SMAS about 3.0 cm horizontally anterior to the tragus of the ear.

50. What are the symptoms or findings of facial nerve (N VII) injury?

By your own examination, determine *exactly* which muscle functions are deficient and to what extent so that you may determine which branch of N VII may be impaired. Ask yourself whether the injury is complete or partial and if it may be caused by cautery, scissors, suturing, or stretching. Weakness can be evaluated by testing the functions of brow raising, blinking, winking, lip puckering, smiling, and lower lip pouting. It is important to observe these functions and to determine the muscle group malfunctions.

Neuromuscular stimulation, administered by the patient several times daily at home, will assist recovery, maintaining muscle function as the motor nerve branches regain function. The motor nerves are stimulated over the locator points with a suitable stimulator. The patient should repetitively put all muscles of expression through a regimen of exercises after each stimulation. Recovery is usually complete within a few weeks to 3 months, either by resolution of a neural injury or through networking with ramifications of adjacent nerve branches.

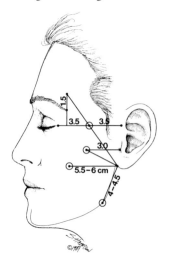

Facial nerve locator points. Lateral diagram illustrating the points where the branches of the facial nerve can be located in reference to the ear. (Copyright © 1987, R.A. Peterson, M.D., F.A.C.S., with permission.)

51. What organisms are the most prevalent in face-lift infection?

Staphylococcus aureus, gram-negative bacilli, streptococci, and *Candida albicans* (yeast).

52. How do you make the diagnosis of postoperative face-lift infection?

Any unexpected localized swelling or inflammation, with or without pain, occurring several days after surgery, is suggestive of infection. Needle aspiration producing purulent fluids yields a diagnosis.

53. Which infections do you consider to be the most difficult to treat? And the most dangerous for tissue viability?

Infections with streptococci and gram-negative bacilli, as they spread rapidly with both abcesses and cellulitis, and effective antibiotics are more difficult to identify.

54. How should a face-lift infection be treated?

Prompt diagnosis and initiation of *adequate* treatment are the keys to rapid improvement and prevention of cicatrix or tissue loss. Once the presence of an infection is established, the *nearest* part of the face-lift incision is opened and a tract is dissected with scissors under the skin to the abscess. One should *not* incise and drain *over* the abscess because tissue loss and scar may well occur.

The drainage is cultured. The abscess is suctioned and irrigated with sterile saline, followed by 3% hydrogen peroxide. A ¼-inch iodoform gauze wick is laid through the incision into the abscess and a dressing is applied. Intravenous antibiotics are administered to cover gram-negative rods, streptococci, and staphylococci. An oral antibiotic is prescribed while awaiting a culture and antibiogram report from the laboratory.

This treatment is repeated at least once daily, and even twice, if necessary. It is our preference to personally treat such patients in our clinics, unless there are systemic symptoms or rapid progression of the infection. Should these occur, hospitalization and consultations would be in order.

Face-lift infections treated by this regimen usually subside within 4–5 days. Tissue loss and scars are rare and usually do not occur if treatment is aggressive. If corticosteroids are given during and after face-lift surgery, the symptoms of infection and abscess may be masked and infection may progress even though antibiotics have been administered.

55. If you are treating a face-lift infection that is not responding, what other organisms may be present?

Yeast *(Candida albicans)*. Yeast infection in a face-lift skin flap appears as a deep-red pustular erythema with multiple surface pustules that enlarge, coalesce, and become tracts into the dermis and subdermis. A creamy white, purulent fluid exudes from many tracts, or follicles, when digital pressure is applied in the area. Topical antibiotic therapy has no beneficial effect and the lesion may progress to ischemia and necrosis. Daily topical *antimycotic* (Nystatin) cream dressings and/or oral antifungal medications (itraconazole) are usually rapidly effective.

56. Is it safe to perform ancillary surgical procedures at the time of a SMAS, deep-tissue, or mid-face suspension face-lift surgery?

Although each ancillary procedure has its own risks and potential problems, *all* are usually safe to do at the same time, *except skin resurfacing*, by abrasion, chemical peel, or laser. It is our opinion that it is risky to resurface the skin of the cheeks at the same time as a face lift because simultaneous skin surface surgery, face-lift dissection, and lifting may jeopardize skin circulation and viability. Lips and chin resurfacing added to the face lift can, at times, cause sufficient excess facial edema to cause ischemia and necrosis of the cheek flaps.

BIBLIOGRAPHY

1. Hamra ST, personal communication, Dallas, April, 1991.
2. Hamra ST: Composite rhytidectomy and the nasolabial fold. Clin Plast Surg 22:313–324, 1995.
3. Millard DR Jr, Garst WP, Beck RL, Thompson ID: Submental and submandibular lipectomy in conjunction with a face lift in the male or female. Plast Reconstr Surg 49:385, 1972.
4. Mitz V, Peyronie M: The superficial musculoaponeurotic system (SMAS) in the parotid and cheek area. Plast Reconstr Surg 58:80, 1976.
5. Peterson RA: Correction of the senile chin deformity in face lift. Clin Plast Surg 19:433–445, 1992.
6. Peterson RA: The custom facelift: Design and maintenance. An opinion. Clin Plast Surg 19:415–423, 1992.

7. Peterson RA: Facelift: Inconspicuous scars about the ears. Clin Plast Surg 19:425–431, 1992.
8. Peterson RA, Johnston DL: Facile identification of the facial nerve branches. Clin Plast Surg 14:785, 1987.
9. Ramirez O: The subperiosteal approach for the correction of the deep nasolabial fold and the central third of the face. Clin Plast Surg 22:341–356, 1995.
10. Skoog T: Personal communication, Uppsala, Sweden, 1967.
11. Skoog T: Tord Skoog Plastic Surgery. Stockholm, Almquist & Wiksell International, 1974, pp 300–330.

56. RHINOPLASTY

George C. Peck, Jr., M.D., and George C. Peck, M.D.

1. Which came first, open or closed rhinoplasty?

A review of late nineteenth and early twentieth century literature indicates that nasal procedures were performed through external incisions.

2. Who was the first surgeon to use the intranasal approach?

Roe appears to the be first surgeon to use the intranasal approach as early as 1887. In 1931 Joseph popularized the closed technique and introduced it in the United States through Aufricht and Safian.

3. What underlying anatomic structures are associated with the proximal, middle, and distal thirds of the nose?

- Proximal third—nasal bones
- Middle third—upper lateral cartilages
- Distal third—lower lateral cartilages

4. List four important nasal angles.

The septal, nasofrontal, tip-columellar, and nasolabial angles (95° in men, 105° in women).

5. Where is the internal nasal valve? What is its function?

The angle formed between the junction of the caudal quadrangular cartilage and the distal upper lateral cartilages, along with its mucoperichondrial lining, constitutes the internal nasal valve, which widens and narrows in its angulation during respiration.

6. How do the upper lateral cartilages relate anatomically to the nasal bones and lower lateral cartilages?

The upper lateral cartilages lie posterior to the nasal bones and lower lateral cartilages. They connect to the cartilaginous septum with fibromembranous tissue.

7. What is the soft triangle?

The soft triangle consists of the two juxtaposed layers of skin separating the dome of the alar cartilage from the nostril border.

8. Describe the internal lining of the nose.

From the nostril opening to the nasal valve, the vestibular lining is composed of squamous epithelium. Cephalad to the nasal valve, a mucous membrane lines the passageway.

9. What is the blood supply to the nasal tip?

The nasal tip receives its blood supply from the angular artery off the lateral nasal artery.

10. Define tip projection and nasal length.

Nasal tip projection is the distance from the nasal spine to the nasal tip. Ideally, the nasal tip should project 1–2 mm beyond the supratip and should be 67% of the nasal length. Nasal length is the distance from the root of the nose (nasofrontal groove) to the nasal tip.

11. What is a Pinocchio tip? A parrot beak deformity?
A Pinocchio tip is excessive nasal tip projection. A parrot beak deformity is a high supratip with inadequate nasal tip projection.

12. What are the most important supports of the nasal tip?
The primary supports of the nasal tip are the septum, the domes of the lower lateral cartilages, and all of their associated attachments.

13. Name the causes of supratip fullness.
The cephalad portion of lower lateral cartilage, the dorsal septum, fibrofatty tissue, scar tissue, and thick sebaceous skin are causes of supratip fullness.

14. Define an open roof. How is it corrected?
An open roof results from lowering the dorsum without nasal bone infracture. The dorsum appears flat and wide. Bilateral infracture of the nasal bones reestablishes the nasal bone pyramid.

15. What is the most important technique to give definition to the nasal tip?
By excising the cephalad portion of lower lateral cartilage with fibrofatty tissue, the surgeon creates a level discrepancy between the tip and supratip, producing an aesthetically pleasing gull-wing highlight.

16. How do you determine adequate septal support of the nasal tip?
Push down on the nasal tip with one finger; if resistance and recoil are good, septal support is adequate. If there is little resistance or recoil, septal support is inadequate.

17. How do you treat inadequate tip projection?
Inadequate nasal tip projection with adequate septal support responds to an onlay graft(s). Inadequate tip projection with inadequate septal support requires an umbrella graft.

18. What is an onlay graft? An umbrella graft?
An **onlay graft** is a 4 × 9-mm, convex cartilage graft from lower lateral, septal, or conchal cartilage that is placed in a horizontal pocket overlying the alar domes. An **umbrella graft** consists of a 3-cm strut of septal, rib, or conchal cartilage that is placed in a vertical pocket between the medial crura from the nasal spine to the nasal tip. This strut is capped with an onlay graft.

19. What are the most common causes of airway obstruction? How are they treated?
- An enlarged inferior turbinate can be treated with bipolar electrocautery or turbinectomy.
- A deviated septum is treated with septoplasty or submucosal resection of the septum.
- Inspiratory collapse of the middle vault secondary to lack of cartilaginous support responds to spreader grafts or cartilage filler grafts.
- Intranasal scarring may require Z-plasties or skin graft.
- A pinched nasal tip with collapse of the alar rims is treated with cartilage grafts.

20. What is a saddle deformity? How is it treated?
A saddle deformity, congenital or traumatic, is a dorsum that is too low. A moderate saddle deformity is corrected with a cartilage graft (septal, conchal). A severe saddle deformity requires a bone graft (iliac, cranial).

21. What is the most common cause of a pinched nasal tip?
The integrity of the lower lateral cartilages is important to maintain the support of the alar rims. Transecting the lower lateral cartilages near the dome causes collapse of the alar rims and a pinched tip. This deformity is corrected with cartilage grafts, reconstructing the lower lateral cartilages.

22. What is a stairstep deformity? How is it avoided?
A stairstep deformity is a prominent ledge of nasal bone after infracture, a step off the narrowed nasal bone. This deformity can be avoided by keeping the infracture low on the maxilla.

23. Should the periosteum be removed from the nasal bones before infracture?

No. Removing the periosteum causes unnecessary trauma, edema, and ecchymosis. The nasal bone may fall into the piriform aperture, creating a depression and skeletalization of the septum.

24. How long should one wait for a secondary rhinoplasty?

Most surgeons agree that a secondary rhinoplasty should not be performed for 1 year.

25. Which preoperative pose accentuates the problems of the nose?

The lateral profile with the patient smiling accentuates the dorsal hump, length of the nose, crowded lip, and inadequate tip projection.

26. What is the relationship between sculpturing the lower lateral cartilages and nasal tip projection?

Excising the cephalad portion of the lower lateral cartilage reduces the volume of the nasal tip pyramid and nasal tip projection. The most common problem after rhinoplasty is inadequate nasal tip projection.

27. What causes a retracted columella? How is it treated?

A retrosee or retracted columella results from overresection of the caudal border of the septum or excision of the nasal spine. This deformity is corrected with rectangular cartilage grafts to the posterior two-thirds of the columella.

28. How do you rotate the nasal tip?

The tip may be rotated by sculpturing the lower lateral cartilages, by excising a portion of the anterior one-third of the caudal septum, or with sutures. Postoperative edema exaggerates tip rotation.

29. Define veiling of the alar rims.

Approximately 1–2 mm of columella should be visualized in profile. Veiling of the alar rims occurs when the alar rims overhang the columella. Treatment, described by Millard, consists of wedge excisions of the alar rims.

30. How do you narrow flaring nostrils?

The general shape of the alar base is an isosceles triangle. A modified Weir's resection of the alar base corrects flaring nostrils and a wide floor. The inferior incision should be kept in the alar groove to minimize the scar.

31. How do you inject the nose preoperatively?

We use a few milliliters of a concentrated solution of epinephrine (1:30,000) with lidocaine and perform a circumferential block of the nose. No local solution is injected into the nasal tip, supratip, or dorsum to avoid distorting the nose.

32. How do you perform septal surgery?

Most important are good hemostasis and visualization. Hydrodissection of the mucoperichondrium with local anesthesia aids in septal surgery. Elevate the mucoperichondrial flaps by starting high on the septal wall, and create a pocket to the end of the septum. Then sweep inferiorly to complete the elevation of mucoperichondrial flaps.

BIBLIOGRAPHY

1. Gruber RP, Peck GC: Rhinoplasty: State of the Art. St. Louis, Mosby, 1993.
2. McCarthy J: Rhinoplasty. In McCarthy J (ed): Plastic Surgery. Philadelphia, W.B. Saunders, 1990, pp 1785–1894.
3. Peck G: Techniques in Aesthetic Rhinoplasty. New York, Gower Medical, 1990.
4. Rees TD: Rhinoplasty. In Rees TD, Latrenta GS (eds): Aesthetic Plastic Surgery. Philadelphia, W.B. Saunders, 1994.
5. Rohrich RJ, Gunter JP, Friedman RM: Nasal tip blood supply: An anatomic study validating the safety of the trans-columellar incision in rhinoplasty. Plast Reconstr Surg 95:795–799, 1995.
6. Sheen JH: Aesthetic Rhinoplasty. St. Louis, Mosby, 1987.
7. Tardy EM: Rhinoplasty: The Art and the Science. Philadelphia, W.B. Saunders, 1997.

57. OTOPLASTY

Jeffrey Weinzweig, M.D., and Norman Weinzweig, M.D.

1. What is a prominent ear?

A prominent ear, also commonly referred to as a lop ear, cup ear, or Dumbo ear, protrudes excessively from the temporal surface of the head. The normal external ear forms an angle of approximately 21–25° with the temporal scalp. A more obtuse angle (> 25°) may cause the ears to appear overly prominent on frontal or posterior view.

2. What are the pathologic characteristics of the prominent ear deformity?

The three major pathologic characteristics of the prominent ear deformity are (1) a poorly defined or absent antihelical fold; (2) conchal excess (> 1.5 cm deep); and (3) a conchoscaphal angle > 90°. Each of these characteristics may exist in varying degrees. Thus, the excessive depth of the concha may be evenly distributed or may affect the upper pole (cymbum) more than the lower pole (cavum). Similarly, the entire antihelical fold may be underdeveloped or just a specific part, such as the superior crus or inferior crus.

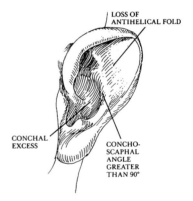

Components of the prominent ear deformity: (1) poorly defined or absent antihelical fold, (2) conchoscaphal angle > 90°, and (3) conchal excess. (From LaTrenta GS: Otoplasty. In Rees TD, LaTrenta GS (eds): Aesthetic Plastic Surgery, 2nd ed. Philadelphia, W.B. Saunders, 1994, pp 891–924, with permission.)

3. What are the embryologic origins of the ear?

The mandibular (first) branchial arch and the hyoid (second) branchial arch each contribute three hillocks of approximately equal size to the formation of the ear. Ultimately, the hyoid arch contributes 85% to the formation of the ear, including the helix, scapha, antihelix, concha, antitragus, and lobule. The mandibular arch contributes the tragus and helical crus only.

4. When does antihelical folding begin in utero?

The ear begins to protrude from the developing face by the third to fourth month of gestation, at which time antihelical folding commences. Incomplete folding of the antihelix results in a conchoscaphal angle > 90°, producing the prominent ear deformity.

5. By what age has the ear attained 85% of adult size? When should otoplasty be performed?

Three years. Therefore, otoplasty is ideally performed in the interval between age 3 and the commencement of school so that the child can avoid the psychological trauma of ridicule by classmates.

6. What is the nerve and vascular supply to the ear?

The auriculotemporal nerve (V_3) provides sensibility to the tragus and crus of the helix only. The great auricular nerve (a branch of the cervical plexus) provides sensibility to the lobule, antitragus, antihelix, scapha, external acoustic meatus, postauricular sulcus, helix, and concha. The external acoustic meatus receives additional sensory supply via auricular branches of the vagal and glossopharyngeal nerves. The vascular supply to the external ear is via the posterior auricular and superficial temporal arteries, both terminal branches of the external carotid artery.

7. What are the normal proportions of the ear?

The ear's width is typically 50–60% of its length with an average width of 3–4.5 cm and average length of 5.5–7 cm. Viewed from the front, the ear extends from the brow superiorly to the base of the columella inferiorly. Laterally, the ear should lie a single ear-length behind the lateral orbital rim.

8. How is ear protrusion defined?

Protrusion of the ear is defined in terms of both distance and angle. The distance from the scalp to the anterior edge of the helix ranges from 1.5–2 cm; the cephaloauricular angle is a mean of 25° in men and 21° in women.

9. What is the average distance of each third of the ear from the head?

The helical rim measures approximately 10% of the vertical height of the ear (7 mm) and protrudes to 10–12 mm at the helical apex (upper third), 16–18 mm at the midpoint (middle third), and 20–22 mm at the lobule (lower third).

10. What is the normal incline of the ear?

The normal ear inclines posteriorly approximately 20° off the vertical, which is slightly less steep than the plane of the nasal dorsum.

11. Should the helix be visible from the frontal view?

Yes. From the frontal view, the helix of both ears should be visible beyond the antihelix.

12. What are the anatomic goals of otoplasty?

The anatomic goals are threefold: (1) production of a well-defined antihelical fold; (2) conchal reduction; and (3) a conchoscaphal angle of 90°. Of course, the extent to which each of these goals is pursued depends on the severity of the specific characteristics of the deformity. In addition, several general guidelines are applicable:

1. The position of the two ears with respect to the temporal surface of the head should match within 3 mm at any specific point.
2. Protrusion of the upper third of the ear must be completely corrected; mild protrusion of the lower two thirds may be acceptable if the upper third is fully corrected.
3. The postauricular sulcus should not be significantly decreased or distorted.
4. The helix should have a smooth and regular contour.
5. The ears should not be placed too close to the head.

13. Who performed the first otoplasty?

Although Dieffenbach is usually credited for having performed the first correction of a prominent ear in 1845, his technique was used for correction of a posttraumatic deformity. The earliest elective otoplasty for prominent ear deformity was reported by Ely in 1881. Dieffenbach's procedure consisted of postauricular skin excision and conchomastoidal suture fixation; Ely's procedure included these techniques as well as conchal strip excision.

14. Can skin excision alone correct the prominent ear deformity?

No. Although skin excision is virtually always performed during otoplasty, it is done to avoid skin redundancy in the postauricular sulcus rather than to maintain the set-back position of the ear. Although some beneficial effect on ear position may initially be attributed to skin excision, over time the elasticity of the skin inevitably results in recurrence of the prominent ear deformity. Even Dieffenbach knew this 150 years ago and included conchomastoidal sutures in his technique (see question 18).

15. What important concept did Luckett contribute to the principles of otoplasty?

In 1910 Luckett introduced the concept of restoration of the antihelical fold for correction of the prominent ear deformity. He used a cartilage-breaking technique that consisted of excising a strip of medial skin and cartilage along the entire vertical length of the antihelical fold. In some cases a sharp edge was created along the antihelical fold, which Luckett attempted to correct with several horizontal mattress sutures.

16. What is Gibson's principle?

Gibson's principle states that cartilage spontaneously bends or warps away from the scored surface by "release of interlocked stresses." A number of cartilage-weakening techniques (e.g., incision, abrasion, scoring) take advantage of this principle to recreate the antihelical fold by interrupting the anterior surface of the auricular cartilage.

17. What is the Stenstrom technique?

Through a small postauricular incision, an otoabrader is used to rasp the anterior surface of the antihelix to recreate the antihelical fold. Stenstrom and Heftner were the first to apply the Gibson principle in otoplasty. Cartilage scoring also may be achieved with a 2-mm anterior skin incision along the inside edge of the helix. After cartilage weakening, 5 or 6 radially oriented Mustardé sutures (4-0 clear nylon) are placed.

18. What is the purpose of conchomastoidal sutures?

Conchomastoidal sutures are simple or mattress sutures that penetrate the full thickness of the cartilage of the posterior conchal wall and the fascia/periosteum of the mastoid process. These sutures anchor the posterior wall of the concha to the mastoid prominence, reducing conchal projection and decreasing the depth of the postauricular sulcus. Before placing these sutures, it is helpful to resect a portion of the soft tissue (muscles and ligaments) in the postauricular sulcus. This resection permits closer approximation of the conchal cartilage to the mastoid fascia/periosteum and facilitates the conchal reduction.

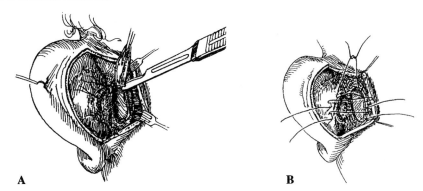

A   **B**

Conchomastoidal sutures. *A,* Resection of postauricular soft tissue. *B,* Several permanent mattress sutures secure the conchal cartilage to the mastoid fascia. (From LaTrenta GS: Otoplasty. In Rees TD, LaTrenta GS (eds): Aesthetic Plastic Surgery, 2nd ed. Philadelphia, W.B. Saunders, 1994, pp 891–924, with permission.)

19. Is there another way to reduce conchal projection?

Conchal cartilage excision. Through an anterior incision, a full-thickness crescent of excessive cartilage may be excised from the prominent conchal rim to reduce its height. Alternatively, a posterior incision may be used to excise a strip of cartilage from the deepest part of the conchal cup.

20. What is the purpose of Mustardé sutures?

Mustardé sutures, also referred to as conchoscaphal sutures, are used to create the antihelical fold. These permanent mattress sutures are placed posteriorly through the full thickness of the scaphal and conchal cartilage on either side of the antihelix. As they are tied, the antihelical fold is created. The cartilage surfaces are approximated only far enough to produce an aesthetic fold. The cartilage surfaces usually do not meet; instead, the sutures span the gap between them. Placement of these sutures is usually facilitated by first making several pairs of ink marks on the concha and outer aspect of the antihelix while pressing medially on the helix. These pairs of marks outline the position of the mattress sutures to be used in the repair. A 25-gauge needle dipped in ink is used to transfer the ink marks through the postauricular skin and tattoo the underlying cartilage. The cartilage can be directly tattooed if the postauricular skin excision has already been performed. The sutures (usually 4-0 clear nylon) are placed as described and tied simultaneously.

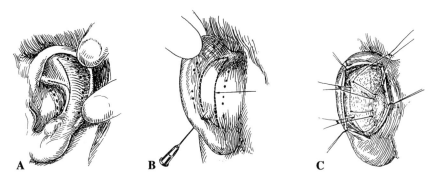

Mustardé (scaphoconchal) sutures. *A*, Several pairs of ink marks are made on the scapha and concha on either side of the antihelix. *B*, Markings are transferred to the postauricular skin and cartilage with 25-gauge needles dipped in ink. *C*, After postauricular skin excision down to cartilage, several permanent sutures are placed in the full thickness of the scaphal and conchal cartilage, piercing the perichondrium of the anterior cartilage. The sutures are tied simul.taneously. (From LaTrenta GS: Otoplasty. In Rees TD, LaTrenta GS (eds): Aesthetic Plastic Surgery, 2nd ed. Philadelphia, W.B. Saunders, 1994, pp 891–924, with permission.)

21. How is a prominent lobule corrected?
Prominence of the lobule, or lower third of the ear, is corrected by a modified fishtail excision extending from the posterior surface of the lobule to the mastoid skin.

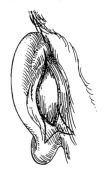

Correction of prominent lobules. A modified fishtail excision is performed in the postauricular sulcus. (From LaTrenta GS: Otoplasty. In Rees TD, LaTrenta GS (eds): Aesthetic Plastic Surgery, 2nd ed. Philadelphia, W.B. Saunders, 1994, pp 891–924, with permission.)

22. Correction of which third of the ear is most important?
The upper third. Although a minor degree of remaining protrusion of the middle or lower third may be acceptable if the top is completely corrected, the reverse is not true.

23. What is a "telephone ear" deformity?
Inadequate correction of a projecting antitragus and lobule may result in a secondary telephone ear deformity in which the upper and lower thirds of the ear appear relatively prominent with respect to a properly corrected middle third. The ear resembles a telephone receiver.

24. What is the difference between cartilage-*molding* and cartilage-*breaking* techniques?
Cartilage-molding techniques, such as those of Mustardé and Furnas, take advantage of the soft, pliable characteristics of cartilage, especially in children. Such techniques use Mustardé conchoscaphal mattress sutures to maintain the new antihelical fold without excising any cartilage. Scoring of the anterior surface of the antihelix is performed as needed.

Cartilage-breaking techniques, such as those of Converse and Wood-Smith, are especially useful for the stiffer cartilage of adults. These techniques use full-thickness incisions or breaks through the cartilage to permit tubing of the antihelix, which is then stabilized with several sutures. The amount of conchal excess is estimated by pressing inward on the newly folded antihelix, and an elliptical conchal strip is excised. The edges of the newly folded antihelix and freshly contoured conchal rim are approximated with several permanent 4-0 mattress sutures. Care is taken not to evert the edges of the cartilage because eversion may cause secondary sharp ridging, the main complication of cartilage-breaking techniques.

25. What is the most common late deformity after otoplasty?

Residual deformity, which is usually identified within 6 months of surgery, may present a problem in as many as 10–24% of patients after otoplasty (according to review of several series). Such problems may result from sharp ridges and irregular contours along the antihelical fold (more common with cartilage-breaking techniques), sinus tracts secondary to the presence of permanent sutures, overcorrection with any cartilage-weakening technique, and a secondary telephone deformity. Despite the potential for residual deformity, in most series fewer than 10% of patients require subsequent otoplasty revision.

26. What is the most likely cause of sudden onset of pain after otoplasty?

Hematoma. Sudden-onset, persistent, or unilateral pain should raise the index of suspicion for hematoma and warrants immediate dressing removal and evaluation. Evacuation of a clot after suture removal often is easily accomplished and should be followed by reapplication of a head dressing with mild compression.

27. What organisms are usually responsible for cellulitis after otoplasty?

Staphylococci or streptococci are usually the culprits, although *Pseudomonas* sp. is occasionally responsible. Intravenous antibiotics are often indicated. Topical mafenide acetate (Sulfamylon) cream is often useful in preventing further spread of the infection and chondritis. Infections must be controlled immediately because long-term sequelae may include the development of residual deformity.

28. Can chondritis occur after otoplasty?

Although rare, chondritis may occur after inadequate treatment of postoperative infection. Chondritis is a surgical infection requiring immediate exploration, debridement of necrotic cartilage, and soft tissue coverage to prevent severe cartilage destruction and resultant deformity.

29. When can prominent ears be treated nonoperatively?

Within the first 72 hours of the neonatal period, the cartilage elasticity is affected by high levels of circulating maternal estrogens, resulting in unusual malleability of the auricular cartilage that permits nonoperative treatment of several congenital ear anomalies, including prominent ear deformity. After 72 hours, these hormonal levels drop and the cartilage becomes stiffer. Splinting materials for nonoperative management of congenital ear deformities include Steri-Strips, rubber-coated electrical wire, and lead-free solder covered by a polyethylene suction catheter. Splinting of the prominent ear to the mastoid surface for 1–2 months often corrects the deformity.

30. Which is the best technique for correction of the prominent ear deformity?

Each patient requires individual assessment to determine which technique(s) is best suited to meet the specific needs of the deformity. Not every prominent ear warrants conchal excision, conchoscaphal (Mustardé) sutures, conchomastoidal sutures, or abrasion of the anterior surface of the antihelix. Most, however, require some combination of these techniques to achieve the desired goals of otoplasty. Most otoplasty procedures (such as the Mustardé technique) include a maneuver to recreate the antihelical fold (see figure in question 20).

31. Describe patient management after otoplasty.

A dressing of mineral oil-soaked cotton and fluffed gauze is applied under a light cotton wrap. This dressing is removed within the first few postoperative days—sooner if signs or symptoms of infection or hematoma are present. The sutures are removed after 7–10 days, and the patient is instructed to sleep wearing an elastic ski band over the ears for 2–3 weeks after surgery.

CONTROVERSY

32. Should postauricular skin excision always be performed during otoplasty?

Not necessarily. Much has been written about various approaches to postauricular skin excision during otoplasty. Some advocate centering the excision over the postauricular sulcus; the excision thus includes skin from the posterior surface of the ear as well as the mastoid region. Others prefer to bring the excision within several millimeters of the postauricular sulcus without actually crossing it or including mastoid skin. Still others contend that skin preservation is necessary to compensate for excessive skin contraction that may obliterate the posterior sulcus or pull the mid-helix into a hidden position on frontal view, creating a telephone ear deformity. Therefore, the excision of postauricular skin is based on the surgeon's experience and preference.

BIBLIOGRAPHY

1. Bauer BS: Nonoperative treatment of congenital deformities of the ear. Oper Tech Plast Reconstr Surg 4:104–108, 1997.
2. Elliot RA: Complications in treatment of prominent ears. Clin Plast Surg 5:479–490, 1978.
3. Ely ET: An operation for prominent auricles. Arch Otolaryngol 10:97, 1881 [reprinted in Plast Reconstr Surg 42:582–583, 1968].
4. Furnas DW: Correction of prominent ears by conchal mastoid sutures. Plast Reconstr Surg 42:189–193, 1968.
5. Furnas DW: Otoplasty. In Aston SJ, Beasley RW, Throne CHM (eds): Grabb and Smith's Plastic Surgery, 5th ed. Philadelphia, Lippincott-Raven, 1997, pp 431–438.
6. LaTrenta GS: Otoplasty. In Rees TD, LaTrenta GS (eds): Aesthetic Plastic Surgery, 2nd ed. Philadelphia, W.B. Saunders, 1994, pp 891–924.
7. Luckett WH: A new operation for prominent ears based on the anatomy of the deformity. Surg Gynecol Obstet 10:635, 1910 [reprinted in Plast Reconstr Surg 43:83–89, 1969].
8. Mustardé JC: The correction of prominent ears using simple mattress suture. Br J Plast Surg 16:170–176, 1963.
9. Stal S, Klebuc M, Spira M: An algorithm for otoplasty. Oper Tech Plast Reconstr Surg 4:88–103, 1997.
10. Stenstrom SJ: A "natural" technique for correction of congenitally prominent ears. Plast Reconstr Surg 32:509–518, 1963.
11. Stenstrom SJ, Heftner J: The Stenstrom otoplasty. Clin Plast Surg 5:465–470, 1978.
12. Tanzer RC: An analysis of ear reconstruction. Plast Reconstr Surg 31:16–30, 1963.
13. Tolleth H: Artistic anatomy, dimensions and proportions of the external ear. Clin Plast Surg 5:337–350, 1978.
14. Weinzweig N, Chen L, Sullivan WG: Recurrence following correction of prominent ears: A histomorphologic study in a rabbit model. Ann Plast Surg 33:371–376, 1994.

58. ABDOMINOPLASTY

Michael Brucker, M.D., and David Barrall, M.D.

1. What is the blood supply of the anterior abdominal wall?

The anterior abdominal wall has superior, inferior, and lateral vascular supply. The superior epigastric artery and the musculophrenic artery, both branches of the internal mammary, feed the upper half of the abdominal wall. The inferior blood supply consists of the inferior and superficial epigastrics medially as well as the deep and superficial circumflex iliac arteries laterally. The skin and subcutaneous tissue derive their blood supply from medial rectus perforators as well as laterally from intercostal and lumbar segmental arcades.

Vascular zones related to abdominoplasty can be separated into superior medial (zone I), inferior medial (zone II), and lateral (zone III) areas. Zone II and most of zone I (depending on the extent of dissection) are devascularized in an abdominoplasty. As a result, the abdominal wall flap is vascularized primarily by the intercostal and lumbar arcades of zone III.

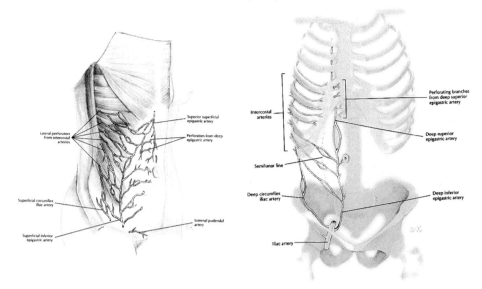

Superficial *(top left)* and deep *(top right)* vasculature supply to the anterior abdominal wall. (From Pitman GH (ed): Liposuction and Aesthetic Surgery. St. Louis, Quality Medical Publishing, 1993, with permission.)

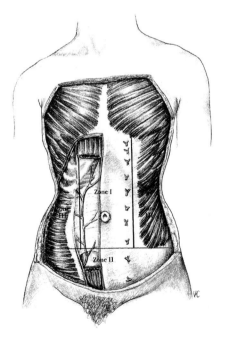

Right, Vascular zones of the anterior abdominal wall. (From Matarosso A: Abdominoplasty. Clin Plast Surg 16:289, 1989, with permission.)

2. What are the layers of the anterior abdominal wall?

The layers of the anterior abdominal wall vary according to location on the wall. The basic layers of the lateral abdomen, from superficial to deep, are (1) skin, (2) Camper's fascia, (3) Scarpa's fascia, (4) external oblique, (5) internal oblique, (6) transversalis fascia, and (7) peritoneum. The arcuate line, which is found below the umbilicus in the mid abdomen, demarcates a change in the thickness of the anterior and posterior rectus sheath. Above the arcuate line (level 1 in the figure on page 312), the external oblique fascia and half of the internal oblique fascia give rise to the anterior rectus sheath. The other half of the internal oblique fascia combines with the transversalis fascia to form the posterior rectus sheath. Below the arcuate line, the internal oblique fascia contributes all of its fibers to the anterior sheath, and the transversalis fascia alone forms the posterior sheath. This may result in a relatively weaker fascial segment below the arcuate line that is more susceptible to laxity. Overlying and closely adherent to the anterior rectus and external oblique fascia is the innominate fascia, or fascia of Gallaudet, which covers a plexus of small arteries and veins. Undermining of the abdominal wall flap in an abdominoplasty should proceed above this layer to preserve the delicate vasculature and reduce the incidence of postoperative seroma formation.

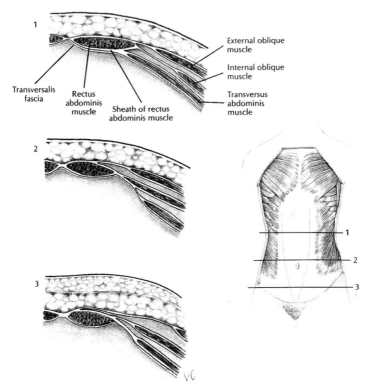

Cross-sectional anatomy of the fascial system of the anterior abdominal wall at three different levels. (From Pitman GH (ed): Liposuction and Aesthetic Surgery. St. Louis, Quality Medical Publishing, 1993, with permission.)

3. What is the superficial fascial system?

The superficial fascial system (SFS) is made up of a horizontal, loose connective tissue layer and its investing vertical and oblique septa. The distinct compartmentalization of the SFS defines the adipose layers of the anterior abdominal wall. The layer of adipose tissue superficial to Scarpa's fascia in the anterior abdominal wall is usually of uniform thickness with a compact septal framework, whereas the deep layer is highly compartmentalized with a globular septal framework. The deep adipose layer is primarily responsible for distinct contouring of the abdomen. In a male or android pattern, this fatty layer is in the upper abdomen and flanks, whereas in a female or gynoid pattern it is in the lower abdomen, hips, and thighs.

4. What are the basic elements of abdominal contour abnormalities?

Most patients seeking abdominoplasty do so because they wish to correct a contour abnormality. The abnormality is often a complex composite of multiple basic problems. Four fundamental areas of concern should direct the plastic surgeon in correction of the abnormality: (1) to evaluate the degree of skin redundancy and flaccidity; (2) to assess the degree of excessive adipose tissue and its location; (3) to evaluate muscle diastasis and aponeurotic laxity; and (4) to assess undesirable scars or striae and their location. These four basic elements direct the surgical approach for optimal correction of anatomic problems.

5. What is the basic surgical approach to abdominoplasty?

One of the most important steps in the basic abdominoplasty begins before the surgery with supine and upright marking of the patient's abdomen. Skin laxity and the area of proposed resection are of most concern at this stage. With the patient properly marked, the appropriate skin incisions are then based on the extent of tissue that needs to be resected. The standard low transverse incision is the most widely used and widely modified of the abdominoplasty incisions. The abdominal skin flap is elevated off the rectus sheath from pubis to zyphoid with preservation of the umbilical stalk and circumferential excision from the skin flap. The lower aspect of the skin flap is then resected, and the rectus sheath and external oblique fascia are plicated as indicated. By tacking the abdominal skin flap into place, liposuction can be used to define and fine-tune the contour of the abdomen. Liposuction is particularly useful for excessive flank adipose tissue not incorporated into the primary dissection. The umbilicus is then resutured into its new location, and the new superior margin of the skin flap is sutured to the original inferior margin.

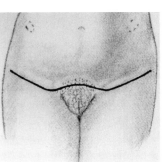

Low transverse or W-type incision. (From Pitman GH (ed): Liposuction and Aesthetic Surgery. St. Louis, Quality Medical Publishing, 1993, with permission.)

6. What is a fleur-de-lis abdominoplasty?

Fleur-de-lis describes the shape of the incision in this inverted T-type abdominoplasty. It is useful in patients with a significant amount of medial obesity or when a large pannus must be excised. The procedure begins with a traditional W-type or Regnault low transverse incision, which is used in conjunction with a vertical wedge component that may be taken as high as the zyphoid as well as inferiorly over the mons pubis, if necessary. This method resects medial tissue and draws the new medial margins into the midline.

7. What is a modified Weinhold or T-excision abdominoplasty?

As its name implies, the T-excision abdominoplasty places the horizontal component of incision at the level of the umbilicus and extends a vertical wedge resection down to the pubis. The skin flap undermining is carried out both inferiorly and superiorly. This technique is used in patients with upper medial obesity and is effective at reducing "love handles" by both elevating and medially displacing the lower lateral skin flaps.

8. What are the indications for the so-called mini-abdominoplasty?

The mini-abdominoplasty employs a shortened low transverse incision and is used primarily in patients with infraumbilical obesity and/or low-midline musculofascial laxity. The same techniques of skin flap undermining, often with the aid of endoscopic equipment, are used as in a standard abdominoplasty. The umbilicus, however, is often left in continuity and simply retracted inferiorly after resection of redundant skin in the superior flap. The rectus sheath and external oblique fascia are then plicated, usually in the midline and laterally, and liposuction is used for flank and upper thigh contouring.

9. What is the role of liposuction in abdominoplasty?

The extent of liposuction used in an abdominoplasty varies greatly, depending on the desired result and amount of tissue to be resected. Suction-assisted lipectomy (SAL) and abdominoplasty are complementary modalities in body contouring and, in general, are used inversely, depending on the severity of the contour abnormality. Typically, liposuction has its greatest role in procedures requiring minimal tissue excision and minimal musculofascial repair; however, it is often used in large abdominoplasties to tailor areas such as the flanks. SAL of the upper and lateral abdomen (zones II and III in the figure in question 1) should be avoided because it may jeopardize blood supply to the abdominal flap.

10. What are the relative contraindications to abdominoplasty?

Contraindications to abdominoplasty focus primarily on conditions that may predispose to poor skin flap viability after dissection. Examples include previous scarring above the umbilicus, which may indicate poor segmental blood flow, and previous skin undermining; a history of smoking; cardiovascular disease; and morbid obesity. Although not true contraindications, considerations such as future pregnancy and unreasonable expectations of outcome should always be discussed before surgery.

11. When is musculofascial repair or plication indicated?

Musculofascial repair is indicated in all patients with musculofascial laxity. The anterior aponeurosis of the abdominal wall is the frame on which the cutaneous flaps are draped, and a significant amount of trunk contouring can be achieved at this level. Different techniques can be used, depending on the type and extent of fascial laxity. Most surgeons use a vertical rectus plication in the midline as a starting point. The external oblique may be further plicated laterally for better waist definition. Some surgeons even advocate external oblique dissection from the rectus and underlying internal oblique with resuturing of the fascia in the midline. An indication for mini-abdominoplasty, particularly in patients with multiple previous pregnancies, is the low-midline fascial laxity that results from stretching in the relatively weaker fascial system below the arcuate line. This laxity generally can be corrected with midline plication of the anterior rectus sheath.

12. What about the umbilicus?

The umbilicus usually lies in the midline at the level of the superior iliac spines; from an anatomic standpoint, these landmarks are used to replace it within the superior skin flap. With musculofascial plication, the umbilical stalk is shortened slightly; this aids in creating an inwardly drawn, aesthetic navel. Freeman and Weimer recommend defatting the umbilical stalk to less than 1.5 cm in diameter and insetting it to a reverse omega incision in the superior skin flap. The reverse omega incision is reported to add hooding to the superior aspect of the umbilicus. The vertical midline of the skin flap is slightly defatted above and below the new umbilicus site to recreate the vertical raphe. The umbilical stalk is then affixed to the skin flap with sutures that both approximate the skin edges and capture the deep fascial margin. This technique not only strengthens the closure but also helps to create the invagination of the umbilicus.

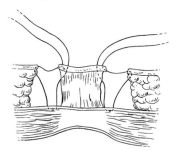

Suturing technique for affixing the umbilicus to the superior skin flap and anterior rectus fascia. (From Pitman GH (ed): Liposuction and Aesthetic Surgery. St. Louis, Quality Medical Publishing, 1993, with permission.)

13. What are the complications of abdominoplasty?

The more common complications of abdominoplasty, in order of decreasing frequency, are wound infections, seromas, hematomas, minor skin edge necrosis, and minor skin edge dehiscence. Together these complications occur in approximately 12% of all abdominoplasties and are responsible for over 98% of all complications reported. Complications such as major skin necrosis requiring reoperation, deep vein thrombosis, or pulmonary embolism are significantly more serious but occur rarely.

BIBLIOGRAPHY

1. Castanares S, Goethel JA: Abdominal lipectomy: A modification in technique. Plast Reconstr Surg 7:378, 1967.
2. Dellin AL: Fleur-de-lis abdominoplasty. Aesth Plast Surg 9:27, 1985.
3. Dubou R, Osterhout DK: Placement of the umbilicus in abdominoplasty. Plast Reconstr Surg 61:291, 1978.

4. Freeman BS, Weiner DR: Abdominoplasty with special attention to construction of the umbilicus: Technique and complications. Aesth Plast Surg 2:65, 1978.
5. Grazer FM, Goldwyn RM: Abdominoplasty assessed by survey with emphasis on complications. Plast Reconstr Surg 59:513, 1977.
6. Hughes WE Jr: The anatomic rationale for abdominal lipectomy. Am Surg 45:612, 1979.
7. Lewis TS: Midabdominoplasty. Aesth Plast Surg 3:195, 1979.
8. Markman B, Barton FE: Anatomy of the subcutaneous tissue of the trunk and lower extremity. Plast Reconstr Surg 80:248, 1987.
9. Matarossa A: Abdominoplasty. Clin Plast Surg 16:289, 1989.
10. Pitanguy I: Abdominal lipectomy. Clin Plast Surg 2:401, 1975.
11. Pitman GH (ed): Liposuction and Aesthetic Surgery. St. Louis, Quality Medical Publishing, 1993.
12. Psillikas JM: Plastic surgery of the abdomen with improvement in the body contour, physiopathology and treatment of the aponeurotic musculature. Clin Plast Surg 11:465, 1984.
13. Regnault P: Abdominal dermolipectomies. Clin Plast Surg 2:401, 1975.
14. Rohrich RJ: Body contouring (overview). Select Read Plast Surg 7:38, 1995.
15. Wilkinson TS: Limited abdominoplasty techniques applied to complete abdominal repair. Aesth Plast Surg 18:49, 1994.

59. BODY CONTOURING

Samuel J. Beran, M.D.

1. What is the anatomic distribution of fat in men and women?

Men and women generally accumulate fat in distinct and predictable patterns, which are genetically and hormonally related. The distribution in men is primarily around the abdomen and torso (android pattern). Women accumulate fat around the hips and thighs (gynoid pattern).

2. Are there differences in the layers of fat?

The subcutaneous fat in the trunk is composed of two layers, superficial and deep. The superficial layer is dense and compact, with multiple fibrous septa. The deep layer is more loose and areolar with few septa. The deep layers are principally located around the umbilical, paralumbar, gluteal, and medial thigh regions.

3. How is cellulite formed?

The fat present in cellulite is no different from ordinary subcutaneous fat. The distinct appearance of cellulite is due to the architecture of the superficial fat in these areas. The presence of dense vertical septa separates the fat into pockets. As the fat hypertrophies or the skin relaxes with age, the septa act as anchor points to the skin. This results in the classic accordion appearance of cellulite.

4. If fat is removed, will it come back?

Fat cells are produced by the body during three different periods: in utero, early childhood, and early adolescence. In general, after reaching maturity, the total number of fat cells in the body will not increase. Fat cells that are removed through liposuction or other techniques will not be replaced by other fat cells. However, the remaining cells may hypertrophy, and the total fat mass in the area may increase. The one exception is morbid obesity, in which the fat cells may become hyperplastic and multiply.

5. What is liposuction?

Liposuction, also known as lipoplasty or liposculpture, is the surgical removal of adipose tissue through the use of small metal cannulas.

6. Who originally developed liposuction? When did it become accepted?

Dujarrier is generally accredited with the first use of liposuction in 1921. He attempted to remove fatty deposits from around the knees of a ballerina but perforated the femoral artery, resulting in an amputation. This set back liposuction for several years. The modern development of liposuction can be traced to such surgeons as Schrudde, Fisher, Meyer, and Illouz in the 1970s and 1980s.

7. What are the indications for liposuction?

Liposuction works best for treating localized fat deposits that do not respond to traditional diet and exercise. The treated areas will retain the new contour unless the patient has large weight gains. Liposuction is not a treatment for obesity. Patients with significant medical problems, patients who have poor skin tone or inelasticity, and patients who are taking anticoagulants should not undergo liposuction.

8. What is the difference between ultrasound-assisted liposuction and traditional liposuction?

Traditional liposuction removes fat cells through the mechanical avulsion of fat. Ultrasound-assisted liposuction (UAL) uses an ultrasound generator and handpiece to produce ultrasound energy to destroy fat cells in vivo through a process known as cavitation. The emulsified fat is then removed through a hollow channel in the cannula using standard suction.

9. What is wetting solution? Why do we use it?

Wetting solution is the delivery of subcutaneous infiltration into the subcutaneous fat before the use of liposuction. It was pioneered by Illouz in the 1970s and later adapted by many surgeons, most notably Klein, who developed the tumescent technique. The use of wetting solution has two advantages: an anesthetic effect secondary to the use of lidocaine and a hemostatic effect due to the use of epinephrine.

Technique	Infiltrate	Estimate of Blood Loss (as % of Volume)
Dry	No infiltrate	20–45
Wet	200–300 cc per area	4–30
Superwet	1 cc infiltrate per 1 cc aspirate	1
Tumescent	Infiltrate to skin turgor	1
	2–3 cc infiltrate per 1 cc aspirate	

10. What are the most common sequelae of liposuction?

The difference between sequelae and complications is what the doctor tells the patient: the patient *will* have the sequelae after the procedure but *may* have the complications. The most common sequelae include contour irregularities, paresthesias, edema, ecchymosis, and discoloration, which occur routinely in almost all patients who undergo liposuction. However, they resolve spontaneously or with minimal treatment such as massage.

11. What are the most common complications of liposuction?

The most common complications of liposuction include significant blood loss, fluid shifts, asymmetries, and contour deformities. The possible complications of skin loss, skin burns, and seroma formation are seen more frequently with UAL than with traditional liposuction.

12. Is it safe to perform liposuction with abdominoplasty?

It is safe to perform liposuction in some areas of the trunk in conjunction with abdominoplasty. These areas include the flanks and anterolateral abdominal wall; however, the central abdomen should not be treated because skin or flap loss may occur.

13. What is the recommended treatment for gynecomastia?

Currently, UAL is an excellent modality for treatment of gynecomastia. It removes the dense fibrous fat of the male breast and contours the area around the central core. Occasionally, resection of the small fibrotic remainder may be needed.

14. Does the excessive skin need to be resected after removal of fat via liposuction?

In general, even despite large amounts of removed fat, skin has good elasticity and will conform to the new underlying volume. However, in patients with inelastic skin or in elderly patients, the skin may not redrape and skin resection may be needed.

15. How do you determine whether a patient will benefit from abdominoplasty vs. liposuction?

The first determinant is the status of the abdominal wall musculature. During examination it is critical to check for the presence of a lax abdominal wall. Diastasis or wall laxity cannot be treated by liposuction. Secondly, if the patient has inelastic skin or severe skin excess, the skin may not redrape; therefore, excisional techniques are more appropriate.

16. What is the treatment for arm ptosis and lipodystrophy?

There are two approaches. In mild-to-moderate cases, liposuction, either traditional or ultrasound-assisted, may be effective. If the deformity is moderate to severe or the patient has inelastic skin, direct excision (brachioplasty) may be performed.

17. How do you prevent complications from a medial thigh lift?

The most common complications from a medial thigh lift are wide scars, vulvar distortion, and relapse. They may be prevented by anchoring the thigh flap to the deep layer of the superficial perineal fascia (Colles' fascia).

18. What is autologous fat transplantation?

In this process fat is harvested from one area of the patient and transplanted to another. Examples include removal of abdominal fat for such procedures as lip augmentation, repair of postliposuction deformities, and facial sculpturing. The survival rate of transplanted fat cells is controversial. In general, if the fat is treated gingerly, rinsed, and centrifuged, the survival rate is 25–50%.

19. What are Autologen and Alloderm?

Autologen is autologous processed dermis, and Alloderm is processed cadaver dermis. Both products can be used for augmentation of the lip, contour deformities, and the nasolabial fold. Although no large long-term studies have analyzed survival rates of the dermis, several reports show no resorption after 1 year.

20. Does the use of Autologen and Alloderm involve any risk?

The significant risks with use of Autologen are infection and resorption. Alloderm is treated by a number of techniques to eliminate viable viral and/or cell structures.

CONTROVERSIES

21. Will ultrasound-assisted liposuction (UAL) replace traditional liposuction?

Although initially greeted as the replacement for traditional liposuction, the clinical applications of UAL are now more apparent. UAL appears to be more effective than traditional liposuction in fibrous tissue such as the buttocks, gynecomastia, and secondary liposuction. There may be increased skin shrinkage with the use of UAL. UAL, however, will not replace traditional liposuction. Instead, it extends the use of liposuction in body contouring.

22. Is fat transplantation the best way to perform lip augmentation or minor contouring procedures where augmentation is required?

The use of fat transplantation is somewhat controversial. Although some surgeons believe that 50% or more of grafts will survive, many believe that the survival rates are too variable and unpredictable for safe use. Alternatives include biologic products such as autogenous dermis, processed cadaver dermis, porcine or bovine collagen, and synthetic products such as Gore-Tex.

23. Does tumescent liposuction have an advantage over other techniques?

Liposuction performed without the use of subcutaneous infiltration has a much higher rate of blood loss than liposuction performed with wetting solutions. However, the exact dosage of subcutaneous infiltration required to provide the beneficial effects has not been thoroughly studied. The risk of true tumescent infiltration is fluid overload.

24. Are there cures for cellulite?

At present a number of modalities are purported either to ameliorate or to cure cellulite. However, no definitive studies show clear results in reducing or eliminating cellulite. Techniques that have been reported to be effective include ultrasound liposuction, Endermologie, massage techniques, and application of creams. None of these has proved to be fruitful.

BIBLIOGRAPHY

1. Dillerud E: Suction lipoplasty: A report on complications, undesired results, and patient satisfaction based on 3511 procedures. Plast Reconstr Surg 88:239, 1991.
2. Guerrerosantos J: Analogous fat grafting for body contouring. Clin Plast Surg 23:619–632, 1996.

3. Klein JA: Tumescent technique for local anesthesia improves safety in large-volume liposuction. Plast Reconstr Surg 92:1085, 1993.
4. Lockwood TE: Fascial anchoring technique in medial thigh lifts. Plast Reconstr Surg 82:299, 1988.
5. Markman B, Barton FE Jr: Anatomy of the subcutaneous tissue of the trunk and lower extremity. Plast Reconstr Surg 80:248, 1987.
6. Rohrich RJ, Beran SJ, Fodor PB: The role of subcutaneous infiltration in suction-assisted lipoplasty: A review. Plast Reconstr Surg 99:514, 1997.
7. Zocchi M: Clinical aspects of ultrasonic liposculpture. Perspect Plast Surg 7:153, 1993.

60. CHEMICAL PEELING AND DERMABRASION

Sheilah A. Lynch, M.D.

1. What is chemical peeling?

Chemical peeling, also called chemexfoliation, chemosurgery, or dermapeeling, is the application of one or more exfoliating agents to the skin, resulting in destruction of portions of the epidermis and/or dermis with subsequent regeneration of new epidermal and dermal tissues. The various agents in use may be categorized according to the depth of wounding that they produce. Superficial or light peeling involves wounding to the papillary dermis; wounding to the upper reticular dermis is considered medium-depth peeling; and deep-depth peeling is to the midreticular dermis.

Chemical Peeling Wounding Spectrum*

Superficial wounding (to the stratum granulosum-papillary dermis)
Very light: TCA, 10–20% (TCA, superficial), resorcin, Jessner's solution, salicylic acid, solid CO_2, α-hydroxy acids, tretinoin
Light: TCA, 35%, unoccluded, single or multiple frost
Medium-depth wounding (to the upper reticular dermis)
Combination CO_2 + TCA, 35–50%, unoccluded, single or multiple frost
Combination Jessner's solution + TCA, unoccluded, single or multiple frost
TCA, 50%, unoccluded (TCA, deep), single frost
Full-strength phenol, 88%, unoccluded
Pyruvic acid
Deep-depth wounding (to the midreticular dermis)
Baker's phenol, unoccluded
Baker's phenol, occluded

* Depth depends on prepeel skin defatting preparation, wounding agent strength or amount applied, and skin thickness or location. Clinical reepithelialization may depend on skin location and the character of the dermal pathology, which may determine the degree of inflammatory response evoked. TCA = trichloroacetic acid.
From Brody HJ: Chemical Peeling. St. Louis, Mosby, 1992, p 21, with permission.

2. What are the indications for chemical peeling?

Chemical peeling may be used for photoaging, including actinic keratoses, solar elastosis, solar lentiges, and rhytids; pigmentary disturbances, including melasma, postinflammatory pigmentary changes, and other pigmentary dyscromias; superficial scarring; acne vulgaris; rosacea; and milia.

3. What agents are most commonly used for chemical peeling? What are the typical concentrations?

Phenol and trichloroacetic acid (TCA) are most commonly used. The Baker formula for phenol is:
3 ml U.S.P. phenol (C_6H_5OH) (88%)
2 ml tap water
8 drops of liquid soap (Septisol)
3 drops of Croton oil
Phenol, a keratocoagulant, denatures and coagulates the surface keratin. Croton oil is a skin irritant that enhances the action of phenol. Soap is added to act as a surfactant to enhance penetration. The

water is a diluent to slow down keratocoagulation and enhance absorption. TCA strength can be varied depending on the depth desired:

Light peeling   10–25%
Intermediate peeling   26–50%
Deep peeling   51–75%

The major advantage of TCA is its versatility. The depth of peeling can be individualized for a particular patient's needs, skin type, and underlying pathology.

4. How do you choose a particular peeling agent to suit your patient's skin type?

Fitzpatrick has classified skin into six types based on color and response to sunlight. Types I–III are ideal for peeling of all varieties, but the line of demarcation between peeled and unpeeled skin is most prominent in actinically damaged type I skin with marked neck poikiloderma. Red-haired, freckled people should forgo the treatment. Type IV skin can be peeled with all peeling agents. If the patient has an eye color other than brown, however, the likelihood of postinflammatory pigmentation is reported to be less. Types V and VI also can be peeled with all peeling agents, but the risk of unwanted pigmentation is greater. Test spots should be performed at the hairline in patients who are at greatest risk (types V and VI), but this test does not guarantee that the remainder of the face will respond identically.

Fitzpatrick's Classification of Sun-reactive Skin Types

SKIN TYPE	COLOR	REACTION TO FIRST SUMMER EXPOSURE
I	White	Always burn, never tan
II	White	Usually burn, tan with difficulty
III	White	Sometimes mild burn, tan average
IV	Moderate brown	Rarely burn, tan with ease
V	Dark brown*	Very rarely burn, tan very easily
VI	Black	Never burn, tan very easily

* Asian, Indian, Oriental, Hispanic, or light African descent, for example.
From Brody HJ: Chemical Peeling. St. Louis, Mosby, 1992, p 36, with permission.

5. Is pretreatment necessary before chemical peeling?

Yes. For patients undergoing TCA peels, tretinoin (Retin-A) and 4% hydroquinone should be used for 4–6 weeks before treatment. Tretinoin decreases the thickness of the stratum corneum, thereby increasing the permeability of the epidermis to chemical peeling. Hydroquinone suppresses melanocyte activity and helps to prevent the tendency toward postpeel hyperpigmentation. For patients who cannot tolerate tretinoin, glycolic acid facial creams, used for 4–6 weeks before peeling, have yielded comparable results.

6. Is taping necessary during chemical peeling?

Use of occlusive adhesive-type tape after phenol-based solutions have been applied is standard procedure. The results are definitely more profound and longer-lasting when tape is used. If a lesser degree of depth of peeling is desired, the peel may be performed without tape, using petroleum jelly occlusive dressing. In contrast, tape occlusion with TCA does not increase penetration.

7. Can peeling be done simultaneously with surgery?

Peeling solution should not be applied to any areas that have been undermined during a surgical face lift. The only areas that may be considered for peeling are those around the mouth that have not been surgically altered. Simultaneous disruption of the blood supply by undermining and the chemical burn produced by the application of the phenol solution are likely to produce irreversible skin changes, perhaps even skin necrosis.

8. Which should be done first—facial surgery or facial peeling?

If both procedures are planned, surgery should be performed first and the peeling 2–3 months later. If the peeling is done first, somewhat more time must elapse before the surgery can be safely performed because of the slower healing after peeling. The choice as to which procedure to do first depends on whether the sagging of the face or the lines of the face are the primary concern of the patient.

9. What complications may be encountered after peeling?

Postoperative changes can be classified into two categories. Category 1 consists of sequelae that are expected as procedural side effects and resolve completely. Examples include pigmentary changes, prolonged erythema (< 3 months), colloid milia, pustulocystic acne, reactivation of latent facial herpes simplex virus infection, and superficial bacterial infection.

Category 2 consists of sequelae that are characteristic of the individual agent, occur regardless of patient setting, may be secondary to poor postoperative care, and are considered true complications. True complications include pigmentary changes, prolonged erythema (> 3 months), hypertrophic scarring, atrophy, and systemic effects such as hepatic, renal or cardiac abnormalities associated with phenol.

Skin depigmentation may occur, and patient selection is important. Patients with multiple freckles and other sun-induced blotches, as commonly seen in people with red hair, should forgo the treatment. Special care should be taken to stop the peel just under the jawline to hide the line of demarcation and to feather, or blend, the edge. Milia, which are small, superficial epidermal inclusion cysts, may occur during the first 6–8 weeks after treatment. In most instances they resolve with vigorous washing and/or scrubbing. Persistent cysts need to be punctured and evacuated.

10. What peeling solution may cause cardiac arrhythmias when it is applied too rapidly to too large an area?

EKG changes, premature atrial or ventricular contractions, bigeminy, and trigeminy may occur in patients who absorb large amounts of phenol through the skin. Trichloroacetic acid is not cardiotoxic. Cardiac arrhythmias have not been reported following its use.

11. Regeneration of the epidermis and upper dermis occurs via dermal appendages. What previous procedures or medications affect the concentration of dermal appendages and consequently regeneration?

Laser procedures for hair removal and electrolysis leave the tissue with a reduced number of appendages and therefore a limited regenerative capacity. Accutane (isotretinoin), used for the treatment of acne vulgaris, inhibits sebaceous gland function. Accutane presents a transient risk for reepithelialization problems, and patients should not undergo peeling or dermabrasion while taking this medication or for 6 months after termination of its use.

12. Discuss Glogau's classification for photoaging and how treatment strategy changes for each group.

Glogau's classification of photoaging divides patients into four groups based on the degree of actinic keratoses, wrinkling, and acne scarring and the amount of makeup worn by the patient. This classification helps to assess the degree of sun damage in patients with and without a history of acne scarring and to make treatment decisions.

Photoaging Groups—Glogau's Classification

Group I—mild (usually age 28–35 yr)
   No keratoses   No acne scarring
   Little wrinkling   Little or no makeup

Group II—moderate (usually age 35–50 yr)
   Early actinic keratoses—subtle skin yellowing   Mild acne scarring
   Early wrinkling—parallel smile lines   Little makeup

Group III—advanced (usually age 50–65 yr)
   Actinic keratoses—obvious skin yellowing   Moderate acne scarring
      with telangiectasia   Wears makeup always
   Wrinkling—present at rest

Group IV—severe (usually age 65–75 yr)
   Actinic keratoses and skin cancer have occurred   Severe acne scarring
   Wrinkling—much cutis laxa of actinic, gravitational,   Wears makeup that does not
      and dynamic origin   cover but cakes on

From Brody HJ: Chemical Peeling. St. Louis, Mosby, 1992, p 38, with permission.

13. What are alpha hydroxy acids?

Alpha hydroxy acids (AHAs), a group of nontoxic organic acids found in natural foods, have been incorporated into a variety of creams, lotions, and cleansers for general use. They include glycolic, lactic, malic, tartaric, and citric acids. Recently the clinical applications of AHAs have expanded to include their use as alternative chemical peeling agents. Glycolic acid is currently the most commonly used AHA. It is frequently applied as a series of peels separated by 1–4 weeks in a 50–70% nonneutralized concentration. TCA peels usually have a longer interval between applications.

14. How do glycolic acid peels compare with standard chemical peels?

Many of the risks and complications associated with the other peeling agents are minimized with the use of glycolic acid. Virtually every patient is a candidate for glycolic acid peels, including Asians, African-Americans, Hispanics and others with deeply pigmented skin. In addition, almost every part of the body can be peeled, including the back, chest, arms, and legs.

15. What is dermabrasion?

Dermabrasion is the surgical process by which the skin is resurfaced by planing or sanding, usually by means of a rapidly rotating abrasive tool such as a wire brush, diamond fraise, or serrated wheel. This process removes the epidermis and superficial dermis to treat a variety of dermatologic conditions.

16. What are the indications for dermabrasion?

Dermabrasion may be used to treat a variety of scars, including traumatic, acne, and surgical scars as well as superficial lentigos, actinic keratoses, both decorative and traumatic dermal tattoos, and, most commonly, fine facial wrinkling, particularly in the perioral region.

17. Compare the effects of dermabrasion in the perioral area with the effects of phenol.

Because dermabrasion is a mechanical process, the depth of peel is more controllable; thus, healing is faster with less discomfort. Erythema following dermabrasion resolves faster than that seen with phenol. For dark-complected patients, dermabrasion has less of a bleaching effect than phenol.

18. Should patients undergoing chemical peel or dermabrasion of the perioral area receive acyclovir prophylaxis?

Yes. For patients with a history of herpes simplex the use of prophylactic acyclovir is warranted. Adequate prophylactic doses of acyclovir have not been clearly established by a randomized, controlled study. Data suggest that 2400 mg/day in three divided doses clinically minimizes postoperative HSV infection rates and also reduces the severity and duration of illness in patients who become infected. Valacylovir (Valtrex), a newer alternative, may be conveniently administered twice a day as 500-mg capsules or tablets.

BIBLIOGRAPHY

1. Baker TJ, Gordon HL, Stuzin JM: Surgical Rejuvenation of the Face, 2nd ed. St. Louis, Mosby, 1996.
2. Baker TJ, Stuzin JM: Chemical peeling and dermabrasion. In McCarthy JG (ed): Plastic Surgery. Philadelphia, W.B. Saunders, 1990, pp 748–786.
3. Brody HJ: Chemical Peeling. St. Louis, Mosby, 1992.
4. Fitzpatrick TB: The validity and practicality of sun-reactive skin types I through VI. Arch Dermatol 124:869–871, 1988.
5. Glogau, RG: Chemical Peel Symposium. American Academy of Dermatology, Atlanta, December 4, 1990.
6. Gross BG: Cardiac arrhythmias during phenol face peeling. Plast Reconstr Surg 73:590, 1984.
7. Murad H, Shamban AT, Premo PS: The use of glycolic acid as a peeling agent. Dermatol Clin 13:285–286, 1995.
8. Perkins SW, Sklarew EC: Prevention of facial herpetic infections after chemical peel and dermabrasion: New treatment strategies in the prophylaxis of patients undergoing procedures of the perioral area. Plast Reconstr Surg 98:428–429, 1996.
9. Resnik SS, Resnick BI: Complications of chemical peeling. Dermatol Clin 13:309–311, 1995.
10. Swinehart JM: Test spots in dermabrasion and chemical peeling. J Surg Oncol 16:557–563, 1990.
11. Stuzin JM, Baker TJ, Gordon HL: Treatment of photoaging: Facial chemical peeling (phenol and trichloroacetic acid) and dermabrasion. Clin Plast Surg 20:9, 1993.
12. Truppman ES, Ellenby JD: Major electrocardiographic changes during chemical face peeling. Plast Reconstr Surg 63:44, 1979.

61. AESTHETIC LASER SURGERY

Gary J. Rosenberg, M.D., F.A.C.S.

1. What does laser mean?
Laser is an acronym for light amplification by stimulated emission radiation. The laser was first developed by Maimon in 1954.

2. How is laser light created?
All light is part of the electromagnetic spectrum. Surgical lasers are found between the near infrared and ultraviolet portions of the electromagnetic spectrum, including visible light. The active medium of a laser is solid, gas, or liquid in which, when excited by absorbing energy, the atom is elevated from a normal ground state to a higher energy state. Then, on spontaneous return to its ground state, the atom releases the absorbed energy—the spontaneous emission of radiation. If the atom is energized, thus interacting with a photon of identical wavelength, the energy emitted (photons) travels in the same direction and in the same phase with the energizing photon—stimulated emission of radiation.

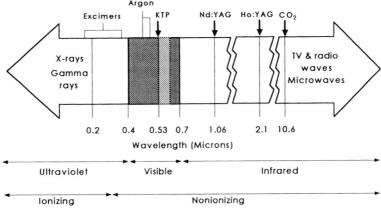

Electromagnetic spectrum.

3. Describe the components of a laser.
An active medium is contained within a resonator. At each end of the resonator cavity, there are parallel mirrors. An energizer pump supplies the source of energy (thermal, electric, or optical). Then the energy is absorbed by the active medium, causing a population inversion of the atoms within the resonator. On reflection, the energy is amplified between the parallel mirrors. A portion of the energy is allowed to escape through one of the mirrors, which is partially reflecting. Escaping light is monochromatic and collimated.

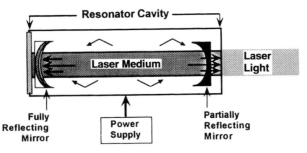

The components of a laser.

4. Describe how laser light interacts with tissue.

On contact with tissue, a small amount of light is reflected, some is scattered, and some is transmitted through the tissue. But the vast majority is absorbed. On absorption into the tissue, the imparted kinetic energy is converted to heat, which coagulates, ablates, or cuts the tissue. The chromophore in the tissue determines which wavelength will be absorbed by the tissue.

5. What is selective photothermolysis?

Selective photothermolysis is the process whereby selective destruction of specific microscopic cellular structures is determined by the duration pulse of the laser. To avoid destruction of the surrounding tissue, there must be a rapid decrease in temperature after the initial exposure to the laser energy, with heating secondary to absorption. The time required for tissue to cool to 50% of the initial temperature is called **thermal relaxation time**. Therefore, high energy of short duration (microseconds) protects the remaining tissue. At the time of vaporization, the surrounding tissues are immediately cooled to 60–70° Celsius. At this temperature collagen shrinks and tightens as it it reconfigures. The initial shrinking and tightening of the skin are visualized as laser resurfacing is performed.

6. What are the long-term effects of the CO_2 laser on the skin?

After the initial inflammatory phase and reepithelialization have been completed, there is an ingrowth of new collagen in the Grenz layer of the dermis (neocollagenesis). Between 6 weeks and 6 months there is a tremendous proliferation of new collagen throughout the entire thickness of the dermis. Studies have shown that proliferation continues up to 1 year and may continue even longer. There is also a simultaneous new formation at 6 months to 1 year. The elastin organizes itself into a tight network, particularly in the deep dermis.

7. How does reepithelialization occur?

The progenitor cells for the reepithelialization remain protected deep within the hair follicles and sweat glands at the time of laser resurfacing. Migration, reproduction, and coalescence of these progenitor epidermal cells reepithelialize the skin. With time, the normal layers of the epidermis reconstitute themselves.

8. Does the pigmentation of a patient's skin influence the results of laser resurfacing?

Patients with lighter, thin skin usually require less aggressive resurfacing. Most often, the rhytids of the skin have the quality of cigarette paper and respond readily to conservative laser resurfacing. Postoperative erythema may last longer than the usual 4–6 weeks. Proper moisturizers, reassurance, and avoidance of agents that may irritate the skin are required. Occasionally, a patient with excessive sensitivity of the skin may require further interventional management. At the other end of the spectrum are patients with dark, olive complexions and thick skin. Such patients tend to hyperpigment after laser resurfacing. This process is self-limiting but can be treated readily with hydroquinone 4% twice daily; hydrocortisone 1% twice daily; and tretinoin 0.0125% twice daily. Patients should be treated for 3 weeks preoperatively and then as soon as the hyperpigmentation appears postoperatively. An honest discussion of hyperpigmentation with patients prior to laser resurfacing is the most important component of treatment.

9. Since the CO_2 laser is in the invisible infrared spectrum, should precautions be taken for protection of the eyes?

The Occupational Safety and Health Administration and common sense dictate that the answer is a resounding yes. There is no excuse for damage to the eye of the patient, plastic surgeon, or staff. Everyone in the operating room must wear protective plastic eyewear. A reflected beam may shatter eyewear made of glass. All patients undergoing laser resurfacing must have frosted metal scleral protectors with lubricating ointment. It is also helpful to place two drops of topical ophthalmic anesthetic drops in each eye before placement of the scleral protectors. Scleral protectors must be frosted on their outer surface.

10. If a patient presents with increased erythema and swelling, itching, and pain 5–10 days postoperatively, what should be done?

Rule out contact dermatitis, especially from topical antibiotic ointments. A diagnostic potassium hydroxide preparation to rule out candidal infection is important, along with a skin culture to rule out topical bacterial infection. Candidal infection is effectively treated with oral antifungal agents as well as a topical antifungal. Bacterial infection should be treated with the appropriate antibiotic revealed by culture and sensitivity.

11. Describe the management of a patient who presents with painful vesicular lesions, with or without low-grade fever.

Most likely the lesions are due to herpes simplex virus and are treated most effectively with valacyclovir, 500 mg 3 times/day, usually for 1 week. As long as the low-grade fever improves or dissipates, this management is all that is needed. Patients with systemic signs such as increasing malaise, increased fever, weakness, or central nervous system symptoms should be admitted to the hospital and receive intravenous antiviral agents.

12. Can laser resurfacing of the face be done simultaneously with face and neck lift?

Most experienced laser surgeons laser the midface at the same time that they perform the face and neck lift but not the full face for fear of necrosis of facial flaps. At present, it is considered high risk to resurface the entire face simultaneously with face and neck lift.

13. Which is preferable for postoperative care—the open or closed technique?

The closed technique, which consists of covering the skin with Flexan, Vigilon, Second Skin, Silon, or another occlusive agent, is preferred by many laser surgeons. Others favor a dressing of only vaseline with regular compresses consisting of hydrogen peroxide 50%/50% water, followed by compresses of Domeboro solution. A recent study by Seckel demonstrated an increased rate of infection with the closed technique.

BIBLIOGRAPHY

1. Anderson R, Parrish J: Selective photothermolysis precise microsurgery by selective absorption of pulsed radiation. Science 220:524–527, 1983.
2. Anderson R, Parrish J: Laser-tissue interactions. In Fitzpatrick RE, Goldman MP (eds): Cutaneous Laser Surgery. St. Louis, Mosby, 1994.
3. Fitzpatrick RE: The Ultrapulse CO2 laser: Selective photothermolysis of epidermal tumors. Laser Surg Med 5(Suppl):56, 1993.
4. Rosenberg GJ: A comparison of the Coherent Ultrapulse and Sharplan Silk Touch lasers. Presented at the Annual Meeting of the American Society of Plastic and Reconstructive Surgeons, Dallas, TX, November 1996.
5. Rosenberg GJ: Discussion of Stuzin J.M., Baker T.J., Baker T.M., Kilgman A.A., Histologic effects of high-energy pulsed CO_2 laser on photoaged facial skin. Plast Reconstr Surg 99:2055, 1997.
6. Rosenberg GJ: The longterm histologic effects of the carbon dioxide laser on skin [submitted for publication].
7. Rosenberg GJ, Gregory RO: Lasers in aesthetic surgery. Clin Plast Surg 23:29–48, 1996.
8. Seckel B: Shrinking effect of CO_2 laser resurfacing of skin. Presented at the Annual Meeting of the American Society of Laser Medicine and Surgery, Phoenix, AZ, April 1997.
9. Sriprachya AS, Fitzpatrick RE, Goldman MP, Smith SR: Infections complicating carbon dioxide laser resurfacing for photoaged facial skin. Dermatol Surg 23:527, 1997.
10. Stuzin JM, Baker TJ, Baker TM, Kligman AM: Histologic effects of the high energy pulsed CO_2 laser on photoaged facial skin. Plast Reconstr Surg 98:2036, 1997.
11. Wheeland RG: Clinical uses of lasers in dermatology. Laser Surg Med 16:2–23, 1995.

62. TATTOOS

Raymond G. Dufresne, Jr., M.D.

1. What is a tattoo?

A tattoo is a foreign material entered into the dermis by needle or some other trauma that results in a visible, indelible mark in the skin. The depth varies with the type of tattoo and has an effect on the choice of removal technique. Professional tattoos from the tattoo parlor are usually placed superficially in the dermis at a fairly uniform layer. As a result, the material is fairly accessible to most removal techniques. However, the amount of dyes may be significant. Homemade tattoos with India ink have a varied depth (1–3 mm), but usually a smaller amount of ink is present. Traumatic tattoos from an abrasion tend to be superficial. Traumatic tattoos from penetrating injuries usually have a deeper component. Historically, newer and professional tattoos were believed to be easier to remove. However, with the Q-switched lasers, older and homemade tattoos seem to respond the best.

Options for Tattoo Removal

Deep destruction	Inflammatory methods
CO_2 laser	Tannic acid
Infrared coagulator	Oxalic acid
Superficial destruction	Urea
Chemical peeling	Surgical methods
Dermabrasion	Excision, including serial excision
Salabrasion	Punch excision
Electrocautery	Excision with grafting
Dermaplaning	Flap
Argon/KTP lasers	Tissue expansion
Cryosurgery	Other
Q-switched lasers	Overtattooing

2. What is the history of the tattoo?

The story of tattoos begins with the desire to decorate the human body. Tattoos certainly existed in ancient Egypt. The Polynesians were known to have had tattoos and, thus, started a naval tradition. In modern times, tattoos have become prevalent in Western society.

3. Why do people get tattoos?

Tattoos have been placed for decoration (personal satisfaction, attention-seeking behavior, identification with groups such as Hell's Angels, gangs, or armed forces), identification (prisoners, Nazi concentration camp survivors), and personal proclamations, including love. Tattoos may be used for cosmetic purposes, such as eyeliner, eyebrows, and nipple reconstruction. Tattoos are used medically for marking radiation ports. Lastly, tattoos may result from trauma. The most common example is an auto accident in which road debris enters the skin. Of course, many of us have a tattoo resulting from running with a pointed pencil.

4. How does motivation affect outcome of removal?

In some circumstances, such as removing a tattoo that says "I Love Sally" from a man who is married to Jill, a quick CO_2 laser removal or excision resulting in a minor scar may be quite acceptable to the patient. However, when a scar is not acceptable, removal with a Q-switched laser may be the better option. Patients with tattoos from trauma or radiation markers may have psychologic problems that the physician must consider and address.

5. Are cosmetic, professional tattoos safe?

Overall, the answer is yes. The dyes are generally selected to have little reaction (i.e., to be inert). This does not mean, however, that the patient cannot become sensitized to a tattoo. The red from cinnabar, for example, is a well-described sensitizer. Usually, the reaction is delayed hypersensitivity, but more serious anaphylactic reactions may occur or even coexist. The delayed hypersensitivity presents as a granulomatous and/or itchy dermatitis-like reaction in the area of a certain dye. At times the reaction may be photoallergic.

The use of a Q-switched laser in a patient with an allergic reaction is dangerous because the dyes are broken up and freed from the macrophages, allowing potential worsening of the reaction. In this situation, excision or possibly the CO_2 laser is a better choice.

Infectious disease transmission is a more serious question. Hepatitis has been associated with tattoos for decades, and the fear of AIDS has raised concern about tattooing in the public health sector. Some states ban tattooing, others regulate and license tattooing, and still others have no oversight at all.

6. Have weird reactions been reported in tattoos?

Of course. Anything arising in a tattoo becomes a case report, including skin cancers, such as melanoma, keratoacanthoma, and sarcoid, and diseases that show kebnerization, such as psoriasis, keloids, discoid lupus, lichen planus, and Darier's disease. Rarely, systemic immune responses such as erythema multiforme and scleroderma may occur in association with tattoos. Reactions of the metal pigments may occur during an MRI. A host of rare infections have been reported in association with tattoos: leprosy, *Treponema pallidum*, papillomavirus, molluscum, and *Mycobacterium tuberculosis*.

7. Why not simply cut out the tattoo?

There is nothing wrong with cutting out a tattoo. This method of removal is fast and direct and may be cost-effective. In some circumstances, cutting out the tattoo is the most prudent treatment and, in cases of allergy, the least risky. Simple punch excisions may be used for small traumatic scars. For larger tattoos, serial excisions, flaps, tissue expansion, or excision with application of a skin graft may be considered. In considering excision, remember that most tattoos occur in sites that tend to heal with problem scars, such as the torso and extremities.

8. What happened to the CO_2 laser?

The CO_2 laser was a popular option before Q-switched lasers, built on the success of other destructive processes and the current love affair with new high-tech approaches to any problem, were developed. CO_2 laser removal was a favored approach due to the bloodless field, ability to view the tattoo particles, and high patient approval. In comparison with other destructive methods, the CO_2 laser vaporizes the tattoo, generally removing it in one session. Larger tattoos are removed in smaller sections ($10 cm^2$) to avoid contraction scars on the extremities.

In the first step, the laser vaporizes or blisters off the epidermis; the tattoo becomes brighter with the loss of the skin cells. The laser is then used to vaporize into the dermis to remove the bulk of the tattoo material. Not all of the material needs to be removed, because some of the tattoo is leached out during the healing phase. Some surgeons use the CO_2 laser like dermabrasion to remove the epidermis and then combine it with other destructive techniques, such as salabrasion or tannic acid. Urea also has been used (50% ointment) as an adjunct to superficial laser abrasion.

The wound is allowed to heal by second intention, usually with some type of occlusive dressing (e.g., Vaseline gauze, Vigilon). Because of the risk of hypertrophied scars, some surgeons use potent topical steroids as soon as reepithelialization occurs. In any case, intervention with intralesional steroids (e.g., 5–20 mg/dl triamcinolone) may still be needed. Although the outcomes are sometimes good, CO_2 laser removal makes sense only if the patient is happy with a scar rather than the tattoo and wants one treatment.

9. What about salabrasion?

If one removes the epidermis and invades the superficial dermis in some manner, some of the dyes will leach out of the dermis and may disseminate during the inflammatory process. Salabrasion was classically done with table salt, abrading the skin and leaving salt on the wound for several minutes; longer periods up to 4 hours or more result in more pigment removal but also more scarring. The longer the salt is present, the greater the injury.

10. How does tannic acid work?

Tannic acid or oxalic acid also has been used after epidermal abrasion to induce an inflammatory reaction and subsequent leaching of pigment. Tannic acid has been used alone in an overtattooing method without dermabrasion.

11. Can dermabrasion be used alone?

In this approach, the epidermis and superficial dermis are abraded. The tattoo brightens with the loss of the epidermis. An occlusive dressing is placed and removed daily; the leaching of dye is noted. The wound can then be abraded with gauze. This approach allows more time for the material to leach out of the dermis. If the response is partial, the procedure can be repeated. The depth of destruction is kept superficial; thus, scarring can be minimized. However, scarring, dyschromia, and partial response are problems.

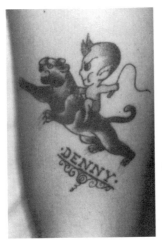 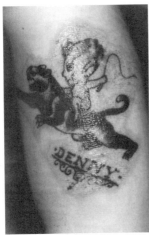 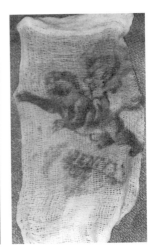

Left, Multicolored tattoo. *Center,* Tattoo immediately after superficial dermabrasion. Note brightening of the tattoo after epidermis removal. *Right,* Tattoo pigment on gauze 24 hours after dermabrasion. (Courtesy of Dr. Louis Fragola.)

12. If dermabrasion works, what about chemical peeling?

Because a chemical peel with trichloroacetic acid (or even phenol) causes epidermal loss and some dermal injury, it may be effective on tattoos. Although a few reports exist, including a large Scottish study, chemical peeling has not been generally used.

13. What about dermaplaning?

In addition to the CO_2 laser and dermabrasion, a dermatome may be used to remove the epidermis and upper dermis. This technique has been reported in a small number of cases. It makes sense that any technique of superficial destruction or removal will work in the same manner.

14. Any other thoughts on nonselective destruction?

Light electrocautery may be used in small tattoos, and the infrared coagulator is effective in the removal of the material in tattoos. The argon laser also has been used, but with scarring and residual pigmentation resulting. As always, the ratio of tissue damage to extent of material removal is the heart of the matter. The Q-switched lasers changed this ratio (and require less skill).

15. What are Q-switched lasers?

Presently, three Q-switched lasers are available: ruby (694 nm), YAG (1064 nm and double-frequency YAG at 532 nm), and alexandrite (760 nm). These lasers operate by giving off short pulses (nanoseconds) that disrupt the tattoo material and cause minimal disruption of adjacent dermis and epidermis (i.e., they demonstrate selective photothermolysis). Q-switched lasers can disrupt the intracellular pigment selectively, alter the pigment, and allow the redistribution and elimination of pigment because the duration of the laser is so short and the energy so high that the pigment is heated and disrupted before the adjacent dermis is injured.

The wavelength must be matched to the color pigment, and multiple wavelengths are needed to treat different colors. All Q-switched lasers work well with black and India ink, but the ruby laser will not remove red, although it is effective in green tattoos. The double-frequency YAG is effective for red but not green. The alexandrite appears to be effective in blue/black, red, and green but does less well with orange and yellow.

16. Any tips for using Q-switched lasers?

• I routinely use a clear polyurethane or Vigilon-like material over the tattoo to keep the splatter, which moves too fast for an evacuator, off my face and out of the air. A cool sheet of Vigilon is soothing and in theory may reduce epidermal damage.

- With treatment, whitening of the epidermis gives you a sense of the endpoint. Heavy bleeding points suggest an overaggressive approach.
- Competitive absorption in a heavily pigmented patient limits effectiveness but may still be used. As one would expect, the less tanned the patient's skin, the better.
- Do not rush. A few months between treatments is not a problem; in fact, it may be beneficial.

17. What kind of complications may occur with the Q-switched laser?

In comparison with other techniques, scarring occurs in a small number of cases and usually responds to time and intralesional steroids. Scarring decreases as the time between treatments is lengthened from 2 weeks to 6–8 weeks. Most patients have temporary hypopigmentation. However, occasionally a white depigmentation may be permanent. Rarely, a tattoo may change color with treatment; a well-described phenomenon is light or natural tones that turn black with treatment. However, unmet expectations are probably the most common problem.

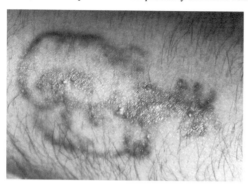 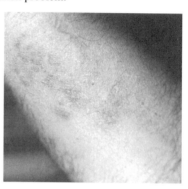

Left, Old, partially faded professional tattoo after two treatments with the Q-switched YAG. Note slight hypertrophic scar at the strings of the gloves. *Right,* Response to four additional laser treatments, with good improvement in tattoo disappearance and resolution of the scar without treatment. Note slight hypopigmentation in the treated area.

18. So the worst problem is that it may not work?

Exactly. Even with the right laser, the number of treatments and final outcome (i.e., how much is removed) cannot be predicted. Imagine the frustration of 10 treatments with only partial response.

19. Are some tattoos easier to remove than others with the Q-switched lasers?

The easiest to remove are clearly the homemade lesions, which use a small amount of India ink. The worst are bright, new, multicolored tattoos. Tattoos overlying other tattoos are hard and unpredictable. Old tattoos respond better than new tattoos.

20. What about traumatic tattoos?

In most tattoos foreign material is introduced on purpose, but material may be entered by trauma, such as road grit from an auto accident, powder from a blast, or pencil point from rushed movements. The best approach is prevention in the acute phase, trying to remove as much material as possible immediately after the incident. Careful cleaning of the wound, including the use of brushes, should be performed. The use of an occlusive dressing may allow further material to leach out, much like a therapeutic dermabrasion.

21. Once you have a traumatic tattoo, are the choices the same as for a decorative tattoo?

Exactly. The choices are excision, spot dermabrasion, laser abrasion, or Q-switched lasers. The depth and materials vary from case to case, and one needs to be creative in treating a tattoo. In addition, patients may have an underlying scar that becomes more apparent after the pigment is gone. Remember to consider the psychologic effects of the trauma when evaluating patient expectations.

22. Does the tattoo have a role in plastic surgery?

The use of medical tattooing procedures is underappreciated. In the past, tattoos were used to hide scars or blend in discolorations, such as port wine stains. Cosmetic tattooing has been used in skin grafts and vermilion enhancement. Although the use of tattooing in port wine stains has been re-placed with better treatments, tattoos are more commonly used in circumstances such as permanent eyeliners, eyebrows, postmastectomy periareolar reconstruction, and covering areas of vitiligo. Low-cost units for this purpose are readily available. Penmark makes a commonly used unit.

The loss of pigment in vitiligo can be stressful and quite obvious, especially in a pigmented pa-tient. By using a unit such as the Penmark enhancer with a multineedle brush, wide areas can be cov-ered. This technique is most helpful in localized areas, such as the hand, that respond poorly to psoralen and ultraviolet A (PUVA) and are difficult to cover effectively.

Cosmetic tattooing may be used to enhance existing eyelids (blepharopigmentation) or eyebrows or to mimic hair for patients with traumatic hair loss or alopecia areata. Ferrous oxide is the common pigment and appears to have a great safety profile with few allergic reactions. Cosmetic tattooing also may be used to create the illusion of an areola and nipple when a formal reconstruction is not desired or possible. It has the advantage of a low invasive approach, and the appearance can be excellent.

Retattooing (i.e., covering a prior tattoo) can be helpful by hiding the offending portion. Examples include tattooing clothes on a naked figure or hiding the name of a loved one from the past.

Medical Uses of Tattooing

Color blending and pigment replacement	Mimicking of lost structures
Port wine stains	Hair loss—eyebrows, eyelids
Skin grafts	Postmastectomy nipple reconstruction
Vermilion—coloration of flaps	Cosmetic enhancement
Scars/burns	Eyebrows, eyelids
Vitiligo	Vermilion
Miscellaneous: radiation ports	

BIBLIOGRAPHY

1. Goldstein N: Tattoo removal. Dermatol Clin 5:349–358, 1987.
2. Guyuron B, Vaughan C: Medical grade tattooing to camouflage depigmentation. Plast Reconstr Surg 95:575–579, 1995.
3. Mazza JF, Rager C: Advances in cosmetic micropigmentation. Plast Reconstr Surg 92:750–751, 1993.
4. Penoff H: The office treatment of tattoos: A simple and effective method. Plast Reconstr Surg 79:186–191, 1987.
5. Piggot TA, Norris RW: Treatment of tattoos with trichloroacetic acid: Experience with 670 patients. Br J Plast Surg 41:112–117, 1988.
6. Zelickson BD, Mehregan DA, Zarrin AA, et al: Clinical, histologic, ultrastructural evaluation of tattoos treated with three lasers systems. Laser Surg Med 15:364–372, 1994.

63. ENDOSCOPIC SURGERY

Oscar M. Ramirez, M.D., F.A.C.S., and W.G. Eshbaugh, Jr., M.D.

1. What technologic advances enabled the rapid proliferation of endoscopic techniques in surgery?

- **Creating an optical cavity.** Techniques such as insufflating the abdominal cavity with nonflam-mable gas (e.g., CO_2), filling synovial spaces with saline, and use of specialized retractors and sleeves for soft tissue endoscopy allow enlargement of the workspace for endoscopic procedures.
- **Electrocoagulation.** The earlier uses of high-frequency currents produced destructive temper-atures and were hazardous with insufflated oxygen in closed body cavities. The modern use of mono- and bipolar electrocautery with nonflammable gases allows hemostasis with much lower temperatures.
- **Light source.** With the advent of fiberoptics and "cold light" (heat shield placed around the bulb) consisting of an incandescent tungsten element in iodine, halogen, or xenon vapor, abun-dant light with minimal heat can be transmitted to the surgical cavity.

• **Imaging.** Coherent bundling of glass fibers, the Hopkins rod-lens system scope, solid-state chip sensor video cameras, of which the charged coupled device (CCD) is the most common, and high-resolution monitors allow mainstream use of endoscopy in surgery.

2. What is the Hopkins rod endoscope?
Named for the British physicist who introduced it, the Hopkins rod greatly improves the optics of endoscopy by using a glass rod with interspersed air spaces rather than the traditional tube of air with interspersed glass lenses.

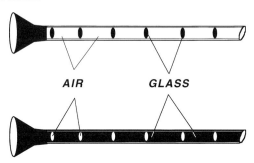

The Hopkins rod endoscope *(bottom)* compared with the traditional glass rod endoscope *(top)*.

3. How is endoscopic surgery different in plastic surgery compared with other specialties?
Most endoscopic procedures in other specialties are performed in naturally occurring, readily accessible body cavities, such as the abdominal, thoracic, synovial, and sinus cavities, or hollow organs, such as the gastrointestinal tract and urinary bladder. In plastic surgery, most endoscopic procedures are performed in surgically created soft tissue planes, which required the development of specialized instrumentation. Lack of natural cavities and incompatibility with existing instrumentation used in other specialties are the main reasons why plastic surgeons were late in developing endoscopic techniques.

4. Which common procedures in plastic surgery are now performed endoscopically?
The endoscopic forehead lift has gained widespread popularity. Endoscopic procedures for harvesting of certain flaps (muscle, jejunum, and omentum), removal of benign subcutaneous tumors, carpal tunnel release, tissue expansion, and rejuvenation of the face and neck have become increasingly common. Breast procedures for augmentation, implant inspection, gynecomastia correction, mammary hypertrophy, and ptosis are performed endoscopically in selected patients. More recent advances in endoscopic plastic surgery are currently used less commonly. Examples include treatment of varicose and incompetent veins, reduction and fixation of facial fractures, neurolysis, tendon and nerve harvesting, and strip craniectomies for craniosynostosis.

5. Which muscles are responsible for forehead animation?
The frontalis, corrugator supercilii, procerus, and orbicularis oculi. Over time, repeated contractions of these muscles lead to prominent wrinkle lines perpendicular to the axis of the muscle.

6. What is the nerve supply to each of these muscles?
The frontalis and corrugators are innervated by the frontal branch of the facial nerve. The buccal branch innervates the procerus, and the orbicularis is innervated by the frontal and zygomatic branches.

7. Which muscles are associated with the vertically oriented glabellar frown lines?
The corrugator supercilii. The corrugators have obliquely oriented fibers within the superomedial portion of the orbicularis oculi. These muscles must be modified to improve the glabellar frown lines.

8. What is the significance of the procerus muscle?

The procerus is a vertically oriented muscle extending from the nasal root superiorly into the glabellum. It pulls down the medial brow and glabellar skin and contributes to the development of horizontal wrinkles at the root of the nose.

9. What are the important components of an endoscopic forehead lift?

The areas to be dissected are infiltrated with lidocaine containing epinephrine. Three to six slit incisions are made behind the hairline in the central, paramedian, and temporal regions if lateral brow dissection is planned. The optical cavity is created with blunt dissection posteriorly as far as the occiput, depending on the amount of skin to be redraped; anteriorly to 3 cm above the orbital rims; and temporally to create a plane between the superficial temporal fascia and temporal fascia proper. With aid of the endoscope, the temporal dissection is continued within 1 cm of the zygomatic arch. The forehead is elevated in the subperiosteal plane across the supraorbital rims to the lateral canthi. The corrugator supercilii, procerus, and orbicularis oculi muscles are modified by transection, disruption, resection, or denervation. The wide undermining of the scalp allows the forehead to be elevated upward without skin excision. Fixation of the redraped scalp is commonly achieved with temporary percutaneous screws or permanent sutures placed into the outer cortex of the skull.

10. The location of which nerves is important during an endoscopic forehead lift?

The **frontal branch of the facial nerve** may be encountered in the temporal dissection. This motor nerve runs in the superficial fat pad above the superficial temporal fascia and crosses the zygomatic arch midway between the tragus and lateral canthus. The **supraorbital and supratrochlear nerves** are sensory branches of the ophthalmic division of the trigeminal nerve. The supraorbital nerve exits the superior orbit adjacent to the periosteum, travels superiorly 2–3 cm, penetrates the frontalis muscle, and continues in a subcutaneous position to the forehead and scalp. The supratrochlear nerve exits the orbit medial to the supraorbital nerve and courses through the corrugator muscles to its subcutaneous location in the scalp.

CONTROVERSY

11. What are the advantages and disadvantages of endoscopic surgery vs. the traditional or open approach?

Advantages. Endoscopic techniques allow small, remote incisions with magnification and illumination of the operative field. Patients often have a shorter convalescence with significant reductions in morbidity and financial costs. Teaching is enhanced with the use of multiple high-resolution monitors that allow many students to view the procedure simultaneously.

Disadvantages. As with any new technique, a learning curve is associated with developing proficient skills in endoscopic procedures. Critics cite the losses of stereoscopic viewing and tactile sensory information with endoscopic surgery. Because of the relatively recent development of many endoscopic procedures performed in plastic surgery, long-term results are unavailable.

BIBLIOGRAPHY

1. Baker TJ, Gordon HL, Stuzin JM: Surgical Rejuvenation of the Face. St. Louis, Mosby, 1996, pp 531–541.
2. Price CI: Equipment and instrumentation. In Ramirez OM, Daniel RK (eds): Endoscopic Plastic Surgery. New York, Springer-Verlag, 1996, pp 10–15.
3. Ramirez OM: Endoscopy in plastic surgery: A myth or reality? In Habal MB (ed): Advances in Plastic and Reconstructive Surgery, vol 15. St. Louis, Mosby, 1998, pp 1–38.
4. Rosenberg PH, Cooperman A: A chronology of endoscopic surgery and development of modern techniques and instrumentation. In Ramirez OM, Daniel RK (eds): Endoscopic Plastic Surgery. New York, Springer-Verlag, 1996, pp 3–6.

64. AUGMENTATION OF THE FACIAL SKELETON

Stephen D. Bresnick, M.D., D.D.S., and John F. Reinisch, M.D.

1. What are the two most common sites in which alloplastic implants are used for facial augmentation in Western cultures?

The chin and cheekbones are the most common sites for alloplastic facial implantation. Western cultures tend to find a strong, muscular jawline and chin extremely attractive. In addition, high cheekbones with associated subtle cheek hollows are considered aesthetically desirable. Chin implants are the most common alloplastic implants in facial aesthetic surgery. Malar implants are the second most common alloplastic implant.

2. In Asian cultures, what is the most common site for placement of an alloplastic facial implant?

The nasal dorsum is the most common anatomic site for placement of an alloplastic facial implant in Asian countries. A defined and sculpted nasal dorsum is considered aesthetically desirable in many Asian cultures.

3. What is the most common material used to make alloplastic facial implants?

Silicone (solid) is by far the most common material used in the construction of alloplastic implants. Silicone implants are biocompatible, stable, modifiable, and easy to work with. Silicone is used to manufacture all types of alloplastic facial implants, including chin, malar, and submalar implants. Polyethylene (Medpor) and hydroxyapatite implants are also used in facial alloplastic implantation but far less commonly than silicone. Polyethylene implants are manufactured for ear reconstruction, nasal augmentation, and other facial augmentation purposes. Hydroxyapatite implants are used for reconstruction of the cranium (cranioplasty), dental alveolar ridges, and other facial bony structures.

4. Compare tissue reaction to a solid, smooth silicone implant and a solid, textured polyethylene implant.

Solid silicone implants used in facial augmentation are smooth and generate the formation of a capsule. Capsules have an inner, smooth, endothelial lining. The capsule does not grow into silicone implants. On the other hand, porous polyethylene implants allow tissue ingrowth; they are made of thousands of tiny polyethylene beads fused together. Pores between the beads allow small blood vessels and collagenous matrix to grow into the interstices of the implant. Thus, polyethylene implants are much more difficult to remove than silicone implants.

5. Is liquid silicone currently used in facial augmentation?

No. In modern practice, liquid silicone has no role as an augmentation material. However, since the 1960s, many patients have undergone liquid silicone injections freely into facial tissues for facial augmentation. Although discontinued in the United States, liquid silicone is still used for facial augmentation in some countries. Liquid silicone is associated with significant long-term complications. Over time, liquid silicone tends to migrate through tissue planes, causing significant inflammatory reactions, tissue calcification, and deformity.

6. Alloplastic implants can augment structures in the head and neck to improve speech function. How can an alloplastic implant be used to improve speech in patients with short or abnormally functioning palates?

Implants can be placed in the posterior pharynx to augment the pharyngeal wall. During certain sounds in normal speech, the soft palate touches the posterior pharyngeal wall. Patients with short or abnormal palates often do not make palatal contact with the posterior pharyngeal wall. Such patients have velopharyngeal incompetence. Nasal escape of air results in hypernasal speech. Alloplastic implants made of Teflon or silicone can be placed beneath the prevertebral fascia in the posterior pharynx to plump up the posterior pharyngeal wall and to help obtain closure with the palate during speech.

7. What anatomic designs are available in facial implants?
    A great variety of implant designs is commercially available. Examples of facial implants include chin, jowl, combination chin-jowl, nasal dorsal, malar, extended malar, submalar, dorsal columella, and mandibular angle implants. Implants also may be custom-manufactured for an individual patient. Most facial implants are constructed of silicone elastomer.

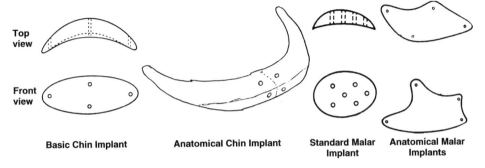

Top view / Front view

Basic Chin Implant   Anatomical Chin Implant   Standard Malar Implant   Anatomical Malar Implants

Various shapes of common facial alloplastic implants.

8. A patient seeking a consultation for facial cosmetic surgery has a large nose, weak chin, and an obtuse cervicomental angle. The plastic surgeon plans to perform rhinoplasty, chin augmentation with a silicone implant, and liposuction of the neck. In what order should these procedures be performed?
    Facial balance and harmony are important concepts in aesthetic surgery. Alteration of the chin and neck significantly alters the appearance of the patient and creates a stronger lower facial appearance. For this reason, chin augmentation should be performed before rhinoplasty. Alteration in the profile of the chin influences the amount of recontouring of the nose. Once chin augmentation has been performed, less extensive nasal reduction is required to create facial balance and harmony. Thus, it would be advisable to perform the procedures in the following order: chin augmentation, neck liposuction, and rhinoplasty.

9. In what ratio (implant projection to soft tissue projection) do facial alloplastic implants augment soft tissues?
    The facial soft tissue response to facial skeletal change is about 0.66. In other words, an implant with 1 cm of projection gives significantly less than 1-cm projection (about 0.66 cm) when it is placed. The difference is due to the thinning of the soft tissues overlying the implant. Most large chin implants provide about 0.8 cm of projection, or about 0.5 cm of soft tissue projection after placement.

10. In what anatomic location are facial alloplastic implants placed in relation to facial soft tissues and bone?
    Alloplastic implants are best placed subperiosteally. Subperiosteal placement with careful pocket dissection is important to minimize complications and give the best results. With a subperiosteal location, most alloplastic implants are stable and non-palpable. Careful dissection to the subperiosteal plane and subperiosteal placement of the implant minimizes soft tissue trauma, decreases possible injury to the facial expression muscles, and minimizes postoperative sensory dysfunction.

11. Ear reconstruction can be performed with alloplastic implants shaped into the normal anatomic configuration of an external ear and require coverage with vascularized fascia. What is the most common fascial layer used to cover an alloplastic ear implant?
    The temporoparietal fascia, which is located just deep to the hair follicles and superficial to the temporalis muscle, is most commonly used to cover alloplastic ear implants. The superficial temporal artery runs through the temporoparietal fascia. This fascial layer can be raised as a flap and transposed downward over an alloplastic ear framework to create a vascularized envelope for the implant. Skin grafts and skin flaps may be used to cover the fascia.

12. Several years after placement of a chin implant, the patient notices that the chin prominence has slightly decreased. No evidence suggests that the implant has been displaced. What is the most likely cause for subtle loss of prominence?

Bone resorption beneath the implant is the most likely explanation. Over time, implants usually cause some resorption of the underlying bone. This is usually not a significant problem; most often, the loss is only several millimeters in bone thickness.

13. What surgical approaches are used for the placement of chin implants?

Chin implants are placed with either an intraoral or a submental approach. The **intraoral approach** has the advantage of rapidity, convenience for the surgeon, and no external skin incision. Disadvantages of the intraoral approach include a higher infection risk, less visualization of the dissection, and possible disruption of the labial sulcus.

The **submental approach** is often used when additional procedures, such as liposuction, direct submental fat excision, or platysmaplasty, are planned. Advantages of the submental approach include better visualization of the dissection, access to neck soft tissues, lower infection risk, and improved preservation of the labial sulcus. Disadvantages of the submental approach include external scar (although it is well camouflaged), more difficult dissection, and longer operating time.

14. What surgical approaches are used for the placement of malar implants?

Malar implants may be placed through either intraoral or extraoral approaches. The **extraoral approaches** include subciliary, preauricular, and transcoronal approaches. The subciliary approach is best used when malar augmentation is combined with lower lid blepharoplasty, because direct visualization of the zygoma and precise implant placement are possible. Care must be taken to avoid the possible complications of eyelid scarring and ectropion. The preauricular approach is useful when malar augmentation is combined with face lift (usually composite or deep-plane face lift). This approach allows sterile placement of the malar implant and lower infection rates, but it is not used when malar augmentation without face lift is desired. Transcoronal placement of malar implants may be used when malar augmentation is combined with forehead lift or subperiosteal face lift.

The **intraoral approach** is preferred by most surgeons. This technique involves placement of an anatomically sized implant in a subperiosteal location over the zygoma with a minimal buccal vestibular incision. Advantages of the intraoral approach include ease and rapidity of placement, no visible scar, and low complication rates.

15. What are common complications after placement of an alloplastic facial implant?

The most common complications include hematoma, infection, extrusion, malposition, sensory nerve dysfunction, and facial muscle weakness. Most complications are related to a postoperative hematoma that causes wound healing problems and infection. The incidence of infection, extrusion, or hematoma has been found to be less than 1% in several series.

16. What is the most common complication after placement of a chin implant? A malar implant?

Hypoesthesia of the lower lip is the most common complication after placement of a chin implant. This problem is usually transient, unless the mental nerve has been inadvertently damaged or the implant is impinging on a nerve. **Malposition** is the most common complication after malar implant placement.

BIBLIOGRAPHY

1. Binder WJ, Schoenrock LD, Terino EO: Augmentation of the malar-submalar/midface. Fac Plast Surg Clin North Am 2:265, 1994.
2. Terino EO: Alloplastic facial contouring by zonal principles of skeletal anatomy. Clin Plast Surg 19:487, 1992.
3. Terino EO, Sofino MV: Facial contouring with alloplastic implants. In Aston SJ, Beasley RW, Thorne CHM (eds): Grabb and Smith's Plastic Surgery, 5th ed. Philadelphia, Lippincott-Raven, 1997, pp 699–703.
4. Tolleth H:Concepts for the plastic surgeon from art and sculpture. Facial aesthetic surgery: Art, anatomy, anthropometrics, and imaging. Clin Plast Surg 14:585, 1987.
5. Whitaker LA: Temporal and malar-zygomatic reduction and augmentation. Clin Plast Surg 18:55–64, 1991.
6. Wilkinson TS: Complications in aesthetic malar augmentation. Plast Reconstr Surg 71:643, 1983.
7. Wolfe SA, Vitenas P: Malar augmentation using autogenous materials. Clin Plast Surg 18:39–54, 1991.

VIII. Trunk and Lower Extremity

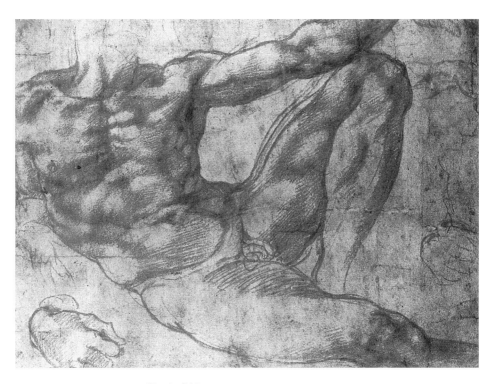

Sketch of Adam
[For the *Creation of Adam* in the Sistine Chapel]
Michelangelo
1511
Red chalk
The British Museum, London
© 1992 Alinari/Art Resource, New York

65. CHEST WALL RECONSTRUCTION

Norman Weinzweig, M.D., and Jeffrey Weinzweig, M.D.

1. When do the skeletal components of the chest wall form embryologically?

The ribs, costal cartilages, and sternum form during the sixth week of gestation. The primitive sternum arises from two lateral mesenchymal bands that fuse by the ninth week of gestation. During this period the thoracic ribs, costal cartilages, and intervening musculature develop independently of the sternum. By the ninth week, the ribs have matured and cartilages 1–7 have joined the sternum. Cartilages 8–10 are incorporated shortly afterward. Congenital chest wall anomalies arise from developmental disturbances during this period.

2. What are the muscular layers of the chest wall?

Between the overlying skin and underlying rib cage are a number of muscles that can be divided into two main groups: **inspiratory** and **expiratory** muscles. The inspiratory muscles serve as elevators of the superior aperture of the rib cage and assist with expanding the chest volume. They include the sternocleidomastoid and scalene muscles, which insert onto the clavicle and the first and second ribs. Major resections of the upper sternum and ribs result in a partial collapse of the ribs inferiorly and a measurable functional loss in ventilation. The expiratory muscles attach to the much larger inferior aperture of the rib cage and constrict the skeletal structure downward, forcing the abdominal contents upward against the diaphragm to assist with expiration, coughing, and sneezing. They include the rectus abdominis, internal oblique, and external oblique muscles. Muscles attached to the clavicle, scapula, and humerus, such as the pectoralis major, trapezius, and latissimus dorsi, are primarily involved in movement of the shoulder and arm.

3. What are the functions of the chest wall?

The chest wall has both structural and functional roles:

1. It provides a bony shell for protection of vital visceral organs, including the heart, lungs, liver, spleen, pancreas, and kidneys.

2. It provides a flexible frame for respiratory movements.

3. Muscular components actively contribute to inspiration and expiration.

4. Chest wall muscles attached to the clavicle, scapula, and humerus contribute to movement of the shoulder and arm.

5. Overall expansion of the rib cage is crucial to creating negative pressure necessary for lung expansion during inspiration; loss of rigid support over a large area of the rib cage results in an inward motion of the chest wall—paradoxical movement.

4. What are the most common indications for chest wall reconstruction?

Defects of the chest wall requiring reconstruction most often result from (1) trauma, (2) tumor resection, (3) infection, (4) radiation ulcers, or (5) congenital defects. These defects may be superficial, involving only the soft tissue of the chest wall, or complex, involving the skeletal framework, thoracic cavity, or mediastinum.

5. What are the principles of chest wall reconstruction?

1. Adequate debridement and resection of all tumor, osteoradionecrotic tissue, or infection
2. Obliteration of intrathoracic dead space
3. Skeletal stabilization if more than four ribs or > 5 cm of chest wall are resected en bloc
4. Adequate soft tissue coverage
5. Aesthetic consideration

6. What type of tissue is most often used for reconstruction?

Muscle and musculocutaneous flaps are the tissues of choice for chest wall reconstruction. Local skin flaps, regional pedicle flaps, and thoracoabdominal tube flaps were used until the popularization of muscle and musculocutaneous flaps in the mid 1970s. The pectoralis major, latissimus dorsi, serratus anterior, and rectus abdominis muscles are most frequently used.

7. What are the indications for free tissue transfer?
Free tissue transfer for chest wall reconstruction is performed infrequently. It is reserved for cases in which regional flaps are unavailable or have already been used. Microvascular anastomoses can be performed using the thoracodorsal, subscapular, or internal mammary arteries as recipient vessels.

8. What options are available for skeletal stabilization?
Stabilization of the sternum for defects encompassing more than four contiguous rib segments is necessary for restoration of normal protective and respiratory function of the chest wall. Various materials can be used in this capacity, including autogenous tissue (rib grafts, fascia, large muscle flaps), synthetic compounds (Teflon, Prolene mesh, Gore-Tex), and composite mesh (a Marlex-methyl methacrylate composite). Muscle flaps can also stabilize large chest wall defects without resulting in flail segments, especially in the radiated chest wall, in which local tissues have stiffened secondary to chronic inflammation from radiation exposure.

9. What is the incidence of median sternotomy infection?
Median sternotomy infection occurs in 0.4–5.0% of cardiac procedures.

10. What is the significance of sternal wound infections?
Postcardiotomy sternal wound infection is a life-threatening complication. Mortality rates range from 5–50%. Infection may extend into the mediastinum, affecting prosthetic valves, bypass grafts, and suture lines.

11. Should serial debridement be performed after sternal wound dehiscence?
Not necessarily. Nahai et al. reported a series of 211 consecutive cases of sternal wound coverage. The pectoralis major muscle flap was used in 56% and the rectus abdominis muscle in 38%. Single-stage debridement with muscle flap coverage immediately on diagnosis of sternal dehiscence was successful in 95% of cases.

12. Is there a correlation between use of the internal mammary artery (IMA) for bypass grafting and the incidence of sternal wound infections?
Yes. Perforators of the IMA are the main blood supply to the sternum. Therefore, use of the IMA for bypass grafting may compromise the vascular supply of the sternum, delaying wound healing and increasing the risk of infection. Cosgrove et al. demonstrated no sternal wound complications in patients in whom saphenous vein grafts were used for bypass, a 0.3% incidence in patients in whom unilateral IMA grafts were used, and a 2.4% incidence in patients in whom bilateral IMA grafts were used.

13. How are sternotomy wound infections classified?
Pairolero classified infected sternotomy wounds into three types:

Type I infected sternotomy wounds occur in the first 1–3 days postoperatively and consist of serosanguinous drainage with negative wound cultures without cellulitis, costochondritis, or osteomyelitis. Wounds require reexploration, minimal debridement, and rewiring of the sternum.

Type II infected sternotomy wounds occur in the first 2–3 weeks postoperatively and consist of purulent mediastinitis with positive wound cultures, cellulitis, costochondritis, and osteomyelitis.

Type III infected sternotomy wounds present months to years after cardiac procedures. Draining sinus tracts result from chronic costochondritis and osteomyelitis. Type II and Type III wounds require thorough debridement and reconstruction.

14. How are median sternotomy wounds reconstructed?
Because of its location on the chest wall, its size, and its arc of rotation, the pectoralis major muscle is the flap of choice for reconstruction of median sternotomy wounds. This muscle originates on the clavicle, sternum, six upper ribs, and aponeurosis of the external oblique muscle and occupies

the anterior chest wall. It inserts on the intertubercular sulcus of the humerus, forming the anterior wall and fold of the axilla. The pectoralis major muscle is a type V muscle supplied by the thoracoacromial artery, its dominant pedicle, and segmental perforators from the IMA.

The muscle is harvested through the sternotomy wound. Wide undermining at the level of the pectoralis fascia is performed, and the muscle is then detached from the ribs and sternum. Dissection proceeds laterally after identification of the thoracoacromial pedicle on the undersurface of the muscle, and the humeral attachment is divided. The muscle is then dissected from the clavicle and advanced medially to cover the defect. Coverage of large defects with exposed heart and great vessels can often be accomplished with bilateral pectoralis major muscle flaps.

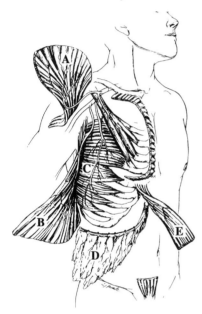

Pedicle flap donor sites for chest wall reconstruction. *A*, Pectoralis major muscle flap. *B*, Latissimus dorsi muscle flap. *C*, Serratus anterior muscle flap. *D*, Greater omentum flap. *E*, Rectus abdominis muscle flap. (From Cohen M: Reconstruction of the chest wall. In Cohen M (ed): Mastery of Plastic and Reconstructive Surgery. Boston, Little, Brown, 1994, p 1250, with permission.)

15. How can the pectoralis major muscle be used as a "turnover" flap?

The pectoralis major muscle can be based medially on the perforating branches of the IMA if it is intact. After the anterior surface of the muscle is exposed, dissection of the muscle from the chest wall is performed from lateral to medial to avoid injury to the IMA perforators. The thoracoacromial pedicle is identified and ligated, and dissection is continued up to 2–3 cm lateral to the midline— again, to protect the perforators. The muscular attachment to the humerus is divided, and the muscle is turned over like a page in a book to cover the defect. When possible, preservation of a partial attachment of the superior portion of the muscle to the humerus provides a better aesthetic result by preserving the anterior axillary fold.

16. When is the rectus abdominis muscle used?

The rectus abdominis muscle can be used to supplement a pectoralis major muscle flap when additional bulk is needed or when the pectoralis major muscle is not available. Based superiorly on the deep superior epigastric artery, a terminal branch of the IMA, this type III muscle can be turned on itself to fill a defect of the chest wall or mediastinum. The rectus abdominis muscle is harvested through a midline or paramedian skin incision. The anterior rectus sheath is incised, and the muscle is divided at the necessary level inferiorly and elevated from the posterior rectus sheath in a caudad to cephalad fashion. The muscle is mobilized on its superior pedicle and transposed into the defect.

17. Can the rectus abdominis muscle be used when the ipsilateral IMA has been harvested for bypass grafting?

Yes. The rectus muscle can be harvested based on the eighth intercostal vessel. However, the distal third of the rectus muscle often has tenuous vascularity.

18. What role does the omentum play?

Weinzweig and Yetman reported the largest series of omental transposition flaps for coverage of infected sternal wounds. In their series of 25 patients, the greater omentum, either alone or in combination with muscle flaps, provided reliable coverage after radical sternectomy for deep infections, including osteomyelitis, chronic chondritis, and mediastinitis, as well as for extensive and lower third sternal wounds. Ninety-five percent of wounds ultimately healed without intraabdominal problems or chest wall instability.

19. What is a sternal cleft?

Sternal clefts, described as early as 1772 by Sandifort, are rare deformities in which a grotesque depression in the middle of the chest may reveal the pulsating heart through the overlying skin. Interruption of sternal fusion may result in these impressive anomalies. A superior sternal cleft occurs secondary to a deficiency in cephalad fusion; a distal sternal cleft results from a premature cessation of fusion.

20. Which congenital anomalies are associated with developmental abnormalities of the ribs?

Developmental abnormalities of the ribs may result in supernumerary ribs or hypoplasia of the costal cartilages, which may be associated with Poland's syndrome. Anomalous rib development also may result in pectus excavatum and pectus carinatum.

21. Which congenital chest wall anomaly is associated with ipsilateral hand deformities?
Poland's syndrome.

22. What is Poland's syndrome?

Described by Alfred Poland in 1841, this congenital anomaly is characterized by partial or complete absence of the pectoralis major muscle and hypoplastic or absent adjacent musculoskeletal components. The deformity consists of a number of unilateral findings, including partial agenesis of the ribs and sternum, brachysyndactyly, mammary aplasia, and absence of the latissimus dorsi, serratus anterior, and pectoralis major muscles in the severe form. In the mildest form of Poland's syndrome, mild hypoplasia of the breast and lateral nipple displacement may be the only findings.

23. Do the reconstructive goals differ in females and males with Poland's syndrome?

Yes. Although the goal in both cases is restoration of a natural contour to the anterior chest wall, reconstruction of a symmetric breast mound, a normal-appearing nipple-areolar complex, and subclavicular fullness are necessary in female patients. In both male and female patients, the best aesthetic result is usually accomplished by a latissimus dorsi muscle transfer to the anterior chest wall. In women, simultaneous insertion of a submuscular mammary prosthesis is usually performed. Depending on the severity of the anomaly, a muscle flap may be performed without the need for a mammary implant; similarly, reconstruction of mild forms of the syndrome may require use of a prosthesis alone.

24. What is pectus excavatum?

Pectus (chest) deformities occur as commonly as 1 in 300 live births. Pectus excavatum (funnel chest) is the most common chest wall deformity. The depression of the anterior chest wall usually begins at the sternal angle (angle of Louis) and reaches its deepest point at the level of the xiphoid. The concave deformity is occasionally so severe that the sternum contacts the vertebral bodies or passes to one side of the vertebral bodies into the paravertebral gutter, accounting for the associated cardiopulmonary and physiologic abnormalities. This anomaly is believed to result from overgrowth of the costal cartilages, which force the sternum posteriorly in the case of pectus excavatum and anteriorly in the case of pectus carinatum (see question 26).

25. How is pectus excavatum treated?

The **Ravitch technique** for reconstruction involves elevation of perichondrial flaps and resection of the involved costal cartilages (usually 4 or 5 on each side) with preservation of the costochondral junction when possible. The xiphoid process is divided to permit elevation of the sternum. A posterior transverse osteotomy of the sternum is performed superiorly, and the sternum is fractured forward. A bone wedge is used to stabilize the sternum at the osteotomy site posteriorly. An anterior transverse osteotomy is then performed inferiorly and stabilized with a bone wedge anteriorly. The sternum is then stabilized with wires to adjacent ribs and bilateral pectoralis flaps are sutured to the sternum in the midline.

The **sternum turnover procedure** involves transection of the ribs and intercostal muscles bilaterally at the costal arches along the margin of the deformity. The sternum is transected above the level of the deformity, removed en bloc, and turned over. The convex side is then flattened by wedge resections and trimmed to fit the chest wall defect. The sternum is sutured in place with wires, and each costal cartilage or rib is sutured with heavy silk.

26. What is pectus carinatum? How is it related to pectus excavatum?

Pectus carinatum (pigeon breast) is a protrusion deformity of the anterior chest wall and is considered the opposite of the pectus excavatum deformity. This condition occurs much less commonly than the excavatum anomaly. Surgical reconstruction for pectus carinatum is similar to that used to correct pectus excavatum. The abnormal costal cartilages are resected through a subperichondrial approach, and the sternum is repositioned to restore the anterior chest wall contour. A substernal metallic strut is used to support the repositioned sternum. Wires are used to secure the strut to the sternum and surrounding ribs.

BIBLIOGRAPHY

1. Arnold PG, Pairolero PC: Chest wall reconstruction: Experience with 100 consecutive patients. Ann Surg 199:725, 1984.
2. Arnold PG, Pairolero PC: Surgical management of the radiated chest wall. Plast Reconstr Surg 77:605, 1986.
3. Boyd A: Tumors of the chest wall. In Hood RM (ed): Surgical Diseases of the Pleura and Chest Wall. Philadelphia, W.B. Saunders, 1986.
4. Carberry DM, Ballantyne LWR: Omental pedicle graft in closure of large anterior chest wall defects. NY State J Med 75:1705, 1975.
5. Cohen M: Reconstruction of the chest wall. In Cohen M (ed): Mastery of Plastic and Reconstructive Surgery. Boston, Little, Brown, 1994, pp 1248–1267.
6. Hester TR, Bostwick J: Poland's syndrome: Correction with latissimus muscle transposition. Plast Reconstr Surg 69:226, 1982.
7. Hugo NE, Sultan MR, Ascherman JA, et al: Single-stage management of 74 consecutive cases of sternal wound complications with pectoralis major myocutaneous advancement flaps. Plast Reconstr Surg 93:1433, 1994.
8. Jurkiewicz MJ, Arnold PG: The omentum: An account of its use in reconstruction of the chest wall. Ann Surg 185:548, 1977.
9. Nahai F, Rand RP, Hester TR, et al: Primary treatment of the infected sternotomy wound with muscle flaps: A review of 211 consecutive cases. Plast Reconstr Surg 84:439, 1989.
10. Pairolero PC, Arnold PG: Management of infected median sternotomy wounds. Ann Thoracic Surg 42:1, 1986.
11. Poland A: Deficiency of the pectoralis muscle. Guy's Hosp Rep 6:191, 1841.
12. Ravitch MM: Congenital Deformities of the Chest Wall and Their Operative Correction. Philadelphia, W.B. Saunders, 1977.
13. Roth DA: Thoracic and abdominal wall reconstruction. In Aston SJ, Beasley RW, Thorne CHM (eds): Grabb and Smith's Plastic Surgery, 5th ed. Philadelphia, Lippincott-Raven, 1997, pp 1023–1029.
14. Seyfer A: Congenital anomalies of the chest wall. In Cohen M (ed): Mastery of Plastic and Reconstructive Surgery. Boston, Little, Brown, 1994, pp 1233–1239.
15. Shaw WW, Aston SJ, Zide BM: Reconstruction of the trunk. In McCarthy JG (ed): Plastic Surgery. Philadelphia, W.B. Saunders, 1990, pp 3675–3796.
16. Weinzweig N, Yetman R: Transposition of the greater omentum for recalcitrant sternotomy wound infections. Ann Plast Surg 34:471, 1995.

66. ABDOMINAL WALL RECONSTRUCTION

Norman Weinzweig, M.D., and Gloria Chin, M.D.

1. What is the functional role of the abdominal wall?
The abdominal wall consists of a well-delineated system of vertically, obliquely, and transversely oriented muscles that play a key role in posture, standing, walking, bending, and lifting. In addition, the abdominal wall muscles protect the abdominal viscera and increase intraabdominal pressure to aid in coughing, vomiting, defecation, micturition, and parturition. These muscles also play a supporting role in normal respiration.

2. What are the anatomic limits of the anterior abdominal wall?
The anterior abdominal wall is bordered superiorly by the lower rib margins and xiphoid process and extends inferiorly to Poupart's ligaments and the pelvic brim.

3. What are the layers of the abdominal wall?
• Skin
• Superficial fascia: superficial fatty layer, Camper's fascia, Scarpa's fascia
• Muscles and their aponeuroses: external oblique, internal oblique, transversus abdominis, rectus abdominis, and pyramidalis
• Properitoneal fat
• Peritoneum

4. What are the origins and insertions of the abdominal wall muscles?
External oblique muscle—most superficial of the three muscles in the lateral aspect of the abdominal wall. It arises from the lower eight ribs and interdigitates with the serratus anterior and latissimus dorsi muscles. It inserts on the anterior half of the iliac crest; inferiorly its aponeurosis forms the inguinal ligament (Poupart's ligament), which extends from the anterosuperior iliac spine to the pubic spine.

Internal oblique muscle—lies beneath the external oblique. Its origin is in the lumbodorsal fascia, anterior two-thirds of the iliac crest, and lateral two-thirds of the inguinal ligament. The lower fibers join those of the transversus abdominis muscle to form the conjoined tendon, which inserts on the pubic crest and spine and on the ileopectineal line. The superior fibers insert as a broad aponeurosis into the linea alba and cartilages of the seventh to ninth ribs.

Transversus abdominis muscle—located deep to the internal oblique muscle. Its origin lies in the lower six ribs, lumbodorsal fascia, anterior two-thirds of the iliac crest, and lateral one-third of the inguinal ligament. It inserts on the linea alba and contributes to the conjoined tendon that inserts on the pubic spine and ileopectineal line.

Rectus abdominis muscle—longitudinal muscle located in the medial aspect of the abdominal wall. It arises from the front of the symphysis and pubic crest and inserts on the xiphoid process and cartilages of the fifth through seventh ribs.

Pyramidalis muscle—small triangular muscle that lies superficial to the rectus muscle. It arises from the front of the pubis and inserts on the linea alba half way between the symphysis and umbilicus.

5. What are the functions of the abdominal wall muscles?
The rectus muscles flex the body anteriorly and are important in climbing in and rising out of bed. The external and internal oblique muscles are involved in rotating the upper body against the lower body. The vertical component of these muscles can substitute for the rectus muscles if they are absent.

6. What is the arterial supply to the abdominal wall?
1. **Superior epigastric artery**—a terminal branch of the internal mammary artery that supplies the upper central abdominal skin through the upper rectus muscle.

2. **Thoracic and lumbar intercostal arteries**—travel between the external and internal oblique muscles with direct lateral skin perforators.

3. **Deep inferior epigastric artery**—a branch of the external iliac artery that enters the lower rectus muscle and supplies it and the accompanying vertical or transverse skin paddle.

4. **Deep circumflex iliac artery**—a branch of the external iliac artery supplying the inner aspect of the ileum and skin over the iliac crest.

5. **Superficial inferior epigastric artery**—a branch of the femoral artery that supplies the skin and subcutaneous tissue of the lower abdomen.

6. **Superficial circumflex iliac artery**—a branch of the femoral artery that supplies the skin and subcutaneous tissue over the anterosuperior iliac spine.

7. **Superficial external pudendal artery**—a branch of the femoral artery that supplies the skin and subcutaneous tissue over the pubis.

7. What is the venous and lymphatic drainage of the abdominal wall?

The venous drainage parallels the arterial supply to the abdominal wall. The upper abdomen is drained by the superior epigastric, intercostal, and axillary veins. The lower abdomen is drained by the superficial inferior epigastric, superficial circumflex iliac, and deep inferior epigastric veins. The superficial lymphatics drain into the groin and axillary nodes. The deep system drains upward toward the internal mammary or deep iliac nodes.

8. What are the most frequent causes of abdominal wall defects?

Trauma (shotgun blasts)	Massive infection (necrotizing fasciitis)
Tumor (primary or recurrent)	Postoperative incisional hernia
Radiation therapy	Congenital anomalies (gastroschisis, omphalocele)

9. What is gas gangrene of the abdominal wall? How do you differentiate it from anaerobic clostridial cellulitis?

Gas gangrene, or clostridial myonecrosis, is a rare but highly lethal postoperative complication that requires early recognition and prompt surgical debridement of *all* involved layers of the abdominal wall. Clinical signs include wound swelling, tenderness, drainage, discoloration that changes from pink to magenta within a few hours, and usually a small amount of crepitation. The patient is toxic out of proportion to the temperature elevation, with signs of tachycardia and hypotension. The wound culture is polymicrobial with at least one species of *Clostridium*, usually *C. oedamatiens* or *C. septicum*. The most important exotoxin is lecithinase. The main difference between anaerobic clostridial cellulitis and clostridial myonecrosis is the relationship of the gas to the signs of toxicity; a small amount of gas with severe toxicity usually represents clostridial myonecrosis.

10. What are the most common congenital defects of the anterior abdominal wall?

Omphalocele and gastroschisis.

11. What is an omphalocele? What causes it?

An omphalocele is a developmental anomaly of the abdominal wall that occurs in 1 in 3,200 to 1 in 10,000 live births, often in association with sternal or diaphragmatic abnormalities, heart defects, or extrophy of the bladder. Large defects, often associated with syndromes, have a high mortality rate. An omphalocele results from failure of the four folds of the abdominal wall (endoderm, ectoderm, inner splanchnic and outer somatic mesoderm) to fuse at the umbilical ring. The sac (yolk sac) of amnion and chorion that covers the eviscerated mass commonly contains liver and midgut. The defect develops during the extracolemic phase, between the sixth and twelfth weeks of intrauterine life, when the entire midgut passes out of the abdomen and into the yolk sac. After a period of linear growth the bowel rotates 270° counterclockwise around the superior mesenteric vascular axis before returning into the abdomen. Defects range from those limited to the umbilicus to those extending from the xiphoid to the pubis. The umbilical cord attachment is most often at the apex of the sac.

12. Is an omphalocele a true hernia?

An omphalocele is *not* a true hernia. No peritoneum lines the sac, and the contents have never truly been in the abdomen.

13. What is a gastroschisis?
A gastroschisis is a full-thickness defect of the abdominal wall that occurs lateral to the umbilical ring with the umbilical cord attached at the normal position. The herniated viscera are *not* covered by amnion.

14. Besides the physical findings of the abdominal wall, what characteristics do patients with gastroschisis have in common?
Nonrotation of the bowel, abnormally short midgut, and small peritoneal cavity.

15. How does a gastroschisis differ from an omphalocele?
A gastroschisis differs from an omphalocele in that it lacks a covering sac and it is rare to see liver or other organs in the defect. The intestines are usually thickened, matted, and shortened because of prolonged contact with the amniotic fluid. Umbilical cord insertion is normal. The abdominal wall defect is lateral to the umbilicus, usually on the right side where the umbilical vein has resorbed, leaving it structurally weaker.

16. What are the major causes of mortality in patients with an omphalocele or gastroschisis?
Sepsis, increased intraabdominal pressure postoperatively, respiratory insufficiency, and catabolic state associated with prolonged intestinal ileus.

17. What other major anomalies are seen in patients with gastroschisis and omphalocele?
Intestinal atresia (20–25% of patients), malrotation, and volvulus.

18. What is the treatment of patients with gastroschisis or omphalocele?
Primary closure, if it does not produce dangerously high intraabdominal pressure. Otherwise, staged procedures are indicated. Silon (silastic-coated Dacron), polyethylene, or Teflon sheets are sutured to the edges of the fascial defect, and the viscera are gradually returned into the abdomen as the wall relaxes and the cavity enlarges. If necessary, local or regional flaps are then placed.

19. What is "prune belly" syndrome?
Prune belly syndrome, also known as triad syndrome or Eagle-Barrett syndrome, consists of a triad of anomalies found almost exclusively in newborn boys: (1) absent or hypoplastic abdominal wall musculature, (2) bilateral cryptorchism, and (3) dilatation of the urinary tract. On physical examination, the muscular deficiency may be limited to one area, ranging from complete absence of muscle to the presence of all muscles as thin but recognizable structures. Complete absence of the lower rectus muscles is most common. The abdomen appears wrinkled or flabby, much like a prune, because of the weakened abdominal wall. As the child grows, the body contour resembles a pear or pot belly more than a prune. Children are often subject to respiratory complications due to impaired diaphragmatic motion. Surgical correction involves a combined approach to correct the urologic and gonadal defects at the same time. Patients are encouraged to develop the available muscle(s). Recent reports describe the transposition of the tensor fascia lata and rectus femoris muscle flaps to strengthen the abdominal wall.

20. What are the most important considerations in the evaluation of abdominal wall defects?
- Underlying disease process—acute or chronic wound? Reconstruction can proceed either immediately, as in the case of tumor ablation or radiation, or in delayed fashion, as in the case of trauma with gross fecal contamination or massive infection.
- Stability of the wound—has all of the necrotic and/or infected tissue been removed?
- Gastrointestinal fistula
- Partial vs. full-thickness defect
- Lower vs. upper vs. entire abdominal wall defect

21. What studies aid in the evaluation of abdominal wall defects?
A CT scan or MRI is helpful in evaluating the extent of tumor invasion or the integrity of potential muscle or musculocutaneous flaps to be used in reconstruction. The vascular status of these flaps can be determined by a color flow duplex Doppler study that combines Doppler ultrasound and B-mode ultrasound to produce images of blood vessels and their surroundings. A fistulogram or an intestinal contrast study may be needed to evaluate for abdominal fistulas.

22. Describe the management of acute losses of the abdominal wall.

Initial management of acute losses of the abdominal wall, as in traumatic injuries with massive fecal contamination or necrotizing fasciitis, begins with the ABCs of resuscitation (airway, breathing, circulation). After stabilization of the patient, aggressive surgical debridement is performed. It is critical that abdominal wounds *not* be closed under tension because of the prohibitive morbidity and mortality. It is also best to avoid closure of acute injuries by elevation of local soft tissue flaps with the intention of later hernia repair. This approach merely opens new tissue planes that may spread infection and unnecessarily increases the operative time. Although exposed viscera can be directly skin-grafted, skin grafts lack the resilience to protect internal organs, promote adhesions, and provide unstable coverage. Moreover, the risk of early enteric fistulas is high. The treatment of choice in the acute setting is the use of synthetic mesh for abdominal support.

23. What are the objectives in abdominal wall reconstruction?

1. The integrity of the abdominal wall must be restored to protect the intraabdominal viscera and to prevent herniation. Abdominal wall support can be reconstituted either by alloplastic materials, such as Marlex or Prolene mesh, or by musculofascial flaps, such as tensor fascia lata or rectus femoris.

2. Soft tissue coverage can be provided by either a skin graft or one of several flaps. Adjacent abdominal soft tissue can be transposed for coverage. Omentum, measuring as much as 25×45 cm in surface area, can be placed either above or below the mesh to prevent adhesions to the viscera and then skin-grafted. Various musculofascial and musculocutaneous flaps or free tissue transfers can be used for definitive coverage. These flaps also may contain a fascial component and can be used to provide both support and soft tissue coverage.

24. How do you treat acquired abdominal wall defects?

1. **Acute traumatic wounds.** Temporizing measures such as packing or a "zippered"mesh may be used to cover viscera while the acute problems are treated and the patient is stabilized.
2. **Infection**
   - Infection limited to the skin and subcutaneous tissue, including abscesses and some synergistic infections, requires drainage and wide debridement with preservation of the underlying muscle and fascia.
   - Infection of the abdominal wall fascia, such as necrotizing fasciitis, requires wide debridement of the involved fascia and overlying infected skin and subcutaneous tissue.
   - Clostridial myonecrosis involves *all* layers of the abdominal wall and therefore requires full-thickness resection.
3. **Tumor resection.** Primary tumors of the abdominal wall include desmoid tumors, sarcomas, and their malignant variants. There also may be primary skin malignancies, malignant degeneration of chronic scars, fistulas, and radiation injury. Secondary tumors result from extensions of carcinoma of the colon, bladder, gallbladder, or other visceral malignancies. The primary goal of treatment is definitive resection. The specimen is examined. If resection is considered, the wound can be managed temporarily with dressings or mesh.
4. **Radiation wounds** involve an area of skin prone to ulceration or infection that does not heal. The treatment is wide resection and examination of the specimen for recurrence. Once the wound margins are tumor-free, definitive reconstruction can be performed while the wound is temporarily covered with dressings or mesh.
5. **Postoperative defects.** Abdominal wall defects after surgery include incisional hernias, parastomal hernias, and local breakdown of catheter and infusion sites. Defects also may result from exposed or infected mesh, skin-grafted viscera, or painful, irregular scars. Reconstruction is considered only when the initial problem and associated complications are resolved.

25. What are the reconstructive options?

1. **Prosthetic materials** are used for abdominal wall support.
2. **Skin grafts** are most often used in cases of massive abdominal trauma. When the wound is stable, they can be removed by dermabrasion or excision. The hernia is repaired with mesh, and the wound is covered with a local or regional flap.
3. **Local flaps.** Skin and subcutaneous flaps can be based laterally on the intercostal vessels, on perforators from the deep circumflex iliac artery, or on axial vessels from the superficial circumflex

iliac, superior epigastric, or superficial external pudendal arteries. The external oblique muscle may be used as a medially based musculofascial turnover flap or a laterally based musculocutaneous flap. The rectus muscle, based on either the superior epigastric or deep inferior epigastric vessels, may be used as a muscle or musculocutaneous flap.

4. **Regional flaps.** The tensor fascia lata and the rectus femoris muscles are most commonly used. The gracilis muscle is much more limited in its application. It originates from the inferior pubic symphysis and inserts as a tendon on the upper medial tibia. The major pedicle is a branch of the profundus femoris artery located 8–10 cm from the adductor tubercle; one or two minor pedicles are located distally from the superficial femoral artery. It may be used as a muscle or musculocutaneous flap that reaches to the inguinal and perineal regions. The skin paddle is often unreliable.

5. **Distant flaps** include the omentum, the extended latissimus dorsi musculofascial flap, or free flaps. Free tissue transfer may be necessary when the defect is large and no adequate local or regional flaps are available.

26. When is prosthetic material used?

Prosthetic material is used for structural support of the abdominal wall in a stable wound or as a temporizing measure in an open acute or infected wound.

27. What are the criteria for synthetic mesh?

Synthetic mesh is often useful both in the acute setting and at the time of definitive reconstruction. However, alloplastic materials should meet certain criteria. Mesh should be resistant to mechanical stress; it should be strong, durable, and of significant tensile strength so that it will not fragment with usage. Mesh should be chemically inert; it should not be modified by tissue fluids or excite an inflammatory body reaction but instead should be capable of incorporation. Mesh should be tolerant to infection and capable of being reentered in the presence of infection for further exploratory surgery. Mesh also should be easy to handle and capable of being fabricated into the desired shape. Lastly, it should be sterilizable.

28. What types of prosthetic materials have been used for abdominal wall reconstruction?

Tantalum, stainless steel, Mersilene, Vicryl, Prolene, Marlex, and Gore-Tex patch.

29. Describe the experience with prosthetic materials.

Different prosthetic materials vary in their indications and efficacy. However, few clinical reports describe large series with long-term follow-up. Both **tantalum** and **stainless steel** were found to fragment easily and to have less pliability than the other materials and were abandoned many years ago.

Marlex mesh (polypropylene [PP]) was originally used during the Vietnam War for open abdominal wounds. Reports of its usage are few, and follow-up is usually incomplete. Most reports showed a 100% incidence of mesh extrusion or fistula formation when the mesh was directly skingrafted. Piecemeal removal of the mesh was required. Thus, although Marlex mesh demonstrated an early benefit in providing abdominal wall support, especially in the presence of infection, there were uniform long-term problems with skin grafting or closure by secondary intention. Despite excellent quality granulation tissue and initial complete skin graft survival, there is inevitable failure with skin graft breakdown and mesh extrusion, usually within the first 3 months. Voyles looked at the short-term benefits vs. the long-term complications of Marlex mesh in emergency abdominal wall reconstruction. He found good short-term results in his series of 31 patients, in 29 of whom the mesh was placed in the presence of gross contamination. Twenty-three of the patients were reoperated through the mesh without subsequent dehiscence. Long-term results, however, were less favorable. Extrusion was observed in all 9 patients in whom a skin graft was applied directly over the mesh. Enteric fistulas were observed in 3 of the 9 patients. In the 3 patients in whom a flap was applied directly over the mesh, no problems were noted with either mesh extrusion or enteric fistulas.

Prolene mesh has shown a somewhat lower incidence of mesh extrusion when covered with a skin graft, but the incidence still hovers around 40%. Prolene has greater pliability than Marlex. **Gore-Tex** promotes fewer adhesions to the viscera and is more easily removed than Marlex. It does not allow incorporation. **Vicryl** mesh is usually absorbed by 8 weeks and provides temporary support. It does not result in more significant bowel adhesions or suffer spatial disorganization and was found to retain its shape.

30. What is the clinical course of prosthetic materials capable of incorporation?

Within 18–24 hours, a fibrous exudate seals the viscera from the mesh. At 5–10 days, there is ingrowth of granulation tissue through the interstices of the mesh. At 14–21 days, the granulation tissue is ready for either skin-grafting or flap coverage.

31. Describe the technique of prosthetic material placement in abdominal wall reconstruction.

Mesh is best applied directly over the omentum, if the omentum is still intact, to prevent adhesions to the underlying viscera. Mesh may be sewn directly to the remaining musculofascial tissue in end-to-end fashion, or the free edge of the mesh may be folded over on itself for 2–3 cm and then sewn to the musculofascial tissue. It is critical that the mesh be sutured under slight tension to avoid wrinkles, folds, or bunching. Tension is adjusted as the mesh is inset.

32. What are the options for lower abdominal wall reconstruction?
1. Tensor fascia lata musculofascial flap
2. Rectus femoris musculofascial flap
3. External oblique muscle and aponeurosis
4. Inferiorly based rectus flap with or without anterior rectus sheath and overlying skin paddle
5. Groin flap

33. What are the options for upper abdominal wall reconstruction?
1. Superiorly based rectus with or without rectus sheath and overlying skin paddle
2. External oblique muscle and aponeurosis
3. Thoracoepigastric flap
4. Extended latissimus dorsi musculofascial flap with pregluteal and lumbosacral fascia—also may be used for large or ipsilateral abdominal defects. For added length and mobility the latissimus muscle may be detached from its humeral insertion.

34. What is the flap of choice for abdominal wall defects?

The tensor fascia lata is the ideal reconstructive option for abdominal wall defects. A dense, strong sheet of vascularized fascia and overlying skin can be transferred as a single unit in a single stage with minimal donor deficit. It is extremely useful in irradiated and contaminated fields. Protective sensation can be maintained by inclusion of the lateral femoral cutaneous nerve (T12), and voluntary control is provided by the descending branch of the superior gluteal nerve. Flaps wider than 8 cm usually require skin grafting of the donor site; narrower flaps can be closed primarily. There is tremendous disparity between the small size of the tensor muscle, originating from the greater trochanter, and the surrounding tensor fascia lata flap. The cutaneous paddle is reliable to approximately 5–8 cm above the knee; the distal portion is essentially a random pattern flap supplied largely by cutaneous perforators from the vastus lateralis muscle. The dominant pedicle—the lateral circumflex femoral vessels arising from the profunda femoris—pierces the medial aspect of the flap 8–10 cm below the anterosuperior iliac spine. The arc of rotation allows the tip of the flap to reach the ipsilateral lower chest wall and xiphoid, especially in a thin patient. The flap may be used to resurface the entire suprapubic region, lower abdominal quadrants, or ipsilateral abdomen.

35. What is the role of the rectus femoris in abdominal wall reconstruction?

Like the tensor fascia lata, the rectus femoris is an excellent flap choice for reconstruction of the ipsilateral or lower abdominal wall. For extensive defects, a larger cutaneous paddle may be incorporated with the adjacent fascia lata in the musculocutaneous flap. The tip of the flap reaches a point midway between the umbilicus and xiphoid. The flap is supplied by the lateral femoral circumflex vessels. It also can cover the entire suprapubic region and extend to the contralateral anterosuperior iliac spine. After transposition, the vastus lateralis and vastus medialis are approximated to prevent a functional deficit resulting in loss of the final 15° of knee extension. Sacrifice of this muscle in ambulating patients may provide some functional debility.

36. What is the "mutton chop" flap?

Described by Dibbell et al., the mutton chop or extended rectus femoris myocutaneous flap allows reconstruction of large full-thickness abdominal wall defects, including the epigastrium, without prosthetic material.

37. What is the "components separation" method for closure of abdominal wall defects?

Elucidated by Ramirez et al., the theory behind the components separation method is that separation of the muscle components of the abdominal wall allows mobilization of each unit over a greater distance than is possible by mobilization of the entire abdominal wall as a block. For example, the compound flap of the rectus muscle attached to the internal oblique-transversus abdominis muscle can be advanced 10 cm medially. The rectus muscle is separated from its posterior rectus sheath. The external oblique can be elevated, leaving the neurovascular supply to the rectus intact in the internal oblique-transversus layer; however, advancement is limited. Large abdominal wall defects can be reconstructed by the functional transfer of these components, overlapping muscle layers while maintaining their innervation and vascular supply. This technique obviates the need for distant flaps or free flaps. It takes advantage of the three muscle layers lateral to the rectus muscles. The different orientation of the muscle fibers and their attachments makes it difficult to advance them en bloc in a given direction.

38. What is the role of the omentum in abdominal wall reconstruction?

The omentum, a double layer of fused peritoneum arising from the greater curvature of the stomach, is supplied by the right and left gastroepiploic arteries. This flap can cover the entire abdominal wall and perineal areas. It may be used with mesh and provides a good bed for a skin graft.

39. What is the role of tissue expansion in abdominal wall reconstruction?

Tissue expansion is a reconstructive option that has been used in congenital abdominal wall defects for extensive soft tissue defects. Expanders can be placed between the external and internal oblique muscles to create an enlarged external oblique musculocutaneous flap or beneath the subcutaneous tissue but above the fascia.

40. What is the incidence of herniation following TRAM flaps?

Kroll and coworkers reported using mesh in 21.4% of free transverse rectus abdominis muscle (TRAM) flaps and in 45.0% of conventional TRAM flaps. The incidence of lower abdominal wall laxity following conventional TRAM flaps ranged from 0.2–16.0%; it was even lower in free TRAM flaps (1.0–5.0%). There was no difference in abdominal wall strength, based on the ability to perform sit-ups, in patients who had a pedicled or free TRAM flap and age-matched controls.

BIBLIOGRAPHY

1. Bleichrodt RP, Simmermacher RKJ, van der Lei B: Expanded polytetrafluoroethylene patch versus polypropylene mesh for the repair of contaminated defects of the abdominal wall. Surg Gynecol Obstet 176:18–23, 1993.
2. Bostwick J, Hill HL, Nahai F: Repairs in the lower abdomen, groin or perineum with myocutaneous or omental flaps. Plast Reconstr Surg 63:186–194, 1978.
3. Boyd WC: Use of Marlex mesh in acute loss of the abdominal wall due to infection. Surg Gynecol Obstet 144:251, 1977.
4. Brown GL, Richardson JD, Malangoni MA: Comparison of prosthetic materials for abdominal wall reconstruction in the presence of contamination and infection. Ann Plast Surg 13:705–711, 1984.
5. Byrd HS, Hobar PC: Abdominal wall expansion in congenital defects. Plast Reconstr Surg 84:347–352, 1989.
6. Caix M, Outrequin G, Descottes B: The muscles of the abdominal wall: A new functional approach with anatomoclinical deductions. Anat Clin 6:101–108, 1984.
7. Caulfield WH, Curtsinger L, Powell G, et al: Donor leg morbidity after pedicled rectus femoris muscle flap transfer for abdominal wall and pelvic reconstruction. Ann Plast Surg 32:377–382, 1994.
8. De Troyer A: Mechanical role of the abdominal muscles in relation to posture. Respir Physiol 53:341–353, 1983.
9. Dibbell DG Jr, Mixter RC, Dibbell DG Sr: Abdominal wall reconstruction (the "mutton chop" flap). Plast Reconstr Surg 87:60–65, 1991.
10. Hui K, Lineweaver W: Abdominal wall reconstruction. Adv Plast Reconstr Surg 14:213–244, 1997.
11. Klein MD, Hertzler JH: Congenital defects of the abdominal wall. Surg Gynecol Obstet 152:805–808, 1981.
12. Kroll SS, Marchi M: Comparison of strategies for preventing abdominal wall weakness after TRAM flap breast reconstruction. Plast Reconstr Surg 89:1045–1051, 1992.
13. Livingston DH, Sharma PK, Glantz AI: Tissue expanders for abdominal wall reconstruction following severe trauma: Technical note and case reports. J Trauma 32:82–86, 1992.
14. Parkas S, Ramakrishman K: A myocutaneous island flap in the treatment of a chronic radionecrotic ulcer of the abdominal wall. Br J Plast Surg 33:138–139, 1980.

15. Peled IJ, Kaplan HY, Herson M, et al: Tensor fascia lata musculocutaneous flap for abdominal wall recon-
    struction. Ann Plast Surg 11:141–143, 1983.
16. Ramirez OM, Ruas E, Dellon AL: "Components separation" method for closure of abdominal-wall defects:
    An anatomic and clinical study. Plast Reconstr Surg 86:519–526, 1990.
17. Shaw WW, Aston SJ, Zide BM: Reconstruction of the trunk. In McCarthy JG (ed): Plastic Surgery.
    Philadelphia, W.B. Saunders, 1990, pp 3755–3796.
18. Suominen S, Asko-Seljavaara S, von Smitten K, et al: Sequelae in the abdominal wall after pedicled or free
    TRAM flap surgery. Ann Plast Surg 36:629–636, 1996.
19. Taylor GI, Watterson PA, Zelt RG: The vascular anatomy of the anterior abdominal wall: The basis for flap
    design. Perspect Plast Surg 5:1–30, 1991.
20. Voyles CR, Richardson JD, Bland KI, et al: Emergency abdominal wall reconstruction with polypropylene
    mesh: Short-term benefits versus long-term complications. Ann Surg 194:219, 1981.

67. RECONSTRUCTION OF THE POSTERIOR TRUNK

Andrew L. Da Lio, M.D., and William W. Shaw, M.D.

1. What are the common reconstructive problems of the posterior trunk?

Thoracic pressure sores, radiation necrosis, spinal/paraspinal tumor resections, and spina bifida.

2. What muscle or fasciocutaneous flaps may be used in reconstruction of the posterior trunk?

Most wounds of the posterior trunk result from trauma, tumor resection, or irradiation. Classically, muscle coverage has been divided into thirds based on the location of the wound: the trapezius muscle for upper-third wounds, the latissimus dorsi for middle-third wounds, and the gluteus
maximus for lower-third wounds. The scapular/parascapular fasciocutaneous flaps also may be used
for small upper-third defects. Paraspinous muscle flaps may be advanced for relatively small vertical
defects of the spine and paraspinal regions.

LATISSIMUS DORSI FLAP

**3. What is the origin and insertion of the latissimus dorsi muscle? What are the external
anatomic landmarks to identify the muscle?**

The latissimus dorsi muscle is a broad, flat, triangular muscle measuring approximately 35 cm
long, 20 cm wide, and 1 cm thick. It originates from the spinous processes of T7–T12, L1–L5, and
the sacrum, posterior superior iliac crest, and ribs 9–12. It inserts on the intertubercular groove on
the anterior aspect of the proximal humerus.

External landmarks include the posterior midline, posterior superior iliac crest, tip of the
scapula, and posterior axillary line. Forceful contraction of the latissimus dorsi muscle may help to
identify the muscle border at the posterior axillary line.

4. What is the function of the latissimus dorsi muscle and the functional deficit after harvesting?

Functions of the latissimus dorsi muscle include shoulder adduction, medial rotation, and extension. It also assists the pectoralis major in pulling the trunk upward and forward when the arm is raised
(as in rock or mountain climbing). Laitung and Peck examined shoulder function after latissimus dorsi
harvest. Objective measurements of muscle donor site shoulder function were compared with the
equivalent dominant or nondominant shoulders in controls. There was no significant difference in
shoulder power. Range of motion after muscle harvest was decreased 5–30° in one-third of patients because of scar contracture. No patients had occupational problems related to shoulder disability.

5. Describe the vascular anatomy of the latissimus dorsi muscle.

The latissimus dorsi muscle has a type V pattern of circulation with one dominant pedicle (thoracodorsal artery) and secondary segmental pedicles (posterior intercostal and lumbar artery perforating branches). The dominant vascular pedicle to the latissimus dorsi muscle is the thoracodorsal
artery, a branch of the subscapular artery. The thoracodorsal pedicle has a mean length of 9 cm but

can be increased to 11 cm by following the dissection to the subscapular artery. The mean diameter of the thoracodorsal artery is 2.7 mm at its origin, whereas that of the subscapular artery ranges from 3.0–4.0 mm. Despite some variability in vascular anatomy, there is usually a single thoracodorsal and subscapular vena comitans measuring 3–4.5 mm in diameter.

In 86% of cadaver dissections, the thoracodorsal artery bifurcates on the inferior surface of the latissimus dorsi muscle at a clearly defined neurovascular hiatus 2 cm medial to the muscular border. The upper branch courses transversely across the muscle 3.5 cm from the superior border, whereas the lateral branch courses vertically toward the iliac crest 2.1 cm from the lateral margin. This vascular pattern allows splitting of the muscle into two distinct components and thus a variety of insetting options. In the remaining 14% of dissections, no major bifurcation was identified.

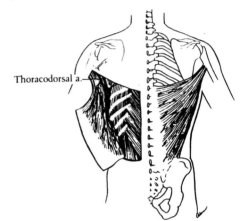

Latissimus dorsi myocutaneous flap with dual blood supply consisting of the thoracodorsal artery and segmental paravertebral perforators, of which there are two rows. (From Vasconez LO, McCraw JB, Camargos AG: Muscle, musculocutaneous, and fasciocutaneous flaps. In Smith JW, Aston SJ (eds): Grabb and Smith's Plastic Surgery, 4th ed. Boston, Little,Brown, 1991, p 1123, with permission.)

6. What is the motor innervation to the latissimus dorsi muscle? Can the latissimus dorsi myocutaneous flap be used as a neurosensory flap?

The thoracodorsal nerve supplies motor innervation to the latissimus dorsi muscle. The nerve arises from the posterior cord of the brachial plexus; descends posterior to the axillary artery, located 3 cm medial to the origin of the subscapular artery; runs with the thoracodorsal artery; and enters the neurovascular hilum with the vessels. The latissimus dorsi myocutaneous flap cannot be elevated as a neurosensory flap.

7. What is the arc of rotation of the latissimus dorsi muscle based on the dominant thoracodorsal pedicle?

Using the dominant thoracodorsal pedicle, the point of rotation is at the neurovascular hiatus. The muscle has a posterior arc of rotation to the neck, occiput, parietal skull, and thoracic vertebrae T1–T12. The anterior arc can reach the ipsilateral hemithorax and sternum, middle and lower third of the face, and superior abdomen.

8. What is the arc of rotation of the latissimus dorsi muscle based on the secondary segmental pedicles?

The point of rotation is along the lateral and/or medial row of minor pedicles, allowing the muscle to reach across the midline for coverage of small defects in the thoracic and upper lumbar vertebral regions.

9. What is the skin territory of a latissimus dorsi myocutaneous flap?

The skin paddle may be raised in various shapes and patterns (oblique, horizontal, vertical skin islands) because of the numerous perforating vessels from the latissimus dorsi muscle to the overlying skin. In general, the perforators are more numerous in the proximal two-thirds of the muscle. Skin paddle widths allowing primary closure range from 8–15 cm, depending on body habitus and skin compliance, and must be individualized. Vertically, the skin paddle may extend downward to the posterior iliac crest, although the most distal aspect may be less reliable in terms of overall vascularity.

10. What are options for coverage of large wounds of the lower back (below T10) in the setting of cancer and/or prior irradiation and infection?

Wounds of the lower back (below T10, lumbar, sacral, and buttock areas) may present difficult problems. Although local flaps (latissimus dorsi muscle reverse flap based on the secondary segmental pedicles, gluteus maximus muscle flap, and transverse back flap) may be considered, they may prove unreliable or inadequate in the face of prior irradiation and fibrosis. In such circumstances, the latissimus dorsi muscle may be transposed inferiorly, using reversed greater or lesser saphenous microvascular vein grafts reliably and with relatively little difficulty, given the large vessel diameters. Although an additional option includes direct anastomoses to the superior gluteal vessels, these vessels are often involved in radiation and fibrosis; furthermore, they are located deep in the wound, making microvascular anastomoses difficult.

11. Can the latissimus dorsi muscle be elevated and transferred based on the serratus anterior branch?

Yes. When the thoracodorsal vessels are divided for whatever reason, the latissimus dorsi muscle may be transposed based on the retrograde flow from the serratus anterior branch into the thoracodorsal artery as the dominant vascular pedicle. Likewise, venous return is preserved through the vena comitans accompanying the serratus branch. Reversal of flow from the serratus anterior branch into the thoracodorsal artery has been clearly demonstrated intraoperatively. Clinically, this finding is significant because the latissimus dorsi myocutaneous flap can be reliably used as a salvage flap for breast reconstruction after failure of free flaps that used the proximal thoracodorsal artery and vein as the recipient vessels.

SCAPULAR/PARASCAPULAR FLAP

12. What are the anatomic landmarks of the scapular and parascapular fasciocutaneous flaps?

The skin territory of the circumflex scapular artery (CSA) may be divided into two regions based on the transverse and descending branches. The scapular flap, based on the transverse branch, is centered on a horizontal line extending from the triangular space (approximately 2 cm above the posterior axillary crease) and the vertebral column. The distal end of the flap may extend to a point midway between the medial border of the scapula and the midline. The parascapular flap, based on the descending branch, is centered on a vertical line extending from the triangular space and posterior iliac spine along the lateral edge of the scapula. The distal end of the flap may extend downward to a point midway between the tip of the scapula and posterior iliac spine. Flap dimensions are highly variable, depending on body habitus and skin laxity, but may reach 10 × 30 cm. An additional variant of the parascapular flap is the IMECS (inframammary extended circumflex scapular) flap, which follows a gradual curve into the inframammary crease, thus improving the location of the scar. This modification is based on the numerous radial vessels from the descending branch of the CSA.

13. What is the triangular space? What is the vascular anatomy of the scapular and parascapular flaps?

The triangular space is bordered by the teres minor and subscapularis superiorly, the teres major inferiorly, and the triceps (long head) laterally. This space marks the exit point of the circumflex scapular artery and vena comitans. Note that the triangular space is *not* the triangle of auscultation, which is formed by the latissimus dorsi, trapezius, and rhomboid major muscles. The CSA is a branch of the subscapular artery, and the dissection may be followed proximally, increasing pedicle length and vessel diameter size.

14. What is the arc of rotation of the (para)scapular flaps?

The point of rotation of the scapular and parascapular flaps is at the triangular space. The arc of rotation includes the shoulder, axilla, and lateral thoracic wall.

GLUTEUS MAXIMUS MUSCLE/MYOCUTANEOUS FLAP

15. What is the Mathes-Nahai pattern of circulation of the gluteus maximus muscle?

Type III: two dominant pedicles (superior and inferior gluteal arteries).

The gluteus maximus muscle is supplied by the superior and inferior gluteal arteries with the piriform muscle separating the two arterial systems. On the left side the muscle has been divided near its insertion along the greater trochanter. (From Vasconez LO, McCraw JB, Camargos AG: Muscle, musculocutaneous, and fasciocutaneous flaps. In Smith JW, Aston SJ (eds): Grabb and Smith's Plastic Surgery, 4th ed. Boston, Little, Brown, 1991, p 1128, with permission.)

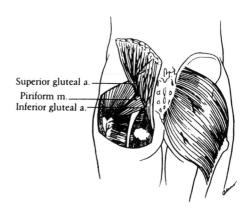

Superior gluteal a.
Piriform m.
Inferior gluteal a.

16. Describe the origin and insertion of the gluteus maximus muscle.

The gluteus maximus muscle originates from the lateral sacrum and posterior superior iliac crest. It inserts into the greater trochanter of the femur and along the iliotibial tract.

17. What is the standard arc of rotation of the gluteus maximus muscle/myocutaneous flap?

The point of rotation based on the superior gluteal vessels is at the lateral border of the sacrum approximately 5 cm below the posterior superior iliac spine. When islanded on these superior gluteal vessels, the myocutaneous flap reaches the ipsilateral ischium and sacrum. This flap is also an important option for coverage of lower lumbar defects.

18. How can you increase the arc of rotation of the gluteal myocutaneous flap?

The skin of the posterior thigh can be raised based on the descending branch of the inferior gluteal artery. The vascular territory of this descending branch can extend 10 x 35 cm, approaching the posterior popliteal crease. When elevated, this fasciocutaneous flap can reach the sacrum, contralateral ischium, perineum, rectum, vagina, groin, trochanter, and anterior thigh. The posterior thigh fasciocutaneous flap can be islanded on the inferior gluteal artery, significantly increasing the arc of rotation. The posterior thigh donor site is usually skin-grafted.

TRAPEZIUS MUSCLE/MYOCUTANEOUS FLAP

19. What are the anatomic landmarks of the trapezius muscle?

The trapezius muscle measures 34×18 cm. It arises from the external occipital protuberance, superior nuchal line of the occipital bone, ligamentum nuchae, and spinous processes of C7–T12 vertebrae and inserts into the lateral third of the clavicle, spine of the scapula, and acromion.

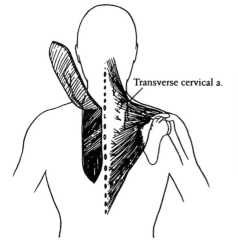

Transverse cervical a.

Trapezius myocutaneous flap with the transverse cervical artery arborizing at the root of the neck. On the left the trapezius myocutaneous flap has been elevated; it usually includes branches that descend inferiorly. (From Vasconez LO, McCraw JB, Camargos AG: Muscle, musculocutaneous, and fasciocutaneous flaps. In Smith JW, Aston SJ (eds): Grabb and Smith's Plastic Surgery, 4th ed. Boston, Little, Brown, 1991, p 1119, with permission.)

20. What is the vascular pattern of the trapezius muscle flap?

The trapezius muscle has a type II pattern of circulation via the transverse cervical artery (dominant pedicle) and minor pedicles supplied by the dorsal scapular artery, perforating posterior intercostal arteries, and a branch of the occipital artery.

21. What is the arc of rotation of the trapezius muscle/myocutaneous flap?

The point of rotation of the trapezius muscle is at the posterior base of the neck at the location of the transverse cervical artery pedicle. The muscle reaches the posterior skull, cervical and thoracic vertebrae, mid to upper face, and neck. It is generally used in reconstruction of the upper third of the back, neck, and head and neck defects. When elevated as a myocutaneous flap, the skin territory can extend beyond the scapular tip into the mid back region with relative safety. One can extend the cutaneous territory by "delaying" the skin portion.

SPINA BIFIDA

22. What are the four variants of spina bifida cystica?

1. Meningocele: no neurologic deficit, with meninges in the cystic herniation.

2. Meningomyelocele: most common form; both meninges and neural elements within the cystic herniation; usually associated with motor and sensory deficits.

3. Syringomyelocele: rare, similar to meningomyelocele but with dilatation of the central canal of the cord.

4. Myelocele: rare; neural elements openly exposed without meningeal or cutaneous coverage.

23. What are the options for wound closure?

Approximately 75% of thoracolumbar and lumbosacral meningomyelocele defects can be closed using wide mobilization and simple primary skin closure. For larger defects, lateral relaxing incisions with bipedicle flap closure and skin grafts, rotation flaps, double rhomboid Z-plasties, composite skin-muscle flaps, and medial advancement of bilateral latissimus dorsi and gluteus maximus muscles have been used with success.

BIBLIOGRAPHY

1. Burns AJ (ed): Trunk reconstruction. Sel Read Plast Surg 7 (31), 1995 [entire issue].
2. Laitung JFG, Peck F: Shoulder function following the loss of the latissimus dorsi muscle. Br J Plast Surg 38: 375, 1985.
3. Mathes SJ, Nahai F: Reconstructive Surgery: Principles, Anatomy, and Technique. New York, Churchill Livingstone, 1997.
4. Nahai F, Hagerty R: One-stage microvascular transfer of a latissimus flap to the sacrum using vein grafts. Plast Reconstr Surg 77:312–315, 1986.
5. Ramirez OM, Ramasastry SS, Granick MS, et al: A new surgical approach to closure of large lumbosacral meningomyelocele defects. Plast Reconstr Surg 80:799, 1987.
6. Smith JW, Aston SJ (eds): Grabb and Smith's Plastic Surgery, 4th ed. Boston, Little, Brown, 1991.
7. Strauch B, Yu HL: Atlas of Microvascular Surgery: Anatomy and Operative Approaches. New York, Thieme Medical Publishers, 1993.

68. RECONSTRUCTION OF THE LOWER EXTREMITY

R. Jobe Fix, M.D., and Tad R. Heinz, M.D.

1. How does a plastic surgeon become involved in lower extremity reconstruction?

Many vascular, surgical, oncologic, and orthopedic wounds benefit from plastic surgical consultation and intervention because of large soft tissue defects and/or combined vascularized bone graft and soft tissue requirements.

2. What types of pathology may require lower extremity reconstruction?

Open fractures of the distal tibia, chronic wounds of the distal third of the leg, unstable scars, defects from sarcoma resections, diabetic ulcers, radiation wounds, osteomyelitis of the tibia, and wounds resulting from ischemia of the lower extremity often require reconstruction.

3. What are common coverage methods for the thigh?

1. Local rotation or advancement flaps of the thigh muscles, with or without skin grafts—in particular, the gracilis, vastus lateralis, and TFL flaps.

2. Fasciocutaneous flaps such as the medial thigh, lateral posterior thigh, or rectus femoris fasciocutaneous flap.

3. More distant flaps such as the rectus abdominis based on the deep inferior epigastric artery and vein.

4. What are the alternatives and considerations for soft tissue coverage of the knee?

Muscle flaps, fasciocutaneous flaps, and free tissue transfer are useful for knee coverage. The gastrocnemius muscle flap is readily available for knee coverage; however, it does not reliably cross the midline to the contralateral aspect of the knee or to the superior aspect of the knee. The distally based vastus lateralis has been described; however, partial necrosis is a frequent occurrence. The saphenous fasciocutaneous flap, as described by Walton and Bunkis, is useful if available. For extensive defects covering the entire surface of the knee, free tissue transfer of a large fasciocutaneous flap or muscle flap is the most reliable.

5. What is appropriate soft tissue coverage for the proximal tibia?

Local muscle flaps include the medial gastrocnemius and lateral gastrocnemius, which is usually shorter than the medial gastrocnemius. Fasciocutaneous flaps include the saphenous flap, a distally based medial or lateral fasciocutaneous flap, or a combination of a gastrocnemius flap with a proximally or distally based fasciocutaneous flap. Free flaps are indicated when the local soft tissue injury contraindicates the use of local muscle or fasciocutaneous flaps and the area is extensive.

6. What are appropriate choices of soft tissue coverage of the mid-tibial region?

For small defects, a turnover flap of the anterior tibialis muscle may be useful. Most defects, however, are larger and may require the soleus muscle, which is readily available and transposes well over this area. Fasciocutaneous flaps from the lateral or medial leg, based distally or proximally, are useful. Of course, free flaps are appropriate when local soft tissue coverage is not available or the defect is extensive.

7. What local coverage is available for ankle or distal tibial exposure?

Small defects < 4 cm² may be covered by the extensor brevis muscle flap, slightly larger defects by the lateral supramalleolar flap, and somewhat larger defects by the dorsalis pedis fasciocutaneous flap. These flaps require a blood supply not compromised by the injury. The distally based soleus flap has been used but with a high incidence of partial necrosis. Distally based fasciocutaneous flaps (based laterally or medially), including the sural neurocutaneous flap, may be safely used with the demonstration of comparable perforators at the respective base of the flap.

8. What are common coverage methods for wounds of the foot?

Several small muscle flaps, such as the flexor hallucis and abductor hallucis brevis, are available but are rarely of practical use given the frequent global injury to the foot and ankle area. The sural artery flap may be of benefit for small or moderate-sized wounds of the ankle and proximal foot as well as the heel area. Most of these wounds, however, require some type of free tissue transfer for satisfactory closure.

9. Why are the wounds of the distal leg so problematic for coverage?

The distal portion of the leg has poor skin elasticity, frequent severe edema, and osseous structures that lie in the subcutaneous tissue and are quite vulnerable. Such wounds also have a high rate of osteomyelitis, which often results in amputation. The distal third of the leg has significant tendinous structures that take skin grafts poorly. Finally, the foot and ankle require good flap durability because they are so frequently exposed to friction and shear by walking and footwear.

10. What are the indications for free tissue transfer to cover the distal lower extremity?

Indications for free tissue transfer include large or circumferential defects exposing fractures, open joints, or the Achilles' tendon; incisions or soft tissue trauma that compromise the lateral or medial fasciocutaneous areas; and compromise of the distal arterial flow, which may prevent the use of lateral supramalleolar or dorsalis pedis flaps.

11. List absolute indications for flap coverage of the lower extremity.

Exposed bypass grafts, open fractures, and tendon and nerve exposure.

12. What is the arterial blood supply to the leg?

The popliteal artery at the knee divides at the infrapopliteal trifurcation into the tibial arteries—namely, the posterior and anterior tibial and peroneal arteries. The posterior and anterior tibial arteries cross the ankle, whereas the peroneal does not but may give branches feeding the two tibial vessels.

13. What are the arterial domains?

The posterior tibial artery tends to predominate in the heel and posterior plantar skin area. The anterior tibial artery supplies the dorsum of the foot after becoming the dorsalis pedis artery and distal portions after bifurcation into the first dorsal metatarsal artery and deep plantar artery. The peroneal artery may fill the anterior or posterior artery systems via its distal branches. Although these distinctions are not hard and fast, they are clinically important because the posterior tibial artery is a frequent target for free tissue transfer by microsurgical techniques.

14. What are special considerations for plantar foot coverage?

Probably the foremost problem in coverage of the plantar foot is the ability of the transferred tissue to tolerate the shear forces involved in walking. Interface problems between the native plantar glabrous skin and the transferred skin are common. Durability, the need to cover fusion or any other osseous work, and, finally, lack of sensation in the transferred tissue are also important. Any insensate tissue transferred is at significant risk for breakdown.

15. What is the most appropriate source of free tissue transfer for coverage of extensive plantar foot defects?

The jury is still out. May et al. present convincing evidence for the use of muscle flaps with skin grafts; however, fasciocutaneous flaps have been used as effectively. Probably the most important criteria are (1) a familiar flap with an adequate pedicle length of sufficient caliber; (2) a flap that is well tailored to the defect, and not excessively thick; (3) muscle flaps to cover deep or irregular defects; and (4) skin flaps for resurfacing superficial degloving tissue defects. Abnormally high pressure points in the plantar surface lead to recurrent breakdowns after reconstruction. Bony abnormalities should be corrected. The patient should be educated about meticulous foot care, and orthotics should be provided.

16. How can abnormal weightbearing in the neuropathic foot be corrected?

Bone spurs and joint dislocation can and must be corrected. For ulceration of the fifth metatarsal head, resection through the metatarsal neck is recommended. The first metatarsal head is debrided only if it is involved in the ulcer base. More commonly the medial or lateral sesamoid bone needs to be removed in the base of the first metatarsal head ulcer. For the second, third, and fourth metatarsal heads, one should perform a metatarsal neck osteotomy. Midfoot bony prominences may require judicious resection around the areas of the metatarsal bases, cuneiform, or navicular bones. Limited midfoot fusions should be considered. Orthotics may be useful to shift weight away from a particular pressure point.

17. Before the development of microsurgical techniques, what treatment was used for lower extremity wounds—especially in the distal third of the leg?

Treatment may have been below-knee-amputation or skin-grafting, which often yielded a poor result. Occasionally success was achieved with local or pedicled flaps and cross-leg flaps in which the limb had to be immobilized for 3–5 weeks before division of the flap pedicle.

18. Why not use a skin graft on lower extremity wounds?

Poor leg skin elasticity, edema, bone close to the skin surface, and a high rate of osteomyelitis and amputation have been associated with inadequate wound coverage in the tibial area, such as with a skin graft. In addition, there are obvious technical problems with getting the skin graft to heal over bone and tendon. It is rarely possible to attain adequate healing in such tissues because of the decreased blood supply in these areas.

19. Can you think of a situation in which a cross-leg flap would be a good choice?

Coverage of a child's heel may be a reasonable indication for a cross-leg flap. The sensate territory of the superior/posterior thigh from the descending branch of the inferior gluteal nerve may be used to perform neurorraphy, and later the pedicled skin flap may be divided. Only a child would tolerate this degree of knee flexion and immobilization for the weeks required without subsequent joint stiffness and contracture.

20. What are the muscle groups and major nerves and arteries of each of the four compartments of the lower leg?

The **anterior compartment**, bounded by the tibia, interosseous membrane, and anterior intermuscular septum, contains the extensor muscles of the foot and ankle with the tibialis anterior, extensor hallucis longus, and extensor digitorum longus muscles. The major artery is the anterior tibial artery, and the deep peroneal nerve courses along with the artery.

The **lateral compartment** is bounded by the anterior intermuscular septum, fibula, and posterior intermuscular septum. The muscles in this compartment are the peroneus longus, peroneus brevis, and peroneus tertius muscles. There is no major artery in the lateral compartment; however, the superficial peroneal nerve runs within it.

The **posterior superficial compartment** is bounded by the deep surface of the soleus muscle and the plantaris tendon. It contains the soleus and gastrocnemius muscles.

The **deep posterior compartment** is bounded by the tibia, interosseus membrane, and fibula. The muscle groups contained within it are the tibialis posterior, flexor digitorum longus, and flexor hallucis longus muscles. This compartment contains the posterior tibial artery, which courses medially between the flexor digitorum longus and soleus muscles, and the peroneal artery, which courses slightly more laterally between the tibialis posterior and flexor hallucis longus muscles. The major nerve in the deep posterior compartment is the posterior tibial nerve.

21. How do you distinguish between diabetic and nondiabetic foot wounds in the nontraumatic setting?

Probably a better distinction is between neuropathic and ischemic wounds, which are treated very differently. Diabetics have no more microvascular or small vessel disease than their aging, arthrosclerosis-matched counterparts. However, diabetics have a tendency toward stocking-and-glove neuropathy, which leads to areas of decreased sensation in the foot that in turn may lead to calluses, fissuring, and infection. The neuropathic wound frequently is on the plantar aspect of the metatarsal heads, where abnormal weight bearing may occur. The patient does not appreciate the risks and continues to walk extensively with eventual deep infection and osteomyelitis. The patient's perfusion, however, may be completely normal. In contrast, the ischemic wound may occur in a patient with arthrosclerosis and typically appears in a location, at the distal toe tips or the heel.

22. Why should we invest significant resources to salvage an ulcerated diabetic limb when the patient can just as well have a below-knee amputation and prosthesis?

The incidence of a second amputation in the contralateral limb approaches 50% within 2 years of the initial amputation. Therefore, within 2 years one may expect a diabetic to have either bilateral below-knee amputations or a combination of below-knee and above-knee amputations, either of which sentences the patient to a wheelchair.

23. What is tarsal tunnel syndrome? What are its clinical findings? How is it treated?

Tarsal tunnel syndrome results from compressing the posterior tibial nerve within a fibro-osseous canal that has for its roof the flexor retinaculum. The classic history includes pain that is usually burning and localized in the plantar aspect of the foot but may radiate up the medial side of the calf. The symptoms are increased by activity and diminished by rest or rubbing the foot. Night symptoms may occur. A positive Tinel's sign may be elicited along the medial or lateral plantar nerve. Sensation to pinprick may be decreased. The diagnosis may be confirmed by nerve conduction velocity studies with prolonged terminal latency to the abductor hallucis or abductor digiti quinti muscle and abnormal potentials with fibrillations. Vascular insufficiency should be absent. When accurately diagnosed, tarsal tunnel syndrome can be treated with release of the fibro-osseous tunnel by lysing the flexor retinaculum.

24. What is compartment syndrome?

In compartment syndrome, muscle and nerve viability is threatened by increased tissue pressure within a fixed, fascially bounded compartment in the body over a prolonged period. There are four compartments in the leg: anterior, lateral, deep posterior, and superficial posterior. The increased pressure results from postischemia reperfusion or direct crush to the limb, as in a tibial fracture. An open wound in the leg does not indicate released or decompressed compartments. Most authors agree that an increase from the normal tissue pressure of 2–7 mmHg to 30 mmHg is concerning and that an increase to 35–40 mmHg is an absolute indication for treatment. A more accurate measurement is differential pressure (diastolic pressure minus compartment pressure); a differential pressure of < 30 mmHg is an absolute indication for treatment. Failure to treat creates a vicious cycle of increasing compartment pressures due to lymphatic and venous obstruction without arterial obstruction. The results are neuropraxia, muscle necrosis, and, finally, axonotmesis and limb ischemia. The tissue injury becomes irreversible in hours with resultant nerve and muscle loss.

25. How is compartment syndrome recognized and treated?

Awareness and early intervention are the keys to treatment. In borderline cases, tingling and increased pain in the limb associated with pain on passive extension of the involved muscle compartment may be treated by major limb elevation and intravenous mannitol. Tissue compartments may be measured by a needle catheter technique. Obvious severe compartment syndrome or expected severe compartment pressure elevation from reperfusion or crush mandates surgical compartment release as an emergency. The urgency cannot be overemphasized.

26. How are the foot sensory nerves evaluated?

Light touch may be used to evaluate the following domains of the foot:

Nerve	Domain
Sural nerve	Lateral midfoot
Posterior tibial nerve	Heel/plantar midfoot
Deep peroneal nerve	First web space
Superficial peroneal	Dorsal distal foot
Saphenous nerve	Medial ankle

27. What are indications for primary amputation in patients with tibial level injury?

The major indication is severe combined injury to bone, skin, joint, nerves, and vessels such that long-term limb survival and function are unlikely. The absence of sciatic or posterior tibial nerve function may be the most important element because meaningful recovery in these patients, even after repair, is poor. Consequences include an insensate plantar surface and almost certain recurrent ulceration, infection, and osteomyelitis. A trade-off must be made with prosthetics that allow high-level function. Other indications include severe infections or contamination, multilevel severe injury, and absent pedal pulses. Scoring systems such as Gustilo's fracture score and the Mangled Extremity Severity Score (MESS) help in decision making. Amputation should be considered seriously in any patient with a limb score greater than seven. The parameters for the MESS include the following:

Skeletal soft tissue injury	Low energy	1
	Medium energy (open fractures)	2
	High energy (military gunshot wound)	3
	Very high energy (gross contamination)	4
Limb ischemia (double score for ischemia > 6 hr)	Near-normal	1
	Pulseless, decreased capillary refill	2
	Cool, insensate, paralyzed	3

Shock	Systolic blood pressure always > 90 mmHg	0
	Transient hypotension	1
	Persistent hypotension	2
Age (yr)	< 30	0
	30–50	1
	> 50	2

From Johansen K, Daines M, Howley T, et al: Objective criteria accurately predict amputation following lower extremity trauma. J Trauma 30:568, 1990, with permission.

Gustilo Scoring for Open Fractures

Gustilo II	Moderate soft tissue injury and stripping
Gustilo IIIA	High energy, adequate soft tissue despite laceration or undermining
Gustilo IIIB	Extensive soft tissue injury and periosteal stripping, usually gross contamination
Gustilo IIIC	Gustilo B with limb ischemia

From Gustilo RB, Mendoza RM, Williams DN: Problems in the management of type III (severe) open fractures.: A new classification of type III open fractures. J Trauma 24:742, 1987, with permission.

28. What are the contraindications to salvage of a Gustilo IIIC injury of the lower extremity?
Preexisting severe medical illnesses, severed limb, tibial loss > 8 cm, ischemic time > 6 hours, and severance of the posterior tibial nerve in adults.

29. What are the indications for lower extremity replant?
For several reasons, lower extremity replantation is not uniformly practiced. The most important limitation is the inability to restore neurologic function to the lower extremity. In addition, prosthetic legs are relatively well accepted and widely used although they have their disadvantages. The loss of a leg is frequently associated with other severe injuries. The provision of a marginally functional replanted lower extremity may create a greater liability with respect to long-term rehabilitation, pain, time lost from employment, and associated risk of replantation surgery. Replantation in a child is expected to have improved neurologic function. Replantation should be considered only when the amputation is a single-level, clean transection without crush or avulsion injury and warm ischemia time is < 6 hours.

30. What are absolute contraindications for lower extremity replantation?
Poor baseline health, multilevel injury to a joint that results in immobility of the knee or ankle, warm ischemic time > 6 hours, and older age.

31. Are there any other considerations for the use of an amputated part?
One should not discard any tissue until considering its possible use in reconstruction of the injured patient. Certainly nerve grafts, skin grafts, and bone grafts can be borrowed from the amputated part to reconstruct other injured extremities. Muscle flaps or foot fillet flaps can be used to cover below-knee amputation stumps that otherwise would need conversion to an above-knee stump.

32. In planning flap coverage of the lower extremity, what considerations are involved for concomitant or future bone reconstruction?
- Shortening of the limb length to decrease the need for intercalary bone graft or the need for flap coverage
- Subsequent bone grafting that may require a posterior lateral approach or reelevation of the soft tissue flap
- Placement of a methylmethacrylate antibiotic-impregnated spacer followed by subsequent bone grafting
- Ilizarov bone transport

33. What is the Papineau technique?
Papineau described staged bone grafting for infected nonunion of the tibial fracture:

Stage I   Complete excision of infected bone and soft tissues with adequate external fixation and packing with topical antibiotic soaked swabs

Stage II   Autologous cancellous bone grafting, again followed by packing with antibiotic-soaked swabs

Stage III   Combination of flaps and skin grafts to achieve soft tissue cover once bony union is complete

34. Can bone transport (Ilizarov technique) be done across or through a free flap?

Yes. The rate of bone transport with movement of wires through a flap at 1 mm/day has not shown to be detrimental to overlying soft tissue coverage, including free flaps.

35. Why may free flaps fail in the leg?

Failure is rare in fresh wounds, which have a flap patency rate of approximately 95%+ and an infection rate of 1.5%. The infection rate, however, is much increased in more chronic wounds (longer than 5 days). The flap survival rate in a chronic wound may be as low as 80% with significant take-back rates. The increased complication and failure rates in more chronic wounds is due to a combination of factors, including contamination, infection, and damaged lymphatics and veins. Significant tissue edema, perivascular fibrosis, and valvular incompetence may contribute to this difficulty. Godina demonstrated good evidence for the benefits of achieving soft tissue wound coverage within 5 days after open fracture. This approach minimizes infection and maximizes flap survival.

36. Provide an appropriate algorithm for primary operative care of lower extremity trauma.

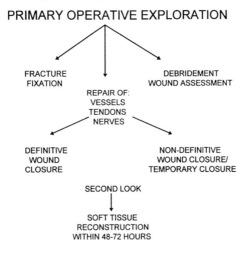

CONTROVERSIES

37. Is a muscle or a fasciocutaneous flap better for open fracture treatment?

Mathes et al. cite better healing and adherence in an infected wound with a muscle flap. Overall, however, the best choice is still unclear. Muscle seems to conform better to regular cavities and to adhere or fibrose better than a fasciocutaneous flap. Fasciocutaneous flaps, however, seem to suit most wounds well and to heal equally well; they also may be transferred as a sensate flap and are much thinner and cosmetically superior. The fasciocutaneous flap has the additional advantage of providing easier reoperations (if necessary), such as for an ankle fusion, bone graft, or nail removal.

38. Which is more expensive—amputation or limb salvage?

Amputation is frequently considered less expensive, but this is true only for the immediate postinjury period. Francel and Williams demonstrated that the initial hospital stay is 50% shorter in the amputation group compared with the salvage group and that the initial treatment costs in the amputation group are approximately 50% of the limb salvage group ($30,000 vs. $59,000). However, when expenses for the prosthetic limb devices and prosthetic care in younger trauma victims are considered, the calculated amount increases to $403,000, which also includes readmissions to the hospital for surgical treatment of stump ulcers. Of course, other factors must be considered, including quality of life, satisfaction with the salvaged limb vs. satisfaction with the prosthesis, return to work, stump pain, phantom pain, and chronic leg pain. Energy also should be considered. Energy expenditure for below-knee amputation may be 20–40% higher than in normal subjects, increasing to 100% higher in hip disarticulations.

BIBLIOGRAPHY

1. Anthony JP, Mathes SJ, Alpert BS: The muscle flap in the treatment of chronic lower extremity osteomyelitis: Results in patients over 5 years after treatment. Plast Reconstr Surg 88: 311, 1991.
2. Arnez ZM: Immediate reconstruction of the lower extremity—An update. Clin Plast Surg 18:449, 1991.
3. Byrd HS, Spicer TE, Cierny G III: Management of open tibial fractures. Plast Reconstr Surg 80:1, 1987.
4. Cierny G III, Zorn KE, Nahai F: Bony reconstruction in the lower extremity. Clin Plast Surg 19:905, 1992.
5. Fix RJ, Vasconez LO: Fasciocutaneous flaps in reconstruction of the lower extremity. Clin Plast Surg 18:571–582, 1991.
6. Fix RJ, Vasconez LO (eds): Reconstruction of the Lower Extremity. Clinics in Plastic Surgery. Philadelphia, W.B. Saunders, 1991.
7. Ger R: The management of open fracture of the tibia with skin loss. J Trauma 10:112, 1970.
8. Godina M: Early microsurgical reconstruction of complex trauma of extremities. Plast Reconstr Surg 78: 285, 1986.
9. Gustilo RB, Mendoza RM, Williams DN: Problems in the management of type III (severe) open fractures: A new classification of type III open fractures. J Trauma 24: 742–746, 1987.
10. Haimovici H: Patterns of arteriosclerotic lesions of the lower extremity. Arch Surg 95: 918, 1967.
11. Johansen K, Daines M, Howey T, et al: Objective criteria accurately predict amputation following lower extremity trauma. J Trauma 30:568–573, 1990.
12. Khouri RK, Shaw WW: Reconstruction of the lower extremity with microvascular free flaps: A 10-year experience with 304 consecutive cases. J Trauma 29:1086, 1989.
13. Mann RA: Tarsal tunnel syndrome. Orthop Clin North Am 5: 109–115, 1974.
14. Masquelet AC, Romana MC, Wolf G: Skin island flaps supplied by the axis of the sensitive superficial nerves: Anatomic study and clinical experience in the leg. Plast Reconstr Surg 89:1115–1121, 1992.
15. May JW Jr, Rohrich RJ: Foot reconstruction using free microvascular muscle flaps with skin grafts. Clin Plast Surg 13: 681–689, 1986.
16. Walton RL, Bunkis J: The posterior calf fasciocutaneous free flap. Plast Reconstr Surg 74:76, 1984.

69. LEG ULCERS

Norman Weinzweig, M.D., and Raymond M. Dunn, M.D.

1. What are the most common chronic wounds seen in our population?
Leg ulcers. They may result in cellulitis, osteomyelitis, gangrene, amputation, and even death. Leg ulcers know no social bounds, crippling all patients, including those in their prime working years, with extraordinary morbidity and costs to society.

2. How often is ulceration the precursor to amputation?
Ulceration is the most common precursor to amputation (84% of cases).

3. What is the differential diagnosis of leg ulcers?
The differential diagnosis of legs ulcers is extensive. The following list is by no means complete.

Vascular disease
- Arterial
  Arteriosclerosis obliterans
  Thrombangitis obliterans
  Hypertension
  Livedo reticularis
- Venous—chronic venous insufficiency
- Lymphatic—elephantiasis nostra
  (lymphedema)

Tumors
- Squamous cell carcinoma (Marjolin's)
- Basal cell carcinoma
- Kaposi's sarcoma
- Lymphoma (mycosis fungoides)

Burns
- Thermal
- Electrical
- Chemical

Metabolic disease
- Diabetes mellitus
- Necrobiosis lipoidica diabeticorum
- Pyoderma gangrenosum
- Porphyria cutanea tarda
- Gout

Vasculitis
- Lupus erythematosus
- Rheumatoid arthritis
- Periarteritis nodosa
- Allergic vasculitis

Hematologic disease
- Sickle cell anemia
- Thalassemia
- Hypercoagulable states (deficiency of antithrombin, protein C, protein S)
- Polycythemia vera
- Leukemia

Infectious disease
- Bacterial
- Fungal (coccidimycosis, blastomycosis, histoplasmosis, sporotrichosis)
- Tuberculosis
- Syphilis

Insect bites
- Brown recluse spider
- Sandfly

Drugs
- Halogens
- Ergotism
- Methotrexate

Radiation

Frostbite

Weber-Christian disease

Lichen planus

Trophic ulcers

Factitial (self-induced)

4. **How should you evaluate a patient with a leg ulcer?**

Begin with a thorough history and physical examination and then order the appropriate lab studies.

History
- Onset, location, size, depth, drainage, infection
- Etiology
- Previous treatment (conservative vs. surgical)
- Ambulatory status
- Shoewear
- Medical history
  Vascular status: claudication? rest pain?
  Diabetes mellitus
  Chronic venous insufficiency
  Collagen vascular disease
  Sickle cell anemia

Physical examination
- Atrophic changes
- Capillary refill
- Skin temperature
- Sensation
- Palpable pedal pulses
- Deformity

Lab studies
- Culture and sensitivities
- Foot films: radiograph, CT scan, MRI, bone scan
- Noninvasive arterial and venous studies
- Ankle/brachial indices
- Pulse volume recordings, photoplethysmography
- Bone biopsy

5. **What are the goals of treatment of leg ulcers?**

Goals include ulcer healing within a reasonable period, return to ambulation as soon as possible, long-term preventative measures against ulcer recurrence, and patient tolerance and compliance with the treatment regimen.

6. **What is the most common cause of leg ulceration?**

Ambulatory venous hypertension is responsible for the overwhelming majority of leg ulcers, accounting for 70–90% of all cases. Twenty-seven percent of the adult population has lower extremity venous abnormalities; 2–5% have clinical manifestations of superficial or deep venous insufficiency; and 1.5% (over a half-million people in the United States) have frank ulceration. Up to 10% of patients with ulcers have concomitant arterial occlusive disease.

7. **What is venous hypertension?**

Venous hypertension occurs when the blood pressure inside the veins, which is normally 15 mmHg in a resting supine position, is elevated to a pathologic level over a prolonged period.

8. **What causes venous hypertension?**

Venous hypertension is caused by incompetent valves in the veins of the legs. The most common cause of abnormally functioning valves is a prior history of blood clots in the legs (thrombophlebitis) and the breakdown of the clots, which damages the delicate valves, particularly their competence or ability to sustain the column of blood from the foot to the heart.

9. How do you diagnose venous hypertension?

There are numerous ways to examine leg veins. In the past the gold standard for evaluation was the **venogram**, an invasive test. Venograms are rarely performed today. Many noninvasive tests can evaluate the anatomy and function of the veins of the leg. The most common and widely used test is **duplex scanning**, which in experienced hands can assess the anatomy as well as function of veins. Other common tests are **photoplethysmography** and **air plethysmography**. These noninvasive tests attempt to measure how quickly blood flows backward or refills the leg when it moves from the supine to the upright position. They are general measures of valvular incompetence and venous hypertension.

10. Name the major veins of the leg.

The major veins of the leg accompany the major arteries: the anterior tibial, posterior tibial, and peroneal veins. These are the deep veins of the leg, or the deep venous system. The greater and lesser saphenous veins make up the superficial system of veins.

11. Describe the anatomy of the veins of the leg.

The deep veins of the leg are paired and travel with the named artery; they are called venae comitantes. The deep veins surround the artery and are connected to each other by small crossing branches, much like the rungs on a ladder. The superficial veins do not travel specifically with significant arteries and are not paired. Both the deep and superficial veins have valves that direct the flow of blood toward the heart and communicate between connecting perforating veins. When the valves of these veins do not function properly, a host of abnormalities may develop in the local area, the most significant of which is an open wound or venous ulcer.

12. What are perforating veins?

Perforating veins connect the superficial and deep systems of venous drainage of the leg. Perforating veins run predominantly between the greater saphenous and posterior tibial veins but are found to a lesser extent throughout the leg between the superficial and deep systems. The perforators on the medial leg (posterior tibial) generally contribute to leg ulceration in this area when they are incompetent or their valves do not work.

13. What are varicose veins?

Varicose veins are dilated, tortuous veins of the superficial system (subcutaneous).

14. What is a varicose ulcer?

Patients with varicose veins who have normal deep veins may develop leg ulceration with prolonged lack of treatment. In such a case, surgical removal of the incompetent superficial veins (ligation and stripping of varicose veins) is an effective treatment for the leg ulceration, which then should respond well to conservative care or simple skin grafting.

15. What are the etiology and pathogenesis of venous ulcers?

The etiology and pathophysiology of venous ulcers are not completely understood. Current concepts include the loss of venous valvular competence in the deep and/or superficial venous systems, which leads to venous hypertension. Prolonged venous hypertension promotes the extravasation of protein-rich edema fluid and red blood cells into the subcutaneous tissues of the lower leg. A pericapillary fibrin cuff functions as a diffusion barrier to oxygen and nutrient exchange at a cellular level. In addition, inflammation caused by chronic red blood cell extravasation and leukocyte trapping in the tissue bed leads to the densely scarred, fibrotic, hyperpigmented skin and subcutaneous tissue changes known as lipodermatosclerosis ("brawny edema"). Lipodermatosclerotic tissue is poorly vascularized, easily traumatized, and prone to slow, poor wound healing with frequent ulcer recurrence.

16. Where are venous ulcers located?

Venous ulcers are generally located in the so-called gaiter region of the leg, which is between the malleoli and gastrocnemius musculotendinous junction. It is thought that perforating veins may transmit excessive pressure to the subcutaneous tissue with contraction of the calf muscle, predisposing to tissue damage. Ulcers also may be located on the foot, between the toes, and on the posterior calf, but these sites are unusual and should encourage consideration of other diagnostic possibilities.

17. Describe conservative management of venous ulcers.
Conservative management of leg ulcers consists of elastic compression, prolonged bed rest with leg elevation, Unna boot application, local wound care with frequent dressing changes, and hygiene. This approach requires a lifestyle change that is often impractical. Moreover, skin grafting is associated with poor long-term results and recurrence rates of up to 43%. None of these modalities corrects the underlying pathophysiology.

18. What is an Unna boot?
Compression bandaging with materials impregnated with various paste substances such as calamine and zinc oxide, wrapped from the toes to the upper calf, including coverage of an open ulcer, was promulgated by Unna in the late 19th century for the treatment of venous ulcers. Any paste bandaging of venous leg ulcers or even dry compression bandaging has come to be known as an Unna boot.

19. How does an Unna boot work?
The value of compression bandaging in the treatment of venous ulceration has been recognized since it was used by Celsus. Various supportive dressing regimens have been developed and promulgated over the centuries. Compression has been shown to enhance fibrinolysis, reducing the pathologic deposition of fibrin in abnormal legs. No clear evidence indicates that the addition of emollients to treat the open wound and surrounding leg skin in patients with lipodermatosclerosis provides greater clinical benefit than compression alone.

20. Describe the surgical management of venous ulcers.
Traditional surgical approaches include varicose vein stripping, subfascial perforator ligation, valvuloplasty, and vein segment transposition and transplantation. Vein stripping usually deals with isolated superficial valvular insufficiency, which rarely causes ulceration. Perforator ligation is associated with frequent wound complications (2–44%) and high recurrence rates (6–55%). Valvuloplasty has demonstrated good results in cases of primary valvular incompetence. Valve transposition and transplantation have demonstrated poor results in cases of postthrombotic recanalization. Although these surgical approaches may improve the regional venous hemodynamics of the lower leg, none addresses the irreversibly scarred lipodermatosclerotic bed.

21. What is a Linton flap?
It is generally believed that perforating veins between the posterior tibial (deep) and saphenous veins (superficial) contribute to venous leg ulceration. In 1938 Linton described an operation to divide the perforating veins in the hope that it would prevent the occurrence of ulceration. Since that time, the ligation of perforating veins has commonly borne the eponym *Linton flap*. The operation consists of an incision parallel and 2 cm posterior to the medial tibial border from the medial malleolus to midcalf prominence (gastrocnemius bulge). The deep muscle fascia is divided, and all perforating veins are ligated. Currently, this operation is performed endoscopically whenever technically feasible to avoid wound-healing complications associated with the original open operation.

22. Who should get a skin graft for a venous leg ulcer?
Patients who have venous leg ulcers should undergo diagnostic evaluation to confirm the status of competence of the deep veins (see question 9). Superficial venous insufficiency with ulceration (about 10% of patients with ulcers) can generally be treated successfully by skin grafting (and removing pathologic superficial and communicating veins). Elderly patients who do not respond to conservative treatment of ulcers may be candidates for skin grafts.

23. What are the goals for long-term cure of recalcitrant venous ulcers?
Despite significant advances in the past 10–20 years in understanding the etiopathogenesis as well as the conservative and surgical management of venous valvular insufficiency and venous ulcers, both remain essentially incurable conditions. Long-term cure of venous ulcers depends on accomplishing the following goals: (1) restoration of normal venous hemodynamics at the level of

and in the region of the venous ulcer and (2) complete removal of the ulcer and *all* surrounding lipo-dermatosclerotic skin and subcutaneous tissue.

24. What is the role of free tissue transfer in the management of venous ulcers?

Recently, Dunn et al. and Weinzweig and Schuler reported their experience with the use of fasciocutaneous and muscle free flaps, respectively, in the treatment of recalcitrant venous ulcers. Both groups found that free tissue transfer provides a long-term cure by replacing the diseased lipodermatosclerotic tissue bed with healthy tissue containing multiple, competent microvenous valves and a normal microcirculation, thereby improving regional hemodynamics. In addition, the transfer can be accomplished in one reconstructive procedure with excellent results. Both groups reported no recurrence of venous ulceration within the flaps. In a few cases, failure to excise all of the liposclerotic tissue led to breakdown and slow healing of the flaps at the margins. Each of these cases eventually healed with conservative measures.

25. Who should get a free flap for a venous leg ulcer?

Patients with deep venous insufficiency, localized recurrent ulceration, and liposclerotic (scarred) tissue benefit from a subfascial excision of the ulcer and scarred tissue and reconstruction with a tissue replacement microvascular flap.

26. What kind of free flap is best for a venous ulcer?

Multiple tissue types have been used successfully to reconstruct leg ulcer defects, including fasciocutaneous flaps, muscle flaps with skin grafts, and omental flaps with skin grafts. Flap selection is commonly based on available donor sites as well as the size and extent of the ulcer defect that is expected after excision.

27. What intrinsic role does the flap tissue play in treatment of venous ulcers?

Fasciocutaneous and muscle free flaps contain multiple valves in their venous systems. These valves are morphologically identical to leg valves and may provide the limited flap area with some long-term protection from reulceration, thus essentially "curing" the chronic condition in the right surgical candidate. Aharinejad et al. and Taylor et al. have done excellent anatomic studies of the microvenous valvular anatomy of the human dorsal thoracic fascia and various muscle flaps, respectively.

28. Describe the scope of the problem with respect to diabetes, arterial occlusive disease, and amputation.

- 50–70% of leg amputations are secondary to diabetes.
- 28% of these amputations fail to heal, resulting in a higher level of amputation.
- 50% of patients undergo amputation of the contralateral leg within 2–5 years.
- The 5-year survival rate after amputation is 40%.

The personal, emotional, economic, and societal consequences are enormous.

29. What is the etiopathogenesis of diabetic foot ulcers?

Diabetic foot ulcers arise primarily from neuropathy (altered proprioception, touch, or pain sensation), vascular disease (with associated ischemia), or both, often complicated by infection. Contributing factors include limited joint mobility, callus formation, high foot pressures, and increasing susceptibility to ulceration.

The **neuropathic foot** (poor sensation, good circulation) is characteristically healthy, well-nourished, and hair-bearing, with good dorsalis pedis and posterior tibial pulses and a high arch. Thick callus formation occurs on pressure points of the soles or toes. Bruising of the subcutaneous tissue and extravasation of blood beneath the calluses leave a rich culture media for local bacteria. The bacteria spread beneath the callus to the underlying joint capsule and metatarsal head, eventually resulting in osteomyelitis.

The **ischemic foot** (poor circulation, acute sensation), on the other hand, is dry, atrophic, scaly, hairless, and undernourished. It is cool to touch with diminished or absent pulses. Infected areas are often painful to touch or pressure. Ulcers often have full-thickness skin necrosis in the center with a surrounding rim of erythema. Seldom is osteomyelitis or a true abscess found with pus located behind the necrotic tissue. Ischemia makes any lesion a serious condition that may quickly become a limb- or life-threatening problem.

30. Discuss two common misconceptions about diabetic foot infections.

1. Small vessel disease—arteriolar occlusive disease may cause ischemic lesions in the presence of normal pulses.

2. Endothelial proliferation in small vessels—thickening of capillary basement membrane but not narrowing or occlusion.

An uncontrolled study by Goldenberg in 1959 indicated that amputation specimens from diabetics showed an increased incidence of arteriolar occlusion due to proliferation of endothelium and deposition of periodic acid-Schiff (PAS)-positive material. In 1984 this misconception was repudiated by LoGerfo and Coffman in a prospective controlled study of amputation specimens from diabetics and nondiabetics, and a similar prospective study using a sophisticated arterial casting technique failed to confirm Goldenberg's theory. No small artery or arteriolar occlusive lesion is associated with diabetes.

31. What is the fate of the contralateral foot in diabetics?

According to the classic study by Kucan and Robson of 45 patients followed for a minimum of 3 years, 22 patients (49%) developed a severe infection of the contralateral foot within 18 months. Fifteen of these patients (68%) required some type of amputation of the contralateral foot (3 toe, 2 ray, 4 transmetatarsal, 6 below-knee). Fourteen of the patients (64%) with severe infections of both feet maintained bipedal ambulation.

32. What is the diabetic Charcot foot?

In 1968 Jean-Martin Charcot first described the neuropathic joint changes associated with the tabes dorsalis, believing them to be a secondary effect of the neurologic deficit related to tertiary syphilis. In 1936 Jordan first described neuropathic arthropathy in diabetics, and in 1947 the Joslin Clinic published the first series of cases. Today diabetes is the most common cause of Charcot joints, which occur in 1 of 680 diabetic feet. Charcot neuroarthropathy of the foot is one of the most devastating consequences of diabetes, occurring in patients with an average duration of diabetes of 12–18 years; 18% of cases are bilateral.

The radiographic findings are characterized by a severely destructive form of degenerative arthritis with simultaneous bone destruction, joint destruction, subluxation or dislocation, and fragmentation in addition to hypertrophic periosteal reaction. Neuropathic arthropathy is a relatively painless, progressive, and degenerative arthropathy of single or multiple joints caused by the underlying neurologic deficits. The most frequent sites of involvement include the tarsometatarsal joints (60%), the metatarsophalangeal joints (61%), and the ankle joint (9%). On examination, the foot is grossly deformed with a typical rocker bottom subluxation of the mid-tarsal region or subluxations of the metatarsophalangeal joints and a high arch with cocked-up toes. The foot is erythematous, warm to touch, and anhidrotic.

The exact mechanism is unknown; however, it is hypothesized that hyperemia from autonomic neuropathy results in ligament laxity and osteolysis. With continued microtrauma due to sensory neuropathy, the bone and joint surfaces are destroyed. Loss of normal protective mechanisms subjects joints to extreme ranges of motion, resulting in capsular and ligamentous stretching, joint laxity with eventual dislocation, fracture, and bone and joint destruction. This process occurs in the presence of bounding pulses and elevated ankle-brachial indices. The hyperemia or increased blood supply promotes resorption of the normal bone, creating a vicious cycle.

33. Describe the status of the arterial system in diabetics.

Not all diabetics have poor circulation. Moreover, many diabetics have absent femoral, popliteal, or pedal pulses yet do not manifest foot problems. This finding suggests that ischemia is usually only one component of the problem. The pathology of atherosclerosis for diabetic and nondiabetic patients is similar, but there are several distinguishing characteristics. Diabetics have a predilection for macrovascular occlusive disease involving the tibial/peroneal vessels between the knee and the foot, as evidenced by the fact that 40% of diabetics presenting with limb-threatening ischemia have a palpable popliteal pulse. The presence of a pulse does not mean that circulation is adequate. No occlusive small vessel disease of the diabetic foot precludes successful revascularization. Occlusive microvascular disease of the foot does *not* exist (see question 30). Revascularization can restore tissue perfusion to the ischemic diabetic foot. Diabetics also have a diminished ability to develop collateral circulation. Calcification involving the intimal plaque and media (medial calcinosis or

Monckeberg's sclerosis) frequently involves arteries at all levels but often spares the foot vessels. Medial calcinosis often gives erroneous ankle-brachial indices and other noninvasive testing results. The classic indications for surgical intervention include incapacitating claudication, rest pain, and threatened limb loss (ulceration or gangrene).

34. Describe considerations in the surgical management of diabetic patients with a foot ulcer.

- General medical condition
- Peripheral circulation
- Local wound status
- Ambulatory status
- Compliance

In addition, one must consider whether amputation is more favorable than revascularization and reconstructive procedures.

35. Describe the management of plantar forefoot ulcers.

Difficult wounds involving the plantar forefoot typically are located over the metatarsal heads. Ulceration often exposes bone and tendon and is usually managed by digital amputations. Forefoot ulcers often require toe fillet, ray, or transmetatarsal amputations. Metatarsal head resections reduce the amount of bone in this area, often allowing the wound to be closed primarily. With respect to the metatarsal head, conservative debridement is performed for the great toe, dorsal free-floating osteotomies for the second through fourth toes, and complete excision for the fifth toe. Soft tissue coverage can be obtained by plantar V-Y advancement flaps, island neurovascular toe flaps or toe fillet flap, and distally based muscle flaps. Free tissue transfer is sometimes necessary to salvage nonhealing transmetatarsal amputation stumps.

36. Describe the management of plantar midfoot ulcers.

Most difficult wounds in the plantar midfoot are associated with Charcot's disease. Fracture-dislocations result in significant architectural changes, collapse of the arch, and alteration of the normal weight-bearing surface. Management often involves extensive resection of the ulcer, including scar tissue, bursal tissue, and underlying bony prominence. The wound is closed by filling its depths with a local muscle flap and a rotation advancement fasciocutaneous flap from the instep based on the medial plantar vessels. The muscle is usually the flexor digitorum brevis or abductor digiti minimi, depending on the location of the ulcer. More extensive defects are managed by free tissue transfers.

37. Describe the management of hindfoot (heel) ulcers.

Hindfoot ulcers often require wide local osseus debridement, especially of the calcaneus. Such ulcers involve defects on the plantar and posterior aspect of the heel. For the plantar aspect, techniques include local rotation or advancement heel-pad tissue flaps, instep island pedicle flaps, turnover muscle flaps, and free tissue transfer. For the posterior heel, where the Achilles tendon is often exposed, skin grafts or local flaps (V-Y advancement, local rotation, and distally based vascularized pedicle flaps) usually suffice. Often the posterior tibial artery is occluded, and free tissue transfer may be necessary with anastomosis to the dorsalis pedis vessels or in situ distal bypass graft. Well-vascularized coverage generally cannot be achieved by local arterialized flaps, such as the lateral calcaneal, dorsalis pedis, and fasciocutaneous instep island flaps. Free tissue transfer is usually required.

38. How are multiple tarsal and metatarsal ulcers managed?

Such ulcers often interfere with ambulation; below-knee amputation is usually indicated.

39. How can foot ulcers be prevented?

- Proper footwear—the most attractive shoes are not necessarily the best fitting
- Proper hygiene—wash feet every day with mild soap and dry thoroughly, especially between toes
- Application of moisture cream everywhere except between toes
- Avoidance of self ("bathroom") surgery
- Avoidance of foot soaking
- Avoidance of heat, heating pads, or sleeping next to the stove or radiator
- Regular physician visits to control blood glucose, weight, and blood pressure
- Avoidance of smoking

- Daily exercise
- Periodic neurologic and vascular examinations

40. What is the bacteriology of foot infections?

Most foot infections (70–80%) severe enough to require hospitalization are polymicrobial (2–6 microorganisms), including gram-positive and gram-negative aerobic (and facultative) organisms as well as anaerobic isolates in 30–80% of cases. *Staphylococcus aureus* is recovered in one-third to one-half of cases. Enterococci are seen in 25–30% of patients, almost always as mixed microbial flora. Among gram-negative organisms are *Proteus* species, *Escherichia coli*, and a variety of *Enterobacteriaceae*. *Pseudomonas aeruginosa* is less common but important because organisms may be resistant to antimicrobials effective against other gram-negative bacilli. Anaerobic species include gram-positive cocci (peptococci, peptostreptococci), bacilli (*Clostridium* species), and gram-negative bacteria (*Bacteroides* species).

41. What are the basic rules for treating any foot infection?

- Absolute bed rest
- Regulation of diabetes
- Adequate wound culture
- Administration of appropriate antibiotics
- Adequate drainage
- Appropriate wound care

42. What is the role of the vascular surgeon and plastic surgeon in salvage of the diabetic foot?

The limb salvage rates in diabetics with difficult foot wounds have increased significantly because of the close collaboration of plastic surgeons and vascular surgeons. This collaboration is largely due to a better understanding of the blood supply in the foot, which allows a wider arsenal of foot flaps as well as more successful revascularization. The recent role of free tissue transfer, which facilitates the closure of wounds of any size in any location, is especially important. The goal is stable wound coverage and bipedal ambulation.

43. Describe the rehabilitation team for the diabetic foot.

- Podiatrist for patient education, preventive maintenance, orthotics, and special shoes
- Physical therapist for return to normal activity, gait training to prepare for a prosthesis, and prophylactic exercises to maintain body tone
- Nutritionist for advice on diet needs
- Surgeon to ensure proper wound healing and proper prosthetics
- Endocrinologist to make the final decision about diabetes management

44. Describe the nature of sickle cell ulcers.

Sickle cell ulcers occur in patients with homozygous sickle cell disease (0.5–3% of the black population in North America). Disabling ulcerations develop in 25.7–73.6% of patients. Ulcerations of the lower extremities are chronic, recurrent, excruciatingly painful, and disabling. They occur in areas of marginal vascularity where minor abrasions become foci of inflammation, which in turn cause decreased local oxygen tension, sickling of red cells, increased blood viscosity, and thrombosis with consequent ischemia, tissue breakdown, and further inflammation. This vicious cycle, initiated spontaneously or by relatively insignificant trauma, results in the replacement of normal tissue by scar tissue, a permanent locus minor resistantiae.

45. What role does skin grafting play in the management of sickle cell ulcers?

Unfortunately, skin grafting is not an answer to this frustrating clinical problem. Skin grafting does not alter the underlying pathophysiology or increase the blood supply to the involved region. Despite adequate wound care, exchange transfusion to lower the percentage of hemoglobin S, and skin grafting, as many as 97.4% of ulcers recur at the same site within 2 years. An average hospital stay of 55 days is required to treat each ulceration.

46. What other reconstructive options are available for patients with homozygous sickle cell disease?

There is a paucity of fasciocutaneous, muscle, or musculocutaneous flaps that are reliable, well-vascularized, and locoregional. Free tissue transfer is the reconstructive procedure of choice for defects of the lower third of the leg. However, the key question is whether the obligate period of ischemia inherent in free tissue transfer inevitably dooms a flap to failure.

47. What is the role of free tissue transfer for limb salvage in patients with homozygous sickle cell disease?

Weinzweig et al. recently reported a series of successful free flaps in patients with homozygous sickle cell disease. Special perioperative measures were taken to optimize the chances of a successful outcome. The obligate period of ischemia did *not* inevitably doom the flap to failure. Perioperative measures include the following:

- Exchange-transfusion to lower hemoglobin S to below 30%
- Maintenance of hematocrit at 31–35%
- Intraoperative flap washout and perfusion with warm heparinized saline-dextran solution
- Administration of dextran and aspirin intraoperatively and postoperatively
- Prophylactic topical and systemic antipseudomonal antibiotics
- Supplemental oxygen
- Warm ambient room temperature

BIBLIOGRAPHY

1. Aharinejad S, Dunn RM, Fudem GM, et al: The microvenous valvular anatomy of the human dorsal thoracic fascia. Plast Reconstr Surg 99:1–9, 1997.
2. Banis JC Jr, Richardson D, Den JW Jr, Acland RD: Microsurgical adjuncts in salvage of the ischemic and diabetic lower extremity. Clin Plast Surg 19:881–893, 1992.
3. Bergan JJ, Yao JST: Venous Disorders. Philadelphia, W.B. Saunders, 1991.
4. Chowdary RP, Celani VJ, Goodreau JJ, et al: Free tissue transfers for limb salvage utilizing in situ saphenous vein bypass conduit as the inflow. Plast Reconstr Surg 75:627, 1985.
5. Cikrit DF, Nichols WK, Silver D: Surgical management of refractory venous stasis ulceration. J Vasc Surg 7:473–477, 1988.
6. Colen LB: Limb salvage in the patient with severe peripheral vascular disease: The role of microsurgical free-tissue transfer. Plast Reconstr Surg 79:389–395, 1987.
7. Dunn RM, Fudem GM, Walton RL, et al: Free flap valvular transplantation for refractory venous ulceration. J Vasc Surg 19:525–531, 1994.
8. Goldenberg S, Alex M, Joshi RA, Blumenthal HT: Nonatheromatous peripheral vascular disease of the lower extremity in diabetes mellitus. Diabetes 8:261, 1959.
9. Hume M: Venous ulcers, the vascular surgeon, and the Medicare budget. J Vasc Surg 16:671–673, 1992.
10. Kozak GP, Campbell DR, Frykberg RG, Habershaw GM: Management of Diabetic Foot Problems, 2nd ed. Philadelphia, W.B. Saunders, 1995.
11. Kucan JO, Robson MC: Diabetic foot infections: Fate of the contralateral foot. Plast Reconstr Surg 77:439, 1986.
12. Lai C-S, Lin S-D, Yand CC, et al: Limb salvage of infected diabetic foot ulcers with microsurgical free tissue transfer. Ann Plast Surg 26:212–220, 1991.
13. LoGerfo FW, Coffman JD: Vascular and microvascular disease of the foot in diabetes. N Engl J Med 311:1615, 1984.
14. O'Donnell TF. Chronic venous insufficiency: An overview of epidemiology, classification, and anatomic considerations. Semin Vasc Surg 1(2):60–65, 1988.
15. Serletti JM, Deuber MA, Guidera PM, et al: Atherosclerosis of the lower extremity and free-tissue reconstruction for limb salvage. Plast Reconstr Surg 96:1136–1144, 1995.
16. Serletti JM, Hurwitz SR, Jones JA, et al: Extension of limb salvage by combined vascular reconstruction and adjunctive free-tissue transfer. J Vasc Surg 18:972, 1993.
17. Shestak KC, Fitz DG, Newton ED, Swartz WM: Expanding the horizons of severe peripheral vascular disease using microsurgical techniques. Plast Reconstr Surg 85:406, 1990.
18. Weinzweig N, Schuler J, Marschall M, Koshy M: Lower limb salvage by microvascular free-tissue transfer in patients with homozygous sickle cell disease. Plast Reconstr Surg 96:1154–1161, 1995.
19. Weinzweig N, Schuler J: Free tissue transfer in treatment of the recalcitrant chronic venous ulcer. Ann Plast Surg 38:611–619, 1997.

70. PRESSURE SORES

Mimis Cohen, M.D., F.A.C.S,. and Sai S. Ramasastry, M.D., F.R.C.S.

1. What is the pathophysiology of pressure ulcers?

Tissue pressures higher than the pressure of the microcirculation (32 mmHg) cause ischemia; if the ischemic period is long enough or repeated frequently, the eventual outcome is tissue necrosis. Thus, the prime mechanism of pressure ulceration is cellular ischemia.

2. Name the primary risk factors for developing pressure ulcers in chair-bound people or people with impaired ability to reposition.

• Immobility
• Incontinence
• Nutritional factors such as inadequate dietary intake and impaired nutritional status
• Altered levels of consciousness

3. What are the Braden Scale and the Norton Scale?

These scales and their modifications are validated risk-assessment tools to identify patients at high risk of developing pressure ulcers. The Braden Scale has been evaluated in diverse sites such as medical/surgical units, intensive care units, and nursing homes; the Norton Scale has been tested with elderly patients in hospital settings.

4. Which areas of the body are more prone to pressure ulcerations?

All areas around bony prominences are at risk. Most pressure ulcers occur on the ischial tuberosity (28%), trochanter (19%), and sacrum (17%). Heel ulcers have the highest incidence (9%) outside the pelvic area.

5. What is the staging system for pressure sores?

Pressure Sore Staging System

Stage I	Nonblanchable erythema of intact skin (heralding lesion of skin ulceration).
Stage II	Partial-thickness skin loss involving epidermis or dermis. The ulcer is superficial and presents clinically as an abrasion, blister, or shallow crater.
Stage III	Full-thickness skin loss involving damage to or necrosis of subcutaneous tissue that may extend down to, but not through, underlying fascia. The sore presents clinically as a deep crater with or without undermining of adjacent tissue.
Stage IV	Full-thickness skin loss with extensive destruction, tissue necrosis, or damage in muscle, bone, or supporting structures (for example, tendon or joint capsule).

From U.S. Department of Health and Human Services: Pressure Ulcers in Adults: Prediction and Prevention. Clinical Practice Guideline No. 3, Publication 97-0047, 1992.

6. In patients with spinal cord injury, what is the pathophysiology of lower extremity spasms?

Spasticity develops because spinal reflex arcs are separated from the controlling influences of higher centers in the nervous system. Incoming fibers from muscle spindles end directly on motor cells as the afferent arm of myotatic or stretch reflexes; activation of such reflexes causes the muscle to contract.

7. How do you manage spasticity in paraplegic patients?

Spasticity can be managed pharmacologically and surgically. The most commonly used drugs include diazepam, 10–40 gm/day, and baclofen, 15–100 gm/day. For spasticity refractory to medications, intrathecal phenol or alcohol is recommended. Neurosurgical alleviation with cordotomy or rhizotomy is indicated for severe cases not responsive to medical care.

8. What is the best modality for evaluation of pelvic osteomyelitis in patients with pressure sores?

The best modality is bone biopsy, which should not be done through the ulcer but rather through healthy skin. Several biopsies from various areas of the pelvis are necessary when generalized pelvic osteomyelitis is suspected.

9. What other tests are helpful in establishing the diagnosis of pelvic osteomyelitis?

Several laboratory and imaging tests can be used, including erythrocyte sedimentation rate, white cell count, plain radiographs, computed tomography, and magnetic resonance imaging. Combined results of plain radiographs, white cell count, and erythrocyte sedimentation rate may have a sensitivity as high as 89%.

10. What is the treatment for pelvic osteomyelitis?

Patients with established pelvic osteomyelitis need to be treated for 6–8 weeks with appropriate intravenous antibiotics. Repeat bone biopsies may be necessary to confirm successful treatment prior to extensive reconstructive procedures.

11. List the surgical steps for pressure sore closure.
  1. Drainage of all collections
  2. Wide debridement of all devitalized and scarred soft tissue
  3. Excision of the pseudobursa
  4. Ostectomy of all involved bone
  5. Careful hemostasis and suction drainage
  6. Obliteration of all residual dead space with well-vascularized tissue (muscle, musculocutaneous, or fasciocutaneous flaps)
  7. Closure without tension

12. What is the blood supply to the gluteus maximus muscle?

The superior and inferior gluteal arteries—branches of the hypogastric artery—supply the superior and inferior portions of the muscle. The piriform muscle is interposed between the superior and inferior pedicles. Both pedicles cross from medial to lateral and enter the undersurface of the muscle.

13. What are the various designs for the gluteus maximus musculocutaneous flap?

The gluteus maximus flap can cover sacral and ischial pressure sores. For coverage of sacral pressure sores, the gluteus maximus flap is usually used as a sliding musculocutaneous flap, as a V-Y musculocutaneous advancement flap, or as a rotation flap. For coverage of an ischial pressure sore, the most common method is to detach the muscle laterally from the greater trochanter and rotate it medially to cover the ischium. With the V-Y advancement, the muscle can be detached completely from the greater trochanter. In nonparalyzed patients, the central portion of the iliotibial tract and the muscle should be left attached to the trochanter to preserve function of the muscle.

14. What is the innervation of the gluteus maximus muscle? Can the gluteus maximus flap be used in nonparaplegic patients without functional deficit?

The gluteus maximus receives innervation from the superior and inferior gluteal nerves. The inferior gluteal nerve is more dominant; it is the strongest external rotator and extensor of the hip. As long as the inferior gluteal nerve is left intact and the muscle is not completely detached from the iliotibial tract and the greater trochanter, function can be preserved in ambulatory patients.

15. What is the blood supply to the gracilis musculocutaneous flap?

The dominant blood supply is the medial circumflex femoral artery, a branch of the profunda femoris. The pedicle courses from medial to lateral. It enters the undersurface of the muscle 10–12 cm inferior to the pubic tubercle.

16. What is the blood supply of the lumbosacral back flap? What are its applications?

The lumbosacral or transverse back flap is based on the contralateral lumbar perforators, usually L1–L5. The flap covers a medium-sized pressure sore of the sacral area; it includes only skin and subcutaneous tissue and does not provide adequate bulk. The lumbosacral flap is a secondary option for sacral pressure sores when other primary options are not available. The donor site needs to be skin-grafted.

17. What is the blood supply to the vastus lateralis muscle?

The descending branch of the lateral circumflex femoral artery, a branch of the profunda femoris. The vessel courses from medial to lateral; after emerging from beneath the rectus femoris muscle, it enters the anterior proximal belly of the vastus lateralis muscle approximately 10 cm inferior to the anterosuperior iliac spine.

18. To the rectus femoris muscle?

The blood supply of the rectus femoris muscle is derived from branches of the lateral circumflex femoral artery. The vessel courses from medial to lateral. Two to three branches enter the undersurface of the muscle at the proximal third.

19. To the gluteal thigh flap?

The blood supply to the gluteal thigh flap is the descending branch of the inferior gluteal artery. The surface landmark for flap design is the midpoint between the greater trochanter and the ischial tuberosity proximally. Distally, the flap can extend to the medial femoral condyle and the posterior border of the tensor fascia lata.

20. To the tensor fascia lata flap?

The blood supply to the tensor fascia lata flap is derived from a terminal branch of the lateral circumflex femoral artery from the profunda femoris artery, which supplies blood to the small tensor fascial lata muscle. The entire lateral thigh skin is vascularized by perforating arteries from this vessel.

21. What flaps can be used to cover perineal pressure sores?

In patients with an intact lower extremity, the gracilis muscle/musculocutaneous flap can be used. In patients with a urethrocutaneous fistula, the urethra should be reconstructed first over a stent with a full-thickness skin graft tube. A gracilis muscle flap can then provide surface coverage. If the lower extremity is not present, the perineal defect can be covered with an inferiorly based rectus abdominis flap using the deep inferior epigastric artery.

22. When is a total thigh flap recommended?

The total thigh flap should not be considered the optimal choice for management of primary sores. It is recommended for recurrent multiple pressure ulcers around the pelvis and perineum. Before reconstruction, coexisting pelvic osteomyelitis must be managed. If a urethral fistula is also present in the perineum, it should be repaired, or urine should be diverted before final reconstruction.

23. What measures does a successful total thigh flap include?

1. Extensive debridement of all devitalized soft tissue and bone
2. Careful planning of surgical incisions to maximize soft tissue use from the thigh and leg
3. Amputation of leg at the appropriate level (if an extensive defect is present, one may extend the thigh leg flap almost to the level of the malleoli)
4. Meticulous hemostasis and placement of multiple suction drains
5. Obliteration of all residual spaces and a tension-free closure

BIBLIOGRAPHY

1. Braden BJ: Clinical utility of Braden Scale for predicting sure sore risks. Decubitus 2:44–46, 50–51, 1989.
2. Colen SR: Pressure sores. In McCarthy JC (ed): Plastic Surgery, vol 6. Philadelphia, W. B. Saunders, 1990, pp 3797–3838.
3. Lewis VL, Bailey H, Pulawski G, et al: The diagnosis of osteomyelitis in patients with pressure sores. Plast Reconst Surg 81:229–232, 1988.
4. Marschall MA, Dolezal RF, Cohen M: Pressure sores. Probl Gen Surg 6:687–698, 1989.
5. Marschall MA, Cohen M: Pressure sores. In Cohen M (ed): Mastery of Plastic and Reconstructive Surgery, vol 2. Boston, Little, Brown, 1994, pp 1371–1386.
6. Mathes SJ, Nahai F: Clinical Applications for Muscle and Musculocutaneous Flaps. St. Louis, Mosby, 1982.

7. Mathes SJ, Nahai F: Clinical Atlas of Muscle and Musculocutaneous Flaps. St. Louis, Mosby, 1979.
8. Mathes SJ, Nahai F: Reconstructive Surgery Principles: Anatomy and Techniques. Vol. 1, pp 499–535, Vol. 2, pp 1173–1206, 1271–1306. New York, Churchill Livingstone–Quality Medical Publishing, Inc., 1997.
9. McGraw JB, Arnold PG: Atlas of Muscle and Musculocutaneous Flaps. Norfolk, VA, Hampton Press, 1986.
10. Norton D: Calculating the risk reflections on the Norton Scale. Decubitus 2:24–31, 1989 [erratum appears in Decubitus 2:10, 1989].
11. Roger J, Pickrell K, Georgiades, N, et al: Total thigh flap for extensive decubitus ulcer. Plast Reconstr Surg 44:108–118, 1969.
12. U. S. Department of Health and Human Services: Pressure Ulcers in Adults: Prediction and Prevention. Clinical Practice Guideline No. 3, Publication 97-0047, 1992.

71. LYMPHEDEMA

Lloyd P. Champagne, M.D., and J. William Futrell, M.D.

1. What is the function of the lymphatic system?

The lymphatic system is a series of endothelial-lined, thin-walled channels that transport fluid, proteins, and particles from the interstitial compartment to the vascular system. Fluid and particles that have escaped from the intravascular system are returned for recycling. The lymphatic system also presents foreign matter to the immune system. When non-self debris such as bacteria are cleared, contact is made with antigen recognition systems. In the intestines, lymphatics have the additional duty of transporting triglycerides and chylomicrons centrally for processing into energy.

2. Where is the lymph system?

A dense system of lymphatic vessels permeates most tissues. In the extremities, the superficial system begins as a cutaneous network of valveless channels that drain into valved collecting vessels in the subdermal layer. These vessels in turn coalesce into larger pathways that follow the major veins. A deeper system exists below the deep muscular fascia, also arranged along the venous system. These pathways drain toward nodal basins in the proximal extremity en route through the trunk to the right and left subclavian vein, the primary sites of reentry of lymph fluid into the venous system. Lymphatics also have been found in most parenchymatous organs with the exception of the interlobular portion of the liver. Lymphatics have yet to be identified in the central nervous system, muscle, tendon, cartilage, bone marrow, and cornea.

3. Define lymphedema.

Lymphedema is the accumulation of protein-rich fluid in the interstitial spaces resulting in an abnormal enlargement of the affected part.

4. What propels lymph through the lymphatic vessels?

Lymphatic flow is facilitated primarily by the compression of lymph channels in contact with surrounding musculature. This mechanism, in concert with a system of valves, promotes the central flow of lymph. As lymph vessels coalesce along major venous and arterial pathways, the pulsations of adjacent vessels intermittently compress the valved channels. The lymph from the extremities then travels toward the neck and is subject to variations in intraabdominal and intrathoracic pressure, again propelling lymph toward the central neck veins. Although the media of larger-caliber lymph vessels contains smooth muscle, this muscle does not directly assist in lymph flow but rather regulates vessel caliber.

5. Where does lymph fluid enter into the circulation?

The extremity lymphatics coalesce into two major lumbar lymph trunks that at the L4 level join to form the cisterna chyli. The cisterna chyli then passes through the aortic hiatus to become the thoracic duct and subsequently empties into the left subclavian vein as it is joined by the left internal jugular vein. Lymph fluid also drains into the circulation from the right lymphatic duct, which drains the right side of the head and neck, upper extremity, thorax, and lung. There are other minor sites of lymph return throughout the body at lymphovenous communications in the lymph nodes.

6. What is the effect of inadequate lymph drainage in the extremities?

As protein and fluid accumulate in the interstitial spaces, lymphatic destruction becomes self-perpetuating. The protein in the interstitium activates the inflammatory cascade. Inflammatory cells permeate the lymphedematous tissues, but the effect of the protein-rich, oxygen-poor environment impairs their phagocytic activity. The decreased capacity for phagocytosis results in net collagen deposition as activated fibroblasts continue to lay down collagen fibrils in response to injury. The end result is thickened, fibrosed channels that have an impaired ability to clear fluid and protein. The adjacent interstitium is similarly changed, showing increased fibrosis and collagen deposition. In addition to the acute injury, chronic injury to smooth muscle causes these cells to transform into fibroblastlike cells, further promoting tissue fibrosis. This cyclic pattern of swelling with tissue injury gradually causes progression of the lymphedema.

7. What is the relationship between bacterial infection and chronic lymphedema?

Considerable morbidity and occasional mortality may occur in patients with lymphedema due to recurring episodes of cellulitis. The stasis of lymph predisposes to infection, and the repeated infection makes the lymphedema worse. Such infections cause permanent alterations in the lymphatic apparatus due to inflammation and fibrosis. Streptococci and staphylococci are the most common causative organisms.

8. What is the most feared consequence of long-standing lymphedema?

Lymphangiosarcoma (LAS) is a rare but highly lethal complication of chronic lymphedema. Most cases have occurred in postmastectomy patients with long-standing obstruction (typically 10 or more years). However, LAS has occurred with lymphedema from other causes. Because these tumors are aggressive and metastasize early, initial radical amputation of the affected limb is believed to offer the best chance of cure. Conservative excision has been associated with a high rate of recurrence and death, and, unfortunately, LAS does not respond to chemotherapy or radiotherapy. Prognosis for LAS is poor with an average survival of 19 months. When the condition occurs in association with arm edema after mastectomy, it is referred to as the Stewart-Treves syndrome.

9. Is lymphedema inherited?

Secondary lymphedema is acquired and therefore cannot be inherited. Primary lymphedema is a diagnosis of exclusion; no identifiable cause is known. Among patients presenting with primary lymphedema, a familial pattern occurs in about 15%.

10. Who is most likely to develop lymphedema? When?

Lymphedema is classified based on the time of presentation and the presence or lack of a defined cause. Primary lymphedema is a diagnosis of exclusion and is classified by time of appearance into congenital, early, and late forms. Lymphedema congenita is present at birth and accounts for about 15% of all patients with primary lymphedema. Milroy's disease is lymphedema congenita that demonstrates a familial pattern of inheritance; it afflicts women twice as often as men and is more likely to involve the lower extremities. Lymphedema praecox or early lymphedema, the most common of the primary edema states, accounts for approximately 75% of primary lymphedema and has its clinical onset from childhood to age 35. Like lymphedema congenita, lymphedema praecox is more common in women and usually affects the lower extremities. Lymphedema tarda or late-onset lymphedema accounts for 10% of primary lymphedema and occurs after the age of 35 years.

Secondary lymphedema is acquired as a result of damage to lymphatics and lymph nodes. In developed countries, metastatic tumor to lymph nodes and surgical removal of nodal basins are the leading causes of secondary lymphedema; therefore, secondary lymphedema is common in older people and postsurgical patients. In tropical and subtropical countries, filariasis, a parasitic infection from the organism *Wuchereria bancrofti*, produces a type of secondary lymphedema that is termed elephantiasis when the swelling reaches gigantic proportions.

11. What disease states are suggested by an enlarged extremity?

The differential diagnosis of an enlarged extremity includes several disorders, each of which should be considered before the condition is labeled lymphedema. Venous edema and obesity are much more likely to be responsible for an enlarged extremity. Extremity obesity, also referred to as lipoedema or lipodystrophy, is common and easily confused with lymphedema. The multiple conditions that contribute to a state of fluid excess, such as renal and cardiac disease, should also be considered early in the differential diagnosis. A partial list of the causes of lymphedema is presented below:

- **Primary lymphedema** (unknown cause but 15% of cases are congenital)
  Lymphedema congenita, praecox, and tarda
- **Acquired lymphedema**
  Malignancy, primary or metastatic
  Extralymphatic compression due to nonmalignant states
  Iatrogenic causes (irradiation or surgery—lymphadenectomy and disruption of lymph channels
    without node removal)
  Trauma
  Inflammation
  Infection—bacterial, fungal, parasitic
- **Disorders not due to lymphedema**
  Lipoedema (obesity)
  Venous edema
  Low protein states (nephrotic syndrome, malnutrition, and cirrhosis)
  Conditions associated with generalized fluid overload (e.g., cardiac, renal)

12. What is the likelihood of extension of lymphedema into another region of the same extremity?

Proximal extension of lymphedema in the same limb is unusual after the first year, occurring in 7% of the patients after the first year and < 1% after 5 years.

13. What is the likelihood of an increase in the girth of an extremity in patients with primary lymphedema of the lower limb?

Although the probability of extension of lymphedema into another region of the lower extremity is low, 35–40% of patients followed for 5, 10, and 20 years experienced increasing girth of the affected extremity. The prognosis for severity of swelling is closely related to lymphographic findings. Proximal obstructive hypoplasia is more likely to be associated with severe edema and progressive swelling.

14. How frequent is bilateral lymphedema?

In Wolfe and Kinmonth's review, contralateral development of lymphedema occurred in only 9% of patients. After diagnosis of the initial lymphedematous state, about 3% developed edema of the other leg between 1 and 5 years; the remaining 6% manifested contralateral disease after 5–20 years.

15. How do lymph fluid and venous edema fluid differ?

The protein content of lymph fluid varies from 1–5 gm/dl, whereas protein in venous edema fluid is below 1 gm/dl. In addition, the ratio of albumin to globulin is higher in lymph fluid.

16. Can lymph channels reestablish continuity after transection?

Transected lymph vessels may reestablish continuity across a gap of approximately 1 mm under optimal healing conditions. In the presence of hematoma, infection, or inflammation, this process is hindered. Delayed healing is an important factor contributing to the development of lymphatic edema after removal of the glands of the axilla or groin. If direct anastomosis does not occur, collateral channels may "enrich" or hypertrophy, or they may reorient to drain lymphedematous areas.

17. When is a confirmatory lymphangiogram indicated?

Lymphangiography is not an innocuous procedure and should be performed only when anatomic detail is needed before a surgical procedure. The procedure is tedious, time-consuming, and potentially dangerous. The most compelling argument against routine use of lymphangiography is its lack of ability to generate information that would alter the treatment strategy.

18. What is the role of CT and MRI in the diagnosis of lymphedema of the lower limb?

CT imaging of lymphedematous compartments reveals a classic feature described as a honeycomb appearance. The honeycomb pattern of the subcutaneous tissues, in conjunction with the size of the subfascial compartment and skin layer, enables examiners to distinguish lymphedema from venous edema and lipoedema (obesity). CT findings in patients with lymphedema also include an increase in skin thickness with maintenance of a normal-sized subfascial muscle compartment. In contrast, deep venous thrombosis causes an increase in the size of the subfascial compartment with a small increase in the thickness of the skin and subcutaneous compartment. The honeycomb pattern of the subcutaneous layer is not seen. CT features of lipoedema include enlargement of the subcutaneous compartment with normal subfascial compartment and skin thickness. Like CT imaging of lymphedema, MRI reveals similar patterns of changes in the soft tissue compartments. Both CT and MRI are useful in delineating nodal architecture. T2-weighted MRI images provide better contrast and resolution between fluid and fibrotic areas and have the additional advantage of imaging tissue without subjecting the patient to ionizing radiation. In most centers MRI is becoming the preferred soft tissue imaging technique.

19. Besides CT and MRI imaging, what other noninvasive means are available for diagnosis of the swollen extremity?

History and physical exam are reliable tools for the diagnosis of lymphedema. Ultrasound may give information about the underlying vasculature as well as detect volume changes in the dermal, subcutaneous, and subfascial compartments; however, it is not widely used. Interstitial lymphangiography with water-soluble dyes and lymphoscintigraphy with technetium-99 radiolabeled colloid offer relatively noninvasive examination without the problems associated with intralymphatic lymphangiography. Lymphoscintigraphy has recently enjoyed increased use as a tool for identifying high-risk nodal basins in patients with potentially metastatic tumor from a primary melanoma.

20. What is the first line of therapy for lymphedema?

Conservative therapy should be attempted before any surgical procedure. The cornerstone of most types of conservative therapies is elevation of the lymphedematous extremity. Standing and even sitting for long periods should be strictly limited. Custom-fitted compression stockings and various mechanical-pump compression devices can assist in lymphedema control, but such devices should not be relied on as the sole means of therapy.

Maintenance of skin hygiene is important because healthy skin prevents entry of bacteria. Chronic dermatophytoses are treated because such infections violate the integrity of the epidermal barrier and may lead to repeated infections. Patients with recurrent cellulitis may benefit from chronic antibiotic therapy for suppression of infection. In obese patients, diet is another part of the treatment regimen; the lymphedema of obesity responds to significant weight loss. In all of these conservative therapies for lymphedema, patient compliance is essential to prevent treatment failure.

21. What surgical options have reproducible, proven efficacy?

No procedures have reproducible, proven efficacy in reversing the pathophysiology of the lymphedematous process. Procedures are classically divided into physiologic procedures that attempt to restore normal drainage patterns and excisional procedures.

22. What are the most common physiologic procedures?

Physiologic procedures attempt to increase lymphatic drainage by augmentation of existing drainage channels or by addition of lymph vessels from transposition of small bowel, omentum, dermal flaps, and skin flaps. Examples include the following:

1. **Lymphangioplasty.** Lymphangioplasty attempts to create new drainage pathways in the subcutaneous tissue. Silk threads, Nylon, Teflon, and rubber tubes are among the materials that have been buried in the subcutaneous tissue in an attempt to wick fluid into healthy areas. The results of such attempts are disappointing, and the procedures are complicated by a high incidence of infection and extrusion of the foreign material.

2. **Buried dermal flaps.** In this bridging procedure a dermal flap is buried in the muscle in an attempt to establish communication between the superficial and deep compartments in the extremity. Studies have failed to prove a functional communication between these compartments. Flap necrosis, wound infection, and dehiscence are troubling complications.

3. **Omental transposition.** The transposition of omentum to an edematous area attempts to establish lymph outflow through the functioning omental lymphatics. Early experience was encouraging, but long-term results have been disappointing, showing no evidence of lymphatic bridging.

Instead, the omentum is surrounded with a fibrous capsule. Complications are similar to those with other procedures; additional problems are associated with the intraabdominal harvest of omentum.

4. **Enteromesenteric bridge.** Transected bowel with denuded mucosa is transposed to an area of transected inguinal lymph nodes. Reports have been encouraging, but larger series from multiple centers are needed to establish the enteromesenteric bridge as a beneficial surgical treatment.

5. **Lymph node–venous anastomosis.** Lymphaticovenous shunts are created by implanting a transected lymph node end-to-side into a vein. Success in patients in the early stages of lymphedematous disease has been reported, but results are transient and may be hindered by fibrous ingrowth and scar formation.

6. **Microlymphaticovenous anastomosis.** Microsurgical lymphovenous anastomosis for treatment of lymphedema has had varied results but appears to work best when two or more anastomoses are performed early in patients with secondary lymphedema.

7. **Microsurgical lymphatic grafting.** Lymphedema due to local blockade of the lymphatic system can be treated by bridging the defect with autologous lymphatic grafts.

23. What are the most common excisional procedures?

At present, ablative or excisional procedures that remove lymphedematous tissues seem to hold more promise of effective therapy for lymphedema. Although these procedures are not curative they offer relief of symptoms. Examples include the following:

1. **Radical excision with skin grafting**, also referred to as the Charles operation, entails the complete removal of skin, subcutaneous tissue, and deep fascia of the extremity. The muscle is then grafted with either split- or full-thickness skin grafts. The procedure is associated with high morbidity, including ulceration, ooze, infection, hyperkeratosis, scar contracture, and an undesirable cosmetic result.

2. **Staged subcutaneous excision** removes most of the subcutaneous tissues while maintaining viable skin flaps for coverage of the defect. The procedure is less radical than the Charles operation and is a reasonable therapeutic choice.

3. **Liposuction** has offered initial volume reduction of 8–23% in both primary and secondary lymphedema. Liposuction is best suited to mild cases in patients with preserved skin elasticity, but it is only a temporary solution; serial suctioning has been required. Liposuction also has been used as an adjunct to surgical excision, enabling larger volumes of skin and subcutaneous tissue to be resected during a single procedure.

CONTROVERSY

24. Should diuretics be part of the conservative regimen for lymphedema?

Adjunctive use of diuretics has been recommended as part of conservative management of the lymphedematous extremity. Although diuretics may be beneficial particularly in the early course of the disease, the improvement is usually transient. Other reports cite long-term maintenance of the lymphedematous extremity with periodic use of diuretics. One reports indicates freedom from swelling for up to 14 years with periodic use of diuretics. The controversy about diuretic use is not limited to efficacy; it extends to the pathophysiology of the disease and potential to cause harm. Foldi states that diuretics "contradict the pathophysiology of the lymphedema" and may be indicated for low-protein edemas accompanied by elevated sodium content of the body. Lymphedema, however, is not due to sodium retention but to retention of proteins and particles in the interstitial space. Diuretic use causes removal of water from the interstitial compartment, further concentrating the remaining proteins. As a result of this concentrating process, interstitial protein levels increase with the possible consequence of increasing fibrosis.

BIBLIOGRAPHY

1. Baumeister RG, Siuda S: Treatment of lymphedemas by microsurgical lymphatic grafting: What is proved? Plast Reconstr Surg 85:64–74,1990.
2. Borel Rinkes IHM, de Jongste AB: Lymphangiosarcoma in chronic lymphedema. Acta Chir Scand 152:227–230, 1986.
3. Campisi C, Boccardo F, Alitta P, et al: Derivative lymphatic microsurgery: Indications, techniques, and results. Microsurgery 16:463–468, 1995.

4. Crockett DJ: Lymphatic anatomy and lymphoedema. Br J Plast Surg 18:12–25, 1965.
5. Foldi E, Foldi M, Clodius L: The lymphedema chaos. Ann Plast Surg 22:505–515, 1989.
6. Gloviczki P, Fisher J, Hollier LH, et al: Microsurgical lymphovenous anastomosis for treatment of lymphedema: A critical review. J Vasc Surg 7:647–652, 1988.
7. Haaverstad R, Nilsen G, Rinck P, et al: The use of MRI in the diagnosis of chronic lymphedema of the lower extremity. Int Angiol 13(2):115–118, 1994.
8. Hadjis NS, Carr DH, Banks L, et al: The role of CT in the diagnosis of primary lymphedema of the lower extremity. AJR 144:361–364, 1985.
9. Louton RB, Terranova WA: The use of suction curettage as adjunct to the management of lymphedema. Ann Plast Surg 22:354–357, 1989.
10. Sando WC, Nahai F: Suction lipectomy in the management of limb lymphedema. Clin Plast Surg 16:369–373, 1089.
11. Stone EJ, Hugo NE: Lymphedema. Surg Gynecol Obstet 135:625–631, 1972.
12. Vaughan BF: CT of swollen legs. Clin Radiol 41:24–30, 1990.
13. Wolfe JHN, Kinmonth JB: The prognosis of primary lymphedema of the lower limbs. Arch Surg 116:1157–1160, 1981.

72. RECONSTRUCTION OF THE GENITALIA

Anthony A. Caldamone, M.D., and Leslie D. Tackett, M.D.

1. Describe the anatomy of the penis, including the fascial layers.

The anatomy of the penis begins with three erectile bodies, two corpora cavernosa and the corpus spongiosum, which surrounds the urethra. The corpora cavernosa, which contain the majority of erectile tissue, are surrounded by the tunica albuginea. The neurovascular bundle, containing the deep dorsal vein, dorsal artery, and paired dorsal nerves, lies between the tunica albuginea and Buck's fascia, which surrounds all three corpora, followed by dartos fascia and skin.

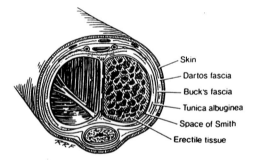

Skin
Dartos fascia
Buck's fascia
Tunica albuginea
Space of Smith
Erectile tissue

Transverse section of the penis at the junction of its middle and distal thirds. The septum is correctly illustrated as strands that interweave with the tunica albuginea both ventrally and dorsally. (From Jordan GH, Schlossberg SM, Devine CE: Surgery of the penis and urethra. In Walsh PC, Retik AB, Vaughn ED, Wein AJ (eds): Campbell's Urology, 7th ed. Philadelphia, W.B. Saunders, 1998, with permission.)

2. Name the origin and branches of the common penile artery.

The common penile artery is a branch of the internal pudendal artery. Its branches are the bulbourethral artery, dorsal artery, and cavernosal artery. The branches of the dorsal artery include the circumflex branches, which contribute to the blood supply of the urethra, and the terminal branches, which supply the glans.

3. What is the role of testosterone in genital development?

The enlargement of the genital tubercle and subsequent elongation of the phallus and developing urethra depend on the presence of testosterone. After conversion to dihydrotestosterone by the 5-alpha reductase enzyme, testosterone is responsible for virilization of the external genitalia.

4. Describe the common features of hypospadias.

1. Dystopic urethral meatus in a ventral position on the penis, scrotum, or perineum
2. Urethral plate distal to the dystopic meatus

3. Dorsally hooded foreskin (97–98%)

4. Ventral chordee (more than 50% of cases)

5. Where is the most common location of the meatus in hypospadias? The least common?

Anterior meatus (glanular, subcoronal, distal penile shaft)	65%
Medial meatus (midshaft)	15%
Posterior meatus (posterior penile shaft, penoscrotal, scrotal, perineal)	20%

6. Name the goals and components of hypospadias repair.

1. Straightening of the penile shaft (orthoplasty)

2. Creation of an adequate caliber urethra (urethroplasty)

3. Repositioning of the urethral meatus to the tip of the penis and creation of a symmetric glans (meatoplasty and glanuloplasty)

4. Achieving a good cosmetic result (skin coverage and scrotoplasty) with normalization of voiding and erection

7. How does one perform an artificial erection?

A tourniquet is placed at the base of the penis. Sterile injectable saline is injected into one corpus cavernosum, either at the base of the penis or via the glans.

8. What are the causes of chordee?

Congenital causes	**Acquired causes**
Fibrosis of the corpus spongiosum	Peyronie's disease
Skin tethering to the corpus spongiosum	Periurethral fibrosis associated with
Deficiency of Buck's fascia or corpora cavernosa	stricture disease
Hypoplastic urethra	
Differential corporal growth	

9. What are the two most common complications of a hypospadias repair?

Urethrocutaneous fistula and urethral stricture complicate approximately 10–15% of all hypospadias repairs.

10. Should one look for other congenital anomalies in a patient with hypospadias?

The most common anomalies associated with hypospadias are cryptorchidism and inguinal hernia; the incidence of each is approximately 9%. Anomalies of the upper urinary tract are infrequent unless other organ system anomalies, such as myelomeningocele or imperforate anus, are present. Therefore, routine screening of the upper urinary tract is not indicated in patients with isolated hypospadias or hypospadias associated with undescended testes or inguinal hernia.

11. What are the classic features of the exstrophy/epispadias complex?

- Divergent rectus with exposed bladder plate
- Low umbilicus
- Widening of the symphysis pubis
- Anteriorly displaced anus
- Short penis with divergent corpora, dorsal chordee, and dorsally displaced meatus (epispadias)
- Short urethra
- Short vagina with stenotic anteriorly displaced orifice
- Bifid clitoris and divergent labia, mons pubis, and clitoris

12. How does exstrophy occur?

Exstrophy results from failure of the cloacal membrane to rupture, which prevents medial mesenchymal ingrowth. Therefore, proper development of the lower abdominal wall is impeded.

13. State the goals of exstrophy reconstruction.

- Abdominal wall closure
- Bladder closure with adequate capacity

• Achievement of urinary continence
• Preservation of renal function
• Functional and cosmetic genital reconstruction

14. What is the most common cause of ambiguous genitalia? What is the most common enzyme abnormality?

Congenital adrenal hyperplasia is the most common cause of ambiguous genitalia; deficiency of 21-hydroxylase is the most common enzyme abnormality.

15. List the categories of ambiguous genitalia.

1. **Female pseudohermaphroditism.** Affected children have a 46XX chromosomal pattern and ovaries. Congenital adrenal hyperplasia is the most common diagnosis.

2. **Male pseudohermaphroditism.** Affected children have a 46XY karyotype and testicular tissue. Defects in androgen synthesis, response to androgens, and failure of müllerian regression are among the many causes of incomplete virilization.

3. **True hermaphrodite.** The most common karyotype in affected children is 46XX, but the 46XY or mosaic karyotype is also found. Both ovarian and testicular tissue are present.

4. **Mixed gonadal dysgenesis.** Most affected children have a 46XY/45XO karyotype with a testis on one side and a dysgenetic or streak gonad on the other. The internal structures are variable.

5. **Pure gonadal dysgenesis.** Affected children, who may have a 45XO, 46XX, or 46XY karyotype, do not usually present with ambiguous genitalia but rather with delayed puberty in adolescence or adulthood. Bilateral streak gonads and müllerian ductal structures are present. Because of high malignant potential, early bilateral gonadectomy is recommended for patients with 46XY karyotype.

16. Describe the considerations that contribute to gender assignment.

A multidisciplinary approach is paramount to successful diagnosis, management, counseling, and gender assignment. Functional anatomic potential, including consideration of phallus size, plays a major role in gender assignment. Less consideration is given to potential fertility and karyotype.

17. What are the anatomic divisions of the urethra?

The **posterior urethra** is the portion proximal to the bulb and includes the prostatic and membranous urethra.

The **anterior urethra** lies distal to entry into the bulb and includes the bulbar, penile, or pendulous urethra and fossa navicularis. The anterior urethra is contained within the corpus spongiosum.

18. Name three causes of urethral stricture disease.

1. Trauma or crush injury
2. Instrumentation such as Foley catheterization or cystourethroscopy
3. Infection (most likely gonorrhea)

19. What studies are involved in the preoperative evaluation of urethral stricture?

As always, one must begin with a history and physical exam. The presence of a stricture is suggested by voiding symptoms such as decreased force of stream, urinary frequency, nocturia, and dysuria. Physical exam may reveal the inability to pass a catheter. Urinalysis and culture should be performed to rule out infection. The stricture must be characterized radiographically using a retrograde urethrogram, voiding cystourethrogram, or both. Ultrasound helps to characterize the length, depth, and density of the stricture. Urethroscopy provides information about the elasticity of the stricture.

20. What tissues are available for reconstruction of the urethra?

1. Preputial, penile shaft, or scrotal skin
2. Free graft of buccal or bladder mucosa
3. Free graft of extragenital skin

21. Who was Peyronie?

François de la Peyronie was a French barber surgeon who commanded the surgical corps for King Louis XIV. Although descriptions of similar penile deformities can be found in ancient Roman literature, Peyronie described the disease that bears his name in a patient who "had rosary beads of scar tissue causing an upward curvature of the penis during erection."

22. What is the cause of Peyronie's disease? What is the most commonly associated physical finding other than penile curvature?

The exact cause of Peyronie's disease is elusive. The most commonly held belief is that the plaque is the end result of an inflammatory response to trauma to the erect penis. Beta-blocking agents also have been associated with the development of plaques. Dupuytren's contracture occurs in approximately 10–30% of patients with Peyronie's disease.

23. If a patient presents with significant penile curvature, what are the important considerations for recommending treatment?

The goal of treatment in Peyronie's disease is to preserve or restore sexual function. Important considerations in the treatment include concomitant erectile dysfunction, penile pain, duration and stability of curvature, and patient satisfaction with sexual function. Treatment should begin with vitamin E until the plaque has matured or the degree of curvature is stable.

24. What materials or tissues have been used in plaque incision or excision and grafting?

Dermis	Dacron	Dura
Tunica vaginalis	Dexon	Vein

25. What additional procedure should be considered in patients with erectile dysfunction and Peyronie's disease?

In patients with erectile dysfunction in addition to penile curvature, one should consider placement of a penile prosthesis at the time of repair of the curvature. Placement of a prosthesis in patients without erectile dysfunction is controversial.

26. After exploration to determine the extent of the injury, how should one manage a degloving injury to the penis?

Currently, most degloving injuries to the penis and scrotum are managed with immediate reconstruction using split-thickness skin grafting. A sheet graft is used on the penis, and a meshed graft reproduces a rugated appearance on the scrotum. Another option is to bury the penis in a subcutaneous abdominal pouch and the testes in thigh pouches for delayed reconstruction.

27. Describe the most common technique for penile reconstruction and phallic construction.

In the past, phallic reconstruction was performed using tubed abdominal flaps in multistaged procedures. Chang and Hwang popularized the use of radial forearm flaps in 1984. Although the technique has undergone many modifications since its original description, the use of the forearm flap remains the standard. Penile rigidity is achieved by the use of an external device or an implanted prosthesis. Prosthesis implantation is delayed at least 1 year from reconstruction to ensure urethral patency and durability as well as viability of the forearm flap.

28. What are the options for construction of a vagina?

1. Bowel (sigmoid colon most commonly)
2. Flaps (pudendal-thigh flap)
3. Split-thickness skin graft or full-thickness skin graft (with or without tissue expanders)
4. Amnion

BIBLIOGRAPHY

1. Canning DA, Koo HP, Duckett JW: Anomalies of the bladder and cloaca. In Gillenwater JY, Grayhack JT, Howards SS, Duckett JW (eds): Adult and Pediatric Urology, 3rd ed. St. Louis, Mosby, 1996.
2. Chang TS, Hwang WY: Forearm flap in one-stage reconstruction of the penis. Plast Reconstr Surg 74:251–258, 1984.

3. Devine CJ, Horton CE: Surgical treatment of Peyronie's disease with a dermal graft. J Urol 43:697–701, 1974.
4. Dunsmuir WD, Kirby RS: Francois de LaPeyronie (1678-1747): The man and the disease he described. Br J Urol 78:613–622, 1996.
5. Hensle TW, Dean GE: Vaginal replacement in children. J Urol 148:677–679, 1992.
6. Jordan GH: Peyronie's disease and its management. In Krane RJ, Siroky MB, Fitzpatrick J (eds): Clinical Urology. Philadelphia, J.B. Lippincott, 1994, pp 1282–1297.
7. Jordan GH, Gilbert DA: Male genital trauma. Clin Plast Surg 15:431–442, 1988.
8. Jordan GH, Schlossberg SM, Devine CE: Surgery of the penis and urethra. In Walsh PC, Retik AB, Vaughn ED, Wein AJ (eds): Campbell's Urology, 7th ed. Philadelphia, W.B. Saunders, 1998.
9. Joseph VT: Pudendal-thigh flap vaginoplasty in reconstruction of genital anomalies. J Pediatr Surg 32:62–65, 1997.
10. Keating MA, Caldamone AA: Current concepts in the management of hypospadias. In Stein BS, Caldamone AA, Smith JA (eds): Clinical Urologic Practice. New York, W.W. Norton, 1995.
11. Mandell J: Sexual differentiation: Normal and abnormal. In Walsh PC, Retik AB, Vaughn ED, Wein AJ (eds): Campbell's Urology, 7th ed. Philadelphia, W.B. Saunders, 1998.

IX. Burns

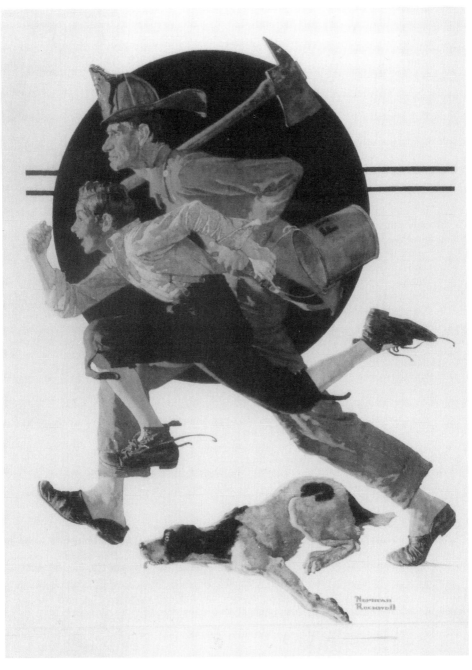

Fire!
Norman Rockwell
1931
The Saturday Evening Post
Cover, 28 March 1931
Reprinted by permission of the Norman Rockwell Family Trust
© 1931 The Norman Rockwell Family Trust

73. THERMAL BURNS

Karen E. Frye, M.D., F.A.C.S., and Arnold Luterman, M.D., F.A.C.S., F.R.C.S.(C)

1. List three functions of the skin that are lost when thermal injury occurs. What are the consequences?

1. Skin (the largest organ of the body) is a barrier to heat loss. In cases of acute burn, care must be taken to keep the patient warm and avoid hypothermia.

2. Skin is a barrier to evaporative losses. Free water losses frequently need replacement in patients with major burn injury.

3. Skin is a barrier to microbial invasion. Thus, the burn patient is highly susceptible to infection.

2. What is the incidence of burn injury in the United States?

Over a million burn injuries occur annually in the United States, of which approximately 100,000 require admission to a specialized burn center. Each year 12,000–15,000 people die of burn injuries.

3. What are the criteria for referring a patient to a specialized burn center?

1. Inhalation injury
2. Burn size > 10% total body surface area (TBSA) in patients < 10 years old or > 50 years old
3. Burn size > 20% TBSA in any patient
4. Full-thickness burns involving > 5% TBSA
5. Burn wound involvement of the face, hands, feet, perineum, or genitalia
6. Associated trauma
7. Comorbid states
8. Special social situations (e.g., child abuse)

4. What are the immediate concerns about the airway of patients with thermal injury?

The airway must be assessed immediately. If the patient has suffered a burn to the upper airway, intubation is necessary to prevent upper airway obstruction due to edema. The airway is assessed most accurately by nasopharyngoscopy. If the exam is performed immediately after injury (0–4 hours) and is normal, it may need to be repeated 6 hours later. Edema may not manifest itself until 6–8 hours after injury. Edema should reach a maximum by 24 hours after injury.

5. What three factors suggest an inhalation injury?

History of the fire occurring in an enclosed space, production of carbonaceous sputum, and elevated carboxyhemoglobin level (COHB > 10%). If all three factors are present, it is highly likely that the patient has suffered an inhalation injury.

6. What diagnostic measures can be used to confirm inhalation injury?

Fiberoptic bronchoscopy may be performed at the bedside. Examination of the lower airway may reveal deposition of carbonaceous particles as well as mucosal edema. If the exam is done soon after injury or if the patient has not been adequately resuscitated, edema may not be evident. Regardless of the findings on bronchoscopy, clinical management of the inhalation injury is initially based on adequate oxygenation and ventilation. A xenon ventilation-perfusion lung scan is the most definitive study for diagnosis of inhalation injury, but it is time-consuming and requires transport of the patient to the radiology department.

7. What are the concerns in transporting a burn victim from a community hospital to a specialized burn center?

The airway must be adequate. If there is any question that the airway may obstruct, the patient should be intubated, preferably via the endotracheal route. Fluid resuscitation should be in progress using the Parkland formula. The patient must be kept warm. Avoid wet dressings, which tend to make the patient hypothermic. The simplest strategy is to wrap the patient in a dry, sterile sheet.

8. How is inhalation injury managed acutely?

The patient must be adequately ventilated and oxygenated. Mechanical ventilation may be required; 100% oxygen should be administered to enhance the off-loading of carbon monoxide from hemoglobin. The half-life of carbon monoxide on room air is 4–5 hours; on 100% oxygen it is reduced to approximately 45 minutes. The patient should be maintained on 100% oxygen until the carboxyhemoglobin level is < 10%.

9. When are prophylactic antibiotics and/or steroids indicated for inhalation injury?

Never. Prophylactic antibiotics for an inhalation injury do not prevent postinhalation pulmonary infectious complications; they only select resistant organisms. Thus, once a pulmonary infection develops, it is more difficult to treat. Steroids should not be used in inhalation injury. They are of no benefit and increase mortality threefold.

10. Describe the resuscitation of thermally injured patients.

Burn wounds involving greater than 20% TBSA typically mount a systemic inflammatory response with resultant capillary leak. Fluid requirements are estimated initially with the Parkland formula:

$$\text{Fluids for first 24 hr} = 4 \text{ cc} \times \text{patient weight in kg} \times \% \text{ TBSA burned}$$

One-half of the fluid is given over the first 8 hours after injury. The second half is given over the remaining 16 hours. The Parkland formula is only an estimate. Some patients require more than the predicted amount of fluid, and some require less. The patient must be continually monitored by repeatedly evaluating heart rate, blood pressure, urine output, and acid-base status. Fluids need to be adjusted accordingly.

11. Describe the initial resuscitation of a child with burn injuries.

Fluid requirements in children are estimated with the Parkland formula, as in adults. In addition, because of a larger body surface area-to-weight ratio, pediatric patients also require additional maintenance fluids, usually administered as D5-1/4NS. In addition to this solution, some carbohydrate is also provided. Because glycogen stores are minimal in young children, hypoglycemia is a potential problem unless exogenous carbohydrate is provided.

12. How is the size of the burn estimated?

The most accurate method is the Lund and Browder chart, which allows for differences in various age groups. The rule of nines is a simpler method but less accurate:

Head and neck = 9% TBSA	Posterior torso = 18% TBSA
Each upper extremity = 9% TBSA	Each lower extremity = 18% TBSA
Anterior torso = 18% TBSA	Perineum = 1% TBSA

For small or scattered burns, a helpful rule is that one patient palm size is approximately 1% TBSA.

13. How is the depth of the wound classified?

Historically, wound depth has been classified as first, second, or third degree. A first-degree wound involves only the epidermis. The classic example is sunburn. A second-degree wound involves the epidermis and dermis but does not extend all the way through the dermis. Second-degree wounds are classified as superficial partial or superficial dermal vs. deep partial or deep dermal injuries. Superficial partial wounds usually heal spontaneously within 3 weeks. Deep partial wounds usually take longer than 3 weeks to close spontaneously. A third-degree burn is a full-thickness injury that involves the entire epidermis and dermis. The classic finding on physical exam is thrombosed vessels.

14. Describe the three zones of a burn wound.

The central area is the zone of coagulation or ischemia and consists of nonviable tissue. Surrounding the zone of coagulation is the zone of stasis or edema, which initially is viable but has decreased blood flow. With hypoperfusion and underresuscitation, the zone of stasis may become part of the zone of coagulation. The outermost area is the zone of hyperemia, which manifests an inflammatory response to the burn wound with increased blood flow.

15. Describe the management of burn wounds involving the extremities.

Any limb with a burn wound requires elevation acutely to minimize edema formation. If wounds are circumferential or nearly circumferential, pulses need to be assessed hourly. Doppler ultrasound may be required for accurate assessment, because palpation of pulses is difficult in the edematous limb. In the upper extremity, the palmar arch pulse, radial pulse, and ulnar pulse should be evaluated. In the lower extremity, the dorsal pedal and posterior tibial pulses should be checked. If a pulse previously detectable by Doppler exam is lost, escharotomies must be performed. The obvious exception is the patient who is not adequately resuscitated (as manifested by a decreased blood pressure, inadequate urine output, and poor perfusion in an uninvolved limb).

16. Why is pain control important in burn patients?

Pain causes a rise in heart rate, blood pressure, and metabolic rate. With adequate pain control, the patient is less hypermetabolic, and heart rate and blood pressure are better controlled. Inadequate pain control also results in an increased incidence of posttraumatic stress disorder during recovery and rehabilitation.

17. What is burn wound anemia?

A patient with a significant thermal injury frequently manifests anemia until the wounds are closed. Anemia results from the shortened half-life of red blood cells in burn patients (40 days vs. normal half-life of 120 days). If blood is taken from a burned victim and transfused into an unburned person, the half-life of the red blood cells returns to 120 days.

18. What is the initial management of the burn wound?

Initially the wound is treated with a topical antimicrobial agent. The most frequently used agent is silver sulfadiazine (Silvadene, Thermazine, SSD). Other available agents include betadine, silver nitrate, and mafenide acetate (Sulfamylon). Mafenide acetate is the only agent that actually penetrates the burn eschar, but it has two disadvantages: it is painful and it is a carbonic anhydrase inhibitor. Therefore, its use over an area of significant size may cause metabolic acidosis. Ears are typically treated with mafenide acetate. It also may be useful in burn wounds with associated cellulitis. Typically, wound care is performed 1 or 2 times/day.

19. What is meant by tangential excision and fascial excision?

Tangential excision refers to a technique used to remove the burn eschar. Basically, the eschar is removed tangentially in layers until all of the necrotic tissue has been excised and a bleeding, viable wound bed is present.

Fascial excision removes the skin and entire subcutaneous layer down to the fascia. It is usually reserved for very deep burn wounds or burn wounds in elderly patients.

20. How and when is a skin graft done?

The first step in grafting a burn wound involves preparation of the recipient site with tangential or fascial excision of the eschar. Once a viable bed is present, a split-thickness graft is harvested from a donor site. The skin graft is usually secured to the recipient site with sutures or staples. This procedure, referred to as excision and grafting, is indicated for any deep partial or full-thickness burn wound and should be performed at the earliest convenient time once the patient has been adequately resuscitated and is stable from a hemodynamic and respiratory standpoint. Indeterminate wounds should be observed initially. Once it becomes evident that spontaneous closure will take longer than 3 weeks, excision and grafting should be performed. Wound closure should be accomplished by day 21 after the burn to avoid contracture and scarring and thereby offer optimal functional and cosmetic results.

21. What are the reasons for graft failure?

- Inadequate vascular perfusion
- Infection
- Accumulation of fluid under the graft
- Residual eschar (necrotic tissue) on the graft bed
- Mechanical shear forces

22. What is a meshed graft vs. a sheet graft?

In a meshed graft holes are created to prevent accumulation of fluid or blood under the graft. Depending on the size of the mesh, a skin graft can be stretched to cover an area significantly larger than the original donor site. Because sheet grafts have no holes, the risk of hematoma formation or fluid accumulation under the graft is increased. Sheet grafts are preferred from a cosmetic standpoint.

23. What is Integra artificial skin? When should it be used?

Integra artificial skin is a matrix of glycosaminoglycan and collagen. It provides a scaffold whereby the body's fibroblasts can lay down collagen in an organized fashion. Thus, a neodermis is formed rather than scar tissue. A sheet of silastic covers the artificial skin, providing barrier function. The burn wound must be excised early. The artificial skin is laid in place and secured with staples. A neodermis is allowed to form; then the silastic is removed and a thin skin graft (0.004 inches) is used to close the wound. With such a thin graft, little dermis is transferred. Thus, donor sites can be used numerous times. The indications for artificial skin are large burn injuries and the need to limit the size of the donor site (e.g., in patients with an associated inhalation injury or geriatric patients).

24. Discuss the use of temporary wound dressings.

Temporary wound dressings or barrier dressings are useful when the wound is free of necrotic tissue and infection. The classic biologic barrier dressings have been allograft (cadaver skin) and xenograft (pigskin).

Allograft is considered by most experts to be the best temporary dressing; it provides good vascularization of the wound bed. A major disadvantage to its use is cost. Recent concerns involve transmission of viral infections. Allograft usually lasts about 2–3 weeks.

Xenograft is less expensive but does not last as long as allograft or provide vascularization of the wound bed.

Various synthetic wound dressings are currently available. **Biobrane**, one of the older synthetic barrier dressings, is a bilaminar material with an outer layer composed of silicone and Nylon fabric and an inner layer of collagen. Other collagen-based dressings are also available. Some hydrogel dressings are 80% water and provide a moist environment to promote migration of epithelial cells. They also provide a wonderful environment in which bacteria can grow if the wound is infected. Obviously the perfect temporary wound dressing has not been found, and new products are continually marketed.

25. How are thermal injuries to the perineum and genitalia managed?

Good local wound care is the mainstay for wounds of the perineum and genitalia. Because this area has an excellent blood supply, most wounds heal spontaneously. Excision and grafting to the perineum and/or genitalia are technically difficult. For these reasons, wounds of the perineum and genitalia usually should not be managed with early excision and grafting. If after 3–4 weeks a red granulating wound results, skin grafting can be performed. Catheterization is not indicated for burns of the perineum or genitalia unless it is needed to monitor fluid status.

BIBLIOGRAPHY

1. Boswick JA (ed): The Art and Science of Burn Care. Rockville, MD, Aspen Publishers, 1987.
2. Goodwin CW, Finkelstein JL, Madden MR: Burns. In Schwartz SI, Shires GT, Spencer FC (eds): Principles of Surgery, 6th ed. New York, McGraw-Hill, 1994.
3. Herndon DN (ed): Total Burn Care. Philadelphia, W.B. Saunders, 1996.
4. Hunt JL, Purdue G, Rohrich RJ: Burns: Acute burns, burn surgery, and post-burn reconstruction. Sel Read Plast Surg 7(12):1–41, 1994.
5. Pruitt BA, Goodwin CW, Pruitt SK: Burns. In Sabiston DC, Lyerly HK (eds): Textbook of Surgery: The Biological Basis of Modern Surgical Practice, 15th ed. Philadelphia, W.B. Saunders, 1997.

74. ELECTRICAL INJURIES

Mahesh H. Mankani, M.D., and Raphael C. Lee, M.D., Sc.D., F.A.C.S.

1. What is an electrical injury?
Lee and Astumian defined electrical injury as tissue injury resulting from exposure to supraphysiologic electric currents or forces.

2. How common are electrical injuries in the United States?
Deaths from electrical injuries typically number 0.5 per 100,000 population per year in the United States. In 1994 the United States suffered 84 deaths due to lightning strikes and 561 deaths due to electrical exposures not related to lightning.

3. What are the mechanisms for electrical injury?
The pathomechanics of tissue damage in electrical injury are complex. However, two mechanisms predominate: (1) current-generated heating with resulting thermal burn and (2) direct electric force denaturation of cell membrane protein and lipids. Passage of electrical current through a solid body results in conversion of electric energy to heat, a phenomenon called **Joule heating**. The heat production (Q) is proportional to the square of the current (I), tissue resistance (R), and time of contact (t):

$$Q \propto I^2Rt$$

The direct effects of the electrical forces on the cell membrane may lead to the creation of large pores, a process referred to as electroporation. These pores may lead to ion leakage, escape of metabolites, and pathologic membrane permeability to macromolecules as large as DNA. Electrical forces also may lead to the denaturation of membrane proteins.

4. Why is the term *electrical burn* imprecise?
The use of the term *burn* implies that the mechanism for tissue injury is entirely thermal in origin. However, electrical injuries arise from both thermal and nonthermal mechanisms.

5. To what does the term *entrance and exit points* refer?
This somewhat archaic term arises from the concept that a direct current travels from a site of higher potential (voltage) to a site of lower potential, with the intervening human body serving as a conductor. The portion of the patient in contact with the higher voltage is considered the *entrance* site, whereas the site of lower potential is the *exit* site. Alternating current is characterized by a reversal of the direction of current flow with each half cycle of the frequency of the power source. Therefore, in most circumstances no particular anatomic contact point is the entrance or exit point. It is more precise to refer to the patient's points of contact with the sites of higher and lower potential.

6. What is the voltage of typical wall outlets in the home?
Wall outlets in American homes are characterized by an alternating current (AC) of 60 Hz (or 60 cycles per second) and a line-to-line voltage of 110 or 120 volts (V) for general use. In addition, most homes have a line-to-line voltage of 240 V for high-power appliances.

7. How can you calculate the current to which a victim may be exposed during an electrical injury?
The current that is involved in an accident may be calculated by using the known voltage from the outlet and estimating the resistance offered by the body, the contact, and the ground. These parameters often are not known because of the use of various types of clothing and protective gear. The resistance offered by the tissues of the human body, excluding resistance at the interface between the skin and the voltage source, is approximately 500–1000 ohms between the two hands, between the two feet, or between a hand and a foot. Thus the maximal current that a person can experience while grounding a home electrical outlet is as follows:

$$I = V/R \; or$$
$$I = 120 \text{ V}/500 \text{ ohms} = 0.24 \text{ A}$$

The actual current that the person experiences is probably much less because of the additional resistance between the skin and the contacts.

8. What is the minimal voltage necessary for soft tissue injury?

The type of current, its frequency, and its magnitude determine the body's response to the injury. For a person to experience ventricular fibrillation after contact with a voltage source, for instance, the necessary magnitude of alternating current is measurably less than that required from a direct current source. Likewise, a 1-kHz source requires a higher current than a 60-Hz source to produce ventricular fibrillation. A 60-Hz current, typical of wall outlets, with a magnitude of 0.5 mA produces a startle response. Current greater than 10 mA through the forearm may not allow the victim to release his or her grip on the contact. This phenomenon is referred to as the "let-go" threshold and is likely due to electrical stimulation of the dominant forearm flexors. Exposure to a current of 50 mA for longer than 2 seconds may induce ventricular fibrillation, whereas a 1-A current can induce immediate asystole as well as lysis of skeletal muscle and nerve.

9. What are the common modes of exposure to damaging electrical fields?

Victims experience electrical injury when electrical contact is established with an electrical power source. Arcs and flames are good electrical conductors and often mediate the contact under high-voltage conditions. Thermal and thermoacoustic blast injury due to heat from the electrical arc also may cause injury. Electrical contact with the voltage source contributes to Joule heating, electroporation, and protein denaturation. Thermal injury from an electrical flash commonly occurs when the victim is in proximity to an electrical arc. The temperature of an electrical arc can approach $5000°$ C. Heat from the arc may cause a thermal injury. Patients may describe being some distance from the site of the electrical disturbance. On exam, they may not have identifiable contact points. Instead they may demonstrate partial- to full-thickness thermal burns similar in character to nonelectrical burns. Secondary injuries from the electrical exposure include falls from elevated high-tension wires and tetanic contractions from the current leading to cervical or long bone fractures.

10. How are electrical injuries classified?

Clinicians divide electrical injuries into high- and low-tension injuries based on the voltage at the point of contact. High-voltage electrical injuries arise from contact with sources greater than 1000 V, whereas low-voltage electrical injuries arise from contact with voltages less than 1000 V.

The clinical classification of high- and low-tension injuries is distinct from an electrical utility industry classification for power lines. Clinically, high-voltage shock differs from low-voltage shock in that arc-mediated electrical current flow may precede mechanical contact under high-voltage conditions. The voltages delivered by three-phase power lines are categorized as low, medium, high, extrahigh, and ultrahigh. Low voltages are less than 600 V, and medium voltages range from 2400 V to 69 kV. High voltages range from 115–230 kV and extrahigh voltages from 345–765 kV. Ultrahigh voltages are above 1.1 MV. The most common injuries from utility lines involve medium-range voltages because of their prevalence among transmission lines. Using this scheme, note that a medium-line voltage may cause a high-voltage injury.

11. What additional aspects of the history of electrical exposure must be explored?

Determine the type of contact and the length of time that the patient had contact with the voltage source. Determine whether the patient experienced mechanical contact with the current source, made electrical contact with an arc, or suffered flash burns. If the patient had direct contact with the voltage source, identify the involved portions of the patient's anatomy and the duration of the contact.

12. What laboratory studies are appropriate at the time of admission?

Blood gases and serum electrolytes, particularly potassium concentration, are important to measure immediately to guide therapy. If high serum potassium and acidosis suggest extensive muscle necrosis, surgical debridement is likely to be needed as soon as feasible. Elevation of serum creatinine and creatine phosphokinase also suggest massive tissue destruction. Urine myoglobin content is more qualitative.

13. What are the findings of compartment syndrome in the extremities? When is treatment appropriate?

In victims of electrical shock the usual symptoms and signs of compartment syndrome are not reliable because sensory and motor nerve injuries resulting from the electrical shock can be indistinguishable from the clinical manifestations of muscle and nerve ischemia. Palpation of the injured compartment for tenseness is also unreliable because few practitioners have enough personal experience. Arterial pulses are usually intact. When suspected, the diagnosis must be confirmed by directly measuring the compartment pressure.

Recommendations vary with regard to the appropriate compartment pressure at which to perform a fasciotomy. Whitesides advocates fasciotomy when the compartment pressure rises to within 10–30 mmHg of the patient's diastolic pressure. Matsen, however, recommends fasciotomy when the compartment pressure exceeds 45 mmHg.

14. What is the role of magnetic resonance imaging (MRI) in the identification of compromised, electrically injured tissue?

MRI with new open architecture magnetics provides rapid and detailed information about the anatomic sites and severity of injury. In addition, technetium-99 pyrophosphate and similar radionuclide scans have been noted to distinguish between uninjured and injured muscle with high specificity and sensitivity after electrical contact. However, in major electrical trauma the radionuclide scans require too much time to provide information to aid clinical surgical interventions and have not been found to reduce hospital stay or decrease the number of operative procedures.

15. How are fluid requirements calculated in electrical injury resuscitation?

Maintenance of an appropriate intravascular volume can be challenging in major electrical injuries. A high degree of tissue destruction may not be reflected by a limited, discrete cutaneous burn. The adequacy of resuscitation must be confirmed by noting adequate renal profusion. When mannitol is used to enhance diuresis in the face of myoglobinuria, urine output cannot be used as a reliable indicator of renal perfusion. In such situations, the central venous pressure (CVP) or pulmonary capillary wedge pressure (PCWP) should be monitored with an intravenous catheter.

16. What is the significance of myoglobinuria?

Myoglobinuria in the face of electrical injury is indicative of rhabdomyolysis and, if left untreated, is associated with intratubular deposition of pigments, which leads to acute renal failure.

17. How are hemoglobinuria and myoglobinuria diagnosed and treated?

The urine characteristically becomes dark red or burgundy. The patient should undergo a forced diuresis, and urine should be alkalized to maintain solubility of the pigments. This is best accomplished by adding sodium bicarbonate, 88–132 mEq/L of IV infusate. Urine output can be maintained through the administration of mannitol, 25–37 gm IV, or furosemide, 40 mg IV.

18. During a lightning storm, what is the safest location to avoid lightning injuries?

Victims of lightning strikes either are struck directly by the lightning or receive the sideflash. The sideflash is a discharge from the primary target through the air or ground to another object. A victim standing beneath a tree during a thunderstorm may receive a sideflash via the tree. The safest place to stay during a lightning storm, therefore, is in a protected shelter with grounded metal fixtures, such as plumbing, which provide a safe path for the lightning to reach ground. Alternatively, remaining in a closed automobile is safe because the person cannot easily serve as a conduit to ground. However, standing next to the automobile leaves one vulnerable to sideflash.

19. Can victims of electrical injury develop delayed neurologic sequelae?

Yes. In a recent study of 90 patients suffering from electrical trauma, 11 developed late neurologic symptoms, including muscle weakness, sensory deficit, paresthesia, and new pain complaints.

20. What advice should you give to the parents of a child with an electrical injury of the oral commissure?

Electrical burns of the oral commissure in children typically result when the child bites down on a live household electrical cord. Tissue loss ranges from superficial ulceration to full-thickness losses of the lips and cheek. In the second and third weeks after the injury, sloughing of devitalized tissue may be accompanied by bleeding from the labial artery. Parents can control this hemorrhage through finger compression of the commissure. They should be advised of this possibility at the time of injury.

BIBLIOGRAPHY

1. Baxter CR: Present concepts in the management of major electrical injury. Surg Clin North Am 50:1401–1418, 1970.
2. Bernstein T: Electrical injury: Electrical engineer's perspective and an historical review. Ann N Y Acad Sci 720:1–10, 1994.
3. Bradley W, Salam-Adams M: Acute and subacute myopathic paralysis. In Petersdorf R, Adams R, Braunwald E, et al (eds): Harrison's Principles of Internal Medicine, 10th ed. New York, McGraw-Hill, 1983, pp 2184–2187.
4. Council NS: Accident Facts. Itasca, IL, National Safety Council, 1997.
5. Dalziel C: Electric shock hazard. IEEE Spectrum 9:41–50, 1972.
6. DeFranzo A: Injuries from physical and chemical agents. In Georgiade G, Georgiade N, Riefkohl R, Barwick W (eds): Textbook of Plastic, Maxillofacial, and Reconstructive Surgery, 2nd ed. Baltimore, Williams & Wilkins, 1992, pp 253–268.
7. Donelan MB: Reconstruction of electrical burns of the oral commissure with a ventral tongue flap. Plast Reconstr Surg 95:1155–1164, 1995.
8. Fontanarosa PB: Electrical shock and lightning strike. Ann Emerg Med 22:378–387, 1993.
9. Grube BJ, Heimbach DM, Engrav LH, Copass MK: Neurologic consequences of electrical burns. J Trauma 30:254–258, 1990.
10. Hammond J, Ward CG: The use of technetium-99 pyrophosphate scanning in management of high voltage electrical injuries. Am Surg 60:886–888, 1994.
11. Hunt JL, Sato RM, Baxter CR: Acute electric burns: Current diagnostic and therapeutic approaches to management. Arch Surg 115:434–438, 1980.
12. Lee R: Injury by electrical forces: Pathophysiology, manifestations, and therapy. Curr Probl Surg 34:677–765, 1997.
13. Lee RC, Astumian RD: The physiochemical basis for thermal and nonthermal 'burn' injuries. Burns 22:509–519, 1996.
14. Matsen FA III, Winquist RA, Krugmire RB Jr: Diagnosis and management of compartmental syndromes. J Bone Joint Surg 62A:286–291, 1980.
15. Robson M, Smith D: Thermal injuries. In Jurkiewicz M, Krizek T, Mathes S, Ariyan S (eds): Plastic Surgery: Principles and Practice. St. Louis, Mosby, 1990, pp 1392–1397.
16. Rowland S: Fasciotomy: The treatment of compartment syndrome. In Green D (ed): Operative Hand Surgery, 3rd ed. New York, Churchill Livingstone, 1993, pp 661–693.
17. Schwab S: Renal diseases. In Orland M, Saltman R (eds): Manual of Medical Therapeutics, 25th ed. Boston, Little, Brown, 1986, pp 177–195.
18. Tsong TY: Electroporation of cell membranes. Biophys J 60:297–306, 1991.
19. Whitesides T, Hirada H, Morimoto K: Compartment syndromes and the role of fasciotomy: Its parameters and techniques. In AAOS Instructional Course Lectures. St. Louis, Mosby, 1977, pp 179–196.

75. CHEMICAL INJURIES

Shalini Gupta, M.D.

1. What are the major categories of agents that cause chemical injuries?

Chemical injuries can be categorized into four groups: acid burns, alkali burns, phosphorus burns, and chemical injection injuries. Mechanisms of injury and methods of treatment differ among the four groups, although some similarities are present. More than 25,000 products that cause serious chemical injuries are available for use in the home, agriculture, and industry.

2. Which body surfaces are most commonly involved?

Because most injuries are incurred during handling of chemical substances, hand and upper limbs are affected most often. However, splash injuries may involve multiple areas, especially uncovered regions such as the face and lower extremities.

3. How are chemical injuries different from thermal burn injuries?

Chemical burns do not actually "burn" like thermal injuries. Instead, the chemical solution co-agulates the tissue protein, causing necrosis. The major difference between thermal and chemical burns is the length of time of destruction. Thermal burn injuries are momentary, whereas chemical injuries continue to cause damage until the offending agent is entirely removed or neutralized. Furthermore, chemical injuries may result in severe systemic toxicity.

4. What is the mechanism of injury of chemical burns?

Acid burns cause coagulation necrosis, whereas alkalines cause saponification followed by lique-faction necrosis. Alkalines in general penetrate much deeper and carry a greater risk of severe systemic toxicity. Desiccant acids cause exothermic reactions, which result in thermal injuries as well as chemical trauma.

Chemical Agents

AGENT	COMMON USE	CHARACTERISTICS	AGENT TO REMOVE OR DILUTE	SYSTEMIC EFFECTS
Oxidizing agents				
Chromic acid	Metal cleansing	Ulcerates, blisters	Water lavage	
Potassium permanganate	Bleach, deodorizer, disinfectant	Thick, brownish purple eschar	Water lavage, eggwhite solution	
Sodium hypo-chlorite	Bleach, deodorizer, disinfectant	Local irritation, inflammation	Water lavage, milk, eggwhite solution, paste, starch	
Corrosive agents				
Phenol	Deodorant, sanitizer, plastics, dyes, fertilizers, explo-sives, disinfectants	Soft white eschar, brown stain when eschar removed, mild to no pain	Copious water lavage, polyethylene gly-col solution, vege-table oil	Minor exposure: tachy-cardia, arrhythmias Significant exposure: depression, hypo-thermia, cardiac depression, respira-tory depression
Phosphorus (white)	Explosives, poisons, insecticides, fertilizers	Necrotic with yellow-ish color, garlic odor, glows in dark, pain	Lavage with 1% copper sulfate, cover with castor oil	Nephrotoxic, hepatic necrosis
Sodium metal, lye KOH, NaOH, NH$_4$OH, LiOH, Ba$_2$(OH)$_3$, Ca(OH)$_3$	Cleaning agent (washing powder, drain cleaner, paint remover), cement	Soft, gelatinous, brown eschar	Sodium metal: oil im-mersion Lye: water lavage	
Protoplasmic poisons				
Salt formers (acids) Tungstic, picric, sulfasalicylic, tannic, cresylic, acetate, formic, trichloroacetic	Industrial	Thin, hard eschar	Water lavage	Nephrotoxic, hepatic necrosis
Metabolic competitor/ inhibitor Oxalic acid	Industrial	Chalky white ulcers	Large volume calcium salts, copious water lavage, intravenous calcium	Hypocalcemia
Hydrofluoric acid	Industrial	Painful, deep ulcera-tions	Water lavage, subcu-taneous calcium, subcutaneous mag-nesium sulfate	Hypocalcemia, hypomagnesemia

5. What is the first aid treatment for chemical injuries?

First, remove any clothing or other sources of contact with the offending agent. Next, and most importantly, copiously irrigate, irrigate, irrigate. Irrigation should be initiated within minutes of con-tact. The continuous flow of water dissipates any heat of dilution produced by the injury and greatly minimizes the extent of injury. Roughly 1–2 hours of continuous irrigation with low pressure is recommended. Nails, hairs, and web spaces should be carefully inspected. Any evidence of ocular or inhalation injury should be explored. Several chemical injuries also benefit from the use of antidotes. A toxicologist should be contacted immediately. It is notoriously difficult to estimate the extent and depth of chemical burns because the burn process is insidious and ongoing. More often than not, extent of injury is grossly underestimated; hence, aggressive overresuscitation is recommended. Urine output is the single most important guiding parameter.

6. Are there any chemical injuries that should *not* be irrigated with water?

Beware of burns caused by elemental sodium, potassium, or lithium, all of which spontaneously ignite when exposed to water. Such burns should be extinguished with a class-D fire extinguisher. Alternatively, sand can be used to smother the fire. The burn then should be covered with mineral or cooking oil to isolate the metal from water. Irrigation is also contraindicated for phenol burns. Unlike other acid burns, phenol, an organic acid, penetrates more in dilute solution and less in a concentrated solution.

Treatment Measures for Specific Chemical Burns

Irrigation with water

Chromic acid	Sulfosalicylic acid	Dichromate salts
Cantharides	Acetic acid	Tungstic acid
Lyes and alkalis	Cresylic acid	Picric acid
Potassium hydroxide	Potassium permanganate	Tannic acid
Sodium hydroxide	Dimethyl sulfoxide (DMSO)	Trichloroacetic acid
Ammonium hydroxide	Sodium hypochlorite	Formic acid
Barium hydroxide	Phenol	Gasoline
Calcium hydroxide	Hydrofluoric acid	

Calcium salts irrigation and/or injection: hydrofluoric acid

Cover burn with oil: sodium metal, lithium metal, mustard gas

Special measures for certain chemicals
Sodium and lithium metals: pieces must be excised
Hydrofluoric acid: calcium gluconate injection
Phenol: Polyethylene glycol wipe
White phosphorus: copper sulfate irrigation
Alkyl mercury agents: debride and remove blister fluid

7. What are the criteria for admission of patients with chemical burns?
- High-risk factors (concurrent illness)
- Burns of the hand, foot, face, eye, or perineum
- Burns involving more than 15% of total body surface
- Most cases of second- or third-degree burns

8. How are tar and grease best removed?

Tars and commercial greases are derived from long-chain petroleum and coal hydrocarbons (except for the few that contain silicone). Neosporin ointment is the ideal choice for tar and grease removal. Its antibiotic aspect helps to control infection, and its petrolatum base dissolves tar. Petrolatum is an oleaginous colloidal suspension of solid microcrystalline waxes in petroleum oil. It is composed of long-chain aliphatic hydrocarbons and found in most tars and industrial greases. In the emergency department, petroleum jelly has proved similarly effective in removing tars and greases from injured body parts.

9. Describe the nature and appearance of acid burns.

Acid burns are generally quite painful, and the patient may require a considerable amount of sedation. Their appearance may range from erythematous, as in a superficial injury, to a yellow-gray or black eschar with a leather-like appearance in deeper burns.

Sulfuric acid	Green-black to dark brown eschar
Nitric acid	Yellow eschar and tissue staining
Hydrochloric acid	Yellow-brown eschar and tissue staining
Trichloroacetic acid	Whitish, soft tissue slough

10. How are acid burns treated?

Begin with copious and continuous irrigation with water, which is most effective if instituted within the first 10 minutes after injury. A dilute solution of sodium bicarbonate should be used for further irrigation. Following these measures, care is similar to that of thermal burns. Full-thickness injuries need to be excised and skin-grafted.

11. How are hydrofluoric acid burns different? What is the mechanism of injury?

Hydrofluoric acid burns are more like alkaline burns than acid burns. First, as with other acid burns, the high concentration of hydrogen ions in the tissue produces a typical caustic skin injury that alters the skin's normal protective barrier. The second mechanism is more subtle and dangerous. Soluble free fluoride ions penetrate the damaged skin and cause liquefaction necrosis of the soft tissues, decalcification of bone, and local dehydration. This process may continue for hours or days, causing extensive local and systemic injuries if left untreated. Free fluoride ions bind with calcium and magnesium and cause severe depletion of intra- and extracellular stores of calcium and magnesium, leading to disruption of many biochemical processes.

12. Where is hydrofluoric acid found?

Hydrofluoric acid is a highly corrosive, inorganic acid of elemental fluorine that is used in the manufacturing of plastics and semiconductors, pottery glazing, glass etching and frosting, and rust removal. It also is found in several household items, including aluminum brighteners and heavy-duty cleansers. It has been widely in use after the discovery in the late 17th century of its ability to dissolve silica. Injuries result from small holes in gloves and failure to take precautionary measures against the virulence of this benign- and watery-appearing acid.

13. What is the treatment of hydrofluoric acid burns?

Treatment consists of prompt water irrigation, followed by clipping of the fingernails to avoid trapping of acid beneath them, and, finally, inactivation of the fluoride ions. Topical application and massage of a 10% calcium gluconate gel into the involved skin control the pain and progression of less severe injuries. If there is no evidence of injury from the contact, exposed skin may be covered for 24 hours with magnesium oxide topical ointment, which inactivates the fluoride ions. Injection of a 10% calcium gluconate solution into the affected area is also recommended to prevent progression of injury and systemic fluoride poisoning. Usually, multiple injections of 0.1 ml or 0.2 ml are given through a 30-gauge needle without anesthesia. Relief of pain is usually dramatic and is the indicator for further treatment. Intraarterial injection of calcium gluconate is also an important adjunctive treatment. Once an arterial catheter is placed, 10 ml of a 10% calcium gluconate or calcium chloride solution mixed with 40–50 ml of 5% dextrose is infused over 4 hours. Treatment is continued until the patient is pain-free for 4 hours. This method avoids direct injection into painful areas.

14. What are other potential complications of acid injuries?

Oxalic acid and hydrofluoric acid may cause severe hypocalcemia and hypomagnesemia. Liver and/or kidney damage may occur with tannic, formic, and picric acids. Inhalation injuries also may follow exposure to strong acids.

15. Describe the nature and appearance of alkali burns.

Alkali burns appear less dramatic than acid burns but cause deeper injury. The tissue usually appears leathery.

16. Where are alkalis commonly found?

Alkalis are the most common chemicals found in homes. They are the active component in products used for unblocking drains and cleaning ovens and in garden lime, fertilizers, and cement. Cement burns and burns from plaster of Paris used for splints and casts are a risk among health care workers.

17. What is the mechanism of injury of alkali burns?

Alkalis produce less immediate danger than acids but ultimately cause more tissue destruction. Alkali burns initially may appear benign but progress to full-thickness injuries if left untreated. Lye burns initially cause saponification of tissue fats, which results in death of fat cells. Unattached alkali molecules are then free to penetrate and cause further injury. The pH change in the damaged tissue is much greater and more prolonged than in acid injuries.

18. How are alkali burns treated?

Because of the greater change in pH of the damaged tissue, copious water irrigation should be administered for at least 1 hour. After irrigation, partial-thickness injuries are treated with occlusive dressings and periodic observation. Topical mafenide acetate (Sulfamylon) has been recommended not only for its bacteriostatic effect but also because it combines with active lye in the wound to form sodium acetate and innocuous mafenide acetate radicals. The sulfate radicals of gentamicin should be avoided, however, because they produce an exothermic reaction that may cause further damage.

19. What is the composition of cement and the mechanism of its burn injury?

Cement is composed of calcium carbonate, silicon dioxide, aluminum oxide, magnesium carbonate, sulfuric acid, and iron oxide. This alkalotic substance is a common cause of burns in industrialized nations. The most common type of burn is abrasion by prolonged contact and rubbing of the skin with cement. Heat burns occur during the manufacture of cement by contact with hot cement powder. Explosive burns result from explosive discharge of powder from a kiln during manufacture. First-line treatment is copious irrigation with water to remove the corrosive substance. Although the dangers of wet cement are known, irrigation to remove the substance is the recommended action.

Chemical	Source
Hydrofluoric acid	Industrial cleaning, tile etching
Desiccants, sulfuric acid	Food industry, assaults, farming
Corrosives	
Black liquor (mixture of sodium carbonate, sodium hydroxide, sodium sulfate, sodium thiosulfate, and sodium sulfite)	Pulp and paper industry
Potassium hydroxide	Cleaning solutions
Sodium hydroxide	Industrial cleaning, film processing, glue industry, environmental detoxification, home and industrial laundry
Phenol	Industrial cleaning, chemical industry
Aqueous ammonia	Refrigeration (meatpacking)

20. Where is phosphorus found?

Although phosphorus products are common in the military (firearms), they are also found in products such as fireworks, insecticides, rodenticides, and fertilizers. Phosphorus is a waxy, translucent solid that spontaneously ignites on contact with air and is usually preserved in water.

21. What is the mechanism of phosphorus injury?

Phosphorus ignites spontaneously when exposed to air and is rapidly oxidized to phosphorus pentoxide. It is extinguished by water but may reignite upon drying. Particles of phosphorus embedded in skin continue to burn in an exothermic oxidation reaction until the products are removed by debridement, neutralization, or complete oxidation.

22. What is the treatment of phosphorus injuries?

Initial treatment is copious water irrigation, followed by debridement of visible particles. The wound should be washed briefly with 1% copper sulfate to form black cupric phosphide and to facilitate the removal of phosphorus particles. However, copper sulfate is not a form of treatment and should be washed off to prevent copper toxicity after all particles have been removed.

23. What causes chemical injection injuries? Where do they most often occur?

Most chemical injection injuries are caused by the interstitial injection of irritating chemicals or medications due to extravasation during intravenous administration. Therefore, most cases occur in the upper limb between the antecubital fossa and dorsum of the hand.

24. What is the mechanism of injury?

An inflammatory reaction is produced initially and may progress to tissue death, sloughing, and ulceration, depending on the amount, concentration, and toxicity of the injected material. Often the problem is recognized early by discomfort in a communicative patient and results in nothing more than temporary local erythema. However, injection injuries may be so severe as to warrant amputation.

25. What are the major agents in injection injuries and their mechanisms of action?

1. **Osmotically active agents.** Hypertonic solutions containing cations such as calcium and potassium in ionized form cause an osmotic imbalance across the cell membrane, disrupt cellular transport mechanisms, and cause cellular death from intracellular fluid imbibition. Other solutions cause desiccating cell death, including solutions of 30% urea, calcium gluconate, potassium, calcium chloride, Renogafin-60, hypertonic parenteral nutrition, and 10% dextrose.

2. **Ischemia-inducing agents** include catecholamines and vasopressin, which cause injury by local ischemia. Epinephrine, norepinephrine, metaraminol, dopamine, and dobutamine have been reported to cause injury.

3. **Agents with direct cellular toxicity** include vesicant antineoplastic drugs, sodium bicarbonate, sodium thiopental, digoxin, nafcillin, and tetracycline. The mechanical compression caused by extravasation and secondary wound infection compound the problem.

26. What are the clinical features of injection injuries?

Osmotically active and cationic solutions are the most unpredictable in estimating extent of injury and cell death. The presence of epidermal blisters is invariably an indication of full-thickness rather than partial-thickness skin loss. Demarcation of nonviable tissue is usually evident within 1 week of injury.

27. What is the most commonly used antitumor drug? Describe its toxicity.

Doxorubicin is an intercalating antibiotic used in the treatment of breast, prostate, bladder, and lung cancers, lymphomas, and many sarcomas. The clinical result is a painful subcutaneous reaction. The cytotoxic effect is perpetuated by the release of the doxorubicin-DNA complex from dead cells, making it available to viable cells. This local reaction spreads into a progressively enlarging area of ulceration surrounded by a zone of indurated inflammation. Continued use of doxorubicin has been known to increase the rate and extent of tissue necrosis at a site of extravasation or to cause breakdown in a previously healed area. Injury caused by doxorubicin can smolder for 15 weeks before an ulcer develops in the spreading, inflamed, indurated, and painful soft tissue mass created by the extravasation.

CONTROVERSIES

28. How should injection injuries be treated?

1. Documentation of the volume of extravasated chemical is useful in predicting the extent of injury.

2. The intravenous line should be immediately moved. However, some authors believe in leaving the line in place to administer an antidote or to withdraw extravasated solution.

3. Cold should be applied over the extravasation site to cause vasoconstriction and to contain the chemical within the area. Cold may have a direct effect on reducing the toxicity of doxorubicin but has been shown to increase the toxicity of vinca alkaloids. Cold may be applied for 15 minutes 4 times/day for 3 days or more aggressively for 50 minutes of each hour for the first 24–36 hours.

4. Warm application also has been recommended to provide vasodilatation and hence increase fluid absorption and reduce concentration of the extravasated drug. Heat, however, has been consistently shown to enhance the toxicity of doxorubicin.

5. Some antidotes are available. Hyaluronidase destroys tissue cement and thereby reduces injury by allowing rapid diffusion of the irritant fluids. It is advocated for extravasation of solutions of 10% dextrose, calcium, and potassium, aminophylline, nafcillin, radiocontrast media, and total parenteral nutrition. Phentolamine is an alpha blocker used as an antidote for vasopressors. Sodium thiosulfate injected in 1/6 M concentration significantly reduces skin ulcerations caused by nitrogen mustard. Topical dimethyl sulfoxide (DMSO) in 90% alpha tocopheral succinate may be of some benefit after doxorubicin extravasation. Corticosteroids have been the most consistently reported antidote for antitumor drug extravasations. The addition of sodium bicarbonate has been shown to augment their effect.

6. The affected limb should be kept elevated to promote free venous and fluid drainage.

7. The affected area should be left open or covered by a light dressing to allow frequent inspection.

8. A light splint should be made to hold the wrist in 30° dorsiflexion and to permit the fingers to fall into full flexion at the metacarpophalangeal joints, allowing free active and passive movements.

29. What is the role of surgery in injection injuries?
Injuries that heal by conservative means should be allowed to do so. But what about injuries that probably will fail medical treatment? It is important to appreciate the many benefits of early surgical treatment of injuries not likely to heal. Early aggressive surgery is indicated for massive extravasations with any suggestion of arterial compromise, muscle compartment syndrome, or rapidly spreading skin necrosis. In patients with a well-demarcated area of slough, generous debridement should be carried out under antibiotic cover. Some believe that the indication for surgery in antitumor drug extravasation is persistent or increasing local pain 1 week after injury. When doxorubicin ulceration is established, excision must be radical, including a margin of normal skin and subcutaneous tissue and extending to healthy tissue on the deep surface. Involved fascia and tendons may have to be sacrificed. Because doxorubicin is fluorescent, ultraviolet light has been used to identify infiltrated areas. Local muscle flaps and skin grafts may be necessary to protect underlying neurovascular tissue and to provide coverage.

BIBLIOGRAPHY

1. Carototto RC, Peters WJ, Neligan PC, et al: Chemical burns. Can J Surg 39:205–211, 1996.
2. Erdmann D, Hussman J, Kucan JO: Treatment of a severe alkali burn. Burns 22:141–146, 1996.
3. Hansborough JF, Zapata-Sirvent R, Dominic W, et al: Hydrocarbon contact injuries. J Trauma 25:250–252, 1985.
4. Herbert K, Lawrence JC: Chemical burns. Burns 15:381–384, 1989.
5. Klein DG, O'Malley P: Topical injury from chemical agents: Initial treatment. Heart Lung 16:49–54, 1987.
6. MacKinnon MA: Hydrofluoric acid burns. Dermatol Clin 6:67–74, 1988.
7. Moran KD, O'Reilly T, Munster AM: Chemical burns: A ten-year experience. Am J Surg 53:652–653, 1987.
8. Mozingo DW, Smith AA, McManus WF, et al: Chemical burns. J Trauma 28:642–647, 1988.
9. Murray J: Cold, chemical, and irradiation injuries. In McCarthy JG (ed): Plastic Surgery. Philadelphia, W.B. Saunders, 1990, pp 5431–5451.
10. Sawhney CP, Kaushish R: Acid and alkali burns: Considerations in management. Burns 15:132–134, 1989.

76. FROSTBITE

James W. Fletcher, M.D., and Jagruti C. Patel, M.D.

1. What are the three common types of cold injury?
Tissue-freezing injury (frostbite), non–tissue-freezing injury (trenchfoot, chilblain or pernio), and hypothermia.

2. What is frostbite?
Frostbite occurs when the temperature falls to 28° F (–2° C) and tissue freezes, resulting in formation of intracellular ice crystals and microvascular occlusion.

3. What is chilblain (pernio)?
Chilblain refers to skin exposed to chronic high humidity and low temperature without tissue freezing. The core body temperature remains normal. Mountain climbers are typically affected.

4. What is trenchfoot?
Trenchfoot develops when the extremities are exposed to a damp environment over long periods at temperatures of 32–50° F (1–10° C). Heat is lost because the extremity is wet, and vascular flow is poor because of vasoconstriction.

5. What are the symptoms of trenchfoot?
Trenchfoot is characterized by numbness, tingling, pain, and itching. The skin is initially red and edematous, then gradually takes on a gray-blue discoloration. After a few days the foot becomes hyperemic. Within 3–6 weeks the symptoms resolve, but the extremity may still be sensitive to cold.

6. What is cold urticaria?

Cold urticaria is a syndrome consisting of urticaria and angioedema due to exposure to cold temperatures (seen especially with aquatic activities). Anaphylaxis may occur, depending on the severity of the disease. There are two types of urticaria: familial and acquired. History and a cold stimulation test confirm the diagnosis.

7. What predisposing risk factors contribute to frostbite?

- Substance abuse (30–50%), especially alcohol
- Psychiatric illness (10–20%)
- Environmental factors (lack of appropriate clothing and weather conditions)
- Peripheral vascular disease (decreased flow)
- Age (elderly and very young)
- Race (African Americans are at greater risk than whites)
- Medications (e.g., aminophylline, caffeine, fiorinal, ergot alkaloids)

8. How is frostbite classified?

Degree of Injury	Clinical Features	Outcome
First degree	White/yellow plaque, hyperemia, edema; causalgia and pain may indicate nerve damage.	Tissue loss and necrosis are rare.
Second degree	Blisters containing clear or milky fluid; erythema and edema are common.	Characteristic recovery without tissue loss.
Third degree	Deep, full-thickness skin necrosis.	Tissue loss is common.
Fourth degree	Cyanosis, gangrene, and necrosis.	Underlying muscles and bone are affected.

9. What is the pathophysiology of frostbite?

Tissue damage may result from direct cellular damage or the secondary effects of microvascular thrombosis and subsequent ischemia. The recognized changes during freezing are (1) extracellular ice formation, (2) intracellular ice formation, (3) cell dehydration and crenation, (4) abnormal electrolyte concentrations due to above, and (5) perturbations in lipid-protein complexes. With rewarming, ice crystals melt and injured endothelium promotes edema. Epidermal blisters form, and free radical formation continues the insult. Elaboration of inflammatory mediators, prostaglandins, and thromboxanes induces vasoconstriction and platelet aggregation, which worsen ischemia (see figure on facing page.)

10. What vascular changes occur with frostbite?

The vascular endothelium is particularly susceptible. Seventy-two hours after freezing and thawing, the endothelium may be completely obliterated and replaced by fibrin deposition. Investigators also have observed electron microscopic evidence of perivascular fluid extravasation and endothelial swelling and lysis.

11. What immunogenic factors play a role in frostbite?

Neutrophil-endothelial cell adhesion mediated by integrins (CD11a/CD18) and selectins (L, P, and E) plays a germane role in modulating cellular dysfunction in frostbite as well as other disorders of interest to the plastic surgeon (ischemia/reperfusion, hemorrhagic shock, allograft rejection). Factors elaborated from pathways set in motion by the recruited immunocompetent cells, such as thromboxane B_2 and prostaglandins E_2 and $F_{2\alpha}$, have been isolated from frostbite blisters. Evidence also suggests that blockade of the inflammatory cascades may influence outcome.

12. How is frostbite treated?

Rapid rewarming is the cornerstone in the acute management of frostbite. Immersion in water heated to 104–108° F (40–42° C) is the standard of care for all degrees of frostbite. This tight range of temperatures should be strictly followed because the benefit to frozen tissues at lower temperatures is reduced and burn injury may occur at higher temperatures. Parenteral analgesia should be administered as needed for pain. Massage of the area is contraindicated because it may exacerbate the injury. After rapid rewarming the standard protocol to prevent progressive tissue/dermal ischemia includes the following:

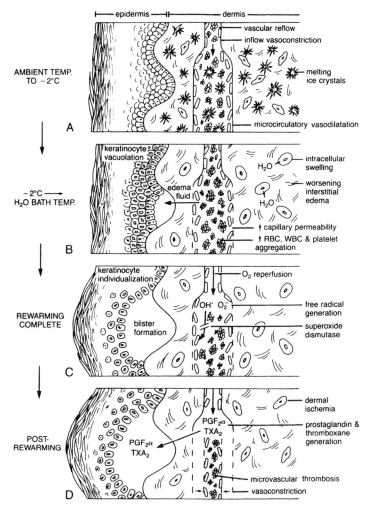

Pathophysiology of frostbite. *A*, As rewarming begins, ice crystals melt. *B*, Injured endothelium promotes edema. *C*, Epidermal blisters and free radicals form. *D*, Inflammatory mediators induce vasoconstriction and platelet aggregation. (Redrawn from Heggers JP, Robson MC, Manavalen K, et al: Experimental and clinical observations on frostbite. Ann Emerg Med 16:1056, 1987.)

- Debride clear blisters.
- Hemorrhagic blisters are left intact and aspirated if infected.
- Elevate affected areas to decrease edema.
- Apply topical thromboxane inhibitor (aloe vera [Dermide]) to injured areas.
- Give systemic antiprostaglandin agent (i.e., aspirin, ibuprofen).
- Give tetanus toxoid prophylaxis when appropriate.
- Whirlpool treatments to decrease the incidence of infection and early mobilization with passive manipulation of injured extremities are advocated when appropriate.

13. What is the role of surgery in the treatment of frostbite?

Reconstruction has no role in the acute phase of frostbite. Attempts to debride aggressively in the early phase of frostbite or amputation may compromise viable tissue. The only indication for early operative intervention is to ameliorate a constricting eschar or to drain a subeschar infection that has failed topical antimicrobials. If tissue injury progresses to gangrene, amputation and/or coverage may be required. Surgery should be delayed until the area is thoroughly demarcated.

14. What other diagnostic modalities are used in determining the extent of frostbite?

Radioisotope vascular and bone imaging, angiography, thermography, and digital plethysmography have been used to assist in making earlier determinations of tissue viability.

15. Is any adjuvant therapy useful in the treatment of frostbite?

1. The use of an intermediate alpha blocker has been advocated as pharmacologic sympathectomy to relieve arteriospasm. Tolazoline HCL and injected reserpine begin to block sympathetic vascular effects in 3–24 hours; their effects may last for 2–4 weeks.

2. Nifedipine in doses of 20–60 mg has been advocated for chilblain to prevent new lesions and to clear present lesions through vasodilatory effects.

3. Free radical scavengers such as dimethyl sulfide, vitamin C, and vitamin E may have potential in treating the reperfusion component of injury. Thrombolytics such as low-molecular-weight dextran, heparin, urokinase, and streptokinase have shown promise in experimental models but require further clinical trials to be considered beneficial.

16. What are the late sequelae of frostbite?

Arthritis is common after frostbite. Pain, hyperasthesias, and cold sensitivity are more infrequent and are seen with more severe cases. Hyperhydrosis and pigment changes may occur as well. Of interest to the hand surgeon is the occurrence of epiphyseal insult in children and subsequent growth deformities.

BIBLIOGRAPHY

1. Blair JR, Schatzki R, Orr ND: Sequelae to cold injury in one hundred patients: Followup study four years after occurrence of cold injury. JAMA 163:1203, 1957.
2. Britt DL, et al: New horizons in management of hypothermia and frostbite injury. Surg Clin North Am 71:345–370, 1991.
3. Brown FE, Spiegel PK, Boyle WE Jr: Digital deformity: An effect of frostbitten children. Pediatrics 71:955, 1983.
4. Demling RH: Cold injury. In Demling RH (ed): Thermal Injury. New York, Scientific American, 1995.
5. Korthuis RJ, Anderson DC, Granger DN: Role of neutrophil-endothelial cell adhesion in inflammatory disorders. J Crit Care 9:47, 1994.
6. McCauley RL, et al: Frostbite: Methods to minimize tissue loss. Postgrad Med 88:67–77, 1990.
7. McCauley RL, et al: Frostbite injuries: A rational approach based on the pathophysiology. J Trauma 23:143, 1983.
8. Porter JM, et al: Intra-arterial sympathetic blockage on the treatment of clinical frostbite. Am J Surg 132:625, 1976.
9. Rustin M, et al: The treatment of chilblains with nifedipine. Br J Dermatol 120:267, 1989.
10. Urschal JD: Frostbite: Predisposing factors and predictors of poor outcome. J Trauma 30:340–342, 1990.

77. METABOLISM AND NUTRITION

Kristine J. Guleserian, M.D., and William G. Cioffi, M.D.

1. What is the hypermetabolic response to burn injury?

The hypermetabolic response to burn injury is characterized by increases in cardiac output, minute ventilation, and core body temperature and a decrease in nitrogen balance. The magnitude of response is directly proportional to burn wound size. In patients with burns > 50% total body surface area (TBSA), the metabolic rate reaches 1.5–2 times the predicted resting energy expenditure.

2. What are the responsible mediators?

Catecholamines are the major mediators of the hypermetabolic response. Catecholamine excretion correlates well with burn size and increased metabolic rate. Increased circulating levels of glucagon and cortisol are also observed with catabolism.

3. Which organ systems are involved?

The systemic pathophysiologic response to burn injury occurs in a biphasic pattern of early hypofunction followed by later hyperfunction. *All* organ systems are affected in this stereotypic manner; however, the magnitude and duration of the response are directly related to the extent of burn.

Biphasic Organ System Response to Burn Injury

ORGAN SYSTEM	EARLY CHANGE (PHASE 1)	LATE CHANGE (PHASE 2)
Cardiovascular	Hypovolemia	Hyperdynamic state
Pulmonary	Hypoventilation	Hyperventilation
Renal	Oliguria	Diuresis
Central nervous	Agitation	Obtundation
Endocrine	Catabolism	Anabolism
Gastrointestinal	Ileus	Hypermotility
Skin	Hypoperfusion	Hyperemia

4. How can the hypermetabolic response be blunted?

With hypermetabolism, heat production is increased and core body temperature rises to a level of maximal comfort and least energy expenditure. Ambient temperatures below thermal neutrality result in catecholamine release and increased metabolic rate. Maintenance of the ambient environment at 88° F to keep the core body temperature at 100.0–100.5° F helps to prevent additional energy expenditure.

5. When does the metabolic rate return to normal?

Once wounds are closed after excision and grafting, the metabolic rate begins to return to baseline. Metabolism does not return to normal until wound remodeling is complete.

6. How is the immune system affected in burn patients?

The cutaneous barrier to invading organisms is the first breakdown of the immune system with burn injury. There is also immediate activation of the complement system, arachidonic acid cascade, and inflammatory cytokine cascade. Circulating levels of immunoglobulins are depressed.

7. What is the goal of nutritional support in burn injury?

Nutritional support should provide adequate calories and protein to match the elevated metabolic needs and nitrogen losses of burn patients and thus prevent the erosion of lean body mass.

8. When should nutritional support be started?

Nutritional support should be instituted as soon as possible.

9. What is the preferred route of administration of nutrition?

Enteral nutrition is the preferred route. It is the safest and most practical means of nutrient provision and is possible in most burn patients. In addition to eliminating the risks associated with central venous catheters, it also helps to maintain gut mucosal integrity and stimulates greater insulin release with subsequent promotion of anabolism. If the oral route of administration is not possible, a naso/oroenteric tube or feeding gastrostomy/jejunostomy tube should be placed.

10. When should parenteral nutrition be considered?

In general, parenteral nutrition should be avoided in burn patients. If adequate nutritional support cannot be provided by the enteral route (e.g., because of severe or prolonged ileus), parenteral nutrition may be used to prevent excessive erosion of lean body mass.

11. What are the complications of parenteral nutrition in burn patients?

The most common and dreaded complication associated with parenteral nutrition is sepsis. Other complications are related to central venous catheter placement, such as pneumothorax, bleeding, thrombosis, foreign body or air embolism, misplacement of catheter, arrhythmias, and local wound infection. Care of central venous catheters must be meticulous to limit complications. Line site changes (every 3–7 days) are necessary to limit catheter-related infection.

12. Who gets an ileus?

Nearly all patients with burns exceeding 20% TBSA develop a paralytic ileus. Narcotic administration, electrolyte derangements, comorbid medical conditions, and older age increase the risk of developing an ileus.

13. How should an ileus be managed?

Paralytic ileus associated with burn injury should be managed with nasogastric decompression to prevent emesis and aspiration. Because ileus is confined to the stomach and colon with normal small bowel function, early enteral feeding can be accomplished with a naso/oroenteric feeding tube. Electrolytes should be replaced and maintained in the normal range.

14. When does an ileus resolve?

Resolution usually occurs between 24 and 72 hours. In severely burned patients an ileus may not resolve until the second week, and parenteral nutrition may need to be implemented.

15. How should nutritional needs be estimated?

The Harris-Benedict equation, specific burn formulas, and nomograms based on body size and age have been used to estimate caloric needs. All are comparable but often overestimate caloric requirements. Indirect calorimetry is the gold standard and should be used in all severe burns (> 40% TBSA). Caloric requirements change as burn wounds are closed and activity level increases; therefore, nutritional support should be adjusted accordingly.

16. What is the optimal calorie-to-nitrogen ratio?

The ideal calorie-to-nitrogen ratio should range between 100:1 and 150:1. Nitrogen losses may be significant, exceeding 40 gm/day.

17. How should you assess the adequacy of nutritional support?

In severely burned patients, nitrogen balance and resting metabolic expenditure should be measured by 24-hour urine collections (for determination of nitrogen balance) and indirect calorimetry at weekly intervals. Daily weights, fluid input/output, and calorie counts should be recorded daily. Measurement of serum visceral protein levels, including prealbumin and retinol-binding protein, is unreliable.

18. What are the consequences of overfeeding?

Overfeeding may lead to lipogenesis, diarrhea, and increased CO_2 production.

19. What nutrients are lost through the burn wound?

All vitamins and micronutrients are lost through burn wounds as well as via urine. Serum levels are invariably low, particularly in burns exceeding 40% TBSA.

20. Should supplemental vitamins and minerals be provided?

Many vitamins and minerals are cofactors for protein metabolism, and deficiencies may result in impaired wound healing from reduced tensile and collagen strength of the burn wound. Guidelines for vitamin and trace element intake after burn injury have no documented basis, and clinical evidence of deficiencies is often obscured by burn wounds. Supplementation of vitamins and micronutrients, particularly 500 mg vitamin C (ascorbic acid), 10,000 IU vitamin A, and 10 mg zinc per day, should be considered in all burn-injured patients.

21. What are the special considerations in children?

Metabolic expenditure is significantly higher in children and must be met with increased nutritional support to prevent permanent growth disturbances.

CONTROVERSIES

22. Does recombinant human growth hormone have a role in burn injury?

Recombinant human growth hormone (rhGH) has been shown to increase protein anabolism and to improve donor site wound healing in severely burned children in a prospective, randomized, double-blinded clinical trial. A dose of 0.2 mg/kg/day resulted in increased protein turnover and protein synthesis and a 2-day decrease in the length of time for split-thickness donor sites to heal.

23. What is the best prophylaxis against stress ulcers?

The resumption of oral intake as soon as possible is the best prophylaxis against stress ulcers. Serious gastrointestinal tract bleeding and gastritis usually can be prevented by maintaining gastric pH > 5. Bacterial overgrowth in an acid-neutralized stomach has been proposed as a risk factor for nosocomial pneumonia; therefore, nonbuffering cytoprotective agents such as prostaglandin E_2 and sucralfate (Carafate) have been proposed for stress ulcer prophylaxis. A randomized study in burn patients, however, showed no difference in the incidence of pneumonia when sucralfate was compared with a regimen of antacids and histamine blockade.

24. Are specialized enteral formulas beneficial?

The use of specialized enteral formulas containing fish oils, glutamine, arginine, fiber, and branched-chain amino acids is of uncertain benefit.

BIBLIOGRAPHY

1. Carlson DE, Cioffi WG, Mason AD, et al: Resting energy expenditure in patients with thermal injury. Surg Gynecol Obstet 174:270–276, 1992.
2. Cioffi WG, McManus AG, Rue LW III, et al: Comparison of acid neutralizing and non-acid neutralizing stress ulcer prophylaxis in thermally injured patients. J Trauma 36:541–547, 1995.
3. Gilpin DA, Barrow RE, Rutan RL, et al: Recombinant human growth hormone accelerates wound healing in children with large cutaneous burns. Ann Surg 220:19–24, 1994.
4. Herndon DN, Barrow RE, Stein M, et al: Increased mortality with intravenous supplemental feeding in severely burned patients. J Burn Care Rehabil 10:309–315, 1989.
5. Herndon DN: Total Burn Care. Philadelphia, W.B. Saunders, 1996.
6. Prelack K, Cunningham JJ, Sheridan RL, Tomkins RG: Energy and protein provisions for thermally injured children revisited: An outcome-based approach for determining requirements. J Burn Care Rehabil 18:177–181, 1997.

78. BURN RECONSTRUCTION

Zahid B. M. Niazi, M.D., F.R.C.S.(Ire), and Jane A. Petro, M.D., F.A.C.S.

1. What are the general principles of rehabilitation?

1. Adequate treatment in the acute injury phase includes preventing infection; timely wound closure; preserving joint mobility, strength, and endurance; promoting independence in self-care; controlling edema; and educating the patient, family, and peers about burn recovery.

2. Prepare the patient for resumption of a normal life, including return to school or work, as soon as possible after healing of wounds.

3. Prevent contractures with exercises, splints, and active physical and occupational therapy.

4. Apply early surgical or therapeutic treatment for contractures.

5. Provide psychological support.

These principles apply to both the acute phase of burn care and to the extended period of outpatient recovery.

2. When does burn reconstruction begin?

It begins as soon as the patient is stable and has been adequately resuscitated. Nutritional support is initiated almost immediately. In patients with large burns, lack of nutrition results in poor or delayed healing with associated complications. The initial surgical steps are as follows:

1. Escharotomy of circumferential full-thickness burns.

2. Early tangential excision for deep partial-thickness or nearly full-thickness burns. Thin slices of burned tissues are removed, and the exposed layer is evaluated to determine whether viable tissue has been reached on which a skin graft can be placed. Early tangential excision minimizes the chances of burn wound infection. The risk of infection increases exponentially from day 5 onward. Tangential excision allows preservation of a maximal amount of tissue.

3. Excision to fascia is limited to the deepest burns in which subcutaneous tissue is nonviable. Split-thickness skin grafts on fascia tend to have a poorer functional and cosmetic outcome. Excision to fascia also results in protracted distal edema in the extremities due to resection of lymphatic channels.

3. What is an escharotomy?

Escharotomy means opening the eschar. The eschar is incised in areas with circumferential third-degree/full-thickness burns. Escharotomy most commonly involves burns of the extremities but also may involve the chest, abdomen, or neck. The procedure is painless and can be carried out by the bedside without anesthesia because you are cutting through nonviable tissue. In the extremities an escharotomy improves circulation to the distal part of the limb and prevents compartment syndrome; in the chest region it improves ventilatory excursion. Burns of the neck requiring escharotomy are nearly always associated with inhalation injuries and result from such severe fire exposure that survival is rare.

4. What features obscure signs of arterial insufficiency in circumferentially burned extremities? How should you monitor such patients?

During the initial 48 hours after a burn injury, a circumferentially burned extremity is at risk of vascular compromise. Evaluation of peripheral circulation is hampered by (1) overlying burned tissue that may be hard and unyielding and (2) tissue edema that accumulates under the burned skin, creating the pressure that leads to vascular compromise. The only reliable method of ascertaining vascular status is a Doppler flowmeter. Other techniques, such as measuring compartment pressures, are generally not needed. Physical exam showing circumferential or nearly circumferential burns with firm and unyielding tissue and Doppler evidence of diminished flow are sufficient clinical signs to justify escharotomy. Performing the release early, before lactic acidosis affects the tissues and venous engorgement becomes problematic, helps to preserve tissues and to maintain satisfactory resuscitation.

5. What are the earliest signs of ischemia in a circumferentially burned extremity?

Alert patients may report numbness and tingling. In sedated or unconscious patients the earliest signs are Doppler findings of diminished or absent digital pulses. If the fingers are unburned, pulse oximetry may be useful. In circumferential upper extremity burns, however, unburned fingers are rare, whereas shoes or boots protect the feet and toes when lower extremities are burned.

6. What underlying pathology results in an intrinsic minus hand in a recently burned upper extremity? How should you treat it?

The pathology that results in an intrinsic minus hand is a compartment syndrome of the deep muscles of the hand. This syndrome is treated by making three radial incisions between the metacarpals on the dorsum of the hand and then dissecting down to the muscle compartments and releasing them.

7. Where do you place the incisions for upper limb escharotomies?

Incisions are placed longitudinally along the medial and lateral aspects of the humerus and the radial and ulnar aspects of the forearm and wrist. Digital escharotomies are also placed on the radial and ulnar borders in the mid lateral line.

8. What reconstructive factors must be considered in the acute phase of the burn?

The reconstructive considerations include (1) prevention of further injury or deepening of the burn by maintaining adequate perfusion during resuscitation; (2) early excision by tangential shave/excision and grafting of the deeper burns to promote prompt healing; (3) prevention of contractures by proper physical therapy; (4) exercises and splinting; and (5) attentive management of healed areas to prevent hypertrophic scar formation. In the management of burns of the face and hands, aesthetic units should be considered to obtain the most desirable cosmetic result.

9. When should burn scar treatment be initiated?

In general, surgical planning is reserved for mature scars. Immature scars (healed for less than 6 months) may respond to conservative treatments such as lubrication with oil-based skin lotions, massage, pressure garments, and exercise. If scar tissue warrants replacement (as in the hand or face if a thickened scar causes significant deformity), the surgeon does not need to wait for the scar to mature. Certain principles guide the categorizing of reconstructive procedures:

Urgent procedures cannot be delayed (e.g., an exposed eye, bone, or cartilage).

Essential procedures are performed to restore function

Desirable procedures are performed to restore a more normal appearance.

10. Which anatomic sites take priority in burn wound management?
The hands and face.

11. When was the first recorded treatment of a burn? What was the treatment regimen?
Circumstantial evidence indicates that herbs were valued by Neanderthal man in Iraq as early as 60,000 B.C. In the Ebers papyrus 482, dated 1500 B.C., the burn wound regimen was as follows:

Day 1   Black mud
Day 2   Dung of calf mixed with yeast
Day 3   Dried acacia resin mixed with barley paste, cooked colocynth, and oil
Day 4   Paste of beeswax fat and boiled papyrus with beans
Day 5   Mixture of colocynth, red ochre, leaves, and copper fragments

Of interest, the burned limbs were supported in copper splints, demonstrating that even then physicians were aware of contractures and tried to prevent them.

12. What options are available for temporary wound cover?
(1) Biologic dressings: cadaver grafts, porcine grafts, amniotic membranes. (2) Synthetic skin substitutes: Biobrane, Kaltostat (calcium alginate or seaweed dressing). Eventually these dressings must be replaced with autografts when donor sites become available. Many new products have been marketed for temporary wound coverage. Most claim a reduction in subsequent scar formation and morbidity and improved survival rates.

13. What are the options for permanent wound coverage?
Permanent wound coverage is usually done by split-thickness skin graft (STSG), which may be applied as a sheet graft or a meshed graft. At specific sites, we sometimes apply a full-thickness skin graft (FTSG) (e.g., around the eyes). Rarely do we perform pedicled flaps or free flaps in the acute phase of treatment, but these options may be needed at a later date to address burn scar contractures. The source of autologous split skin grafts is generally the patient's own body. When the burn wound involves a disproportionate percentage of the whole body (> 60% total body surface area), a small section of skin taken from the patient is grown independently into sheets of cultured epithelial cells before being applied as a skin graft. Recent research has developed a nonantigenic cultured epithelium, which is harvested and grown from infant foreskin and soon will be commercially available. Ongoing work has focused on dermal replacement in conjunction with cultured skin that is applied at the time of burn excision and then dermabraded and overgrafted when the cultured skin becomes available.

14. What is the difference between excision to fascia and tangential excision?
Excision to fascia decreases blood loss and is often faster to perform (applicable only to third-degree burns). However, the cosmetic and functional results of skin grafts on fascia are poorer. The use of excision to fascia is confined to cases in which the burn is very deep or very large surface areas are deeply burned. **Tangential excision** and skin grafting, on the other hand, preserve unburned tissue and yield better cosmetic and functional results. Patients have less protracted edema compared with patients who have undergone excision to fascia. Blood loss may be minimized with the use of tourniquets or sequential surgery.

15. What are the late complications of a burn injury?
(1) Pigment changes in the skin (darker or lighter), (2) texture changes (hypoplastic or hyperplastic), (3) sleep deprivation caused by a combination of disturbed circadian rhythms, severe burn scar itching, and posttraumatic stress syndrome, (4) scar contracture resulting in physical deformities, (5) aesthetic concerns, (6) psychological consequences, and (7) heterotopic bone formation.

16. What is the best form of burn reconstruction?
Prevention of the development of excessive scars and scar contractures.

17. What are the general rules of burn reconstruction?

Apply sheet grafts on the hands, face, and neck following aesthetic facial units. Also apply thicker grafts in areas more likely to contract (i.e., perioral and periorbital regions and neck) so that graft contraction is decreased. Thin STSGs contract most, whereas thicker STSGs contract less. FTSGs do not contract. A meshed graft has interstices that take longer to heal, and the cosmetic result is poor. Splints are applied to prevent contractures. An occupational or physical therapist should be involved from the start to maximize mobilization and to prevent contractures while maintaining range of motion. Splints to the hands, neck braces, and extension splints to the elbows, knees, and axilla reduce scar contracture. Devices to maintain the feet in dorsiflexion, whether they are burned or not, are also useful if any length of bedrest is likely. Patients are fitted with Jobst pressure garments as soon as healed deep partial-thickness/deeper grafted or ungrafted burns are stable, thus decreasing scarring. Follow-up should continue until the end of the growth period in children so that growth restrictions can be recognized early and treated. Adults should be followed until the sequelae of burn injury, both functional and emotional, are resolved.

18. What are functional reconstructions?

Reconstructions that restore normal function of a part are referred to as functional reconstructions. The regions most frequently requiring functional reconstruction are (1) head and neck area, (2) axilla, (3) hands and elbows, (4) anterior chest wall in pubescent girls, and (5) joint release of other areas to allow normal range and growth.

19. How can hypertrophic scars be prevented? How can they be treated?

Hypertrophic scars can be prevented or minimized by the following techniques:

1. Early application of pressure on healed or grafted skin. Custom-made garments (called Jobst garments for the company which first manufactured them), with 25–30 mmHg pressure worn 22–24 hours/day, have been used for this purpose. Their use was first popularized by Sally Abston at the Galveston Shriner Children's Burn Center. The one drawback of pressure in a child may be retardation of growth and the need for frequent remeasurements and new garments during periods of rapid growth.

2. The use of silicone sheets or silicone gel

3. The use of Haelan tape (steroid-impregnated tape) or steroid injections

4. Surgical release or excision of a hypertrophic scar and coverage of the area with a skin graft or by local or distant flaps

There is no overnight cure for disabling scars and contracture. They are a frustrating complication for recovering patients. Surgical reconstruction to correct functional impairment is often needed before wound maturation is complete.

20. What is the classic deformity following a hand burn? How is it treated?

The classic deformity of a burned hand is a claw deformity. Normal hand function is limited by pain, sensitivity, and decreased strength and leads to a dysfunctional position. The burn claw develops as a contracting scar pulls the metacarpophalangeal joints into hyperextension, flexing the interphalangeal joints, adducting the thumb, ulnarly rotating the fifth digit, and flattening the longitudinal and transverse arches of the hand. If the contracting scar is unopposed, thickening and contracture of the joint capsule and ligaments, joint subluxation, and shortening and/or adhesions of the tendons may result.

Palmar burn scars may impair function if contracture of the first web space limits thumb and finger abduction and extension. Spheric grip is reduced by scarring of interdigital spaces. Prehension may be limited by scarring that maintains the thumb in extension. The thumb represents 40% of hand function. Contracture of the thumb or thenar web space may restrict function and needs to be released by thick STSGs, FTSGs, Z-plasty, or a combination of local flaps and skin grafts. Postoperative splinting maintains the thumb in extension. Night wear is continued for 6–9 months. When dorsal hand scarring is extensive, complete scar excision and regrafting are a good choice, followed by long-term splinting.

21. How are neck contractures treated?

Scarring and contracture of the neck region may severely limit function, cause alterations of normal posture, and make intubation for surgery difficult. Neck contractures make driving unsafe.

When a burn scar extends toward the face, eating and swallowing may be restricted and facial distortion may develop as the scar pulls down the mouth and perhaps even the lower eyelids. When it extends to the shoulder, axilla, and pectoral region, shoulder motion is affected. Breast tissue can be pulled upward or displaced or may move abnormally with motion.

After the hand, the neck is the most common site affected by contracture. The method chosen for contracture release depends on the severity of scarring and extent of involvement. Excising the scar and regrafting the neck require long-term postoperative care to prevent recurrent contracture. Splitting the scar and adding skin graft are also acceptable. In either case, splints are applied postoperatively to prevent recurrence of neck flexion contracture.

Compression garments may be started 1 week after the postoperative dressing is removed. For scar remodeling of the superior chest, anterior shoulders, and pectoral region, flexible inserts of a silastic elastomer and/or prosthetic foam are used to distribute the pressure of compression jackets. Silicone gel also may be used under the splint and/or garment. Aesthetic units must be considered. The average time for wearing the splint or garment is about 1 year; use may be discontinued when the graft is flat and no longer hyperemic.

22. What surgical procedure was developed to manage severe neck contractures?

The Chinese flap, or radial forearm free flap, was developed by Chinese surgeons to provide a thin vascularized flap to cover the neck area once the scar tissue was excised. Guofan et al. first described its use in 1978.

23. What is microstomia?

Microstomia is a contracture of the mouth, particularly the oral commissure, caused by perioral facial burns. The most common burns resulting in this deformity are electrical burns sustained by toddlers chewing on electric cords. More rarely, deep burns of the face or burns caused by ingesting lye may cause microstomia. The tissue loss from this injury may lead to cosmetic and functional impairment, oral dysfunction with eating, and impaired oral hygiene, dental care, facial expression, and speech. A microstomia prevention appliance (MPA) is commercially available. Patient compliance is fair. Surgical reconstruction of the perioral area with use of an appropriate splint postoperatively is an early priority.

24. Why do axillary contractures need to be treated?

The shoulder is the most mobile joint; scar contracture may restrict functional independence. Upper body dressing, eating, and posture may be affected if significant scarring extends to the trunk; elbow motion may be restricted if it extends down the arm. Preventing axillary contracture is often difficult with deep burns of this region. Regular exercise and range of motion maneuvers are important. The type of surgical procedure depends on the degree of scarring of adjacent skin and involvement of the hair-bearing area of the axilla. The timing of axillary reconstruction remains controversial. The airplane splint is the primary orthosis used after most surgical procedures. Initially, it is worn constantly, then at night for 3–6 months. For band contracture release (e.g., Z-plasty), only 30–45° of shoulder abduction is needed; in such cases an airplane splint is not necessary. Sometimes molds are used with compression. Even continuous passive motion (CPM) may be needed after release of long-term contractures to stretch ligaments and muscles and disrupt adhesions.

25. Why is it important to treat young girls with anterior chest burn scars?

Burn scars of the skin overlying the breasts restrict breast enlargement during puberty, causing significant cosmetic deformity.

26. Why must an ectropion be corrected early?

Contracture by eversion of eyelid skin may result in a pulling away from the globe and prevent adequate closure of the eyelids. The resultant dryness of the cornea leads to ulceration and corneal opacity. Ectropion should be corrected early to prevent corneal damage. Careful attention to the eye in patients with severe facial burns is imperative.

27. What is burn alopecia?

Burn alopecia is baldness of scalp skin caused by deep burns.

28. How is burn alopecia treated?

Initially scalp burns are treated by debridement and STSGs. The hair follicles in the scalp lie beneath the dermis and may be spared even in full-thickness injury. If alopecia develops, the affected area can be excised serially. If a large area is involved, tissue expansion may be used. Areas involving as much as 50% of the scalp can be covered if sufficient undamaged hair-bearing tissue is available.

29. What options are available for treating burn scars?

(1) Revision of scars, (2) Z-plasty, W-plasty, and other local transposition flaps, (3) skin grafts for larger areas of contracture or hypertrophic scars, (4) tissue expansion, and (5) pedicled or free flaps.

CONTROVERSY

30. Which temporary dressing is better: biologic or synthetic?

Both biologic and synthetic dressings are available off the shelf. Synthetic dressings tend to be more expensive than cadaver skin, which is more expensive than pig skin. Synthetic skin limits the use of local creams and solutions, whereas with pig or cadaver skin such treatments can be continued. Cadaver and pig skin result in an immune rejection if they are left in place long enough. Patients rarely develop an allergy to synthetic dressings. Synthetic dressings do not substitute for skin function (evaporative barrier, bacterial and fungal barrier) as effectively as biologic dressings, although newer products may have better properties. The cost, efficacy, and safety of different techniques have not been compared in sufficient clinical trials to prove that one is vastly superior to the other.

BIBLIOGRAPHY

1. Hunt JL, Purdue GF, Pownell PH, Rohrich RJ: Burns: Acute burns, burn surgery, and postburn reconstruction. Sel Read Plast Surg 8:1–37, 1997.
2. Feller I, Grabb WC (eds): Reconstruction and Rehabilitation of the Burned Patient. Dexter, MI, Thomson-Shore, 1979.
3. Grossman JAI: Burns of the upper extremity. Hand Clin 6:163–354, 1990.
4. Salisbury RE: Burn rehabilitation and reconstruction. Clin Plast Surg 19:551–756, 1992.
5. Salisbury RE, Bevin AG (eds): Atlas of Reconstructive Burn Surgery. Philadelphia, W.B. Saunders, 1981.
6. Scarborough J: On medications for burns in classical antiquity. Clin Plast Surg 10:603–611, 1983.

X. Tissue Transplantation

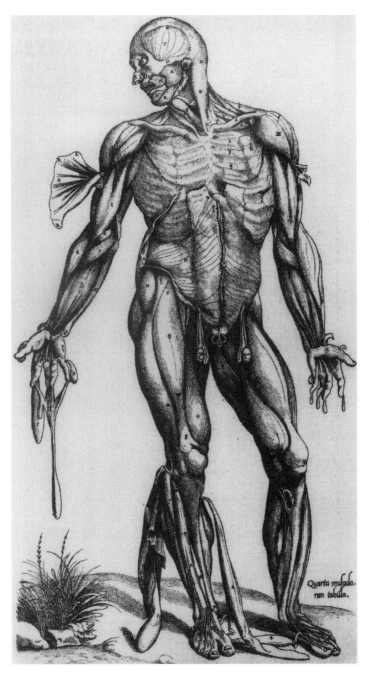

Fourth Muscle Plate
Jan Stefan van Calcar
1543
Woodcut
From Andreas Vesalius
De humani corporis fabrica [Venice, 1543]
© 1998 The Wellcome Institute Library, London

79. PRINCIPLES OF SKIN GRAFTS

Jane H. Kim, M.D., and Kyoung C. Kim, M.D.

1. What are the different types of skin grafts?
Skin grafts can be classified as either split-thickness or full-thickness grafts. Split-thickness grafts consist of the entire epidermis and a portion of the dermis with an average thickness of 0.012–0.015 inches. Full-thickness skin grafts include the entire thickness of the skin, both epidermis and dermis.

Skin grafts are also classified according to their donor sites: autograft = self, allograft = same species, xenograft = different species, isograft = allograft between genetically identical people.

2. Which epithelial appendages are present in the skin? What is their function?
Cells of the developing epidermis in the third month of fetal life invade the dermis and form the hair follicles, sebaceous glands, and sweat glands.

3. How do hair follicles and sebaceous glands affect skin grafts?
In transplanted skin, the growth of hair in an area that should be hairless can be a problem, especially in children. Furthermore, because hairs do not grow vertically but on a slant, incisions should be made obliquely to follow the direction of the hair follicles. On the fourth postgraft day, the original hair shafts are sloughed, and the original follicles begin to produce new hair. Fine hair is present by the 14th postgraft day.

Sebaceous glands, which are appendages of hair follicles, are largest and found in greatest density in the skin of the forehead, nose, and cheeks. They secrete oily sebum, which lubricates the hair and keeps the skin supple.

4. How do sweat glands affect skin grafts?
Apocrine sweat glands tend to be concentrated in the eyelids and axillae, whereas eccrine glands are generally found throughout the body except in the lips and certain parts of the external genitalia. The two types of eccrine glands are those located in the palms of the hand and soles of the feet and those located on the rest of the body surface; the latter function in temperature regulation. Apocrine glands become active at puberty, secrete continuously, and produce an odor due to bacterial decomposition. The sweating pattern of a skin graft will follow that of its recipient site because sweat gland function is directed by sympathetic nerve fibers within the graft bed. Transplanted skin lacks the lubrication supplied by sweat glands because they are temporarily disconnected from their nerve connections. As a result, creams should be applied to grafted skin until the glands are reinnervated.

5. What are the advantages and disadvantages of split-thickness vs. full-thickness grafts?
Split-thickness
    Advantage: take under less favorable conditions
    Disadvantages: shrink considerably; abnormal pigmentation; highly susceptible to trauma
Full-thickness
    Advantages: resist contraction; potential for growth; texture and pigment more similar to
        normal skin
    Disadvantage: require well-vascularized bed

6. What happens to the epithelium in the postgraft period?
Split-thickness skin grafts show a great deal of mitotic activity by the third postgraft day, whereas there is much less mitotic activity in a full-thickness graft. The graft "scales off," and the epithelium doubles in thickness. Increased mitotic activity is accompanied by swelling of the nuclei and cytoplasm of the epithelial cells. In addition, epithelial cell migration toward the surface of the graft contributes to the apparent thickness. Between days 4 and 8, there is rapid turnover of cells and

the epithelium thickness increases up to 7-fold. Desquamation of the epithelium is accompanied by upward migration of follicular epithelium. In fact, not until approximately the end of the fourth week after grafting is epidermal thickness back to normal. Also of note, enzymatic activity progressively decreases in split-thickness grafts over the first few days, but by the fourth day, with host-vessel ingrowth, enzymatic activity increases greatly.

7. Describe the cellular and fibrous components of the dermis.

The source of fibroblasts in a skin graft is still debated. They may be derived from mononuclear cells in the blood or from local perivascular mesenchymal cells. In the first 3 days after grafting, the fibrocyte population decreases. After day 3, fibroblast-like cells appear in the graft and increase in number and enzymatic activity by the 7th and 8th days. Levels return to normal in the following few weeks. The fat of collagen in skin grafts is also debated. Experiments have shown that the collagen persists through 40 days after grafting. Collagen also undergoes replacement, which continues to the 21st day. By the end of the sixth week, all of the old dermal collagen is replaced; the peak occurs in the first 14–21 days after grafting. Also of note, the collagen turnover time is 3–4 times faster than collagen turnover in unwounded skin. Although full-thickness and split-thickness grafts lose the same amount of collagen, a split-thickness graft replaces only half of its original collagen compared with a full-thickness graft. Also included in the fibrous component are elastin fibers, which provide skin resilience. Elastin also has a high turnover rate with continued degeneration through the third week until new fibers emerge at 4–6 weeks after grafting.

8. What is the function of the extracellular matrix (ECM)?

The ECM passively supports the cells and regulates cell-to-cell interaction. The ECM of skin is composed of proteins of both fibroblast and keratinocyte origin. These proteins are involved in directing the communication between keratinocytes and fibroblasts, i.e., in regard to cell proliferation, differentiation, migration, and attachment. For example, fibroblasts within the ECM respond to keratinocytes by producing a basement membrane zone, rich in collagen type IV and laminin. The basement membrane zone then promotes keratinocyte attachment, proliferation, and differentiation.

9. What happens during the healing process of a graft?

Initially the skin graft is white on removal from the donor site. Over the next few days a pink hue develops, and good capillary refill is elicited. By the 14th–21st days, the graft surface, which was originally depressed, becomes level with the surrounding skin. Collagen replacement begins by the 7th day and is nearly complete by the 6th week after grafting. A large number of polymorphonuclear cells and monocytes remain in the dermis for a length of time. Vascularization and remodeling may take many months and result in numerous newly formed vessels with greater arborization than the vessels of normal skin. Finally, by the 5th–6th postgraft days, lymphatic drainage becomes established through the connection of the host and graft lymph channels. As a result, the graft rapidly loses fluid weight until its original pregraft level is reached by the 9th day.

10. How does a skin graft take?

Skin graft take occurs in three phases. During the first 48 hours, the process of **plasmatic imbibition** allows the graft to survive the immediate postgraft period before circulation is established. The imbibition, or diffusion, of exudate from the host bed allows access for nutritive materials and disposal of metabolic waste products. After 48 hours, fine vascular networks form at the interface between the graft and recipient bed. During this period of **inosculation**, anastomotic connections are made between host and graft vessels. Simultaneously, **capillary ingrowth** occurs, during which new vessels grow into the graft from the host bed and actively invade the graft to form its definitive vasculature. How these events actually occur is debated. Some believe that preexisting graft vessels act as nonviable conduits through which the endothelium of the host vessels grow; others believe that new endothelial channels are created.

11. What are the three most common causes of autologous skin graft failure?

The most common cause of autologous skin graft failure is hematoma. The clot inhibits direct contact of the graft with the endothelial buds of the recipient bed so that revascularization cannot occur. The second most common cause of graft loss is infection, which can be avoided by carefully preparing the wound bed. Fluid beneath the graft also may cause graft necrosis. A light pressure dressing minimizes the risk of fluid accumulations. Shear force also prevents graft take, and care should be taken to immobilize the grafted area. Properties of the skin graft itself can determine its survival. For example, grafts taken from a highly vascularized donor site predictably heal better than grafts from a less vascular site.

12. What sensory changes occur as a graft becomes reinnervated?

Graft sensation is regained as nerves grow into the graft. Skin grafts are initially hyperalgesic and slowly regain normal sensation. Sensory recovery begins at around 4–5 weeks and is completed by 12–24 months. Studies show that pain, light touch, and temperature return in that order. Patients need to be warned of thermal insensitivity to avoid injury.

13. What are the choices for donor sites?

Split-thickness skin grafts can be taken from any area of the body. However, because harvesting leaves a scar, scar visibility as well as color match should be considered in choosing a donor site. Split-thickness grafts for the face should be harvested from the "blush" zone, such as the supraclavicular area and scalp. Skin grafts for the extremity and trunk are harvested from the upper thighs and buttocks.

Full-thickness skin grafts are usually harvested where the skin is thin: upper eyelid, postauricular area, or supraclavicular region for facial grafts. Other sites used for full-thickness graft harvesting include the hairless groin, dorsum of the foot, distal forearm, antecubital fossa, and prepuce.

14. What is a dermatome?

A dermatome is a cutting instrument used for harvesting split-thickness grafts. Air- or electric-powered dermatomes are usually used in harvesting split-thickness skin grafts. The width of the graft is determined by the width setting on the dermatome; however, thickness can also be judged by the type of bleeding observed at the donor site. Superficial grafts leave behind many small punctate bleeding points; harvesting of deeper grafts leaves fewer bleeding points that bleed more.

15. When are meshed grafts used?

Meshed grafts are useful when insufficient donor skin is available, when a highly convoluted area must be covered, when the recipient bed is less than optimal, or when moderate drainage is anticipated. However, mesh grafts are absolutely not indicated for covering a joint or the back of the hand because of significant contraction or scarring during healing. Graft meshing is usually performed in 1:1.5 or 1:2 ratios.

16. What are the advantages and disadvantages of meshing?

Advantages: (1) covers a larger area, (2) contours easily and adapts to fit an irregular bed, (3) allows blood and exudate to drain freely, and (4) provides increased edges from which reepithelialization occurs.

Disadvantages: (1) leaves much of the wound to be healed by secondary intention, potentially resulting in wound contracture and (2) yields an unaesthetic cobblestone appearance. Leaving a meshed graft unspread enhances some of its advantages and avoids the cobblestone appearance after healing of the interstices.

17. What methods of graft expansion are available besides meshing?

1. **Pinch grafts** are made by breaking up a graft of skin into small pieces to increase the edge area; they are effective in treating chronic venous stasis ulcers, pressure sores, radiodermatitis, and small chronic traumatic wounds.

2. In **relay transplantation** a graft is cut into 3–6-mm strips, which are laid down 5–10 mm apart. After 5–7 days when the epithelial growth is apparent, the original strips are removed and transplanted, leaving the epithelial remnants in place. This process may be repeated a number of times.

3. **Meek island sandwich grafts** involve using a specialized dermatome and prefolded gauzes to expand graft squares from small pieces of split skin graft. The ratio of expansion is reportedly 1:9. This method is useful for coverage of granulating wounds that have poor grafting conditions.

18. Define primary and secondary contraction.

Primary contraction refers to the immediate elastic recoil of the graft as it is cut. As a result, a full-thickness graft loses about 40% of its original area, and a thin split-thickness graft contracts by approximately 10%. In contrast, secondary contraction occurs as the graft wound heals and is clinically more significant. Full-thickness grafts demonstrate minimal secondary contraction, whereas split-thickness grafts demonstrate significant secondary contraction, depending on the amount of the dermis in the graft. The less dermis, the more the graft will contract secondarily.

19. Which cell is responsible for graft contraction?

The interaction between a graft and its bed can be explained in terms of the life cycle of the myofibroblast. Application of a skin graft appears to check the stimulus of a wound to myofibroblast formation, function, or both. Split-thickness grafts cause a rapid decline in the number of myofibroblasts in a given wound; thus, wounds contract less than comparable nongrafted sites. Full-thickness grafts trigger an even faster decrease in the myofibroblast population; thus, wounds show minimal contraction. It is hypothesized that full-thickness skin grafts do not prevent the formation of myofibroblasts but instead speed up completion of their life cycle, thereby reducing wound contraction.

20. Why is proper preparation of the wound bed so important?

Most skin graft failures can be ascribed to factors associated with the recipient sites. Skin graft survival depends on blood supply from the wound bed. Therefore, exposed bone, cartilage, and tendon do not accept graft because they have limited blood supply. However, periosteum, perichondrium, and paratenon are graftable surfaces. In addition, cortical bone can be debrided, allowing vascular granulation tissue to proliferate. Chronic granulation tissue must be resected down to healthier vascular tissue, which appears red and beefy. The bed must be free of pus and necrotic tissue.

21. What is the maximal allowable bacterial load on a recipient bed site?

All granulation tissue contains bacteria, but not all granulation tissue is infected. If there are more than 10^5 organisms per gram of tissue, the graft will not take. The high bacteria count must be reduced with antibiotic and local wound therapy.

22. What is the optimal dressing for a skin graft?

In most cases, a bolus or tie-over dressing is the best dressing for a skin graft. It improves survival rate by promoting adherence of the graft on the wound. On an extremity skin graft, this technique involves a circumferential compression dressing, often with a splint to immobilize a nearby joint.

23. How can the problem with pigment mismatch be addressed?

Pigmentation changes as a graft heals, depending on the area from which it was harvested. Grafts harvested from the thigh, buttocks, and abdomen become darker as they heal. In contrast, skin grafts from the palm lighten. The skin above the clavicle provides the best color match for grafting facial areas.

Regardless of the donor site, split-thickness grafts often develop darker pigmentation than full-thickness grafts from the same site. Sunshine is also thought to play a role in graft pigmentation and should be avoided for 6 months after grafting. Hyperpigmented grafts are best treated by dermabrasion; the best results are achieved when dermabrasion is done after the graft becomes reinnervated.

24. What are the best types of dressings for donor sites?

Commonly used donor site dressings can be categorized into four groups: open, semiopen, semiocclusive, and occlusive. Biologic dressings are also used. The open wound technique is certainly the cheapest. However, it is associated with prolonged healing time and increased pain. Semiopen dressings, which allow egress of fluid and bacteria, include Biobrane and fine mesh gauzes impregnated with scarlet red, Vaseline, or Xeroform. Xeroform is easy to use, inexpensive, and infection-free; it also allows reepithelialization in approximately 10 days. Biobrane is more comfortable for the patient, but is quite expensive and has been associated with an increased number of donor site infections.

Semiocclusive dressings, such as Op-Site and Tegaderm, are bacteria- and liquid-impermeable but permeable to moisture. They promote faster and less painful healing but are more labor-intensive because fluid tends to collect under the dressings and needs to be drained frequently. Occlusive dressings such as Duoderm are oxygen-impermeable. Duoderm enhances the rate of epithelialization and collagen synthesis and reduces the bacteria count by decreasing the pH of the exudate. Furthermore, because it does not adhere to the bed, it does not cause irritation or pain.

25. How many times can a split-thickness graft be harvested from the same site?

A single donor site can be harvested a number of times. However, although the epithelium always regenerates, the dermis does not. This leads to progressive thinning of the dermis after each split-thickness graft harvesting.

26. What is dermal overgrafting?

In dermal overgrafting, a surface epithelium is replaced with a split-thickness skin graft after the epithelium is removed by dermabrasion or sharp dissection. This process is commonly applied to scar tissue that is extensive, hypertrophic, or pigmented. Mature scars have capillary circulation capable of vascularizing an overlying skin graft.

27. When are allografts indicated?

Allografts are highly effective as temporary biologic dressings and function much like autografts. They are especially useful when skin loss exceeds 50% of the total body surface area (TBSA), resulting in insufficient autograft donor sites. However, although allografts will take on the recipient site and even become vascularized, they are rejected in approximately 10 days or later if the patient is immunosuppressed (e.g., patients with extensive burns). To avoid a rejection response, allografts applied as biologic dressings should be changed every 2 or 3 days. One of the risks of allograft use is transmission of the HIV virus.

28. When are xenografts used?

Xenografts also have been used as biologic dressings. The advantages of xenografts are their low cost, availability, easy storage, and easy sterilization. However, unlike allografts, xenografts are rejected quickly before they become vascularized and have the potential to induce a significant inflammatory response, delaying host healing.

29. What is the clinical significance of human amniotic membrane?

Human amniotic membrane can be used as a temporary dressing and is composed of an inner membrane (amnion) and an outer membrane (chorion). These membranes have a mesenchymal surface in addition to their epithelial (amnion) and decidual (chorion) surfaces. They have been effectively used as temporary dressings for leg ulcers, contaminated or infected raw surfaces (e.g., burns, pilonidal cyst sinuses), and coverage of donor sites. Recent use of freeze-dried, gamma-sterilized amniotic membrane has avoided the problem of bacterial and viral contamination from donors.

30. What are the advantages and disadvantages of amniotic membrane dressings?

Advantages
- More effective than human skin in minimizing bacterial count in burn wounds
- Reduce pain and protect raw surfaces until more permanent coverage is available
- Neovascularization does not occur, and the amnion may be removed in 7–10 days as the wound begins to close

Disadvantages
- Unable to promote healing
- Increased hyperemic reactions
- Hypertrophic scarring

31. What is tissue-cultured skin? What are the clinical uses of cultured keratinocytes?

Tissue-cultured skin is composed of human epidermal cells grown in vitro that are stable enough for grafting. The technique of cultivating keratinocytes was introduced by Rheinwald and Green, who successfully cultured a single keratinocyte to produce an epithelial sheet.

Whole skin is enzymatically digested with trypsin to produce a single-cell suspension of keratinocytes that are then grown on a monolayer of lethally-irradiated mouse fibroblasts in a culture flask. Keratinocyte auto- or allografts are now used in the treatment of burns, leg ulcers, ulcers of epidermolysis, degloving injuries, oral mucosal defects, and after excision of giant congenital nevi in children. From a postage stamp-sized section of skin, a 1 × 1 meter sheet of keratinocyte can be cultured in 3–6 weeks. In burn patients, surgeons can apply cadaver allografts to stabilize the patient while cultivating an autograft.

A disadvantage to their use is the presence of hyperkeratosis for relatively long periods. It is postulated that the newly formed epidermis remains in a hyperproliferative state due to the absence of a modulating dermal factor. Of greater importance, a major disadvantage of cultured keratinocytes is the potential risk of malignancy after grafting because keratinocytes are cultured in the presence of mitogens, leading to possible spontaneous transformation. Other hindering factors to the use of cultured keratinocytes are their high expense, fragility, and sensitivity to infection.

32. What are unilaminar and bilaminar skin substitutes?

Skin substitutes act as artificial skin and are designed to be left in place for a long period, unlike temporary dressings. They have unilaminar or bilaminar membranes and are composed of synthetic and/or biologic materials. **Unilaminar membranes** include hydrogels, hydrocolloid dressings, or vapor-permeable membranes. They provide no mechanical protection but effectively debride the wound, decrease bacterial count, and stimulate granulation tissue growth.

Bilaminar skin substitutes include completely synthetic, biologically inert materials, autologous tissue, and collagen-synthetic composite materials:

- Levine devised a totally synthetic bilaminar membrane consisting of an inner layer of nylon fabric (dermis) with an outer layer of polytetrafluoroethylene (PTFE) membrane (epidermis). The membrane attaches to the bed of a wound within 5 days. It allows passage of water vapor, protects the host from infection, and increases patient survival in large surface area burns. Autograft take has proved to be successful after application of the synthetic membrane.
- Autogenous skin substitutes combine allogeneic fibroblasts with collagen, which acts as a neodermis "sponge" onto which a suspension of autologous epidermal cells (cultured keratinocytes) are added. Studies show that they appear to heal like normal skin 8 months after grafting, and hypertrophic scarring has not been found even 1½ years after grafting. The use of allogeneic fibroblasts reduces the time required to produce the skin substitute (4–7 days), whereas it takes at least 1 month to construct a bilaminar membrane with autologous fibroblasts.
- An example of a collagen-synthetic composite material consists of dermis of bovine collagen attached to a Silastic epidermis, which acts to control moisture. When the dermal component (i.e., matrix of collagen and glycosaminoglycans) is placed on a granulating bed, it becomes a synthesized connective-tissue matrix that acts as dermis within 2–3 weeks. Fibroblasts and blood vessels invade this artificial dermis, and the surface is later replaced by meshed split-thickness autograft or cultured keratinocyte sheets.

33. What are the applications of fibrin glue in skin grafting?

Fibrin glue prepared from fibrinogen concentrates is useful as a biologic adhesive. Its hemostatic properties help to reduce blood loss and to secure the graft in place. The results are decreased hematoma formation and decreased motion of the graft, both of which enhance graft survival as well as cosmetic result. Fibrin glue, whether derived from an autologous, single-donor, or multidonor source, does not interfere with the healing process and does not increase the incidence of infections. With the development of autologous preparation technique, the danger associated with multidonor preparations is eliminated.

34. What is an FDFG?

FDFG stands for free dermal-fat graft. FDFGs provide a lasting and effective source of implant material for repair of soft-tissue contour defects and are often used in the reconstruction of defects of the face. In implanting an FDFG, overcorrection of approximately 20–30% is necessary to compensate for graft shrinkage. One of the risks is epithelial cyst formation. However, this risk is acceptably low when adequate deepithelialization of the FDFG is performed.

35. How effective are parental allografts in treating burns in children?

Large burns covering over 50% of TBSA leave insufficient skin for autologous skin graft coverage even after meshing. One way of dealing with this problem is serial autografting and use of cadaver allograft to cover the remaining areas temporarily while awaiting healing of autograft donor sites for reharvesting. Another option is the use of parental allografts intermingled with the autograft. The parental skin persists for a longer time without rejection even in the absence of deliberate immunosuppression. Although the cellular elements of the parental skin do not survive, the parental dermis contributes to the final skin. Other benefits include psychological benefits to the parent, who feels that he or she is contributing to the child's care, and elimination of the risk of HIV transmission with other allografts.

36. What is the role of skin grafting in the treatment of vitiligo?

Stable vitiligo that is refractory to conventional treatment can be effectively treated with a very thin split-thickness skin graft followed by PUVA treatment. However, the success rate depends on the site of the lesion. The forehead yields the most favorable result, whereas the lip, nose, neck, and bony prominences are difficult to treat in this manner.

BIBLIOGRAPHY

1. Fabre J: Epidermal allografts. Immunol Lett 29:161–165, 1991.
2. Hull BE, Finley RK, Miller SF: Coverage of full-thickness burns with bilayered skin equivalents: A preliminary clinical trial. Surgery 107:496–501, 1990.
3. Kelton P: Skin grafts. Sel Read Plast Surg 8:1–23, 1995.
4. McKay I, Woodward K, Wood HA, et al: Reconstruction of human skin from glycerol-preserved allodermis and cultured keratinocyte sheets. Burns 20(Suppl):S19–S22, 1994.
5. Place MJ, Herber SC, Hardesty RA: Basic techniques and principles. In Aston SJ, Beasley RW, Thorne CHM (eds): Grabb and Smith's Plastic Surgery, 5th ed. Philadelphia, Lippincott-Raven, 1997, pp 17–19.
6. Rudolph R, Klein L: Healing processes in skin grafts. Surg Gynecol Obstet 136:641–651, 1973.
7. Rudolph R, Ballantyne DL: Skin grafts. In McCarthy JG (ed): Plastic Surgery. Philadelphia, W.B. Saunders, 1990, pp 221–274.
8. Saltz R, Sierra D, Feldman D, et al: Experimental and clinical applications of fibrin glue. Plast Reconstr Surg 88:1005–1015, 1991.
9. Waikakul S, Chumniprasas K, Setasubun S, Vajaradul Y: Application of freeze-dried amniotic membrane: A control trial at the donor site of split-thickness skin grafting. Bull Hosp Joint Dis Orthop Inst 50:27–33, 1990.

80. PRINCIPLES OF SKIN FLAP SURGERY

Mitchell A. Stotland, M.D., and Carolyn L. Kerrigan, M.D.

1. How do main distributing arteries reach the cutaneous circulation of a flap?

Arteries that perfuse a surgical flap pass into the skin component in one of two fundamental ways:

1. **Musculocutaneous arteries** travel perpendicularly through underlying muscle bellies into the overlying cutaneous circulation of the skin. They are most prevalent in the supply of skin covering the broad, flat muscles of the torso (e.g., latissimus dorsi, rectus abdominis).

2. **Septocutaneous arteries**, arising originally from either segmental or musculocutaneous vessels, pass directly within intermuscular fascial septae to supply the overlying skin. This arrangement is most common between the longer, thinner muscles of the extremities (e.g., radial forearm flap, dorsalis pedis flap).

2. What are the three main characteristics of skin-containing flaps?

Composition, blood supply, and method of movement.

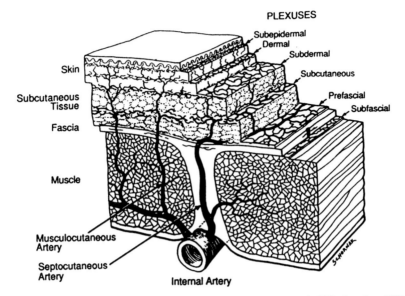

The cutaneous microcirculation. (From McCarthy JG: Plastic Surgery. Philadelphia, W.B. Saunders, 1990, p 282, with permission.)

3. Classify skin-containing flaps in terms of their composition.

Based on which tissues are contained within a flap, one can describe them as cutaneous, fasciocutaneous, myocutaneous, osseocutaneous, or innervated (sensate) cutaneous.

4. Classify skin-containing flaps in terms of their blood supply.

The blood supply of a flap originates from either a musculocutaneous or a septocutaneous artery. The flap is then designed so that the skin is nourished via randomly or axially oriented feeder vessels.

1. **Musculocutaneous artery as main source**
   - **Random flaps:** supplied by one or more musculocutaneous perforating arteries that penetrate the overlying cutaneous circulation specifically at the flap's anatomic base. Their incorporation into the flap base occurs on a random basis.
   - **Axial flaps:** supplied by a named musculocutaneous vessel that is axially oriented within the underlying muscle. By including the muscle in the flap, the overlying skin is supplied by a series of musculocutaneous perforating arteries that exit the muscle and penetrate the overlying cutaneous circulation at multiple points along the course of the flap's axis. With this configuration, the vascular pedicle (i.e., the main musculocutaneous artery) is said to be cantilevered far beyond the flap's anatomic base, providing greater length and reliability.
2. **Septocutaneous artery as main source**
   - **Random flap:** supplied by one or more branches off the septocutaneous system that penetrate the overlying cutaneous circulation specifically at the flap's anatomic base. Their inclusion in the flap base occurs by random selection.
   - **Axial flaps:** supplied by a named septocutaneous vessel that runs longitudinally along the axis of the flap. The vessel may be located deep and incorporated into the flap via a fascial/septal attachment that provides segmental perforators (e.g., radial artery in the forearm flap), or it may be located in a more superficial position free of a fascial association (e.g., superficial circumflex iliac artery in the groin flap).

5. Classify skin-containing flaps in terms of their method of movement.

Flap transfer is commonly described in the following ways:
1. Local transfer: advancement, pivot (rotation), and interpolation (transposition).
2. Distant transfer: direct, tubed, and microvascular.

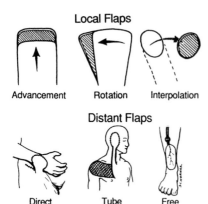

Local Flaps

Advancement   Rotation   Interpolation

Distant Flaps

Direct   Tube   Free

Classification of skin flaps by method of movement. (From McCarthy JG: Plastic Surgery. Philadelphia, W.B. Saunders, 1990, p 277, with permission.)

6. **Classify the following flaps according to their three major characteristics.**
   1. **Limberg flap**
      Composition: cutaneous
      Blood supply: musculocutaneous artery (random)
      Movement: local pivot
   2. **Abbé flap**
      Composition: myocutaneous
      Blood supply: musculocutaneous artery (axial: labial artery)
      Movement: distant direct
   3. **Groin flap**
      Composition: cutaneous
      Blood supply: septocutaneous artery (axial: superficial circumflex iliac artery)
      Movement: distant direct, tubed or microvascular
   4. **Radial forearm flap**
      Composition: fasciocutaneous
      Blood supply: septocutaneous artery (axial: radial artery)
      Movement: local interpolation or distant microvascular
   5. **Cross-finger flap**
      Composition: cutaneous
      Blood supply: septocutaneous artery (random)
      Movement: distant direct
   6. **Forehead flap**
      Composition: myocutaneous
      Blood supply: musculocutaneous artery (axial: supratrochlear with or without supraorbital artery)
      Movement: distant direct or local interpolation
   7. **TRAM flap**
      Composition: myocutaneous
      Blood supply: musculocutaneous artery (axial: superior and/or inferior epigastric artery)
      Movement: local interpolation or distant microvascular

7. **In what year did plastic surgeons successfully introduce free tissue transfer as a reconstructive option? What type of procedure was performed?**
   In 1973 a new era of reconstructive plastic surgery was inaugurated with the publication of a series of reports describing the use of island skin flaps from the abdomen and groin region. These flaps were based variably on the superficial inferior epigastric or superficial circumflex iliac arteries. The initial reports described the use of these flaps for coverage of posttraumatic soft tissue defects of the lower extremity. A subsequent period of widespread experimental and anatomic investigation soon led to an explosion of donor site options and flap compositions for use by the reconstructive surgeon.

8. What is an angiosome? What is its significance in flap design?

Analogous to a sensory dermatome, which is an area of skin innervated by a named sensory nerve, an **angiosome** is a composite block of tissue supplied by the same source artery. The source artery (i.e., a segmental or distributing artery) supplies the skin and underlying structures within the given three-dimensional block of tissue. The entire skin surface of the body, therefore, is perfused by a multitude of angiosome units. Adjacent angiosomes are linked by intervening reduced-caliber vessels referred to as **choke vessels**. In principle, a flap can support one angiosome supplied in a random cutaneous fashion. Moreover, an axial-pattern flap can carry with it an additional angiosome of tissue that is perfused via an intervening choke vessel in a random cutaneous fashion (beyond the domain of the main flap pedicle). Examples include (1) a Bakamjian deltopectoral flap designed with a lateral, random cutaneous extension existing beyond the domain of the medially based intercostal perforating vessels and (2) a TRAM flap incorporating cutaneous extensions lateral to the perforators arising through the underlying rectus abdominis muscle (zones 3 and 4).

9. What is the delay procedure? What is the delay phenomenon?

The **delay procedure** is a preliminary surgical intervention wherein a portion of the vascular supply to a flap is divided before the definitive elevation and transfer of the flap. The resulting benefit, termed the **delay phenomenon**, is that the longitudinal reach of a flap's vascular pedicle is extended, creating a greater flap area due to the survival of a more extended random cutaneous component distally. The mechanism of this phenomenon is somewhat controversial. Explanations include sympathectomy-induced enhancement in vascularity, longitudinal vascular reorientation, vascular enlargement, improved tissue tolerance to hypoxia (metabolic adaptation), and dilatation of choke vessels between vascular territories, allowing capture of adjacent angiosomes.

10. What does the term *critical ischemia time* mean?

Critical ischemia time (CIT) refers to the maximal period of ischemia that a given tissue can withstand and still remain viable after resumption of vascular flow. One may also look at CIT_{50} values, which refer to ischemia time that results in flap necrosis in 50% of cases (analogous to the median lethal dose or LD_{50} of a pharmacologic agent). Critical ischemia is a temperature- and tissue-dependent parameter. Skin grafts can tolerate up to 3 weeks of complete ischemia when stored at 3–4° C. Clinical reports have described the survival of human free flaps and amputated human digits after more than 24 hours of ischemia when they were preserved at hypothermic conditions. Experimental studies in a normothermic skin flap model have shown a CIT_{50} of 9 hours. Muscle, because of its metabolic requirements, is relatively more sensitive than skin to the stress of ischemia. Other metabolically demanding organs (e.g., brain, heart, kidney) are even more vulnerable to the stress of hypoxia and energy depletion, as reflected by much shorter CIT_{50} values.

11. What is primary vs. secondary ischemia?

In microsurgery, the term **primary ischemia** refers to the obligatory interval between pedicle division at the donor site and removal of the vascular clamps after microanastomosis at the recipient site. **Secondary ischemia** occurs postoperatively when the flap pedicle is compromised by either extrinsic or anastomotic obstruction.

12. What does the term *ischemia-reperfusion injury* mean?

Ischemia-reperfusion injury refers to the finding that postischemic reestablishment of vascular perfusion may result in tissue damage above and beyond that directly resulting from the ischemia itself. The distinction between ischemic injury and reperfusion injury has been characterized as **cellular death of attrition** vs. **cellular death by bombardment**. Ischemia results in a death of attrition through processes such as oxygen deprivation, adenosine triphosphate/energy depletion, calcium depletion, and cell membrane dysfunction. Reperfusion results in death by bombardment through processes such as neutrophil respiratory burst with free radical formation; upregulation of cell adhesion molecules, which results in neutrophil diapedesis and degranulation; and leukocyte, platelet, and endothelial cell release of peptide and lipid proinflammatory mediators. Therefore, the experimental and clinical approaches to improving flap survival must consider the implications of both ischemia and reperfusion.

13. What mechanisms may lead to the failure of a pedicled flap? A free flap?

Tissue loss after the transfer of a **pedicled flap** typically results from distal necrosis. In such a situation, the flap is designed too large for its inherent vascular supply and an associated random cutaneous component exists beyond the flap's zone of perfusion. Alternatively, mechanical trauma, a compressive dressing, or an adjacent hematoma may compromise the flap pedicle and result in more extensive tissue loss. **Free flaps**, in contrast, have classically been described as exhibiting an all-or-none survival pattern. In reality, segmental free flap loss is occasionally seen in distal flap zones that represent random extensions of the axially supplied flap (e.g., zones 3 and 4 in a free TRAM flap). Occurring more commonly than extrinsic, mechanical compromise of the pedicle, intraluminal problems arising directly at the level of the microsurgical anastomosis may lead to vascular thrombosis and complete flap loss.

14. How can one optimize the viability of a pedicled flap?

With the use of pedicled flaps, segmental loss is usually due to distal necrosis. In contrast to the early, vigilant surveillance of free flaps, which allows salvage of anastomotic complications by emergent reexploration, there is little need for the use of sophisticated techniques to monitor pedicled flap viability. Rather, proper flap design based on an adequate knowledge of relevant anatomy and published clinical experience are critical to the prevention of distal flap necrosis. Avoidance of (1) extrinsic pedicle compression, (2) undue tension upon wound closure, and (3) excessive flap dependency, with attendant venous congestion, are essential principles. The delay procedure, based on the rationale provided above, also may be used to improve flap viability or to extend flap area. Intravital dyes (e.g., fluorescein) occasionally are used to help determine the zone of perfusion in a pedicled flap. The management of distal flap necrosis is typically conservative or expectant, involving conventional wound care and possible secondary, delayed revision. Clinical observation alone is generally sufficient to identify the rare instance in which a correctable, mechanical disturbance results in impending, total pedicled flap failure.

15. What methods are used to monitor the viability of a free flap that contains a cutaneous component?

More than 20 years after the clinical introduction of microsurgical free tissue transfer, monitoring of free flap viability remains controversial. All experts agree, however, that flap monitoring is crucial in the early postoperative period because of the possibility of total free flap failure secondary to microanastomotic thrombosis. Early flap reexploration rates, depending on the series, may be upward of 15%, although ultimate free flap success is typically achieved in 95% of cases. These figures clearly indicate a significant chance for free flap salvage if secondary ischemia is promptly detected before the onset of the no-reflow phenomenon.

In general, viability is easier to evaluate in skin-containing free flaps than in flaps containing only muscle, bone, or viscera. Clinical observation of skin color, capillary refill, or postpuncture dermal bleeding is a simple and valuable method of flap assessment. A multitude of more sophisticated methods have been used, including intravenous fluorescein (either conventional bolus technique or via low-dose sequential dermatofluorometry), surface Doppler monitoring, temperature probes, laser Doppler flowmetry, tissue pH readings, pulse oximetry, and direct tissue oxygen measurement (via transcutaneous or implantable PO_2 electrodes). Depending on the particular setting, strong arguments can be made on behalf of some or all of these techniques. Yet in experienced hands, clinical observation of *skin-containing* free flaps remains the most useful and reliable monitoring technique.

BIBLIOGRAPHY

1. Daniel RK, Kerrigan CL: Principles and physiology of skin flap surgery. In McCarthy JG (ed): Plastic Surgery. Philadelphia, W.B. Saunders, 1990, p 275.
2. Daniel RK, Taylor GI: Distant transfer of an island flap by microvascular anastomoses. Plast Reconstr Surg 52:111, 1973.
3. Jones NF: Intraoperative and postoperative monitoring of microsurgical free tissue transfers. Clin Plast Surg 19:783, 1992.
4. Kerrigan CL, Stotland MA: Ischemia reperfusion injury: A review. Microsurgery 14:165, 1993.
5. Khouri RK: Avoiding free flap failure. Clin Plast Surg 19:773, 1992.
6. O'Brien BM, Macleod AM, Hayhurst W, Morrison WA: Successful transfer of a large island flap from the groin to the foot by microvascular anastomoses. Plast Reconstr Surg 52:271, 1973.

7. Picard-Ami LA, Thomson JG, Kerrigan CL: Critical ischemia times and survival patterns of experimental pig flaps. Plast Reconstr Surg 86:739, 1990.
8. Stotland MA, Kerrigan CL: Discussion on "Ischemia reperfusion injury in myocutaneous flaps: Role of leukocytes and leukotrienes" by Kirschner RE, Fyfe BS, Hoffman LA, Chiao JC, Davis JM, and Fantini GA. Plast Reconstr Surg 99:6, 1997.

81. PRINCIPLES OF FASCIA AND FASCIOCUTANEOUS FLAPS

Geoffrey G. Hallock, M.D.

1. Define the term fasciocutaneous flap.

According to Tolhurst, any flap that contains fascia with the intent to augment its circulation is a fasciocutaneous flap. Lamberty disagrees with so simplistic a viewpoint, arguing that a specific known "septocutaneous" perforator that discretely supplies the fascia must be included. A broader yet reasonable definition comes from Foad Nahai, who states that fasciocutaneous flaps are skin flaps made more reliable by inclusion of the deep fascia, which usually ensures preservation of the skin circulation.

2. Fascial perforators can be grouped into what two basic types according to their pathway from underlying source vessels?

The chaotic nomenclature for skin flaps uses descriptive terms such as "axial," "random," "direct cutaneous muscle branch," and "septocutaneous" to name vessels that ultimately reach the skin. It can be vastly simplified by considering that skin perforators are either direct or indirect. **Direct** perforators (e.g., axial or septocutaneous) course from the source vessel of a given angiosome to the skin without first supplying some other deep structure. **Indirect** perforators (e.g., musculocutaneous), on the other hand, are minor, terminal branches of vessels that primarily nourish deep structures such as bone or muscle; they have only a secondary role in contributing to skin circulation.

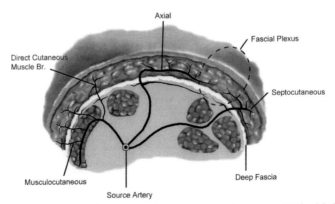

Pathways of the various cutaneous perforators that pierce the deep fascia to supply the fascial plexus. (Courtesy of Carol Varma, Medical Illustrator, The Lehigh Valley Hospital, Allentown, PA.)

BASIC ANATOMY

3. Describe the vascular contributions to the fascial plexus.

The fascial plexus represents the confluence of multiple, adjacent vascular networks and their branches emanating from direct or indirect skin perforators. Intercommunications among these networks exist at the subfascial, fascial, suprafascial, subcutaneous, and subdermal levels.

4. What is the role of the deep fascia in most fasciocutaneous flaps?

Although the deep fascia has an intrinsic microcirculation, for all practical purposes it is avascular. Its real value, when included as part of a fasciocutaneous flap, may be to prevent injury to the more vascular suprafascial portion of the fascial plexus.

5. Can a fasciocutaneous flap be neither fascial nor cutaneous?

Because the deep fascia adds little to the overall circulation of a fasciocutaneous flap, it may be excluded as long as the vasculature within the overlying tissues is kept intact. This vasculature normally is more than enough to ensure viability of what then would be a non-fasciocutaneous flap. The skin as the end-organ of the fascial perforators is actually superfluous and also may be excluded without affecting flap reliability.

6. Describe the composition of the subcutaneous flap and the adipofascial flap.

If both the skin and deep fascia are excluded from a fasciocutaneous flap, the result is a subcutaneous flap. Similarly, retaining the deep fascia without the skin component creates an adipofascial flap. Because a major portion of the fascial plexus remains intact in both, they are simply variants of fasciocutaneous flaps, differing only in their composition.

7. Name the three subtypes of fasciocutaneous flaps using the Cormack-Lamberty and Nahai-Mathes schemas.

Both major classification schemas categorize fasciocutaneous flaps into three subdivisions according to the origin of their fascial perforators.

Cormack-Lamberty Classification of Subtypes:

Type A: Multiple perforators (with no discrete origin; may be a combination of direct or indirect (more common) perforators

Type B: Solitary perforator (single, usually direct, perforator)

Type C: Segmental perforators (multiple, but arising periodically from the same underlying source vessel)

Nahai-Mathes Classification:

Type A: Direct cutaneous perforator (similar to the older term axial)

Type B: Septocutaneous perforator (courses along an intercompartmental or intermuscular septum)

Type C: Musculocutaneous perforator (indirect)

Cormack & Lamberty

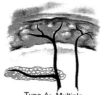
Type A: Multiple

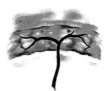
Type B: Solitary

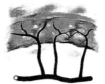
Type C: Segmental

Nahai & Mathes

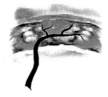
Type A: Direct Cutaneous

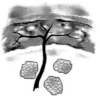
Type B: Septocutaneous

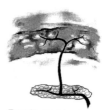
Type C: Musculocutaneous

The two major classification schemas for fascia flaps according to their source of fascial perforators. (Courtesy of Carol Varma, Medical Illustrator, The Lehigh Valley Hospital, Allentown, PA.)

8. Discuss similarities of the subtypes of the Cormack-Lamberty and Nahai-Mathes classification schemas.

Cormack-Lamberty type A has multiple perforators, often including indirect musculocutaneous perforators, and thus resembles Nahai-Mathes type C.

Cormack-Lamberty type B has a single perforator that may go directly to the skin, like Nahai-Mathes type A, as exemplified by the groin flap (superficial circumflex iliac perforator). If the perforator also passes between muscles in a septum, it is equivalent to Nahai-Mathes type B, as exemplified by the inferior cubital artery, which traverses the lateral intermuscular septum before supplying the antecubital forearm flap.

Because segmental perforators usually emanate from a source vessel within an intercompartmental septum (e.g., branches of the posterior radial collateral vessels in the lateral intermuscular septum that supply the lateral arm flap), such Cormack-Lamberty type C flaps are identical to Nahai-Mathes type B flaps.

9. In what body regions do direct fasciocutaneous perforators predominate compared with musculocutaneous perforators?

Because most perforators strictly associated with the fasciocutaneous system arise from intercompartmental or intermuscular septa, they are more prevalent wherever long, slender muscles are found, as in the extremities. In contrast, musculocutaneous perforators are more numerous, arising from the broader and flatter muscles associated with the trunk, where muscular septa are few and far apart.

BASIC PHYSIOLOGY

10. How does the axis determine the proper orientation in designing a fasciocutaneous flap?

The predominant direction of blood flow within a given fascial plexus determines its axis. For the most part the flow is longitudinal in the extremities and somewhat oblique or transverse in the torso. A flap designed or oriented along the direction of this axis maximizes its potential length by encompassing the greatest potential blood supply.

11. Explain the robustness of sensate fasciocutaneous or so-called neurocutaneous flaps.

Suprafascial paraneural vessels, arising either directly from regional source vessels or secondarily from the surrounding fascial plexus, supply not only the given cutaneous nerve but also the skin along the course of the nerve via the formation of "choke" or even true anastomoses between networks of fascial perforators. Thus, the predominant direction of flow or axis follows the course of the nerve. Any flap (skin + nerve = neurocutaneous) oriented along the same course as the nerve probably has the potential to capture the maximal blood flow of any similar flap from that region.

12. What landmarks can be used to determine the appropriate orientation of neurocutaneous flaps in the extremities?

The major superficial venous channels in the extremities serve as the means for outflow from the paraneural plexus and thus tend to parallel the cutaneous nerves. The sural flap (lesser saphenous vein, medial cutaneous sural nerve) and cephalic flap (cephalic vein, lateral antebrachial cutaneous nerve) are two examples in which inclusion of the anatomically obvious vein automatically incorporates the nerve within the flap.

13. What is the arc of rotation of a fasciocutaneous flap?

The distance from the base of the vascular pedicle to the maximal safe length of the flap determines the range of coverage or arc of rotation through which the local fasciocutaneous flap can be transposed.

14. How can the pedicle of each type of fasciocutaneous flap be lengthened to increase its arc of rotation?

Cormack-Lamberty type A. Dissect indirect perforators proximally, usually through muscle. For example, the periumbilical perforator flaps are sustained by and include the deep inferior epigastric vessels, but they are notable for possibly incorporating no portion whatsoever of the rectus abdominis muscle. This technique can be tedious.

Cormack-Lamberty type B. Enter the intercompartmental or intermuscular septum and follow the perforator to its origin from its nonexpendable regional vessel. For example, trace the circumflex scapular artery (scapular flaps) back to the subscapular artery, ending at the latter's origin from the axillary artery.

Cormack-Lamberty type C. Include the entire source vessel with the flap, as is often done with the radial artery of the radial forearm flap, which ends at the bifurcation of the brachial artery.

15. How do you determine the maximal length of a fasciocutaneous flap?

Safe limits, such as length-to-width ratios of 2:1 for the lower extremities, have been determined only by trial and error. There are no set rules because perforators to the fascial system are frequently anomalous not only among individuals but also for opposite sides of the same individual. Whereas a safe or expected range for a local fasciocutaneous flap can be extrapolated from the experience of other surgeons, the maximal arc of rotation remains conjectural.

16. Who was Pontén? What were his superflaps?

Bengt Pontén of Sweden is generally credited with reintroduction of the concept of the fasciocutaneous flap. He found that undelayed, cutaneous flaps in the lower leg, if oriented longitudinally with retention of the deep fascia, have extraordinary viability, even with a 3:1 length-to-width ratio. Historically, only 1:1 flaps (without the fascia) were considered safe. Such flaps were proximally based and sensate; no discrete perforator was identified (i.e., Cormack-Lamberty type A). They may be considered identical to neurocutaneous flaps of the lower extremity, which have a robustness that has proved to be more than just a coincidence.

17. Define a distal-based fasciocutaneous flap.

For muscle flaps, distal-based implies that the vascular pedicle enters the boundary of the flap farthest from the heart or its dominant vascular supply. The former condition is more relevant to fasciocutaneous flaps, because flow in the fascial plexus may be multidirectional. Therefore, distal fascial perforators can be individually selected so that they are just as dominant as a proximal perforator to the same donor territory.

18. Name the primary advantage of a distal-based fasciocutaneous flap.

Proximal skin territories known to be reliable can be transposed on a distal pedicle for potential coverage of acral defects of extremities; otherwise a free flap may be the only acceptable option.

19. Are distal-based flaps and retrograde-flow flaps different?

Sometimes they can be the same. Retrograde-glow flaps usually are distal-based flaps in which both arterial inflow and venous outflow to the proximal skin territory is in a reverse direction from normal. For example, in a distal-based radial forearm flap the radial artery is perfused via the ulnar artery through an intact superficial palmar arch. Yet the distal perforator sustaining a distal-based flap, if appropriately selected, may still have an orthograde pattern of flow; for example, the radial recurrent artery supplying the distal-based lateral arm flap. Suffice it to say that a distal-based flap may be the same as but is not synonymous with a retrograde-flow flap. Furthermore, reverse flow does not necessarily mean retrograde flow.

20. How does venous regurgitation occur in a retrograde-flow flap?

Normally, reversal of venous outflow is obstructed by valves. There are two current hypotheses to explain the clinical observation of venous regurgitation in retrograde-flow flaps despite the valves: (1) the **bypass theory**, which postulates some alternative anatomic structure for venous flow that has no valves, and (2) the **incompetent valve theory**, which suggests that some intrinsic or extrinsic physiologic factor overcomes the normal function of the valve and renders it nonfunctional. The next time you dissect a major limb artery, carefully check the two venae comitantes and note that numerous communicating branches cross over the artery between them. Instead of being a mere nuisance that hinders dissection of that artery, these branches may be an important avenue for circumventing the valves in that segment of veins.

Mechanisms that Allow Reversal of Venous Outflow in Retrograde Perfused Fasciocutaneous Flaps

Bypass via alternative venous pathways
1. Macrovenous (involving the venae comitantes)
   • Interconnecting communicating branches between comitantes
   • Collateral branches that go proximal and distal to the valve to rejoin the same comitante
2. Microvenous (avalvular veins accompanying the venae arteriosae)
3. Avalvular vein segments

Valve incompetency
1. Intrinsic (alterations in valve structure)
   • Structural anomalies preventing cusp contact
   • Intrinsic smooth muscle contractions
2. Extrinsic
   • Intraluminal factors
      Excessive luminal distension
      Overcome by increased proximal/distal pressure gradient
   • Extraluminal factors: external pressures opening the valve

21. How is Allen's test relevant to the Chinese flap?

Because the radial forearm flap initially was developed by the Chinese, it is referred to as the Chinese flap. If the radial artery is included with the flap, the ulnar artery must maintain satisfactory collateral circulation to the hand. Compression of both arteries at the wrist followed by release only of the ulnar artery must demonstrate complete perfusion of the hand (a negative Allen's test). Otherwise, sacrifice of the radial artery is too dangerous.

22. What is the superficial ulnar artery trap?

The superficial ulnar artery trap is an excellent example of potentially disastrous complications due to anomalies that plague the fasciocutaneous system of flaps. Normally, the ulnar artery lies deep within the medial intermuscular septum of the forearm. However, in about 9% of individuals it may lie superficial to the deep fascia; thus, the unsuspected inclusion of all suprafascial structures within a radial forearm flap would totally devascularize the hand.

23. What is the least reliable subtype of fasciocutaneous flaps?

Flaps based on indirect perforators (Cormack-Lamberty type A or Nahai-Mathes type C) are expected to have the least predictable perfusion. All other flap subtypes are more reliable.

APPLIED ANATOMY

24. What is Becker's flap?

The territory of the Becker flap (named after the noted anatomist) corresponds to the dorsal ulnar border of the forearm. Becker described a fairly constant dorsal branch of the ulnar artery that supplies this region. Because its point of piercing the deep fascia is only a few centimeters proximal to the pisiform, it can be used as a distal-based island flap (with orthograde perfusion) by taking the proximal ulnar forearm skin to provide hand coverage without sacrificing the ulnar artery.

25. Why has the groin flap fallen into disfavor?

Although the groin flap is still valuable as a broad-based type B Cormack-Lamberty pedicled fasciocutaneous flap, its use as an island or free flap is hampered by the high frequency of vascular anomalies. The groin flap is an important example of this not-so-uncommon and major problem with the fascia flaps as a group. The groin is nourished medially by both the superficial circumflex iliac (SCIA) and superficial inferior epigastric (SIEA) arteries and laterally by contributions from the deep circumflex iliac artery. Reciprocal relationships in size or variation even in the presence of these vessels is the norm. In 48% of cases, the SIEA and SCIA share a common origin, the common femoral artery. They may be inversely related or equal in diameter, or one may be missing altogether.

26. Name the muscles that define the boundaries of the triangular space.

The teres minor superiorly, the teres major inferiorly, and the long head of the triceps muscle laterally form a potential triangular opening located just superior to the posterior axilla.

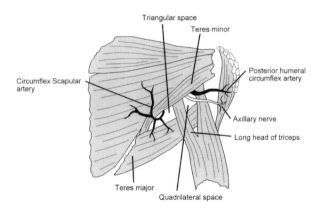

The boundaries of the triangular and quadrilateral spaces. (Courtesy of Carol Varma, Medical Illustrator, The Lehigh Valley Hospital, Allentown, PA.)

27. The anatomic importance of the triangular space is due to what direct fascial perforator that emanates from it?

The largest branch of the subscapular artery usually is the circumflex scapular, which in turn passes through the triangular space and terminates in cutaneous branches that radiate like spokes of a wheel to supply many named upper back fasciocutaneous flaps. Examples include the ascending scapular, scapular (transverse branch), parascapular (descending branch), and inframammary extended circumflex scapular flap (unnamed branch).

28. The dorsal thoracic fascia more commonly is known as the source of what fasciocutaneous flaps?

The upper back fascia is synonymous with the dorsal thoracic fascia and is mainly supplied by the cutaneous branches of the circumflex scapular vessels. Thus, portions of this fascia can be grouped with the better known grouped scapular or parascapular flaps.

29. Name the muscles that define the boundaries of the quadrilateral space.

The long head of the triceps forms the medial side, the teres major the inferior side, and the teres minor the superior border. The humerus defines the lateral side. (See figure above.)

30. What important structures that traverse the quadrilateral space form the neurovascular pedicle to a sensate upper-arm fasciocutaneous flap?

The posterior circumflex humeral vessels and axillary nerve pass through the quadrilateral space. A cutaneous branch of the former and the lateral brachial cutaneous nerve from the latter supply the deltoid flap, which is a potentially sensate flap from the upper outer arm.

31. Perhaps the most notorious liability of the fasciocutaneous flap is potential morbidity of the donor site, especially if a skin graft is needed. How can this risk be minimized?

Any flap variants not incorporating the cutaneous component (such as the subcutaneous, fascial, or adipofascial flaps) leave behind the original skin with its intact subdermal plexus, which can be used to close its own donor site. In patients with local skin redundancy, primary closure may still be possible with fasciocutaneous flaps if the desired flap is small or pretransfer or posttransfer tissue expansion is chosen. Its geometric design may intentionally allow a local flap to close the defect with simultaneous closure of the donor site, such as with a V-Y advancement or a bilobed fasciocutaneous flap.

32. Name several advantages of fascia flaps compared with muscle flaps.

Most importantly, no functioning muscle has to be expended. Fascia flaps are readily accessible because they are near the skin surface; thus, dissection does not usually risk morbidity to important underlying neurovascular structures. If a cutaneous nerve can be incorporated into the design, true sensate flaps can be transferred.

Fascia vs. Muscle Flaps: Advantages and Liabilities

	FASCIOCUTANEOUS	MUSCULOCUTANEOUS
Accessibility	+	–
Compound or composite flaps	=	=
Coverage of the infected or irradiated wound	–	+
Donor site morbidity	–	+
Dynamic transfer	–	+
Expendability	+	–
Malleability	–	+
Potential no. of donor sites	=	=
Reliability	±	+
Sensate	+	–
Size	=	=
Use as free flap	=	=

(+) = asset; (–) = deficiency; (=) = same.

33. Identify the source vessel and classify by subtype these 10 commonly used fascia flaps.

Fascia Flap	*Source Vessel*	*C-L Type*	*N-M Type*
1. Temporoparietal	Superficial temporal	B	A
2. Lateral arm	Posterior radial collateral	C	B
3. Radial forearm	Radial	C	B
4. Ulnar forearm	Ulnar	C	B
5. Groin	Superficial circumflex iliac or inferior epigastric	B	A
6. Saphenous	Descending geniculate	C	A
7. Peroneal*	Peroneal	C	B
8. Scapular parascapular	Circumflex scapular	B	B
9. Posterior interosseous	Posterior interosseous	C	B
10. Gluteal thigh	Inferior gluteal	B	A

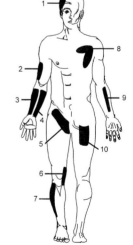

C-L = Cormack-Lamberty schema, N-M = Nahai-Mathes schema.
* Usually raised as part of a composite fibular flap.

BIBLIOGRAPHY

1. Cormack GC, Lamberty BGH: The Arterial Anatomy of Skin Flaps, 2nd ed. Edinburgh, Churchill Livingstone, 1994.
2. del Pinal F, Taylor GI: The deep venous system and reverse flow flaps. Br J Plast Surg 46:652–664, 1993.
3. Elliott LF, French JH Jr, Grotting JC, et al: Flaps: Decision Making in Clinical Practice. New York, Springer, 1997.
4. Hallock GG: Fasciocutaneous Flaps. Boston, Blackwell Scientific, 1992.
5. Hallock GG: Evaluation of fasciocutaneous perforators using color duplex imaging. Plast Reconstr Surg 94:644–651, 1994.
6. Hallock GG: "Microleaps" in the progression of flaps and grafts. Clin Plast Surg 23:117–138, 1996.
7. Hallock GG: Distally based flaps for skin coverage of the foot and ankle. Foot Ankle Int 17:343–348, 1996.

8. Lin SD, Lai CS, Chiu CC: Venous drainage in the reverse forearm flap. Plast Reconstr Surg 74:508–512, 1984.
9. Mathes SJ, Nahai F: Reconstructive Surgery: Principles, Anatomy, and Technique. New York, Churchill Livingstone, 1997.
10. Serafin D: Atlas of Microsurgical Composite Tissue Transplantation. Philadelphia, W.B. Saunders, 1996.
11. Strausch B, Vasconez LO, Findley-Hall EJ: Grabb's Encyclopedia of Flaps. Boston, Little, Brown, 1990.
12. Taylor GI, Caddy CM, Watterson PA, Crock JG: The venous territories (venosomes) of the human body: Experimental study and clinical implications. Plast Reconstr Surg 86:185–213, 1990.
13. Taylor GI, Gianoutsos MP, Morris SF: The neurovascular territories of the skin and muscles: Anatomic study and clinical implications. Plast Reconstr Surg 94:1–36, 1994.

82. PRINCIPLES OF MUSCLE AND MUSCULOCUTANEOUS FLAPS

Geoffrey G. Hallock, M.D.

BASIC ANATOMY

1. When can a muscle be used as a flap?

Any organ with a discrete, intrinsic arteriovenous network can be used as a means for vascularized tissue transfer, and muscle is no different. Of course, the size of the muscle nourished by the desired vascular pedicle must be taken into consideration according to the reconstructive needs; and, as with any tissue used as a vascularized flap, sacrifice of its normal function must be acceptable.

2. Where do the vascular pedicles enter muscles?

The motor nerve(s) of a muscle is always accompanied by a vascular pedicle, which typically is the major source of circulation. However, the reverse is not necessarily true. Virtually every muscle has multiple other vascular sources perhaps serving as collaterals, often at the site of muscle origin or insertion. These may be highly variable, usually overlooked in most anatomy textbooks, and frequently insignificant from a surgical standpoint.

3. Compare the terms dominant, minor, and segmental in reference to the vascular pedicle of a muscle.

The **dominant** pedicle to a muscle usually can sustain the entire muscle when all other collateral sources have been eliminated. A **minor** pedicle can also be of reasonable size, but can maintain only a portion of the given muscle. Previously, the dominant pedicle of a muscle that has other minor pedicles was termed the major pedicle, an important distinction—often the portion of that muscle supplied by the minor pedicle would become precarious when only the major pedicle was left intact. Many muscles have multiple, independent sources of blood supply that each only nourish small portion or segments of the muscle, and hence these have been termed **segmental** pedicles.

4. Based on pedicle type, which muscles are most or least likely to be versatile as muscle flaps?

Muscles with a single, dominant pedicle that can sustain the entirety of a large muscle will be the most useful. Although immediately adjacent segments of a muscle may survive based on their neighbor's segmental pedicle, only a relatively small portion of that muscle could be expected to retain viability if the majority of segmental pedicles were divided. Predictably, these muscles have the most limited role.

5. Why are secondary segmental pedicles important?

In addition to a dominant pedicle, some muscles have a supplemental source of vascularization via an array of pedicles that each independently supply only a segment of the muscle, but if retained as a group can often also sustain the entire muscle if the dominant pedicle were ligated, creating a "reverse" muscle flap that still maintains orthograde flow through the segmental pedicles.

6. Classify muscle flaps according to their mode of innervation.

Taylor has developed a schema to classify muscles according to an increasing complexity of innervation, and concomitant diminished suitability for dynamic muscle transfer:

Type I: Single, unbranched nerve enters muscle
Type II: Single nerve, branches just prior to entering muscle
Type III: Multiple branches from the same nerve trunk
Type IV: Multiple branches from different nerve trunks

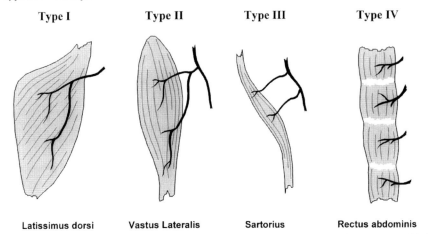

Classification of muscle flaps according to their mode of innervation. (Courtesy of Carol Varma, Medical Illustrator, The Lehigh Valley Hospital, Allentown, PA.)

7. Classify muscle flaps according to their source of vascular supply.

Just as the nerve supply to muscles is highly variable, so is the circulation. The now classic schema of Nahai and Mathes has divided muscles into groups according to their principal means of blood supply:

Type I: Single pedicle
Type II: Dominant pedicle(s), with minor pedicle(s)
Type III: Dual dominant pedicles
Type IV: Segmental pedicles
Type V: Dominant pedicle, with secondary segmental pedicles

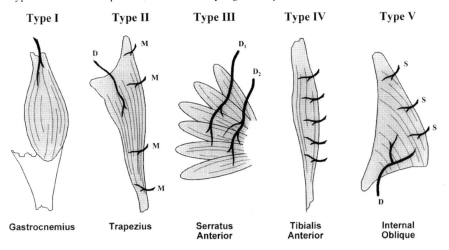

Classification of muscle flaps according to their vascular supply. (Courtesy of Carol Varma, Medical Illustrator, The Lehigh Valley Hospital, Allentown, PA.)

8. Name the most common vascular pattern of muscle flaps.

Most muscles fall into the type II group. When dissected clinically, type I and type III muscles often have anomalous collateral branches (very minor) that probably evolved as a safety feature in case the dominant pedicle were ever disturbed. By definition, this would make both these classes type II muscles as well.

BASIC PHYSIOLOGY

9. According to their vascular pattern, which muscle types would be most or least reliable?

Those with a recognized dominant pedicle would be most reliable, i.e., types I, III, V, as complete muscle viability could be sustained by a single vessel. Sometimes the muscle territory of a minor pedicle is poorly captured by the dominant pedicle in a type II muscle. Due to their segmental means of perfusion, type IV muscles would potentially allow only small flaps that have limited application.

10. Describe the standard arc of rotation of a muscle flap.

When used as a local flap, the range or extent of reach of the muscle when transposed about its point of rotation or dominant vascular pedicle is its standard or usual arc of rotation.

11. What is the arc of rotation of a reverse muscle flap?

If the muscle circulation is based on secondary pedicles instead of the dominant pedicle, and since this array is often on the opposite side of the muscle, a so-called distal–based flap can be elevated with a more distal or reverse area of coverage. The reverse direction of transposition of the muscle would then be restricted by the group of secondary pedicles as the new point of rotation. This should not be confused with a reverse flow flap, such as a latissimus dorsi muscle perfused retrograde via the serratus branch of the thoracodorsal, where the range will be slightly less than the standard arc of rotation as the point of rotation remains virtually unchanged.

12. Explain the concept of function preservation.

If a portion of a muscle is left at its donor site with intact origin, insertion, and innervation, some function will be preserved while the remainder of the muscle is used elsewhere as a flap. This can be achieved by splitting the muscle into segments, each served either by a different dominant pedicle (e.g., hemisoleus) or by individual secondary segmental pedicles (e.g., reverse latissimus dorsi), or if separated at the bifurcation of a major branch of the dominant pedicle to maintain a distinctly separate means of circulation throughout all parts of the muscle.

13. How are arterial territories linked within a muscle flap that has multiple pedicles?

Arterial connections within a given muscle between disparate regions controlled by double dominant pedicles, major or minor pedicles, etc., are via so-called small caliber "choke" arteries that allow bidirectional flow. An important example is the lower transverse rectus abdominis musculocutaneous (TRAM) flap where the superior epigastric pedicle captures the territory of the deep inferior epigastrics via choke anastomoses at the level of the umbilicus.

14. What is the relationship of veins to corresponding arteries in muscles?

Fortunately, a "mirror image" of venous territories paralleling that of the arteries is present. Venous outflow typically is directed toward the major arterial pedicle in the given arterial territory.

15. How are venous territories linked within a given muscle?

Just as arterial territories in a given muscle are linked by bidirectional choke arteries, venous flow from one territory to another can occur through "oscillating" veins which are devoid of valves. Thus in the lower TRAM flap, venous outflow normally directed toward the groin, if regurgitant, can proceed in a reverse direction cephalad across the oscillating veins into the superior epigastric system.

MUSCULOCUTANEOUS FLAP PHYSIOLOGY

16. How are myocutaneous flaps different from musculocutaneous flaps?

Both are composite flaps in which the muscle serves as the vascular carrier of the overlying skin, fat, and fascia. The terms are used interchangeably.

17. By what means does the skin paddle of a musculocutaneous flap normally obtain its blood supply?

Although direct cutaneous branches from the major vascular pedicle of a muscle flap can pass directly to the skin, more typically this nourishment occurs via small terminal branches or musculocutaneous perforators that pass first through the muscle to ultimately supply the skin paddle.

18. Can any configuration of skin attached to a muscle always be expected to survive?

Since musculocutaneous perforators can have random origins, be sparse in number, or spread widely apart throughout a muscle, if none happen to be included within the desired skin paddle it will die. Also, if based distally or far from the dominant pedicle (i.e., on the other side of a series of choke arteries or oscillating veins), although arterial circulation may be adequate, venous outflow could be obstructed by valves leading to necrosis secondary to venous congestion.

19. Name some indirect methods to ensure viability of the skin paddle when raising a musculocutaneous flap.

A. Include as many musculocutaneous perforators as possible:
1. The cutaneous component should be broad–based;
2. Bevel the subcutaneous portion outward from the skin over as wide an area overlying the muscle as possible.

B. Avoid distal skin paddles, especially those distal to the intersection of several territories in a given muscle, as valves can potentially obstruct outflow and cause venous congestion.

20. Can musculocutaneous perforators be identified directly nonoperatively to ensure their inclusion?

Color duplex ultrasound can identify musculocutaneous perforators, from which a map of their location can be created. Not only can their size be calibrated, their directionality and magnitude of flow can also be determined to establish a hierarchy of dominance in that skin territory. An audible Doppler may be more accessible for bedside use, but is more subjective for finding the location and estimating dominance of a given perforator.

21. It has been postulated that the "delay" of a muscle/musculocutaneous flap is achieved through alteration of what venous physiology?

The venous valves in the affected territory after delay maneuvers become regurgitant. For example, division of the deep inferior epigastric vessels 2 weeks prior to elevation of a superior–based lower TRAM flap may ensure greater skin paddle survival, as venograms have shown that the direction of venous outflow is redirected away from the groin unencumbered as the venous valves have become incompetent.

22. Will a transposed muscle flap or musculocutaneous flap undergo neovascularization more rapidly to allow pedicle independence?

Neovascularization or the ingrowth of new vasculature from any recipient site depends on the quality of its bed and tissues at the perimeter. If either is marginal, no neovascularization may occur, and the flap remains permanently dependent on its original pedicle for survival. However, neovascularization at the skin level occurs more rapidly due to the ubiquity of small vessels of the dermal and subdermal plexus, so a musculocutaneous flap would become pedicle-independent more quickly.

23. When compared to fascia flaps, what are some major advantages of muscle flaps?

1. Muscle flaps, perhaps because of superior blood flow rates, are the better choice for wounds compromised by infection or irradiation.
2. Muscle flaps are more malleable and conform better to multidimensional wounds.
3. The vascular anatomy of muscles is generally more reliable because anomalies are less common, which simplifies intraoperative decision making.
4. Dynamic, functioning transfers are possible.

24. While never a problem with a fascia flap, what is the greatest liability of a muscle flap?

In spite of using function preservation techniques, the selection of a muscle flap always sacrifices some function. The given muscle must be expendable; otherwise, it cannot be a flap option.

Attributes and Liabilities of Muscle vs. Fascia Flaps

	FASCIOCUTANEOUS	MUSCULOCUTANEOUS
Accessibility	+	–
Compound or composite flaps	=	=
Coverage of the infected or irradiated wound	–	+
Donor site morbidity	–	+
Dynamic transfer	–	+
Expendability	+	–
Malleability	–	+
Potential number of donor sites	=	=
Reliability	±	±
Sensate	+	–
Size	=	=
Use as a free flap	=	=

(+) = asset, (–) = deficiency, (=) = same.

APPLIED ANATOMY

25. The rectus femoris, vastus lateralis, and tensor fascia lata (TFL) muscles are supplied by which branches of the lateral circumflex femoral artery?

Three-quarters of the time the lateral circumflex femoral artery arises from the profunda femoris, or the femoral artery directly. Its terminal or ascending branch supplies the TFL, and a descending branch goes to the rectus femoris and vastus lateralis muscles, as well as a transverse branch to only the latter.

26. What are the two workhorse muscle flaps of the leg and their corresponding range?

The medial and lateral heads of the gastrocnemius muscle can independently cover the knee and upper third of the leg. The soleus muscle is the muscle of choice for the middle third. Lower third leg and foot defects are often "free flap country," as no large muscle units are available nearby.

27. Which gastrocnemius muscle has the longer reach?

The medial head, because the lateral head must pass around the head of the fibula to reach any proximal leg defect. In addition, the medial head is normally several centimeters longer at its insertion to begin with—check some bare calves to prove this point.

28. What important structures help demarcate the two heads of the gastrocnemius muscle?

Just proximal to their insertion into the Achilles tendon, the two heads of the gastrocnemius muscle may decussate together requiring sharp dissection for their separation. The lesser saphenous vein and median cutaneous sural nerve typically pass in the midline between these two muscle heads, and are important landmarks to preserve.

29. What does the internal oblique muscle have in common with the pectoralis major and latissimus dorsi muscles?

All are type V muscles on the basis of their blood supply. The dominant pedicle to the internal oblique muscle is the ascending branch of the deep circumflex iliac artery, with secondary segmental pedicles from the thoracic and lumbar arteries.

30. For a defect at the given site, provide the local muscle flap of choice for coverage if available.

1. Orbit   _____
2. Upper sternum _____
3. Xiphoid   _____

4. Cervical spine _____
5. Thoracic spine _____
6. Sacrum   _____

7. Perineum _____
8. Hip   _____

Answers: see next page.

31. Name the blood supply and corresponding type of these 10 commonly used muscle flaps.

Muscle Flap	Source Vessel	N-M Type
1. Pectoralis major	Thoracoacromial internal mammary	Type V
2. Rectus abdominis	Superior and deep inferior epigastric	Type III
3. Tensor fascia lata	Lateral circumflex femoral	Type I
4. Rectus femoris	Lateral circumflex femoral	Type II
5. Gracilis	Medial circumflex femoral	Type II
6. Trapezius	Transverse cervical	Type II
7. Latissimus dorsi	Thoracodorsal, lumbar, and posterior intercostal	Type V
8. Gluteus maximus	Superior and inferior gluteal	Type III
9. Gastrocnemius	Sural	Type I
10. Soleus	Popliteal, posterior tibial, peroneal	Type II

Answer to question 30: (1) Temporalis; (2) Pectoralis major; (3) Rectus abdominis; (4) Trapezius; (5) Latissimus dorsi (reverse); (6) Gluteus maximus; (7) Tensor fascia lata; and (8) Gracilis.

BIBLIOGRAPHY

1. Cormack GC, Lamberty BGH: The Arterial Anatomy of Skin Flaps. Edinburgh, Churchill Livingstone, 1994.
2. del Pinal F, Taylor GI: The deep venous system and reverse flow flaps. Br J Plast Surg 46:652–664, 1993.
3. Elliott LF, French JH JR, Grotting JC: Flaps: Decision Making in Clinical Practice. New York, Springer, 1997.
4. Gosain A, Chang N, Mathes S: A study of the relationship between blood flow and bacterial inoculation in musculocutaneous and fasciocutaneous flaps. Plast Reconstr Surg 86:1152–1162, 1990.
5. Hallock GG: Getting the most from the soleus muscle. Ann Plast Surg 36:139–146, 1996.
6. Hallock GG: "Microleaps" in the progression of flaps and grafts. Clin Plast Surg 23:117–138, 1996.
7. Mathes SJ, Nahai F: Reconstructive Surgery: Principles, Anatomy, and Technique. New York, Churchill Livingstone, 1997.
8. McCraw JB, Arnold PG: McCraw and Arnold's Atlas of Muscle and Musculocutaneous Flaps. Norfolk, Virginia, Hampton Press Publishing, 1986.
9. Millican PG, Poole MD: Peripheral neovascularization of muscle and musculocutaneous flaps. Br J Plast Surg 38:369–374, 1985.
10. Serafin D: Atlas of Microsurgical Composite Tissue Transplantion. Philadelphia, W.B. Saunders, 1996.
11. Taylor GI, Caddy CM, Watterson PA, Crock JG: The venous territories (venosomes) of the human body: Experimental study and clinical implications. Plast Reconstr Surg 86:185–213, 1990.
12. Taylor GI, Gianoutsos MP, Morris SF: The neurovascular territories of the skin and muscles: Anatomic study and clinical implications. Plast Reconstr Surg 94:1–36, 1994.
13. Strausch B, Vasconez LO, Findley-Hall EJ: Grabb's Encyclopedia of Flaps, 2nd ed. Boston, Little, Brown, 1998.
14. Watterson PA, Taylor GI, Crock JG: The venous territories of muscles: Anatomical study and clinical implications. Br J Plast Surg 41:569–585, 1988.

83. PRINCIPLES OF MICROVASCULAR FREE TISSUE TRANSFER

Rudolf F. Buntic, M.D., and Harry J. Buncke, M.D.

1. What is a microvascular free tissue transfer?

A microvascular free tissue transfer (also known as a microvascular transplant) involves transplanting expendable donor tissue from one part of the body to another. The tissue must be able to survive on a single-pedicled blood supply with an artery and draining vein. With microsurgical techniques the transplanted part is reanastomosed to recipient site vessels to reestablish blood flow. It is essentially an autotransplant.

2. What are the indications for a microvascular free tissue transfer?

Microsurgical transplants have multiple indications, often to reconstruct complex wounds with complex tissue loss. Common indications include reconstruction after tumor ablation, reconstruction of congenital defects, reconstruction of chronic wounds, and reconstruction after trauma.

3. What are the success rates of microsurgically transplanted tissues?

Tissue survival rates in microvascular free flaps were around 80% in the 1970s and have now improved to over 95%. Survival rates of 98–100% for some transplants is common.

4. Which donor tissue should be chosen?

The choice of donor site in microsurgery requires multiple considerations and planning. Size of the donor tissue, type of wound, pedicle length, and location of wound and donor deformity play a role in selecting the appropriate flap. The size of the donor tissue must adequately cover the wound. Different types of wounds require different donor tissues. Wounds on the hand may require pliable tissues with tendon or even bone to complete the reconstruction. For instance, loss of a thumb is best reconstructed by a toe, whereas osteomyelitis of the tibia is best treated by a muscle transplant. The donor tissue must have a pedicle length that can reach appropriate vessels in the recipient area. Long vascular pedicles may be required if appropriate recipient vessels are not near the wound. The donor deformity also needs to be considered to minimize scarring and potential loss of function.

5. Who should perform microsurgery?

Microsurgical procedures should be performed under the direction of a skilled microsurgeon. Meticulous technique and experience play the greatest role in success. Fine handling and dissecting of small blood vessels should be learned in the laboratory while clinical operative responsibility is gradually increased.

6. What role do anticoagulants play in microsurgery?

The role of routine postoperative anticoagulation in microsurgery has not been determined precisely. In elective microvascular transplants there are no definitive indications for anticoagulation. Surgeon preference plays a role in the choices made. Anticoagulation is believed by some to reduce the chance of postoperative thrombotic complications at the anastomosis site. However, anticoagulation may increase the chance of hematoma at both the donor and recipient sites, and, in rare circumstances, anaphylaxis has been reported with the use of dextran. If postoperative clotting becomes evident and requires reexploration, anticoagulation is usually indicated if the flap is salvaged. The most common pharmacologic agents used in routine postoperative care are aspirin and dextran. Intravenous heparin is generally used when problems such as postoperative thrombosis are encountered. A survey of 73 centers in 22 countries revealed equal success rates for transplants performed with or without anticoagulation.

7. What is the no-reflow phenomenon?

Failure to reperfuse an ischemic organ after reestablishing blood supply is known as the no-reflow phenomenon. The mechanism is believed to be related to endothelial injury, platelet aggregation, and leakage of intravascular fluid. The severity of this effect is correlated with ischemia time.

8. What methods can be used to minimize ischemia?

Generally muscle does not tolerate warm ischemia well for more than 2 hours. Skin and fasciocutaneous flaps can tolerate longer ischemia times (4–6 hours). Meticulous planning is the most important factor to minimize the effects of ischemia because planning decreases ischemia time. All structures in the recipient site should be ready for the flap when the pedicle is divided so that time is not wasted after blood flow to the donor tissue has stopped.

Cooling increases the tolerance of tissue to ischemia. Some surgeons cool the transplant on the operative field with cold wraps and ice. Pharmacologic manipulation of donor tissue has been investigated in the laboratory to prevent formation of free radicals and tissue destruction on reperfusion. Ischemia preconditioning with cyclical clamping and reperfusion of tissues has had laboratory success. These methods are not yet routinely used clinically.

9. Which is more successful—end-to-end or end-to-side arterial anastomosis?

Both end-to-end and end-to-side anastomoses in appropriately selected cases have a similar patency rate in most studies. End-to-side anastomosis may be advantageous in cases with significant vessel size discrepancy or cases in which only one artery is available and required for downstream flow.

10. What is the benefit of coupled anastomoses?

The microvascular coupler is a ring device that allows repair of vessels without hand sewing. Coupled (stapled) anastomoses appear to have patency rates similar to hand-sewn anastomoses when used in appropriate cases. Often, stapled anastomoses can be performed more quickly than those sewn by hand. Staples tend to be easier to use on veins than on arteries because their thinner, more pliable walls make veins simpler to evert around the configuration of the coupler. Vessel size must be precisely matched, and vessel mobilization requirements may be greater for use of the device.

11. How can you tell if a flap is failing?

Clinical evaluation of free flaps postoperatively is crucial to prevent flap loss. Often it is difficult to tell if a flap has a circulatory problem. Flap failure can be divided into arterial insufficiency and venous insufficiency. If there is an arterial circulatory problem the flap usually looks pale and lacks capillary refill. Muscle flaps can be particularly difficult to judge—color change with loss of a beefy red appearance is most common. If venous clot is the cause of flap failure, the flap generally becomes congested and bluish in color. Capillary refill is brisk. Sometimes poking a flap with an 18-gauge needle (away from the pedicle site) helps to judge flap circulation. If there is no bleeding, the problem is inflow. If there is rapid exit of dark red blood, venous congestion is the likely problem.

12. What factors lead to free flap failure?

Failure in microsurgery is most often due to technical factors and poor planning. Technical factors are too numerous to list, but a few examples illustrate their importance. If sutures are tied too loosely, media can be exposed and result in clot. If sutures are tied too tightly on small delicate vessels, they can tear all layers of a vascular repair and distort the intimal surface and result in clot. Too many sutures can lead to increased subendothelial exposure and clot formation.

Other factors leading to flap failure include anastomosis in the zone of injury (poor planning), excessive tension (poor planning), external compression on the pedicle, hematoma formation (which causes compression on the pedicle), and vessel spasm. Twisting of the arterial or venous pedicle leads to clotting at the point where the twist migrates to a fixed branch.

13. How long is it before new endothelium covers the anastomosis site?

After a microvascular repair is performed, a pseudointima is formed within the first 5 days of healing. By 1–2 weeks after repair, new endothelium covers the anastomosis. At the time of repair platelet deposition occurs at sites where intima has been lost or injured. Platelets begin to disappear over the course of 1–3 days, and pseudointima appears. Platelet deposition does not lead to fibrin deposition and thrombosis unless intimal damage is more severe and media are exposed more extensively. Significant damage to vessel walls may result from imprecise and traumatic technique. Traumatic suturing with excessive needle puncture and forceful pull-through of needles without following their natural curvature may damage endothelium.

14. What methods help to relieve spasm?

Topical lidocaine may be used to relieve spasm. The safe topical dose in microsurgery has not been established. Topical papaverine dilates small vessels with a strong local effect. Adventitia can be mechanically stripped, resulting in dilatation of blood vessels and relief of spasm. Hydrostatic dilatation may be used, usually in vein grafts where heparinized saline can be squirted into the vessel under pressure to relieve spasm. Epidural, spinal, or stellate ganglion blocks interrupt the sympathetic fibers near the spinal cord and inhibit sympathetically mediated spasm.

15. What is the order of vessel repair in a free flap? Artery or vein first?

Usually intraoperative anatomic factors come into play. If repair of the artery first will result in poor exposure of the veins, venous repair should be done first. The reverse is also true.

16. Should both arterial and venous repairs be completed before clamps are removed and flow is reestablished?

Some surgeons prefer to perform both arterial and venous repairs before removing the clamps and reestablishing blood flow. Others prefer to repair the artery, release the arterial clamp, and then clamp the vein of the flap before repairing it. The advantage of the latter approach is that inflow is reestablished sooner and ischemia time is minimized. Filling of the vein after this maneuver also helps to judge the excision of redundant vein (a redundant tortuous vein may lead to thrombosis). Some argue that the blood stagnates in the flap and leads to sluggish arterial flow and a higher chance of clot. Usually the flap bleeds through its open edges, however, and flow continues when the vein is clamped. The advantage of repairing both artery and vein before removing the clamp is that blood in the field is minimized and blood does not stagnate in the flap.

17. Does smoking increase the risk of free flap failure?

Numerous studies have shown that wound healing is impaired in smokers. Flap failure does not appear to be increased significantly in smokers; however, wound healing complications at the recipient site appear to be more frequent.

18. Name several choices for skin/fasciocutaneous flap reconstruction.

There are over 33 donor areas from which to choose free flaps, and multiple combinations of flaps are possible. You should consult an atlas of microvascular surgery for a more complete armamentarium. Below is a partial list of the more popular flaps:

- Transverse rectus abdominis myocutaneous flap (TRAM)—most common flap used for microvascular breast reconstruction; based on the deep inferior epigastric vessels.
- Radial forearm—based on the radial artery.
- Scapular, parascapular—based on the circumflex scapular vessel.
- Dorsalis pedis—based on the first dorsal metatarsal artery and dorsalis pedis.
- Lateral arm—posterior radial collateral artery.
- Groin flap—less popular at present, but one of the originals; based on the superficial circumflex iliac artery.
- Bilateral inferior epigastric artery flap (BIEF)—based on the bilateral superficial inferior epigastric arteries.
- Deltoid flap—based on the posterior circumflex humeral artery.
- Superior gluteal flap—rarely used for breast reconstruction now; based on the superficial and deep branches of the superior gluteal vessels.

19. Name several free muscle flaps. Which muscles can be transplanted as functional muscles?

- Rectus—based on the deep inferior epigastric vessels.
- Latissimus—based on the subscapular-thoracodorsal vessels.
- Serratus—based on the subscapular-thoracodorsal vessels.
- Gracilis—branch to gracilis off the medial femoral circumflex artery.
- Extensor brevis—branch to extensor brevis off the dorsalis pedis artery.

The latissimus, serratus, and gracilis muscles are most commonly used as functional transplants; i.e., the nerve is repaired and they are used as a motor. Rectus and extensor brevis also may be used functionally, but this practice is less common.

20. Name several osseous flaps.

- Great toe—based on the first dorsal metatarsal artery.
- Second toe—based on the first dorsal metatarsal artery.
- Rib—a tough dissection; based on the intercostal neurovascular pedicle.
- Fibula—used most often in mandible reconstruction; based on the peroneal vessels.
- Radial forearm—based on the radial vessels.
- Iliac crest—based on the deep circumflex iliac system.
- Scapula—based on the circumflex scapular vessels.
- Calvarium—based on the superficial temporal artery.
- Lateral arm—based on the posterior collateral radial artery.
- Second metatarsal—based on the first dorsal metatarsal artery.

21. Are there any other types of free flaps?

Fascial flaps are less common; the most popular is the temporoparietal fascial flap based on the superficial temporal vessels. Jejunum can be transplanted for esophageal reconstruction, and omentum, one of the first microvascular transplants ever performed, can be used to cover large defects. The main disadvantage of the omentum is the requirement for a laparotomy.

22. Which free flaps are used for facial reanimation?

Gracilis and serratus flaps are most commonly used for reconstruction in facial paralysis. They provide a good vascular pedicle with a suitable single nerve. There is also enough excursion to reconstruct a smile. Their main disadvantage is bulk. The latissimus also may be split into two separate muscle units.

CONTROVERSY

23. Do you need a microscope to perform a free tissue transfer?

Many surgeons believe that increased comfort and magnification make microsurgical repair with a microscope superior to repair performed with loupe magnification. Some authors argue that loupe magnification is cost-effective and portable and results in success rates comparable to those reported with use of the microscope. Loupe magnification up to 6 × is available, whereas the microscope can go from 6–40 ×.

BIBLIOGRAPHY

1. Buncke HJ (ed): Microsurgery: Transplantation-Replantation. An Atlas Text. Philadelphia, Lea & Febiger, 1991.
2. Khouri RK: Avoiding free flap failure. Clin Plast Surg 19:773, 1992.
3. Reus WF, Colen LB, Straker DJ: Tobacco smoking and complications in elective microsurgery. Plast Reconstr Surg 89:490, 1992.
4. Shenaq SM, Klebuc JA, Vargo D: Free tissue transfer with the aid of loupe magnification: Experience with 251 procedures. Plast Reconstr Surg 95:261, 1995.
5. Weinzweig N, Gonzalez M: Free tissue failure is not an all-or-none phenomenon. Plast Reconstr Surg 96:648, 1995.

84. FREE FLAP DONOR SITES

Mahesh H. Mankani, M.D., and Julian J. Pribaz, M.D.

1. What is a composite free flap?

A composite free flap, like a composite graft, is derived from two or more germ layers and contains at least two layers of tissue.

2. What is the quadrangular space? Which structures traverse it?

The quadrangular space is bounded by the teres minor muscle above, the teres major muscle below, the long head of the triceps muscle medially, and the humerus laterally. It is traversed by the posterior circumflex humeral vessels, which perfuse the deltoid free flap.

3. What is the triangular space? Which structures traverse it?

The triangular space lies medial to the quadrangular space and is bounded by the long head of the triceps muscle laterally, the teres minor muscle above, and the teres major muscle below. It is traversed by the circumflex scapular vessels, which perfuse the scapular free flap.

4. Describe the Mathes and Nahai classification of muscle circulation and list examples of muscles used for free transfers from each group.

Type I   One vascular pedicle
Type II   One dominant pedicle and minor pedicles

Type III   Two dominant pedicles
Type IV   Segmental vascular pedicles
Type V   One dominant and secondary vascular pedicles

Type I
- The tensor fascia lata is perfused solely by the transverse branch of the lateral femoral circumflex artery.
- The extensor digitorum brevis is perfused by a branch of the dorsalis pedis artery.

Type II
- The major pedicle of the gracilis muscle is a terminal branch of the medial femoral circumflex artery; one or two minor pedicles from the superficial femoral artery enter the muscle distally.
- The soleus muscle is perfused by branches of the popliteal vessels; the distal 4–5 cm of muscle are perfused by segmental perforating vessels from the posterior tibial artery.

Type III
- The rectus abdominis is perfused by two dominant pedicles. The superior arises from the superior epigastric artery, and the inferior arises from the deep inferior epigastric artery.
- The serratus anterior is perfused by the lateral thoracic artery superiorly and the thoracodorsal artery inferiorly

Type IV—no type IV muscles are appropriate for free tissue transfers.

Type V
- The latissimus dorsi is perfused predominantly by the thoracodorsal artery. The muscle also receives a segmental blood supply medially from branches of the intercostal and lumbar arteries.
- The pectoralis major receives its major blood supply from the thoracoacromial artery. It is also perfused by the lateral thoracic artery, internal mammary artery, and intercostal artery.
- The pectoralis minor is predominantly perfused by the lateral thoracic artery; a direct branch of the axillary artery and the pectoral branch of the thoracoacromial artery provide secondary vascularization.

5. What are the advantages and disadvantages of including a skin paddle with a muscle flap?

Inclusion of the skin paddle with a muscle flap transfer (transfer of a myocutaneous flap) has two major advantages. The skin island serves as a method for monitoring the viability of the flap, and the quality of the skin is often superior to that of a skin graft placed on the muscle. On the other hand, inclusion of the skin paddle may make the flap excessively bulky, an issue of concern in obese patients and recipient sites of limited depth.

6. Which muscles are suitable for facial reanimation because of their size and segmental innervation?

The gracilis and pectoralis minor muscles. The gracilis is innervated by a single motor nerve with multiple fascicles to different portions of the muscle. The pectoralis minor muscle is innervated by the medial and lateral pectoral nerves.

7. Name a reliable donor muscle for coverage of large defects.

The latissimus dorsi muscle provides the largest available transfer, with a size of 25×35 cm^2.

8. Name four muscles that are appropriate for functional free tissue transfers.

Latissimus dorsi	Serratus anterior
Pectoralis minor	Gracilis

9. What are the uses and advantages of the gracilis flap?

The gracilis muscle is a thin, strap-shaped muscle with a consistent pedicle and straightforward harvest; it also allows inclusion of a cutaneous component. Its loss is associated with minimal morbidity. The donor site can be closed primarily with a reasonable appearance. Inclusion of the anterior branch of the obturator nerve provides functionality. The flap can be used for facial reanimation.

10. What portions of the serratus anterior muscle can be safely harvested without risk of inducing winging of the scapula?

To avoid winging of the scapula, it is recommended that the middle and lower 4–5 digitations of the muscle be used.

11. What sensory deficit may result from injudicious harvest of the lateral gastrocnemius muscle?

The common peroneal nerve lies superficial to the lateral head of the gastrocnemius muscle. Traction on the nerve during dissection of the muscle impairs the deep and superficial peroneal nerves. Patients may experience paresis of the dorsiflexor and eversion muscles of the foot and numbness along the dorsum of the foot and in the first web space.

12. What is one of the primary uses of the pectoralis minor flap?

Because of its shape, small size, flatness, and dual nerve supply, the muscle is suited for facial reanimation. In addition, removal of the muscle is not associated with disability or significant scar.

13. List ten sensate cutaneous flaps and their innervation.
   More commonly used flaps
   • Lateral arm flap, innervated by the posterior brachial cutaneous nerve
   • Radial forearm flap, innervated by the medial and lateral antebrachial cutaneous nerves
   • Dorsalis pedis flap, innervated by the deep branch of peroneal nerve in the first web space and
     by the superficial peroneal nerve over the remainder of the flap
   Less commonly used flaps
   • Transverse cervical artery flap, innervated by the supraclavicular nerves
   • Deltoid flap, innervated by a cutaneous branch of the axillary nerve
   • Gluteal thigh flap, innervated by the posterior cutaneous nerve of the thigh
   • Medial thigh flap, innervated by the medial femoral cutaneous nerve
   • Lateral thigh flap, innervated by the lateral femoral cutaneous nerve
   • Saphenous flap, innervated by the medial femoral cutaneous and saphenous nerves
   • Posterior calf flap, innervated by the medial or posterior cutaneous nerves of the thigh and the
     sural nerve

14. What are the advantages of the anterolateral thigh free flap?

The anterolateral thigh free flap is a septofasciocutaneous or musculocutaneous flap perfused by the descending branch of the lateral femoral circumflex artery. Advantages include its long vascular pedicle, its capacity to perform as a flow-through flap, the option for keeping the flap sensate, ease of harvest, the option for simultaneous donor and recipient site dissections, and minimal donor site morbidity.

15. What are the advantages of using the radial forearm flap in reconstruction of the face or hand?

The radial forearm flap is a thin, supple, hairless, and sensate septofasciocutaneous flap that is innervated by the medial cutaneous nerve of the forearm.

16. Under what circumstances can donor site appearance be improved with use of the cutaneous lateral arm flap?

Although the size of the flap can reach 14 × 20 cm, harvest of so large a flap requires closure of the donor site with a skin graft. If the width of the flap is reduced to 6 cm, the donor site can be closed primarily.

17. What are the limitations of one of the earliest free flaps—the groin flap?

The groin flap suffers from variations in vasculature, a small-caliber pedicle, short pedicle length, and difficult harvest.

18. What are two of the most common free bone flaps? What are their advantages and disadvantages?

The vascularized fibula graft and the vascularized iliac crest graft are the two most common free bone flaps. The **free fibular graft** has several distinct advantages, including a length approaching 26 cm, a thick cortex that gives the bone profound structural strength, and minimal donor site morbidity. The flap suffers from a short pedicle and necessary sacrifice of the peroneal artery, which is of particular importance in patients with lower extremity arterial insufficiency. The **iliac crest bone graft** has a long pedicle, a curvature appropriate for mandibular reconstruction, and the possibility for inclusion of overlying muscle and skin with minimal morbidity. However, the mass of transferable bone is limited, the patient is left with a profound contour deformity, and abdominal herniation is a documented consequence of the harvest.

19. With which pedicles can the iliac crest osteocutaneous flap be harvested?

The available pedicles include the superficial circumflex iliac artery (SCIA), deep circumflex iliac artery (DCIA), and dorsal branch of the fourth lumbar artery. The deep branch of the superior gluteal artery typically can supply an osseous flap but is not amenable to creation of an osteocutaneous flap.

20. What morbidity is associated with harvest of the vascularized iliac crest bone graft?

Abdominal herniation remains a significant risk.

21. What are the advantages of using the great toe for thumb reconstruction?

Patient grip strength is greater with use of the great toe than with use of the second toe. Reconstruction involves transfer of two phalanges and a large nail, similar to the thumb. However, use of the great toe impairs the appearance of the foot much more than use of the second toe.

22. What is the most common free fascial flap? What are its advantages and disadvantages?

The free temporoparietal fascia flap, like other fascial flaps, offers thin, nonbulky, supple, and highly vascularized tissue. The flap has been draped over denuded auricular cartilage and has been used to restore a gliding surface for tendon reconstruction in the hand. Particular advantages of the temporoparietal fascia flap include a size up to 14 × 17 cm, an inconspicuous donor site scar, the option for simultaneous donor and recipient site dissections, and the capacity for inclusion of bone from the outer table of the calvarium. Unfortunately, dissection of the flap is tedious, and the harvest is associated with alopecia.

23. Is patient positioning important in deciding on an appropriate donor site?

Extremely important. Some flaps, such as the gracilis muscle, are considered extremely versatile because recipient site preparation and flap harvest can be completed simultaneously. Other flaps, such as the latissimus dorsi muscle, often require patient repositioning between dissection of an anterior recipient site and flap harvest.

BIBLIOGRAPHY

1. Banis J, Abul-Hassan H: Cutaneous free flaps. In Georgiade G, Georgiade N, Riefkohl R, Barwick W (eds): Textbook of Plastic, Maxillofacial, and Reconstructive Surgery, 2nd ed. Baltimore, Williams & Wilkins, 1992, pp 997–1008.
2. Levin L, Pederson W, Barwick W: Free muscle and myocutaneous flaps. In Georgiade G, Georgiade N, Riefkohl R, Barwick W (eds): Textbook of Plastic, Maxillofacial, and Reconstructive Surgery, 2nd ed. Baltimore, Williams & Wilkins, 1992, pp 1009–1020.
3. Manktelow RT, Zuker RM, McKee NH: Functioning free muscle transplantation. J Hand Surg 9A: 32–39, 1984.
4. Mathes SJ, Nahai F: Classification of the vascular anatomy of muscles: Experimental and clinical correlation. Plast Reconstr Surg 67:177–187, 1981.
5. Mathes SJ, Vasconez LO: Myocutaneous free-flap transfer: Anatomical and experimental considerations. Plast Reconstr Surg 62:162–166, 1978.
6. McCraw J, Arnold P: McGraw and Arnold's Atlas of Muscle and Musculocutaneous Flaps. Norfolk, Hampton Press, 1986.
7. Moore K: Clinically Oriented Anatomy, 3rd ed. Baltimore, Williams & Wilkins, 1992.

8. Musgrave R, Lehman J: Composite grafts. In Georgiade G, Georgiade N, Riefkohl R, Barwick W (eds): Textbook of Plastic, Maxillofacial, and Reconstructive Surgery, 2nd ed. Baltimore, Williams & Wilkins, 1992, pp 47–51.

9. Nunley J, Barwick W: Free vascularized bone grafts and osteocutaneous flaps. In Georgiade G, Georgiade N, Riefkohl R, Barwick W (eds): Textbook of Plastic, Maxillofacial, and Reconstructive Surgery, 2nd ed. Baltimore, Williams & Wilkins, 1992, pp 1021–1032.

10. Pribaz JJ, Orgill DP, Epstein MD, et al: Anterolateral thigh free flap. Ann Plast Surg 34:585–592, 1995.

11. Robinson DW: Microsurgical transfer of the dorsalis pedis neurovascular island flap. Br J Plast Surg 29:209–213, 1976.

12. Strauch B, Yu H: Atlas of Microvascular Surgery. New York, Thieme, 1993.

13. Terzis JK: Pectoralis minor: A unique muscle for correction of facial palsy [see comments]. Plast Reconstr Surg 83:767–776, 1989.

14. Whitney TM, Buncke HJ, Alpert BS, et al: The serratus anterior free-muscle flap: Experience with 100 consecutive cases. Plast Reconstr Surg 86:481–490; discussion 491, 1990.

85. LEECHES

Stephen P. Daane, M.D.

1. What are leeches? Sneeches?

Leeches are worms of the Annelid phylum that feed on blood extracted from a host. Because of the practice of leeching in the middle ages, the word "leech" was derived from the English word "laece," which meant physician. Leeches were used extensively in 19th century European medicine for bloodletting, a practice believed to cure virtually any ailment. Consumption of leeches reached a peak in the 1830s, when tens of millions were used annually in France, England, Germany, and the United States.

Sneeches live on beaches and were created by Dr. Seuss. They have nothing to do with plastic surgery.

2. How long have leeches been used in medicine?

The first known use of leeches dates to 3,500 years ago in Egypt, where a tomb painting depicts the application of leeches by a barber-surgeon. Detailed documentation of leeching also dates to 3,300 years ago in India. In the West, leeches were first used for medicinal bloodletting 2,200 years ago by Nicander of Colophon, Greece.

3. How long have leeches been used in plastic surgery?

The modern use of leeches in flap surgery began in 1960 with a report of 70% complete salvage and 30% partial salvage in 20 threatened flaps treated with leeches. They were used in hand surgery in 1981, with a report of 60% survival of 10 artery-only digital replantations treated with leeches. This was a marked improvement over the survival of artery-only replants treated by systemic anticoagulation alone.

Current survival estimates for threatened replanted digits treated with leeches are 60–70%; salvage estimates for threatened pedicle flaps treated with leeches are also 60–70%. *Hirudo medicinalis,* the leech endemic to Southeast Asia and Europe, is the most commonly used species.

4. What are the indications for using leeches?

Venous congestion is a recognized complication of digital replantation that may lead to a sequence of edema, capillary and arterial slowing, venous and arterial thrombosis, flap ischemia, and, finally, necrosis. Leeches are not a panacea for poor flap design or technical problems with vascular anastomoses, but they are indicated as an adjunct for salvage.

Leeches have been used successfully to decongest replanted parts, including completely avulsed ears and digits and partially avulsed segments of the lip, penis, nose, and scalp. They also have been used on threatened digits in purpura fulminans, ear and periorbital hematomas, traumatically degloved tissues, and in the salvage of nipple necrosis in breast reduction procedures.

5. What are the signs of arterial occlusion vs. venous occlusion?

Signs of venous congestion include cyanotic skin color, cool temperature, rapid capillary refill, increased tissue turgor, and rapid dark bleeding in response to a pinprick. Doppler imaging should be the first tool used postoperatively to document arterial circulation because leeches will not be helpful in cases of insufficient arterial inflow. Venous congested tissues may be salvaged if arterial blood flow is maintained until new venous ingrowth occurs; venous competence is usually restored by postoperative day 4 or 5 for replanted digits and by postoperative day 6–10 for free flaps.

	Arterial Occlusion	Venous Occlusion
Color	Pale	Blue-purple
Tissue turgor	Decreased	Increased; engorged and tense
Capillary refill	Slow, absent	Brisk, instantaneous
Temperature	Low	Low

In the absence of overt signs of threatened tissue loss, early detection of complications is aided with temperature monitoring, fluorescein dye injection, or laser Doppler flowmetry, although it is difficult to distinguish between arterial or venous occlusion with any of these modalities.

6. How do leeches work?

The leech front sucker conceals cartilaginous cutting plates that make a 2-mm incision. In 30 minutes a single hirudo leech can ingest up to 10 times its body weight or 5–15 cc of blood. However, the primary therapeutic benefit is derived from an anticoagulant, hirudin, injected from the leech salivary glands. The effect of the anticoagulant may last several hours after the leech detaches, permitting the wound to ooze up to 50 cc of blood.

Hirudin is a polypeptide that inhibits the thrombin-catalyzed conversion of fibrinogen to fibrin. Hirudin also blocks platelet aggregation in response to thrombin and may inhibit factor X. Because factor II (thrombin) is believed to be the final common pathway in all causes of thrombosis, hirudin is regarded as the most potent natural anticoagulant known. Hirudin has two advantages over heparin: (1) it does not require antithrombin III to inactivate thrombin, and (2) it is not bound by heparin-neutralizing platelet factor 4. Clinical trials are in progress to compare the efficacy of heparin and recombinant hirudin in preventing acute coronary closure after angioplasty, in the treatment of unstable angina, and in prophylaxis of deep venous thrombosis (DVT).

Other pharmacologic agents within leech saliva include (1) a local anesthetic; (2) hyaluronidase, a spreading factor; and (3) a histamine-like vasodilator that increases regional blood flow.

7. What are the possible complications of using leeches? What precautions are necessary?

The main complications in using leeches are infection and blood loss. *Hirudo medicinalis* relies on a symbiotic relationship with *Aeromonas hydrophila* within its gut. *A. hydrophila* is a gram-negative rod that causes infection at rates varying from 0–20% within 1–10 days after leech use. Some authors recommend an empiric aminoglycoside or third-generation cephalosporin. Leeches are not natural carriers of viruses, but they can transmit hepatitis B to humans if infected. Universal precautions (handling leeches with gloves and a forceps) must be followed.

A potential result of prolonged leech therapy is a significant drop in hematocrit. Transfusions are often required because of systemic anticoagulation and continuous oozing from leech bites, which may contraindicate leech therapy for Jehovah's Witnesses.

8. How are leeches administered?

The skin is cleansed and isolated with an Op-Site dressing or saline-soaked sponge. The leech's head (narrow end) is directed to the area needing treatment. A leech may be induced to feed by keeping it in a beaker held over the attachment site or by pricking the feeding site with a needle to produce a drop of blood. It is also important to protect the area of the anastomosis with a gauze. Observe the leech frequently until it drops off the patient (usually in 30 minutes). If bleeding stops after the leech is removed, wiping the leech-bite area with a heparin-soaked gauze pledget may promote rebleeding.

Leech rejection is failure of the leech to attach rapidly to a replanted part, poor sucking, or consumption of less than a full meal. These findings have been suggested as poor prognosticators of tissue survival because of arterial insufficiency, despite a favorable tissue color.

For disposal leeches are placed in a container of alcohol and discarded with infectious waste. Leeches may never be reused.

9. How many leeches should you use?

The desired venous outflow of a flap or replanted digit is tailored to the needs of the specific patient by adjusting the number and frequency of leeches applied. In some published reports, leeches were used on venous congested parts as infrequently as 1 leech/day, or as frequently as 1 leech 6 times/day for a duration of 5–10 days.

When the wound does not continue to bleed after leech application, fresh leeches may be reapplied to a digit or flap as frequently as every 30 minutes.

10. Where do you get leeches in the middle of the night?

Because venous congestion may arise suddenly in the immediate postoperative period, an immediately available supply of at least 5–10 leeches is desirable. In the United States, hirudo leeches are available from two vendors on the East Coast who advertise prominently in plastic surgery journals. However, even under the best circumstances, obtaining leeches may take 12–14 hours. Tissue bleeding caused by abrasion of the nailbed of the replanted digit with heparin-soaked sponges every hour usually maintains tissue viability until leeches are available. Telephone calls to the pharmacies of neighboring hospitals may yield an available supply of "loaner" leeches.

Leeches vary in price but are approximately $7 each. In comparison with the costs of an operation and postoperative ICU monitoring, leeches are one of the least expensive parts of a patient's hospitalization. The expense is usually covered as a medication by insurance companies.

BIBLIOGRAPHY

1. Daane S, Zamora S, Rockwell WB: Clinical use of leeches in reconstructive surgery. Am J Orthop 25:528–532, 1997.
2. Dabb RW, Malone JM, Leverett LC: The use of medicinal leeches in the salvage of flaps with venous congestion. Ann Plast Surg 29:250–256, 1992.
3. Kraemer BA: Use of leeches in plastic and reconstructive surgery: A review. J Reconstr Microsurg 4:381–386, 1988.
4. Lineaveaver WC, Hill MK, Buncke GM, et al: *Aeromonas hydrophila* infections following use of medicinal leeches in replantation and flap surgery. Ann Plast Surg 29:238–244, 1992.
5. Smoot CE, Ruiz-Inchaustegui JA, Roth AC: Mechanical leech therapy to relieve venous congestion. J Reconstr Microsurg 11:51–55, 1995.
6. Wells MD, Manktelow RT, Boyd JB, et al: The medicinal leech: An old treatment revisited. Microsurgery 14:183–186, 1993.

XI. The Hand and Upper Extremity

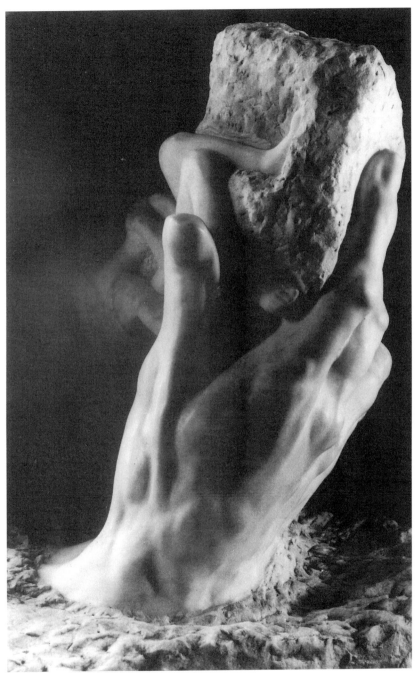

The Hand of God
Auguste Rodin
1897–1989
Marble
Museé Rodin, Paris
© 1998 Museé Rodin

86. ANATOMY OF THE HAND

Lee E. Edstrom, M.D.

1. What is the thickest skin in the hand?
The palmar skin has the thickest epidermis due to the stratum corneum, but the dermis is as thick on the dorsum as the palm.

2. Why can we get away with single layer closure in the palm?
The thick stratum corneum hides the ingrowth of epithelium down the suture into the dermis; thus, sutures can be left in place for over a week without leaving stitch marks.

3. How is the palmar skin so firmly fixed in place?
The palmar fascia is a unique structure, fixed proximally and distally, from side to side, and to the underlying metacarpals by its vertical fibers. The palmar skin is closely attached to the palmar fascia by a tight network of its own vertical fibers. Hence, edema cannot collect as easily on the palmar side of the hand.

4. Does the palmar fascia extend into the fingers?
Yes. The longitudinal fibers of the palmar fascia extend into the fingers and in the web spaces; the natatory ligaments are part of the palmar fascia. In the proximal and middle phalanges, however, Cleland's (dorsal) and Grayson's (volar) ligaments are the stabilizing structures. On the sides of the fingers, dorsal and palmar to the neurovascular bundles, they are attached to the phalanges along the ridge giving rise to the fibroosseous tunnel. In the distal phalanx vertical fibers are attached directly to the underlying distal phalanx and form a honeycomb series of compartments, similar to that in the palm between the skin and palmar fascia.

5. Name two unique types of infection on the palmar side of the hand that are due to the firm fixation of the skin to underlying structures.
A **collar-button abscess** in the palm starts as a tiny infection between the palmar skin and the palmar fascia. It then erodes through the palmar fascia into the underlying loose space, forming a dumbbell- or collar button-shaped abscess, which may be inadequately drained if the anatomy is not appreciated.
A **felon** in the distal phalanx starts in the same way as the collar-button abscess, but it is inhibited from side-to-side spread by the tight network of vertical fibers attaching the skin to the distal phalanx. Spread occurs by erosion through the walls formed by the vertical fibers, adding to the abscess compartment by compartment.

6. How does the unique anatomy of the fingertip shape the development of a paronychia?
A paronychia is an infection of the nail fold and seldom exists without the presence of a nail, which is first a foreign-body irritant and then the roof of the abscess.

7. Can a felon spread around the distal phalanx and become a paronychia? Can a paronychia spread around the nail plate into the palmar pulp and become a felon?
Both events are highly unlikely because of the anatomy of the fingertip. The paronychia spreads around the nail plate and may lift the entire nail plate off the bed but ultimately drains dorsally. The felon spreads on the palmar side, ultimately breaking through the skin. It may spread proximally into the soft tissue of the middle phalanx—or even into the bone and distal interphalangeal (DIP) joint—but not dorsally to the nail fold.

8. Which tissues contribute to growth of the nail plate?
The entire nail bed, including the overlying eponychial fold, contributes material to the developing and growing nail. The proximal nail bed (germinal matrix) forms the early developing nail, the

overlying fold contributes the smooth surface, and the distal bed (sterile matrix) continues to add bulk so that the nail plate does not become too thin from wear.

9. What is the lunula?
The white arc just distal to the eponychium, called the lunula, is a result of persistence of nuclei in the cells of the germinal matrix as they flow distally, creating the nail. As the nuclei disintegrate distal to the lunula, the nail becomes transparent.

10. What is the safe position for splinting the hand?
It is useful to think of joints as having certain positions that tend to produce stiffness and other positions that can be maintained for long periods without developing stiffness. The metacarpophalangeal (MP) and interphalangeal (IP) joints are good examples of this concept. The MP joints recover well from flexion, and the IP joints recover well from extension. The thumb should be abducted and the wrist maintained in mild extension. This is the position from which it is easiest to regain mobility of the joints after prolonged immobilization.

11. Why is flexion the safe position for the MP joint?
The MP joint is characterized by variable tightness of the collateral ligaments, depending on the position of the joint, because of the unique shape of the metacarpal head and the origin of the collateral ligaments dorsal to the axis of rotation of the joint. The head is ovoid in the sagittal plane (creating a cam effect) and possesses a palmar flare in the transverse plane, which requires the collateral ligaments to span a greater distance in flexion than extension. Therefore, the collateral ligaments are stretched tight in flexion but are lax in extension. Because ligaments tend to shorten when maintained in a lax position, prolonged extension leads to shortening of the collateral ligaments, rendering them unable to accommodate the joint in flexion and thus producing an extension contracture.

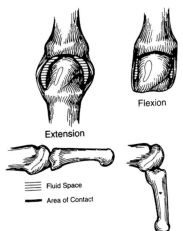

Anatomy of the metacarpophalangeal joint. In extension the collateral ligaments are loose; the joint is relatively unstable and the ligaments are at risk for shortening. In flexion the collateral ligaments are tight secondary to a cam effect; the joint is stable and the ligaments are protected. (From Watson HK, Weinzweig J: Stiff joints. In Green DP (ed): Operative Hand Surgery, 4th ed. New York, Churchill Livingstone, in press, with permission.)

12. Why is extension the safe position for the IP joints?
The collateral ligaments of the IP joints tend to have the same tightness in flexion and extension and thus are not as important in consideration of safe splinting. Two other points are important instead: (1) the extensor mechanism in the region of the proximal interphalangeal (PIP) joint and (2) the volar plates. The volar plate overlies the cartilaginous surface of the phalangeal condyles in extension but in flexion slides proximal to the condyles, where it readily becomes adherent to the filmy soft tissue between the tendon sheath and periosteum. Maintenance of this position produces a flexion contracture. The other consideration is that the extensor mechanism is highly stable in extension but under stress in flexion. This problem is particularly significant when the PIP joint is injured, as in a burn injury. Inflammation may cause attenuation of the delicate extensor mechanism, resulting in disruption of the transverse retinacular ligaments when the joint is stressed in flexion. The lateral bands then slip volarly, creating a boutonnière deformity.

13. The IP joint can be thought of as a box, with the articular surfaces of the phalanges forming the proximal and distal ends. What forms the other sides?

The volar plate forms the bottom and the collateral ligaments the sides. The collateral ligaments extend from their points of origin into a broad, fan-shaped insertion into the phalanx distally and the sides of the volar plate volarly. The volar portion of the collateral ligament is referred to as the accessory collateral ligament. The top or lid of the box is formed by the extensor mechanism, which contributes little to the structural stability of the joint.

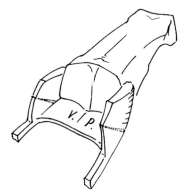

Anatomy of the interphalangeal joint. The three-dimensional ligament-box complex provides strength with minimal bulk. At least two sides of this box must be disrupted for displacement of the joint to occur. (From Dray GJ, Eaton RG: Dislocations and ligament injuries in the digits. In Green DP (ed): Operative Hand Surgery, 3rd ed. New York, Churchill Livingstone, 1993, p 768, with permission.)

14. Which is the most mobile carpometacarpal (CMC) joint?

The CMC joint of the thumb is a saddle joint with motion in three axes, giving the thumb unique mobility.

15. Which are the least mobile CMC joints?

The second and third metacarpals are bound firmly to the trapezoid and capitate, forming a stable structure known as the fixed unit of the hand. Thus, the second and third CMC joints are the least mobile.

16. What is the last muscle innervated by the ulnar nerve as it courses through the palm?

The first dorsal interosseus is the last muscle to receive motor fibers from the ulnar nerve after it passes through the adductor of the thumb, which is next to last.

17. What major peripheral nerve is responsible for extension of the thumb IP joint?

The **median nerve** innervates the radial side of the thenar eminence, which is responsible for MP joint flexion and IP joint extension from the radial side. The **ulnar nerve** innervates the adductor pollicis and ulnar head of the short flexor, which is responsible for the same actions from the ulnar side. The **radial nerve** innervates the extensor pollicis longus (EPL), which is responsible for central IP joint extension. Thus, all three major peripheral nerves contribute to extension of the thumb IP joint.

18. How can you test for function of the EPL?

The EPL has the unique function of lifting the thumb dorsal to the plane of the palm. Ask the patient to place the palm on the table and lift up the thumb.

19. There is much crossover of sensory innervation in the hand. Where do the median, ulnar, and radial sensory nerves supply sensibility with the least chance of crossover from neighboring territories?

The median nerve is alone on the index tip, the ulnar nerve on the little finger tip, and the radial nerve over the dorsal surface of the first web space.

20. Where is the one place on the hand where all three sensory nerves may be expected to provide maximal crossover innervation?

On the dorsal surface of the middle phalanx of the ring finger, the digital nerves from median and ulnar nerves course dorsally, whereas the radial nerve sensory branch courses distally, along with the ulnar nerve dorsal sensory branch on the ulnar side.

21. What three vascular arches provide anastomotic connections between the radial and ulnar blood supplies?

The superficial palmar arch courses palmar to the flexor tendons, gives off the digital vessels, and is a direct continuation of the ulnar artery. The deep palmar arch, which is deep (dorsal) to the flexor tendons, gives off the volar metacarpal arteries and is a direct continuation of the radial artery after the take-off of the princeps pollicis. The dorsal carpal arch travels dorsally over the proximal carpal row, linking the radial and ulnar systems dorsally and giving off the dorsal metacarpal arteries.

22. Despite proper tourniquet application, the wound begins to bleed during repair of a spaghetti wrist. Why?

Blood is shunted down to the hand via nutrient vessels in the humerus. This process may take an hour or even longer. The ascending branch of the humeral circumflex artery enters the bone in the bicipital groove, perfuses the bone through the medullary cavity with connections to the periosteal vessels, and may exit inferiorly at the elbow. Control under these circumstances may be obtained by wrapping an Esmarch or Ace bandage around the elbow at moderate pressure.

23. How can one test the integrity of the vascular anastomotic connections between the two sides of the hand?

Allen's test is performed by occluding both radial and ulnar arteries at the wrist, emptying the hand of blood by repeatedly making a fist, and releasing one of the arteries. The hand should fill with blood immediately, with no significant delay on the side still occluded.

24. What are the boundaries of the carpal tunnel?

The transverse carpal ligament (TCL), in addition to providing a pulley mechanism for the flexor tendons, spans the volar aspect of the proximal palm to form the roof of the carpal tunnel. The TCL courses from the scaphoid tubercle and the crest of the trapezium on the radial side to the pisiform and hamate on the ulnar side.

25. How many structures traverse the carpal tunnel?

Ten. Nine flexor tendons (four flexor digitorum superficialis [FDS] tendons, four flexor digitorum profundus [FDP] tendons, and the flexor pollicis longus [FPL]) and the median nerve pass through the carpal tunnel.

26. What are the boundaries of Guyon's canal?

The TCL forms the floor, the volar carpal ligament (VCL) the roof, and the pisiform the ulnar wall of the canal of Guyon.

27. What are the six dorsal extensor compartments of the wrist?

The six well-defined tunnels through which the extrinsic extensor tendons pass are numbered from radial to ulnar (see figure at top of next page). The first compartment contains the abductor pollicis longus (APL) and extensor pollicis brevis (EPB) and is located on the surface of the radial styloid. Both the APL and EPB may contain several slips; tenosynovitis in this compartment is known as de Quervain's disease. The second compartment contains the two radial extensors of the wrist (extensor carpi radialis longus [ECRL] and brevis [ECRB]), which course through the floor of the anatomic snuffbox on the way to their insertions on the bases of the second and third metacarpals, respectively. Lister's tubercle separates the second compartment from the third compartment, which contains the EPL. The fourth compartment contains the tendons of the extensor digiti communis (EDC) and the extensor indicis proprius (EIP), whereas the fifth compartment contains the extensor digiti quinti (EDQ). The sixth dorsal compartment is located on the head of the ulna and contains the extensor carpi ulnaris (ECU).

28. When is the ECU not primarily an extensor of the wrist?

The sixth dorsal compartment is fixed on the ulnar head. When the radius pivots around the ulnar head in pronation and supination, the ECU assumes different positions relative to the wrist. In full pronation it is ulnar to the wrist and thus primarily an ulnar deviator.

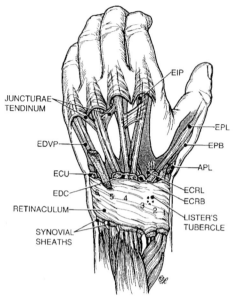

The six dorsal extensor compartments of the wrist. (From Doyle JR: Extensor tendons—acute injuries. In Green DP (ed): Operative Hand Surgery, 3rd ed. New York, Churchill-Livingstone, 1993, p 1927, with permission.)

29. Name the four insertions of the extrinsic extensor tendon.

The extrinsic extensor tendon inserts into (1) the base of the proximal phalanx, (2) the base of the middle phalanx, (3) the base of the distal phalanx (via the slips to the lateral bands; see question 43), and (4) the transverse metacarpal ligament and volar plate.

30. How do you identify the proprius tendons of the index and little fingers?

The proprius tendons (extensor digiti minimi [EDM] and extensor indicis proprius [EIP]) usually lie on the ulnar side of the communis tendon (EDC) and allow independent extension of the little and index fingers, respectively. However, significant variability of the extensor tendons to the index and little fingers, including radial EIP and EDM tendons and supernumerary tendons, has been reported in up to 19% of specimens in anatomic studies.

31. What is the anatomic snuffbox?

It is the hollow on the radial side of the wrist bordered by the contents of the first dorsal compartment on the palmar side, the EPL dorsally, the radial styloid proximally, and the base of the thumb metacarpal distally. The radial artery courses through the snuffbox on its way to the dorsal first web space; in the depths of the snuffbox is the scaphoid. Injury to the scaphoid produces tenderness in the snuffbox.

32. What is the primary flexor of the MP joint?

The intrinsic muscle tendons course volar to the MP joint axis of rotation and are the primary flexors of the MP joint.

33. What is the primary extender of the MP joint?

The extrinsic system extends the MP joint.

34. Which extends the IP joint—the extrinsic or intrinsic system?

The intrinsic system extends the IP joint when the MP joint is in hyperextension; the extrinsic system extends the IP joint when the MP joint is in flexion.

35. When the intrinsic muscles are paralyzed, how is the finger affected?

Because the primary flexor of the MP joint is lost, the MP joints tend to develop a posture of hyperextension—the position from which the paralyzed intrinsics are needed to extend the IP joints (see question 32). Thus, the IP joints fall into flexion, especially with intact profundus tendons, producing the claw deformity.

36. Which interosseous muscles are innervated by the median nerve?

An easy way to remember the answer is the mnemonic **LOAF: L** stands for the two radial lumbricals, **O** for opponens pollicis, **A** for abductor pollicis brevis, and **F** for the superficial head of the flexor pollicis brevis (FPB). The rest of the intrinsic muscles are innervated by the ulnar nerve. The radial side of the thenar eminence is innervated by the median nerve, the ulnar side by the ulnar nerve (adductor pollicis and deep or ulnar head of the FPB).

37. Which of the interosseous muscles abduct the fingers? Which adduct them?

The four dorsal interossei, which arise from the adjacent surfaces of the shafts of the first, second, third, and fourth metacarpals and insert on the proximal phalanges of the index, middle, and ring fingers, abduct the digits from the midline of the hand. The three volar interossei, which arise from the second, fourth, and fifth metacarpals and insert on the respective proximal phalanges, adduct the digits toward the midline. The tendons from these muscles lie volar to the axis of MP motion but dorsal to the transverse metacarpal ligament (TMCL).

38. What does the oblique retinacular ligament (ORL) do?

It controls and coordinates flexion and extension between the IP joints. It courses beneath the PIP joint and over the distal interphalangeal (DIP) joint. As the DIP begins to flex, the ORL tightens, delivering flexor tone to the PIP joint; and when the PIP begins to extend, the ORL tightens, delivering extensor tone to the DIP joint. It thus ensures smooth, modulated, coordinated flexion and extension to the IP joints. It has been called the "cerebellum" of the finger.

39. What happens to the ORL in a boutonnière deformity?

With the PIP joint in flexion and the DIP joint in extension (the boutonnière position), the ORL is lax. Therefore, the ORL shortens (as do all ligaments in a lax position) and helps to maintain the deformity.

40. What is the smallest extrinsic flexor tendon?

The FDS to the little finger not only is the smallest tendon, but also is frequently nonfunctional or even missing. Its consistently small size helps to identify the individual cut ends in the spaghetti wrist.

41. Which interosseous muscles have insertions into the bases of the proximal phalanges?

The first, second, and fourth dorsal interosseus muscles have bony insertions from their superficial bellies/medial tendons.

42. Where else do the interosseous muscles insert?

All of the interosseous muscles have deep bellies/lateral tendons, which travel superficial to the sagittal bands into the aponeurotic expansion as transverse (dorsally across the proximal phalanges) and oblique fibers (parallel to the lateral bands).

43. Which individual structures are maintained in dorsal position by the transverse retinacular ligament of Landsmeer?

Seven tendons are held in place in the region of the PIP joint: the central slip of the extrinsic extensor, the two lateral bands, the two slips from the central slip to the lateral band, and the two slips from the lateral bands to the central slip.

44. Which are the most important pulleys in the fibroosseous tunnel?

The finger flexor unit functions well if the A2 and the A4 pulleys are preserved. Both are needed to prevent tendon bowstringing. The A2 and A4 pulleys are located at the proximal portion of the proximal phalanx (proximal proximal) and the middle portion of the middle phalanx (middle middle), respectively.

45. Why do the profundus tendons usually not retract into the palm after transection in the fingers?

The profundus tendons are tethered by the lumbricals in the palm and by their adjacent profundus tendons, with which they have a common muscle belly. In addition, they may not have avulsed their vincula and thus still may be attached to either the DIP or PIP volar plates.

46. Why can you not pull a superficialis tendon out through a palmar incision if you release it from its insertions in the middle phalanx?

The superficialis tendon does not simply divide when the profundus passes superficial to it; it reconstitutes itself beneath the profundus (the chiasm of Camper) before dividing finally to its two insertions. This structure prevents the superficialis from being pulled out, because it completely encircles the profundus tendon.

47. How is the long vinculum of the profundus tendon related to the short vinculum of the superficialis?

The vincula are folds of mesotenon carrying blood supply to both tendons. Normally, each of the profundus and superficialis tendons has a short vinculum (breve) and a long vinculum (longum). The vinculum longum of the profundus tendon traverses the vinculum breve of the superficialis tendon.

48. Where in the tendon is the longitudinal intrinsic blood supply?

It is concentrated in the dorsal (deep) aspect of the tendon, where the vincula enter.

49. How are the flexor tendons arranged in the carpal tunnel?

The profundus tendons lie side by side on its floor. The FPL is the radialmost member of this group; the superficialis tendons lie on the profundus tendons arranged two by two; the middle and ring finger tendons (third and fourth) are superficial; the index and small finger tendons (second and fifth) lie between them and the profundus row. Remember, 34 (third and fourth) is higher (more superficial) than 25 (second and fifth).

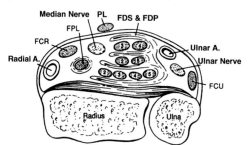

Cross-section through the carpal tunnel. (From Ariyan S: The Hand Book. New York, McGraw-Hill, 1989, p 10, with permission.)

50. How often is the palmaris longus tendon absent?

Approximately 15% of patients do not have a palmaris longus tendon.

51. What is the second most useful tendon for grafting in the hand?

If the palmaris longus tendon is absent, if a longer tendon is necessary, or if additional tendons are needed, the plantaris tendons are excellent sources of graft material.

BIBLIOGRAPHY

1. Ariyan S: The Hand Book. New York, McGraw-Hill, 1989.
2. Green DP: Operative Hand Surgery, 3rd ed. New York, Churchill Livingstone, 1993.
3. Landsmeer JMF: The anatomy of the dorsal aponeurosis of the human finger and its functional significance. Anat Rec 104:31, 1941.
4. Landsmeer JMF: The coordination of finger-joint motions. J Bone Joint Surg 45A:1654, 1963.
5. Lister G: The Hand: Diagnosis and Indications. New York, Churchill Livingstone, 1984.
6. Netter FH: Atlas of Human Anatomy. New Jersey, CIBA-Geigy Corporation, 1990.
7. Warfel JH: The Extremities: Muscles and Motor Points. Philadelphia, Lea & Febiger, 1993.

87. PHYSICAL EXAMINATION OF THE HAND

Christian A. Dumontier, M.D., and Raoul Tubiana, M.D.

1. It takes two months for a complete nail plate to grow. True or false?

False. Nail plate growth is highly variable among individuals and may be modified by numerous factors. However, it takes about 6 months for a complete nail plate to grow. At 2 months after avulsion, the nail plate is visible only at the level of the proximal nail fold.

2. Is it useful to have a proximal nail fold?

Kligman's experiences have shown that the nail matrix is responsible for almost all production of the nail plate but is unable to control its shape. The proximodistal growth of the nail plate is, in part, controlled by the proximal nail fold, which limits the growth in height and forces the nail plate to grow distally. The proximal nail fold is also useful to protect the nail plate, which, at this level of the finger, is thin, fragile, and poorly adherent to the matrix.

3. What is the Hutchinson's sign? What does it mean?

Hutchinson's sign is a dark discoloration of the nail plate and the proximal or distal nail fold. It is highly suggestive of a subungual melanoma.

4. What is the function of nails?

Early medical descriptions state that nails were made for scratching, especially of the small animals that live on our body. Science has since shown that this is not their only function. Nails contribute to thermoregulation because of their richness in neurovascular glomi. Their main function is to serve as a counterpressure for the pulp that enhances discrimination. Patients without nails are unable to button their shirt. Nails also serve to pick up small objects and protect against trauma. Finally, they also have a cosmetic function. Since nails are so useful, maybe you should stop biting them before exams.

5. What is the best test to appreciate the functional sensibility of the hand?

Many sensory tests have been described, but most of them are useful only to appreciate central or medullar neurologic lesions. To pick up and hold small objects correctly, the hand must be able to discriminate and to recognize various forms or textures. The best way to appreciate the functional sensibility of the hand is to test its discrimination.

6. How can you appreciate the sensory discrimination of a finger pulp?

By using the two-point-discrimination test described by Weber. The points of calipers are held against the skin at different distances from each other. The test determines the minimal distance at which the patient can distinguish whether one or two points are in contact with the skin. The patient must be comfortable, and the examiner must avoid pushing against the calipers with his or her fingers, thereby artificially increasing the pressure. The higher the pressure, the wider the area of skin that is deformed and stimulated. One or two points are touched in a random sequence along a longitudinal axis in the center of the finger tip. The American Society for Surgery of the Hand recommends 7 correct answers out of 10 for two-point-discrimination.

7. What is the normal value for the two-point-discrimination test at the pulp of the finger?

Values vary according to fingers and individuals. In most patients, normal values vary between 2–3 mm at the pulp of the finger. In patients employed in heavy labor, normal values are closer to 5–6 mm. In patients with congenital or acquired blindness it may be as low as 1–2 mm.

8. Why do patients with a low ulnar nerve palsy often have permanent abduction of the small finger? What is the name of this deformity?

This acquired deformity is known as Wartenberg's sign. Blacker et al. have shown that the extensor digiti minimi tendon has two bundles. The radialmost tendon passes over the center of the axis of abduction-adduction of the metacarpophalangeal (MP) joint or slightly radial to it. The ulnar tendon, which is the thicker of the two, passes ulnar to the axis in most patients and gains a firm attachment to the tendon of the abductor digiti quinti. By means of these slips, the extensor digiti minimi has acquired a bony attachment to the tubercle of the proximal phalanx. The extensor digiti minimi thus has the potential to abduct the little finger through this indirect insertion.

9. How do you test the flexor digitorum profundus (FDP) tendons?
Tendons of the FDP insert on the volar aspect of the distal phalanx of the fingers. The FDP tendon is the only tendon that allows flexion of the distal phalanx onto the middle phalanx. To test this tendon, the examiner should immobilize the proximal interphalangeal (PIP) joint in complete extension and ask the patient to flex the distal phalanx. In patients with limited strength or mobility, it is easier to appreciate even a small amount of motion if you place the wrist and MP joint in complete extension.

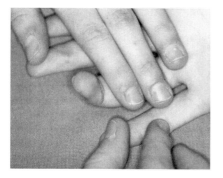

The FDP tendon allows flexion of the distal phalanx onto the middle phalanx. To test the FDP tendon, immobilize the PIP joint in complete extension and ask the patient to flex the distal phalanx.

10. How do you test the flexor digitorum superficialis (FDS) tendons of the fingers?
Tendons of the FDS insert on the volar aspect of the middle phalanx and flex the middle phalanx on the proximal phalanx. However, to examine the FDS tendon, it is mandatory to block the action of the FDP tendon, which is also able to flex the PIP joint after flexing the distal interphalangeal (DIP) joint. To block the FDP, the tendons of which arise from a common muscle belly, you need only to block the DIP joint of two or three fingers in extension. In doing so, you prevent the action of the FDP on the finger you wish to test. You obtain only flexion of the middle phalanx on the proximal phalanx without flexion of the DIP joint. During flexion of the PIP joint, the extensor mechanism glides distally. Patients are unable to control the motion of the distal phalanx from this position. This phenomenon, known as the "floating" distal phalanx, does not always hold true for the index finger, in which the FDP muscle belly is often independent of the three ulnar fingers.

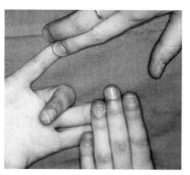

When the patient is asked to flex the finger, you obtain flexion only in the PIP joint if the FDS tendon is blocked. Patients are unable to control the motion of the distal phalanx in this position. This phenomenon is known as the "floating" distal phalanx.

11. If I try to test the FDS of the little finger as described above, why does the patient flex only the MP joint and not the PIP joint?
1. About 15% of people do not have an FDS tendon for the little finger.
2. Another group (also about 15%) has a tendon that is not functional.
3. Some people have an FDS tendon for the little finger that is functional but highly adherent to the FDS tendon of the ring finger, which is maintained in extension. If you allow the PIP joint of the

ring finger to flex, the patient will flex the PIP joint of the little finger. MP joint flexion of the little finger is provided by the flexor digiti quinti and the abductor digiti minimi.

12. How can you determine whether there is an FDS in the index finger if the FDP of the index is independent?

There is only one test to determine whether the FDS of the index finger is present. Ask the patient to hold a sheet of paper between the pulp of the thumb and index. The examiner pulls on the paper while the patient tries to resist. Because flexion strength is provided by the FDS, in a normal finger the digit will be slightly flexed at the PIP joint and extended at the DIP joint as in a "pseudo-boutonnière" deformity. In a patient without an FDS tendon, the DIP joint will flex to resist the traction and the PIP joint will stay in extension in a "pseudomallet" deformity.

13. In patients with rheumatoid arthritis who are unable to extend the ulnar three digits, what are the possible diagnoses?

1. Rupture of the extensor tendons must be suspected. Extensor tendons usually rupture after attrition on a dorsally subluxated ulnar head. In such cases, if you ask patients to extend the fingers, you will see no bowstringing of the extensor tendons beneath the skin.

2. In patients with ulnar deviation of the fingers, extensor tendons may dislocate in the intermetacarpal valleys. In such cases, if the MP joints are not stiff, passive extension of the fingers will allow the patient to maintain the extension.

3. The rarest cause is compression of the posterior interosseous nerve at the elbow. Usually in such cases, extension is weak but still possible, and wrist flexion will draw the fingers into extension as a result of the tenodesis effect.

14. How can you determine that the extensor pollicis longus tendon is intact and functional?

The extensor pollicis longus (EPL) tendon inserts on the dorsum of the distal phalanx of the thumb and is responsible for active extension of the distal phalanx. In most patients, its rupture leads to a flexion deformity of the IP joint and inability to extend the distal phalanx actively. However, extension of the intrinsic muscles of the thumb and adhesions between the EPL tendon and the extensor pollicis brevis (EPB) tendon give some patients the ability to achieve complete active extension of the IP joint even if the EPL tendon is ruptured. To be sure that the EPL tendon is intact, ask the patient to place his or her hand flat on a table. The patient is then asked to raise the thumb off the table (retropulsion). The EPL muscle is the only muscle responsible for this movement. You can also see and palpate the bowstringing of the tendon beneath the skin. Rupture of the EPL tendon was first described in drum players of the Prussian army, but you will probably see it more often in patients with Colles' fractures.

15. If flexion of the MP joint is limited, how can you determine whether the extensor tendons are adherent at the dorsum of the hand or at the wrist level?

By using the tenodesis effect. As most tendons cross several joints, it is possible to contract or relax them by changing the position of these joints. In the case of adhesion at the wrist level, wrist extension adds some flexion at the MP joint, whereas MP joint flexion does not change if the adhesion is located on the dorsum of the hand. This test is valid only if there is no ligamentous retraction at the MP joint.

16. What is Allen's test? How do you perform it?

Allen's test evaluates the patency of the radial and ulnar arteries at the level of the wrist. The patient is asked to raise and clench his or her hand to exsanguinate the cutaneous vascular bed. The examiner compresses the radial artery in the radial groove and the ulnar artery in Guyon's canal. The patient opens the hand without hyperextending the fingers. The palm appears pallid. The examiner releases one compressed artery and notes the time required for the palm to recover its normal color. The maneuver is then repeated to evaluate the other artery.

17. How do you determine a rotational deformity of the finger—in flexion or in extension?

In flexion. The only way to determine a rotational deformity is to ask the patient to flex his or her fingers. Because of the orientation of the MP and PIP joints, all of the fingers converge in flexion toward the scaphoid tubercle. Thus, even a minor rotational deformity that may not be apparent in extension becomes obvious. (See figure at top of next page.)

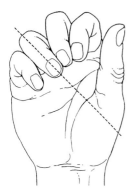

In the case of rotational deformity (fracture, malunion), flexion of a finger causes overlapping of one finger upon another in either a radial or an ulnar direction. (From Tubiana R: The Hand, Vol. I. Philadelphia, W.B. Saunders, 1985, with permission.)

18. Why is DIP joint flexion more important when the PIP joint is flexed than when the PIP joint is extended?

This clinical test is called the Haines-Zancolli test. Limited flexion of the DIP joint, when the PIP joint is maintained in extension, is due to the retaining action of the oblique retinacular (Landsmeer's) ligament. Landsmeer's ligament inserts on the proximal phalanx and digital sheath, volar to the axis of flexion-extension of the PIP joint. It ends on the extensor tendon, dorsal to the axis of flexion-extension of the DIP joint. As a result, there is more stress on Landsmeer's ligament in extension of the PIP joint than in flexion; thus, DIP joint flexion is easier with the PIP joint in flexion than in extension. Landsmeer's ligament coordinates the movement of the IP joints. It is placed under tension by flexion of the DIP joint, which causes simultaneous flexion of the PIP joint. The ligament is also placed under tension by extension of the PIP joint, which in turn causes extension of the DIP joint. Contraction of the oblique retinacular ligament has been described in the boutonnière deformity and Dupuytren's disease.

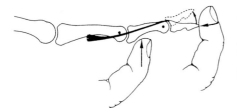

The Haines-Zancolli test is considered positive if flexion of the distal phalanx is not possible when the middle phalanx is maintained in extension; it is possible only if the middle phalanx is flexed. A positive test is the result of contraction of the oblique retinacular ligament. (From Tubiana R: The Hand, Vol. III. Philadelphia, W.B. Saunders, 1988, with permission.)

19. In patients experiencing stiffness with extension of the PIP joint, which clinical test identifies contracture of the interosseous muscles?

The Finochietto-Bunnell test. When the MP joint is in extension, the contracted interosseous muscles impede flexion of the PIP joint because of the traction exerted on the extensors. Flexion of the MP joint relaxes the extensors, and flexion becomes possible at the PIP joints.

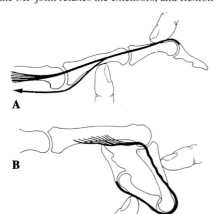

A

B

A positive Finochietto-Bunnell test in a swan-neck deformity of the finger with intrinsic muscle contracture. When the proximal phalanx is maintained in extension, it is impossible to flex the middle phalanx. In cases of contraction of the intrinsic muscles, flexion of the proximal phalanx allows flexion of the middle phalanx. (From Tubiana R: The Hand, Vol. III. Philadelphia, W.B. Saunders, 1988, with permission.)

20. Which clinical test is specific for de Quervain's tenosynovitis? How is it performed?

Finkelstein's test. De Quervain's tenosynovitis affects the first dorsal extensor compartment as its contents (APL and EPB tendons) pass over the radial styloid. Ask the patient to flex the thumb into the palm and to maintain it with the other fingers. The wrist is then placed in ulnar deviation, which causes a sharp pain at the radial styloid due to tension on the APL and EPB tendons.

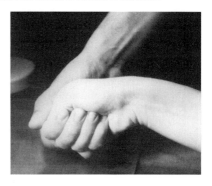

Finkelstein's test for de Quervain's tenosynovitis. The test is positive if the patient experiences sharp pain on the radial styloid when you suddenly place the wrist in ulnar deviation. (From Tubiana R, Thomine JM, Mackin E: Examination of the Hand and Wrist. London, Martin Dunitz, 1996, with permission.)

21. Which clinical signs are suggestive of flexor carpi radialis tendinitis?

Although it has been described only recently (Fitton et al., 1968), flexor carpi radialis (FCR) tendinitis is not a rare disease. As in most cases of tendinitis, pain is the most frequent complaint and is increased by resisted active contraction and passive stretching of the muscle-tendon unit. In FCR tendinitis, pain is localized on the volar aspect of the wrist and frequently radiates to the forearm. Pain is increased by resisted wrist flexion and passive extension of the wrist. Swelling is sometimes present along the tendon of the FCR and must be differentiated from a wrist ganglion. Some patients complain of diffuse pain and paresthesias on the base of the thenar eminence secondary to irritation of the palmar cutaneous branch of the median nerve.

22. If the IP joint of the thumb is flexed, why does the DIP joint of the index finger flex simultaneously?

This anatomic variation, known as Linburg's sign, is present in about 30% of people. It is due to adhesions in the carpal tunnel between the FPL and FDP tendons of the index finger. Flexion of the thumb sometimes causes other fingers to flex. This variation usually causes no functional impairment but has been described as a source of problems in some musicians who lack independence of the fingers.

23. In a patient who has sprained an MP joint, how can you diagnose a ligamentous rupture with instability?

To appreciate instability you must apply stress to the collateral ligament in adduction or abduction. However, abduction-adduction laxity of the MP joint in extension is normal because the collateral ligaments are not under tension. If you place the MP joint in complete passive flexion, because of their eccentric insertion and the shape of the metacarpal head, the collateral ligaments will be under tension without laxity in either abduction or adduction in normal patients. It is then easy to appreciate abnormal laxity in patients with ligamentous ruptures.

24. What are the etiologies of a swan-neck deformity of the fingers?

In swan-neck deformity, the PIP joint is in extension and the DIP joint in flexion. Swan-neck deformity is due to excessive traction by the extensor apparatus inserted on the base of the middle phalanx and is favored by laxity of the PIP joint.

Etiologies of Swan-neck Deformity

ORIGIN	CAUSES	EXPLANATION
PIP joint	Volar plate deficiency	Severe sprain of anterior volar plate; sequela of dorsal PIP dislocation; progressive stretching of volar plate due to synovitis, as in rheumatoid arthritis

Table continued on next page.

Etiologies of Swan-neck Deformity (Continued)

ORIGIN	CAUSES	EXPLANATION
Anterior structures of the PIP joint	Rupture of FDS tendon	Rupture may be traumatic or secondary to synovitis, as in rheumatoid arthritis
Intrinsic muscle contracture	Primary muscle contracture	Spasticity, compartment syndrome
	Secondary muscle contracture	Volar dislocation of MP joint, as in rheumatoid arthritis, brings intrinsic tendons into position dorsal to axis of MP joints; their force acts to increase forces of extensor apparatus
Extrinsic tendons	Chronic mallet finger	To extend distal phalanx, patients increase tension on extensor tendon, which results in increased tension on central slip of extensor tendon
	Increased tension on extensor apparatus	Wrist flexion deformity, as in rheumatoid arthritis, or destruction of proximal insertion of extensor communis at MP level

BIBLIOGRAPHY

1. Hunter JM, Schneider LH, Mackin EJ, Callahan AD: Rehabilitation of the Hand, 3rd ed. St. Louis, Mosby, 1990.
2. Landsmeer JMF: Atlas of Anatomy of the Hand. Edinburgh, Churchill Livingstone, 1976.
3. Lister G: The Hand: Diagnosis and Indications, 3rd ed. Edinburgh, Churchill Livingstone, 1993.
4. Tubiana R, Thomine JM, Mackin E: Examination of the Hand and Wrist. London, Martin Dunitz, 1996.
5. Tubiana R: The Hand, Vol. III. Philadelphia, W.B. Saunders, 1988.
6. Zancolli E: Structural and Dynamic Bases of Hand Surgery, 2nd ed. Philadelphia, J.P. Lippincott, 1979.

88. RADIOLOGIC EXAMINATION OF THE HAND

Wilfred C. G. Peh, M.B.B.S., D.M.R.D., F.R.C.R., and Louis A. Gilula, M.D.

1. Who performed the first radiograph of the hand?

Wilhelm Conrad Roentgen, the discoverer of x-rays, performed the first radiograph of the hand in 1895. Roentgen, then Professor at the University of Würzburg in Germany, was subsequently awarded the first Nobel Prize for Physics in recognition of his great discovery. He obtained an image of his wife's hand using a photographic plate. This radiograph is widely accepted as the first radiograph of a human.

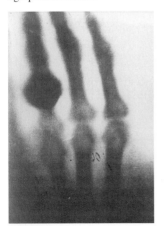

First radiograph of the hand, performed in 1895 by Wilhelm Conrad Roentgen. (Reproduced with permission of Siemen's Medical Systems, Inc., Iselin, New Jersey.)

2. Name some of the most common causes of diagnostic errors in interpreting radiographs of the hand after trauma.
- Inadequate clinical history and physical examination
- Acceptance of poor quality radiographs
- Failure to recognize an abnormality that is actually present
- Failure to obtain or insist on an adequate number of proper radiographic projections
- Missing a second significant finding, such as another fracture, dislocation, or foreign body

3. What is Brewerton's view?

A radiographic projection described by D.A. Brewerton in 1967 for demonstrating involvement of the metacarpal heads in rheumatoid arthritis. This projection aims at profiling the second through fifth metacarpophalangeal (MCP) joints with no overlapping of adjacent cortical surfaces. It is sensitive for revealing early erosions due to synovial arthritis and occult fractures of the metacarpal heads that may not be seen on routine views.

4. Why is Rolando's fracture considered a significant injury?

Rolando's fracture is a Y-shaped or comminuted fracture of the proximal phalanx of the thumb that involves the carpometacarpal (CMC) joint and commonly requires internal fixation. Proper alignment may otherwise be difficult to maintain because of the strong thumb adductors at the base of the proximal phalanx.

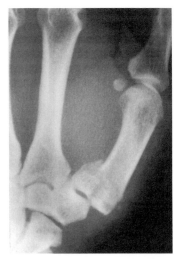

A 49-year-old man with Rolando's fracture of the left thumb. The comminuted fracture involves the CMC joint, and the major shaft fragments are displaced radially. Internal fixation was required for stabilization.

5. How are intraarticular fractures of the base of the phalanges classified?

Steele's classification consists of three categories. Type I is a nondisplaced marginal fracture. Type II is a comminuted, impaction fracture. Type III is a displaced intraarticular fracture with subluxation of the fracture fragments.

6. List the radiographic hallmarks of rheumatoid arthritis. (See figure, top of p. 458.)
- Periarticular osteoporosis
- Periarticular soft tissue swelling
- Marginal erosions
- Joint space narrowing
- Proximal and bilateral symmetric disease distribution

7. How can the ulnar deviation deformity of rheumatoid arthritis be explained?

The pathogenesis is not fully understood. It appears to be initiated by inflammatory arthritis of the metacarpophalangeal joint with a rise in intraarticular pressure. Destruction of the ligamentous and capsular tissues results in instability of the joint. Another contributory factor may be instability and ulnar displacement of extensor tendons. Ligamentous laxity of the fourth and fifth CMC joints, resulting in metacarpal volar descent, also may play a role.

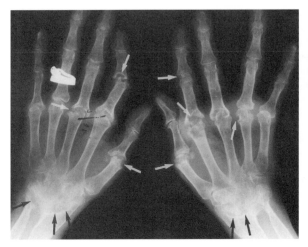
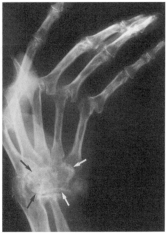

Left, A 65-year-old woman with rheumatoid arthritis. Erosions *(arrows)* of MCP and PIP joints as well as the distal forearm bones are present bilaterally. Note soft tissue swelling around all MCP joints and joint space narrowing at all affected joints. *Right,* Advanced rheumatoid arthritis in a 44-year-old woman. Note ulnar deviation at MCP joints of all digits. Bony ankylosis involves the intercarpal bones *(arrows)*, and ulnar translation of the carpus is present, other features of rheumatoid arthritis.

8. What is the pattern of involvement of primary osteoarthritis?

Primary osteoarthritis affects the distal and proximal interphalangeal joints of the digits and the CMC joint of the thumbs in a bilateral symmetric fashion. It is found predominantly in the hands of middle-aged and older women. Its major features include bone production or osteophytes around narrowed joints.

9. Which is the most common benign bone tumor of the hand?

Enchondroma. In fact, about 50% of enchondromas are found in the hand and wrist. Radiographically, the tumor is seen as a well-defined lucent lesion in the diaphysis or metadiaphysis and may have a well-defined sclerotic rim. It is often expansile with a preserved cortex. The endosteal cortex typically is scalloped or has multiple small concavities. The presence of internal chondroid-type calcifications is considered characteristic.

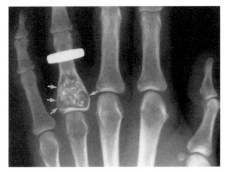

Enchondroma of the proximal phalanx of the left ring finger in a 58-year-old woman. The lesion contains typical punctate internal calcifications and expands the bone with preservation of the cortex. Scalloping *(arrows)* involves the endosteal surface of the overlying cortex.

10. Why is the finding of multiple enchondromas significant?

The condition of multiple enchondromas is named Ollier's disease. When found in combination with soft tissue hemangiomas, the entity is known as Maffuci's syndrome. Radiographically, phleboliths and soft tissue masses may be seen at the sites of hemangiomas. Malignant degeneration of enchondroma to chondrosarcoma may occur in up to 25% of patients with Ollier's disease by the age of 40 years. Maffuci's syndrome is associated with an even higher frequency of malignant transformation of enchondromas.

11. Which is the most common malignant bone tumor of the hand?

Metastases. Metastases and myeloma should be considered whenever a lytic lesion is detected in anyone over the age of 40 years, especially if the lesion has ill-defined margins and/or cortical breakthrough. Bronchogenic carcinoma is the most common origin for metastases to the bones of the hand.

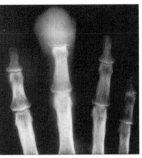

12. Besides metastases and enchondromas, list the other differential diagnoses for multiple lytic bone lesions.

Fibrous dysplasia, eosinophilic granuloma, myeloma, hyperparathyroidism (brown tumor), and infection.

13. What disorder typically produces well-defined erosions with overhanging margins?

Gout. In chronic advanced gout, tophaceous deposits are associated with intra- or periarticular erosions. These erosions are well-defined, have overhanging edges, and may have sclerotic margins. Tophi calcification is unusual and may reflect a coexisting abnormality of calcium metabolism.

Distal phalangeal metastasis in a 67-year-old man. Note bony destruction with associated soft tissue mass, normal mineralization of the adjacent phalanx, and relatively preserved DIP joint (or "adjacent interphalangeal joint").

14. Which disease is characterized by the combination of periarticular soft tissue calcification and subperiosteal bone resorption?

Hyperparathyroidism secondary to renal failure. Subperiosteal resorption is most frequently seen at the radial aspects of the middle phalanges of the hand and is considered a classic finding for hyperparathyroidism. In severe disease, terminal phalangeal resorption also may be present. When the serum calcium-phosphorus ion product is elevated, metastatic calcification may occur within normal tissues, particularly around joints. Chronic renal failure with secondary hyperparathyroidism is the most common cause of metastatic calcification and is usually seen in patients on long-term dialysis. The calcification may decrease or disappear with correction of the metabolic abnormality.

15. List the major causes of a short fourth metacarpal.

Trauma, infarction (e.g., sickle-cell anemia), Turner's syndrome, pseudohypoparathyroidism, pseudopseudohypoparathyroidism, idiopathic shortening, and multiple exostoses.

16. What is classically described as the best way to image reflex sympathetic dystrophy (RSD)?

Three-phase bone scintigraphy. All phases should have abnormal increased uptake. The 3-hour delayed images of bone scintiscans have a 96% sensitivity and 97% specificity in the diagnosis of RSD. There is diffuse increased isotope uptake around the radiocarpal, intercarpal, carpometacarpal, metacarpophalangeal, and interphalangeal joints. Radiographically, RSD may manifest as severe osteoporosis and soft tissue swelling.

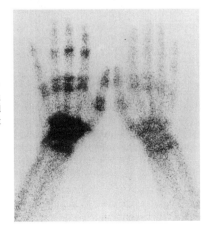

Bone scintiscan (3-hour delay) of a 30-year-old man with reflex sympathetic dystrophy of the left hand. Note diffuse increased isotope uptake at the wrist and proximal finger joints. The first two phases also displayed increased isotope uptake.

17. Does ultrasound have a role in imaging tendons?

Most definitely. By using a high-frequency linear transducer with a stand-off pad, high-resolution images of the tendons can be obtained. The tendons have a general hypoechoic appearance with multiple longitudinal internal fibers. Flexing and extending the finger allow identification and dynamic evaluation of the individual tendons. Indications include tenosynovitis, localized tendinitis, tendon rupture, and functional assessment of repaired tendons.

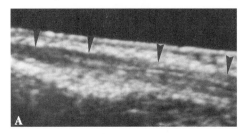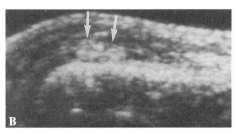

Longitudinal ultrasound scans of the finger extensor tendons in two different patients. *A,* A normal tendon in a 64-year-old man has a smooth regular outline *(arrowheads)* with fine linear internal echoes. *B,* A repaired tendon in a 23-year-old man shows an echogenic focus *(arrows)* at the repair site. Range of motion was normal.

18. Is magnetic resonance imaging (MRI) useful in staging soft-tissue tumors?

Yes. In fact, MRI is currently the modality of choice for tumor staging because it provides exact information about the location and extent of the tumor and its relationship to the surrounding tissues, particularly the neurovascular structures. This information is important for treatment planning.

CONTROVERSIES

19. Can MRI provide a specific tissue diagnosis of soft-tissue tumors?

Most soft-tissue tumors in the hands are benign. From the combination of signal characteristics on different pulse sequences and morphologic appearances, certain benign tumors can be diagnosed with confidence on MRI, including lipoma, giant-cell tumor of the tendon sheath, hemangioma, arteriovenous malformation, and ganglion cyst. For benign tumors with atypical appearances or lesions that do not fit into the above list, malignancy cannot be excluded. Plain radiographs should always be evaluated in conjunction with MR images because calcifications, ossification, and cortical abnormalities may be missed on MRI.

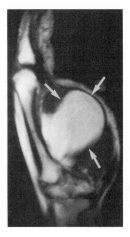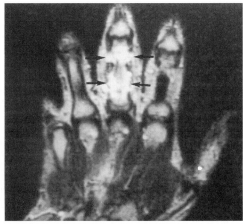

Left, Lipoma of the first web space in a 53-year-old woman. Sagittal T1-weighted MR image shows the typical homogeneous high-signal intensity of a well-defined fatty lesion *(arrows).* The lesion signal intensity is similar to that of the subcutaneous and marrow fat. *Right,* Acute synovitis and synovial hyperplasia of the left long finger in a 52-year-old woman. Coronal T2-weighted MR image shows increased signal of the thickened synovium of the tendon sheath *(arrows).*

20. Does MRI have a role in monitoring the treatment response of inflammatory arthropathies?
    Perhaps. The role of MRI is still evolving. Inflamed synovium can be demonstrated on T2-weighted images (see figure on bottom right of previous page). Subtle changes in the synovium, articular cartilage, and bone can be detected before they are apparent radiographically. The use of dynamic gadolinium-DTPA enhancement to identify active pannus appears to be a promising technique.

BIBLIOGRAPHY

1. Berquist TH: Hand and wrist. In Berquist TH (ed): MRI of the Musculoskeletal System, 3rd ed. Philadelphia, Lippincott-Raven, 1996, pp 673–734.
2. Resnick D, Pettersson H (eds): Skeletal Radiology. London, Merit Communications, 1992.
3. Gilula LA, Yin Y (eds): Imaging of the Hand and Wrist. Philadelphia, W.B. Saunders, 1996.
4. Helms CA. Fundamentals of Skeletal Radiology, 2nd ed. Philadelphia, W.B. Saunders, 1995.
5. Libson E, Bloom RA, Husband JE, Stoker DJ: Metastatic tumors of the bones of the hands and feet. Skel Radiol 16:387-392, 1987.
6. Peh WCG, Truong NP, Totty WG, Gilula LA: Magnetic resonance imaging of benign soft tissue masses of the hand and wrist. Clin Radiol 50:519–525, 1995.
7. Poznanski AK: The Hand in Radiologic Diagnosis, 2nd ed. Philadelphia, W.B. Saunders, 1984.
8. Resnick D. Diagnosis of Bone and Joint Disorders. Philadelphia, W.B. Saunders, 1995.
9. Van Holsbeeck M, Introcaso JH (eds): Musculoskeletal Ultrasound. St. Louis, Mosby, 1991.
10. Winalski CS, Palmer WE, Rosenthal DI, Weissman BN: Magnetic resonance imaging of rheumatoid arthritis. Radiol Clin North Am 34:243–258, 1996.

89. ANESTHESIA

Rosemary Hickey, M.D., and Somayaji Ramamurthy, M.D.

1. Describe the relevant anatomy for upper extremity brachial plexus blocks.
    The brachial plexus is formed by the anterior primary divisions of the fifth to eighth cervical nerves and the first thoracic nerve, with frequent contributions from the fourth cervical and second thoracic nerves. The cervical nerve **roots** reorganize into superior, middle, and inferior brachial plexus **trunks**. The trunks undergo a separation into anterior and posterior **divisions**. As these divisions enter the axilla, they give way to **cords**. The posterior divisions of all three trunks unite to form the posterior cord; the anterior divisions of the superior and middle trunks form the lateral cord; and the medial cord is the anterior division of the inferior trunk. At the lateral border of the pectoralis minor muscle, the three cords reorganize to give rise to **peripheral nerves** of the upper extremity, including the musculocutaneous, radial, median, and ulnar nerves.

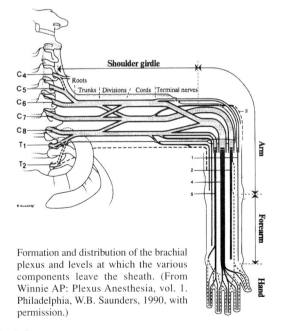

Formation and distribution of the brachial plexus and levels at which the various components leave the sheath. (From Winnie AP: Plexus Anesthesia, vol. 1. Philadelphia, W.B. Saunders, 1990, with permission.)

2. What is the concept of plexus anesthesia?
    Plexus anesthesia provides a system of single-injection techniques for blocking the brachial plexus. The concept is based on the fact that a fascial envelope, which extends continuously from the

intervertebral foramina to the distal axilla, invests the brachial plexus. This fascial sheath may be entered with a single injection of a local anesthetic; the extent of anesthesia depends on the level of injection and the volume of local anesthetic injected at that level.

3. What parts of the brachial plexus are anesthetized by the interscalene, subclavian perivascular, and axillary techniques of brachial plexus block?

The interscalene block anesthetizes the roots, the subclavian perivascular technique the trunks, and the axillary technique the cords of the brachial plexus.

4. What is the interscalene groove? How is it located?

It is located between the anterior and middle scalene muscles. The block needle is inserted in this groove at the level of C6 (which is determined by extending a line laterally from the cricoid cartilage) in performing an interscalene or subclavian perivascular block. To locate this groove, the patient is placed in the supine position with the head turned opposite to the side to be blocked. The patient is instructed to raise his or her head slightly to make the sternocleidomastoid muscle prominent. The anesthesiologist then palpates the posterior border of the sternocleidomastoid muscle and asks the patient to relax. The palpating fingers are then rolled laterally across the belly of the sternocleidomastoid muscle until the interscalene groove is located.

5. Although the block needle enters the interscalene groove for both interscalene and subclavian perivascular blocks, the needle direction differs. Describe the needle direction for each.

For the interscalene block, the block needle is inserted into the interscalene groove perpendicular to the skin in every plane, with a slight caudad direction. For the subclavian perivascular block, the block needle is inserted in the interscalene groove in a directly caudad direction.

6. How is the correct location of the needle in the interscalene or subclavian perivascular space identified?

Elicitation of a paresthesia in the distribution of the brachial plexus roots (interscalene block) or trunks (subclavian perivascular block) indicates the correct needle position within the brachial plexus fascia. The patient may describe the paresthesia as an electric shock sensation in the arm or hand. A nerve stimulator also may be used to identify correct needle placement. The negative terminal of the nerve stimulator is attached to the block needle, and the positive electrode is attached to an electrode on the side of the chest opposite to the arm that is being anesthetized. The needle is advanced until a muscle contraction in the arm or hand identifies the part of the brachial plexus being stimulated. The needle is then advanced until the maximal contraction is identified.

7. What is the "plumb bob" technique of brachial plexus block?

The block needle is introduced at the midpoint of the clavicle and directed perpendicular to the skin in a posterior direction. With the patient supine, this direction is directly toward the floor, following the line of insertion that a plumb bob would generate. If necessary, the needle can be rotated in small steps through an arc of approximately 30° in a more cephalad or caudad direction until a paresthesia is elicited.

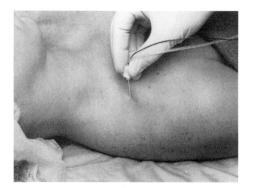

Blockade of the brachial plexus via the plumb bob supraclavicular technique. (From Mulroy MF, Thompson GE: Supraclavicular approach. In Hahn MB, McQuillan PM, Sheplock GJ (eds): Regional Anesthesia: An Atlas of Anatomy and Techniques. St. Louis, Mosby, 1996, pp 101–106, with permission.)

8. Describe the axillary technique of brachial plexus block.

The patient is placed in the supine position. The arm is abducted to 90°, and the forearm is flexed, with the dorsum of the hand lying on the table next to the patient's head. The axillary artery is palpated and followed proximally until it disappears under the pectoralis major muscle. With the index finger over the pulse, the brachial plexus sheath is penetrated with the block needle, and the needle is advanced until one of four endpoints is achieved:

1. A distinctive click is felt as the needle penetrates the brachial plexus sheath, with the short bevel of the block needle contributing to the perception of the click.

2. Paresthesia is elicited in the distribution of the median, radial, or ulnar nerves.

3. Arterial blood is aspirated, indicating puncture of the axillary artery. When arterial blood is aspirated, the block needle may be advanced and the injection made behind the artery; alternatively, half of the local anesthetic can be injected behind the artery and half after withdrawing the needle to the front of the artery.

4. A nerve stimulator may be used to localize nerves within the axillary sheath. The specific muscle twitch response that is elicited identifies the nerve being stimulated. A contraction of an appropriate muscle group in the hand or forearm at a current of 0.5 amps or less indicates proper placement of the block needle within the brachial plexus sheath.

9. What is the multiple compartment concept?

Thompson and Rorie described the presence of septae that extend inward from the brachial plexus sheath and create multiple compartments around the neurovascular bundle. These septae inhibit the spread of local anesthetic when it is deposited in a single injection technique (as popularized by Winnie). Other authors, however, have not observed septae or have found them to be thin and incomplete.

10. What is the advantage of using a catheter technique for brachial plexus block? How is it done?

The insertion of a catheter allows repeated injections of local anesthetic for long surgical procedures. In addition, continuous infusions of analgesic concentrations of local anesthetic may be continued for postoperative pain relief. A blunt-tip needle and catheter set (Contiplex) may be used; identification of a fascial click signifies entrance into the brachial plexus sheath. The proper position of the catheter may be tested by injecting 2–4 ml of cold (refrigerated, 4–6° C) normal saline through the catheter. The saline elicits a short but distinct cold paresthesia into the arm and/or hand, indicating correct position of the catheter. Alternatively, paresthesia or nerve stimulator techniques may be used to identify correct placement of the advancing needle.

11. What determines the choice of local anesthetic for brachial plexus block?

The choice of local anesthetic is based on desired duration of anesthesia, necessity of motor block, and any history of local anesthetic allergy. Lidocaine and mepivacaine are useful for outpatient surgical procedures when the desired duration of anesthesia is 2 hours or less. For longer procedures, a combination of mepivacaine and tetracaine (made by adding 60 mg of tetracaine crystals to 40 ml of 1.0% mepivacaine) is useful. Cockings used 1.5% mepivacaine in a volume of 50 ml and reported a 99% success rate with a transarterial technique. The addition of epinephrine in a concentration of 1:200,000 is useful in prolonging the duration of lidocaine or mepivacaine. It is also useful for the early detection of an intravascular injection, particularly in a technique such as transarterial axillary block, in which the axillary artery is deliberately punctured. Bupivacaine and the new local anesthetic ropivacaine are useful for long procedures (> 4 hours) or when prolonged postoperative anesthesia is desirable.

12. What is ropivacaine? What is its advantage over bupivacaine?

Ropivacaine is the only local anesthetic prepared as the pure s-isomer rather than a racemic mixture. Toxicity studies show that ropivacaine is less cardiotoxic than bupivacaine, although ropivacaine possesses some dysrhythmogenic potential. In a concentration of 0.5%, it has been shown to be an effective agent for brachial plexus block with an onset and duration similar to bupivacaine. Both are long-acting agents that produce profound sensory and motor block.

13. What is the purpose of alkalinization of a local anesthetic?

It has been used to improve onset time and with brachial plexus blocks has produced conflicting results. The principle is that raising the pH increases the percentage of the nonionized free-base form of the anesthetic. This form crosses the nerve cell membrane to reach the site of action of local anesthetics. Although not all studies have demonstrated a benefit of alkalinization, one recent study noted that alkalinization shortened the onset of anesthesia in several nerve distributions.

14. What potential complications are associated with interscalene block?

Some of the main complications of interscalene block include subarachnoid injection, epidural injection, injection into the vertebral artery, pnuemothorax, cervical sympathetic block (Horner's syndrome), recurrent laryngeal nerve block (hoarseness), and phrenic nerve block. Complications that may occur with each technique of brachial plexus block include local anesthetic overdose, allergic reaction to the local anesthetic, intravascular injection, hematoma formation, and nerve trauma.

15. What is the mechanism of phrenic nerve block? How can it be diagnosed? How common is it after interscalene block?

Phrenic nerve block may result from diffusion of local anesthetic cephalad to involve the more proximal cervical roots (C3, C4, and C5) or from an improperly performed block with local anesthetic deposited outside the brachial plexus sheath, anterior to the anterior scalene muscle. Ultrasonography or conventional x-ray technique may be used for diagnosis. Chest radiographs are taken in inspiration and expiration, and the position of the diaphragm is compared. A phrenic nerve block is indicated by little or no movement between inspiration and expiration. Alternatively, a double-exposure technique may be used. The patient is instructed to take a full, deep inspiration, and the first image is taken. The patient is then asked to perform a complete expiration, and a second image is recorded on the same film, thus allowing evaluation of diaphragm movement between inspiration and expiration. One study noted a 100% incidence of ipsilateral hemidiaphragmatic paresis diagnosed by ultrasonography in a group of patients receiving interscalene blocks. Although generally no treatment is required for phrenic nerve block, decreases in pulmonary function (approximately 25% decrease in forced vital capacity and forced expiratory reserve volume at 1 second) may occur. Interscalene blocks should be avoided, therefore, in patients who cannot tolerate reduction in pulmonary function, particularly patients in whom the opposite hemidiaphragm is already paralyzed.

16. How is injection into the vertebral artery and epidural or subarachnoid spaces avoided with an interscalene block?

Careful aspiration before injection and a slightly caudad needle direction lessen the likelihood of inadvertent injection into the vertebral artery and epidural or subarachnoid spaces.

17. If the subclavian artery is punctured in performing a subclavian perivascular block, the block needle should be redirected in which direction to locate the brachial plexus trunks?

The needle should be redirected more dorsally, because the subclavian artery lies anterior to the trunks of the brachial plexus.

18. How is the risk of pnuemothorax minimized in performing a subclavian perivascular block?

The principal cause of this complication is a needle direction that drifts medially toward the cupula of the lung; this direction should be avoided.

19. How is a pnuemothorax treated if it develops as a complication of interscalene or subclavian perivascular brachial plexus block?

If the pneumothorax is small, the patient is given oxygen and observed, provided that positive pressure ventilation does not have to be initiated for general anesthesia with a failed block. If the pneumothorax is larger than 20%, aspiration through a small-gauge catheter followed by patient observation is often all that is necessary. In rare cases, a chest tube is required for reexpansion of the lung.

20. What nerve distribution is frequently missed when an interscalene block is performed?

The ulnar nerve distribution may be difficult to anesthetize with an interscalene block because the block is performed at the level of C6, which is cephalad to the derivation of the ulnar nerve (C8–T1).

21. What are the advantages of an axillary block compared with an interscalene or subclavian perivascular block?

An axillary block is performed remote from the neck and thorax; thus, the site-related complications of blocks above the clavicle (interscalene and subclavian perivascular) are avoided. Such complications include cervical sympathetic block, phrenic nerve block, recurrent laryngeal nerve block, and vertebral, epidural, and subarachnoid injection. The location of the nerves of the brachial plexus is superficial in the axilla, leading to relatively easy identification of anatomic landmarks. One disadvantage is that a larger volume of local anesthetic is required for an axillary block than for an interscalene or subclavian perivascular block.

22. Which nerves are frequently missed with an axillary block? Why?

The musculocutaneous nerve is frequently missed with an axillary block because the musculocutaneous nerve leaves the brachial plexus high in the axilla, which may be proximal to the insertion of the block needle. Thus, the local anesthetic may not reach the nerve, particularly if a low-volume technique is used. If it is necessary to block the musculocutaneous nerve, a separate injection is made by reinserting the needle superior to the axillary artery and injecting 5–8 ml of local anesthetic into the substance of the coracobrachialis muscle. The intercostobrachial nerve is derived from T2, which is not a part of the brachial plexus and must be blocked separately. This nerve is blocked by a subcutaneous skin wheal superficial to the axillary artery pulse, from the anterior to the posterior axillary fold. This injection also blocks the medial brachial cutaneous nerve, which also leaves the brachial plexus high in the axilla. Block of the intercostobrachial and medial brachial cutaneous nerves provides analgesia of the upper inner aspect of the arm and allows more comfortable use of a pneumatic tourniquet.

23. If a postoperative nerve deficit may have been caused by the anesthetic, what should be done?

A careful neurologic exam should be performed, and its results should be documented. An EMG, if done within 3 weeks of injury, may help to establish preexisting pathology if there is evidence of denervation of muscles. The EMG should be repeated 3 weeks after the block and surgery. If a patient had a normal preoperative study or a normal EMG soon after surgery but developed an abnormal EMG 3 weeks after the performance of the block, the block or surgical procedure (the procedure itself or some other incident at the time of surgery, such as improper positioning or tourniquet use) may be the cause of the nerve damage. Early performance of electrodiagnostic studies, along with thorough neurologic evaluation, is of great benefit in establishing the cause of the problem.

24. Describe how the ulnar, median, and radial nerves can be blocked around the elbow.

The **ulnar nerve** is blocked behind the medial epicondyle, where it is palpable, using a 1.5-cm, 25-gauge needle and 5 ml of the local anesthetic agent. Avoid impaling the nerve on the bone to prevent damage to the nerve.

The **median nerve** is blocked by introducing a 3.8-cm, 22-gauge short-beveled needle medial to the artery, slightly above the level of a line drawn between the epicondyles. The nerve is identified by paresthesias or a nerve stimulator, and 5–10 ml of local anesthetic is injected.

The **radial nerve** is blocked 3–4 cm above the lateral epicondyle, where it is close to the distal humerus, after piercing the lateral intermuscular septum. A 3.8-cm, 22-gauge needle is introduced at this level, and 5–10 ml of local anesthetic is injected after the nerve is identified by paresthesias or a nerve stimulator.

25. How are wrist blocks performed?

The **median nerve** is blocked by inserting a 1.5-cm, 25-gauge needle between the palmaris longus and flexor carpi radialis tendons at the level of the ulnar styloid process or the proximal crease of the wrist. In the absence of the palmaris longus, the needle is inserted on the ulnar side of the flexor carpi radialis tendon. After paresthesia is obtained, 5 ml of local anesthetic is injected, taking care to inject the anesthetic around the nerve rather than directly within the substance of the nerve.

The **ulnar nerve** is blocked by inserting a 1.5-cm, 25-gauge needle at the level of the proximal crease of the wrist, just radial to the flexor carpi ulnaris tendon, which is made prominent by active flexion of the wrist. After obtaining paresthesia, 5 ml of local anesthetic is injected, again taking care not to inject directly within the substance of the nerve. The dorsal cutaneous nerve can be blocked by subcutaneous infiltration of approximately 5 ml of local anesthetic, beginning at the site where the ulnar nerve was blocked and extending the infiltration to the midpoint of the dorsum of the wrist.

The **superficial branch of the radial nerve** is blocked by subcutaneous infiltration with 5–7 ml of local anesthetic, starting radial to the radial artery and extending around to the midpoint of the dorsum of the wrist.

26. Why should a ring block be avoided to anesthetize a digit?

A circumferential block around the base of the digit may result in gangrene secondary to compression of the digital arteries, even if no vasopressor drug has been added to the local anesthetic.

27. How can a digital block be obtained?

In the **volar approach** a skin wheal is made directly over the flexor tendon just proximal to the distal palmar crease, and 2–3 ml of local anesthetic without epinephrine is injected on each side of the flexor tendons where the digital neurovascular bundles are located.

In the **dorsal approach**, which is a less painful method of blocking the digital nerves, the needle is inserted to the side of the extensor tendon, just proximal to the web. A skin wheal is made, and 1 ml of local anesthetic is injected superficial to the extensor hood to block the dorsal nerve. The needle is then advanced toward the palm until its tip is palpable beneath the volar skin at the base of the finger, just distal to the web. Another 1 ml of local anesthetic is injected at this site to block the volar digital nerve. Before the needle is removed, it is redirected across the extensor tendon to the opposite side of the finger, and a small skin wheal is made overlying the other dorsal digital nerve. The needle is then withdrawn and reintroduced into the skin wheal on the opposite side of the finger, and the same technique is repeated. Care should be taken to use small amounts of local anesthetic to avoid creating a circumferential ring block, which may result in vascular impairment of the digit.

28. Describe the technique for performing a Bier block.

A dual tourniquet is placed on the upper arm of the side to be blocked. An intravenous line is placed with a 20-gauge plastic cannula and a heparin lock attached. The arm is elevated and exsanguinated with an Esmarch bandage, starting from the fingers and proceeding all the way to the tourniquet. The proximal tourniquet is then inflated, and the Esmarch bandage is removed. The local anesthetic is then slowly injected through the cannula. Lidocaine, 3 mg/kg given as 0.5% without preservative, provides anesthesia within 4–6 minutes and lasts as long as the tourniquet is inflated. The proximal tourniquet is left inflated for 20 minutes or until the patient notices discomfort. The distal tourniquet is then inflated, and when its inflation is confirmed, the proximal tourniquet is deflated. Because the distal tourniquet is applied over an anesthetized area, the patient is not likely to experience discomfort for about 40 minutes. At the completion of the surgical procedure, the tourniquet is deflated for 15 seconds, reinflated for 30 seconds, and deflated again, especially if the duration of anesthesia was 20 minutes or less. If the procedure lasts longer than 40 minutes, the tourniquet can be safely deflated without reinflation.

29. What are the advantages of a Bier block?

The Bier block is technically easy to perform and suitable for outpatient surgery. Bilateral blocks can be done safely. Rapid return of motor function enables the surgeon to evaluate the results.

30. List the major disadvantages of the Bier block technique.

1. **Tourniquet pain.** Even with the use of the double cuff, pain due to the tourniquet limits use of this procedure in operations lasting more than 1 hour.

2. **Problems with tourniquet release.** When the tourniquet is released, a large bolus of anesthetic enters the systemic circulation. This brief elevation of anesthetic level in the blood may produce systemic toxic reactions, including convulsions and cardiac irregularities. The longer the tourniquet remains inflated, the lower the anesthetic blood level. If the cuff is released for 15 seconds, reinflated, and then released again, the peak blood level is lowered and the possibility of systemic reaction is decreased. However, if the tourniquet pressure is decreased gradually, when it reaches a level below arterial and above venous pressure, local anesthetic enters the circulation, producing toxic blood levels.

3. **Loss of anesthesia after cuff deflation.** The duration of postinflation anesthesia is only 5–10 minutes, which may be inadequate in some procedures if the surgeon wants to attain hemostasis and then close the wound.

4. **Equipment problems.** Equipment must be tested and the tourniquet calibrated before use. Once the tourniquet is inflated, the local anesthetic is injected only after the absence of the radial pulse is confirmed. If the proximal and distal cuffs are not properly identified and labeled as such, tourniquet pain is likely to be a problem. Constant vigilance is necessary to make sure that the equipment is in working order and to avoid accidental disconnection and deflation of the cuff.

BIBLIOGRAPHY

1. Brown DL, Cahill DR, Bridenbaugh DL: Supraclavical or nerve block: Anatomic analysis of a method to prevent pnuemothorax. Anesth Analg 76:530–534, 1993.
2. Cockings E, Moore P, Lewis RC: Transarterial brachial plexus blockade using 50 ml of 1.5% mepivacaine. Reg Anesth 12:159–164, 1987.
3. Hickey R, Hoffman J, Ramamurthy S: A comparison of ropivacaine 0.5% and bupivacaine 0.5% for brachial plexus block. Anesthesiology 74:639–642, 1991.
4. Hickey R, Ramamurthy S: The diagnosis of phrenic nerve block on chest x-ray by a double exposure technique. Anesthesiology 70:704–707, 1989.
5. Quinlan JJ, Oleksey K, Murphy Fl: Alkalinization of mepivacaine for axillary block. Anesth Analg 74: 371–374, 1992.
6. Ramamurthy S, Hickey R: Anesthesia. In Green DP (ed): Operative Hand Surgery, 3rd ed. New York, Churchill Livingstone, 1993, pp 25–52.
7. Thompson GE, Rorie DK: Functional anatomy of the brachial plexus sheaths. Anesthesiology 59:117–122, 1993.
8. Urmey WF: Upper extremity blocks. In Brown DL (ed): Regional Anesthesia and Analgesia. Philadelphia, W.B. Saunders, 1996, pp 254–278.
9. Urmey WF, McDonald M: Hemidiaphragmatic paresis during interscalene brachial plexus block: Effects on pulmonary function and chest wall mechanics. Anesth Analg 74:352–357, 1992.
10. Winnie AP: Plexus Anesthesia. Philadelphia, W.B. Saunders, 1990.

90. METACARPAL AND PHALANGEAL FRACTURES

Norman Weinzweig, M.D., and Mark H. Gonzalez, M.D.

Hand fractures can be complicated by deformity from no treatment, stiffness from overtreatment, and both deformity and stiffness from poor treatment.

A.B. Swanson (1970)

1. Describe the epidemiology of fractures of the metacarpals and phalanges.

Fractures of the metacarpals and phalanges are the most common fractures of the skeletal system, accounting for 10% of all fractures in several large series. They are most common in men in the second and third decades of life. Depending on the patient population, fractures are most likely due to either industrial accidents or personal trauma.

2. What is the distribution of fractures according to location?

The distal phalanx is the most commonly fractured bone in the hand (not even considering nailbed injuries), followed by the metacarpals. The middle phalanx is the least commonly fractured because of its protected position and the higher proportion of cortical to cancellous bone. Metacarpals of the border digits are more exposed and sustain more fractures than the central digits. On the other hand, phalanges of the central digits are longer and sustain more fractures than the border digits. In adults, metacarpal fractures are more common than phalangeal fractures, whereas in children the converse is true. In children, one-third of fractures are epiphyseal and 80% Salter II. Fracture stability is seen in three-fourths of phalangeal fractures, one-third of metacarpal fractures, and two-thirds of fractures in children. Approximately 20% of metacarpal and phalangeal fractures are intraarticular.

3. How are fractures classified?

- Bones involved: distal, middle, or proximal phalanx, metacarpal
- Location within bone: base, shaft, neck, head
- Pattern: transverse, spiral, oblique, comminuted
- Displaced or nondisplaced
- Intraarticular or extraarticular
- Closed or open
- Stable or unstable
- Deformity: angulation, rotation, shortening
- Associated injuries: skin, tendon, nerve, vessel

4. Describe the initial evaluation of patients with hand fractures.

Crucial to diagnosis and treatment of hand fractures are a thorough history and physical examination. History should include handedness, occupation, avocation, mechanism of injury (e.g., crush injury with compartment syndrome), time since injury ("golden period"), and place of injury (e.g., home, farm, industry). Physical examination often provides the diagnosis and should include local tenderness, swelling, deformity (angulation, rotation, shortening), alignment (all fingertips must point toward the scaphoid), range of motion (active/passive flexion and extension, intrinsics), and neurovascular status.

5. How is rotation of a finger fracture evaluated?

With the fingers partially flexed, the fingernails should form a gentle arc. The digits should point toward the scaphoid without overlap.

6. What type of radiographs should be obtained?

Radiographs should include anteroposterior (AP) and lateral views of the individual digit, oblique views when the fracture is close to or involves a joint, pre- and postreduction views, and special views as indicated, such as a Brewerton view for clarification of ligament-avulsion injuries of the metacarpal head, a Robert view (true AP of thumb metacarpal with hand in maximal pronation) for the first metacarpal-trapezium joint (Bennett's fracture), and a reverse Robert view for the fifth metacarpal-hamate joint.

7. What is the Salter-Harris classification of epiphyseal injuries in children?

Salter-Harris I: occurs in early childhood when the growth plate is thick with large hypertrophying chondrocytes and a weak zone of provisional calcification. The fracture occurs through the plate itself, with separation of the epiphysis from the metaphysis, usually by a pure shear mechanism. Prognosis is good.

Salter-Harris II: usually occurs after age 10, through the plate and metaphysis. The epiphysis is separated, and a small fragment of metaphysis is broken off with it. Tension by shear or avulsion with an angular force causes cartilage failure, whereas compression causes metaphyseal failure.

Salter-Harris III: usually occurs after age 10. An intraarticular fracture of the epiphysis occurs secondary to an avulsion force, without involvement of the epiphyseal plate. This type of fracture is associated with a poor prognosis unless accurate reduction is performed.

Salter-Harris IV: occurs at any age; rare in the hand. Fracture occurs from the articular surface through the epiphysis plate and metaphysis by compression loading of a portion of the articular surface. Prognosis is poor without anatomic alignment.

Salter-Harris V: occurs at any age; extremely rare in the hand. A compression fracture occurs with damage confined to the epiphyseal plate by severe axial load. The prognosis is poor because of potential growth arrest.

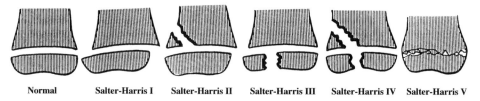

| Normal | Salter-Harris I | Salter-Harris II | Salter-Harris III | Salter-Harris IV | Salter-Harris V |

The Salter-Harris classification of epiphyseal fractures. (From Lister G: The Hand: Diagnosis and Indications, 2nd ed. Edinburgh, Churchill Livingstone, 1984, p 50, with permission.)

8. Describe the general principles for management of hand fractures.

First and foremost, treat the patient, *not* the radiograph. In general, a force of sufficient magnitude to fracture bone can cause significant injury to enveloping structures such as the intrinsic muscles, tendons, ligaments, and neurovascular structures. In some cases (e.g., roller or crushing injuries), decompression must be performed in a timely fashion.

Most fractures can be treated successfully by nonoperative means. They are functionally stable before or after closed reduction and do well with splintage and early mobilization. The goal is restoration of normal function with the three Rs: reduction, retention, and rehabilitation. After accurate fracture reduction, the hand should be immobilized in the intrinsic plus or safe position with extremity elevation to minimize edema. Movement of the uninvolved fingers should be permitted to prevent stiffness. An exercise program should be directed toward the specific fracture with early mobilization of the injured finger. Do not forget that the proximal interphalangeal joint is the most important joint in the hand.

9. How are stable fractures managed?

Stable fractures can often be treated by buddy taping and/or splinting. Repeat radiographs are performed at 7–10 days to check the reduction.

10. What is an unstable fracture?

Unstable fractures cannot be reduced with a closed method or, if reduced, cannot be held in the reduced position without supplemental fixation. Closed or open reduction and internal fixation are required to provide stability and allow early mobilization.

11. How are unstable fractures managed?

Initially unstable fractures can be reduced and converted to a stable position by external immobilization (cast, cast with metal outrigger splint, anteroposterior plaster splint), closed reduction and percutaneous pinning (CRPP), or open reduction and internal fixation (ORIF).

12. What is the safe position for immobilization of the hand? Why is this important?

The metacarpophalangeal (MCP) joints of the digits are maintained in maximal or near maximal flexion. The head of the MCP is cam-shaped, and flexion maintains the collateral ligaments at maximal length. When splinted in extension, the collateral ligaments can shorten, causing a loss of flexion. The interphalangeal (IP) joints of the digits are splinted in near full extension. Splinting in flexion allows the development of checkrein ligaments, causing volar plate contracture and permanent loss of flexion at the IP joints.

13. Describe the different methods of internal fixation.

Fracture Stabilization Techniques

	INDICATIONS (FRACTURE TYPES)	ADVANTAGES	DISADVANTAGES
Kirschner pins	Transverse Oblique Spiral	Available and versatile Easy to insert Minimal dissection Percutaneous insertion	Lacks rigidity May loosen May distract the fracture Pin tract infection Requires external support Splint/therapy awkward
Composite wiring	Transverse Oblique Spiral	More rigid than Kirschner pins Low profile Simple and available	Pin/wire migration Secondary removal (sometimes) Exposure may be significant
Intramedullary device	Transverse Short oblique	No special equipment Easy to insert No pin protrusion Minimal dissection	Rotational instability Rod migration
Interfragmentary fixation	Long oblique Spiral	Low profile Rigid	Special equipment Little margin for error
Plate and screws	Multiple fractures with soft tissue injury or bone loss Markedly displaced shaft fractures (especially border metacarpals) Intra- and periarticular fractures Reconstruction for nonunion and malunion	Rigid fixation Restore/maintain length	Exacting technique Special equipment Extensive exposure May require removal Refracture Bulky
External fixation	Restore length for comminution and bone loss Soft tissue injury/loss Infected nonunion	Preserves length Allows access to bone, soft tissue Percutaneous insertion Direct manipulation of fracture avoided	Pin tract infections Osteomyelitis Overdistraction: nonunion Neurovascular injury Fractures through pin holes Loosening

From Green DP (ed): Operative Hand Surgery, 3rd ed. New York, Churchill Livingstone, 1984, p 705, with permission.

14. What is the apex dorsal bending rigidity (Newton-meters^2) for the different internal fixation techniques in metacarpal fractures?

Dorsal plate and lag screw (0.55), dorsal plate (0.50), and crossed K-wire, K-wire and intraosseous wire, or intraosseous wire (0.07–0.08). Although the latter three techniques do not allow true rigid fixation, they do allow bony union and thus fracture treatment.

15. What are the indications for internal fixation?
- Uncontrollable rotation, angulation, or shortening
- Multiple digit fractures that are difficult to control
- Displaced intraarticular fractures involving more than 15–20% of the articular surface
- Fracture-subluxations of the thumb and little finger carpometacarpal joints
- Unstable fractures: failure of closed manipulation, as in spiral fractures of the proximal phalanx or transverse metacarpal fractures
- Metacarpal head fractures
- Open fractures

16. What are the advantages of K-wire fixation?
- Easiest technically
- Requires minimal dissection
- Universally available
- Much more forgiving than other methods
- Early motion without rigid fixation
- Supplements other methods of fixation
- "Bail-out" after failure of more complex techniques

17. What are the disadvantages of K-wire fixation?
- K-wires may loosen
- K-wires may distract fracture fragments
- Lateral bands may be skewered
- Cannot obtain true compression or rigid fixation
- Multiple attempts may convert a simple closed fracture to a comminuted open fracture that is impossible to fixate
- Pin tract infection

18. How soon can motion be started?
For nondisplaced fractures treated in closed fashion, motion can be started within 3 weeks if the fracture is stable. Midshaft proximal phalangeal fractures require 5–7 weeks for complete bony healing. Midshaft middle phalangeal fractures require 10–14 weeks for complete bony healing of the exceedingly hard cortical portion of the bone (same as scaphoid fractures).

19. How long do fractures requiring open reduction or severely comminuted fractures with disruption of the periosteum take to heal?
Twice as long as simple fractures.

20. Describe the treatment of extraarticular fractures of the distal phalanx.
The distal phalanx is the most commonly fractured bone in the hand. The middle finger and thumb are most frequently involved in fracture. The mechanism of injury is usually a crush injury with significant soft tissue involvement. Comminuted distal phalangeal fractures generally demonstrate twice as many fragments intraoperatively as on radiographs. Anatomic reduction is usually not necessary unless the articular surfaces are involved. Splinting is performed for protection and pain control and discontinued after 3–4 weeks. The two more proximal joints are mobilized to prevent stiffness. Epiphyseal plate injuries are treated by closed reduction with hyperextension. Associated nail matrix injuries are treated by drainage of the subungual hematoma, fracture reduction, and nailbed repair with 7-0 chromic suture using loupe magnification.

21. What are the deforming forces in extraarticular fractures of the middle phalanx?
Fragments are displaced by the forces of the central slip, terminal extensor tendon, and flexor digitorum superficialis (FDS) insertion. Fractures proximal to the FDS insertion angulate dorsally, whereas fractures distal to the FDS insertion angulate volarly.

22. What are the deforming forces in extraarticular fractures of the proximal phalanx? How are they treated?
Proximal phalangeal fractures angulate volarly with the interossei flexing the proximal fragment and the central slip extending the distal portion. Stable, nondisplaced, or impacted middle and proximal phalangeal fractures are treated by temporary protection with a splint followed by

dynamic splinting (buddy taping). Closed reduction and immobilization of the forearm, wrist, and injured digit as well as the adjacent digit(s) in a cast, cast with metal outrigger, or gutter splint are usually adequate. Internal fixation may be used. Various traction techniques or external fixation methods are used for markedly comminuted fractures or bone loss. Avoid excessive traction, which may prevent bony union.

23. How are closed diaphyseal fractures of the phalanges treated?

Acceptable angulation of diaphyseal fractures of the proximal and middle phalanges is 10° in any plane. No malrotation can be accepted, and allowable shortening is less than 5 mm. If a fracture is minimally displaced, it may be splinted with the MCP joints in full flexion and the IP joints in near full extension. Active motion should be started in 3–4 weeks to avoid stiffness. If the fracture is displaced, closed reduction can be performed. A fracture than cannot be maintained with acceptable displacement in a splint is considered unstable. An unstable fracture can be treated with closed reduction and percutaneous pinning or open reduction and internal fixation. Options for internal fixation include intraosseous wiring, compression screws, plates, and intramedullary fixation. Diaphyseal fractures of the distal phalanx can generally be treated with closed reduction and splinting.

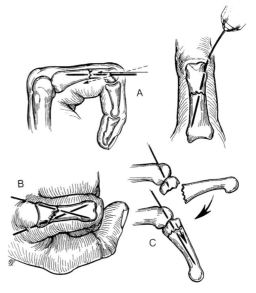

Three methods of closed reduction and percutaneous pinning of a transverse phalangeal fracture. *A*, The fracture is reduced, and a Kirschner pin is placed in the proximal phalanx in retrograde fashion. *B*, An alternative method of percutaneous pinning for fractures of the proximal one-half of the shaft; the pins are driven in anterograde fashion. *C*, Technique for closed reduction and percutaneous pin fixation useful for extraarticular fractures near the base of the proximal phalanx in which Kirschner pins cross the MP joint. (From Green DP (ed): Operative Hand Surgery, 3rd ed. New York, Churchill Livingstone, 1993, p. 732, with permission.)

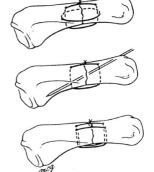

Intraosseous wire configurations. *Top*, 90-90 wires. *Center*, Single loop with supplemental Kirschner pin. *Bottom*, Parallel loops. (From Green DP (ed): Operative Hand Surgery, 3rd ed. New York, Churchill Livingstone, 1993, p. 738, with permission.)

24. What are the complications of phalangeal fractures?

1. Loss of motion results from tendon adherence at the fracture site and contracture, especially at the proximal interphalangeal (PIP) joint level. Extensor tenolysis rarely improves active PIP

joint extension. With flexor adherence, either excise the FDS or resort to PIP fusion as a salvage procedure for severe flexion contracture.

2. Malunion secondary to volar angulation after fractures near the base of the proximal phalanx. Treatment consists of an opening wedge osteotomy and bone graft.

3. Malrotation after spiral or oblique proximal and middle phalangeal fractures. Treatment consists of an osteotomy at the metacarpal or phalangeal levels.

4. Pin tract infection

5. Nonunion results from either bone loss, soft tissue interposition, inadequate immobilization, or distraction at the fracture site. Treatment involves resection of nonviable bone and bone grafting.

25. What is the best view for diagnosing metacarpal head fractures?

Metacarpal head fractures are often difficult to diagnose. Brewerton views should be obtained if a metacarpal head fracture is suspected.

26. How are metacarpal head fractures treated?

1. Comminuted or oblique fractures with displacement require ORIF with K-wires or small screws.

2. Comminuted fractures limited to the metacarpal head distal to the ligament require early mobilization after protection for several weeks. Displaced fractures proximal to the origin of the ligament may require ORIF.

3. Collateral ligament avulsion fractures require ORIF if displaced and/or more than 20–30% of the joint surface is involved. Obtain Brewerton views.

4. Small osteochondral fracture fragments are generally excised.

27. What are possible complications of metacarpal head fractures?

• Avascular necrosis of the metacarpal head may occur after horizontal fractures.

• Epiphyseal arrest may result in shortening of the metacarpal, usually without functional loss.

28. What is a boxer's fracture?

A boxer's fracture is a metacarpal neck fracture, usually resulting from a direct blow with comminution of the volar cortex and dorsal angulation. Boxer's fracture is a misnomer because most metacarpal neck fractures involve the little and ring fingers, whereas a professional boxer is most likely to injure the middle or index fingers with a more direct central impact of the punch. This results in angulation with the apex dorsal because of the pull of the intrinsic muscles. Malunion results in loss of prominence of the metacarpal head, diminished range of motion, and a palpable metacarpal head in the palm, which causes pain with grip.

29. What is the Jahss maneuver?

The Jahss maneuver is a technique for closed reduction of metacarpal neck fractures. Sixty years ago Jahss recognized that flexing the MP joint to 90° relaxed the deforming intrinsic muscles and tightened the collateral ligaments, allowing the proximal phalanx to exert upward pressure on the metacarpal head. He applied a cast in two parts, first immobilizing the proximal metacarpal fragment and then flexing the MP and PIP joints, pushing upward on the flexed PIP joint while applying the second part. The Jahss maneuver remains the best technique for closed reduction of these fractures; however, fingers should never be maintained in the Jahss position (MP and PIP joints both flexed at 90°). Instead, after reduction the fingers should be held in an intrinsic plus splint.

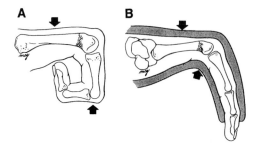

The Jahss maneuver for reduction of a metacarpal neck fracture. *A*, Arrows indicate the direction of pressure application for fracture reduction. *B*, After reduction, the fingers are held in an intrinsic plus position in an ulnar gutter splint with molding as indicated by arrows. (From Green DP (ed): Operative Hand Surgery, 3rd ed. New York, Churchill Livingstone, 1993, p. 701, with permission.)

30. How much angulation can be accepted in metacarpal neck fractures? How are they treated?

The amount of angulation that should be accepted is controversial. Angulation is unacceptable if it involves pseudoclawing of the finger on distal extension. Pseudoclawing is compensatory MCP joint hyperextension and PIP joint flexion on attempted extension of the digit. Up to 40° of angulation can be accepted in the mobile ring and little metacarpals. Closed reduction should be attempted for more than 15° of angulation. No more than 10–15° of angulation is acceptable for the index and middle metacarpals. These fractures are often associated with a lack of compensatory carpometacarpal motion. ORIF is required; crossed K-wires or tension band wiring may be used. For less than 15° of angulation, an ulnar gutter splint is applied for 10–14 days. For 15–40° of angulation, reduce and apply an ulnar gutter splint for 3 weeks. For greater than 40° of angulation,

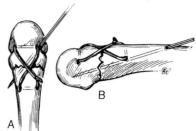

Tension band wiring *(A)* and single Kirschner pin fixation *(B)* of a metacarpal neck fracture. (From Green DP (ed): Operative Hand Surgery, 3rd ed. New York, Churchill Livingstone, 1993, p. 703, with permission.)

volar comminution, extensor lag, or unacceptable reduction, treat with percutaneous pinning. ORIF is usually not necessary. Angulation exceeding the recommended degrees can lead to a prominent metacarpal head in the palm and painful grasp. Any rotational deformity is unacceptable.

31. How are metacarpal shaft fractures treated?

Transverse fractures are usually caused by direct blows (axial loading). They demonstrate dorsal angulation secondary to the strong volar force exerted by the interosseous muscles. The more proximal the fracture, the less the angulation that can be tolerated. Oblique and spiral fractures result from torsional forces acting on the finger as a lever arm. No rotation is acceptable because as little as 5° of rotation in a metacarpal fracture may cause up to 1.5 cm of digital overlap. Up to 5 mm of shortening is acceptable. The intermetacarpal ligaments minimize the degree of shortening. Closed reduction and plaster immobilization are usually adequate. Placing a patient in a "clamdigger" or intrinsic plus splint prevents contractures. If closed reduction is unsuccessful, perform an open reduction with percutaneous pinning or another method of internal fixation, such as plating or lag screw compression. Immobility is the chief cause of stiffness.

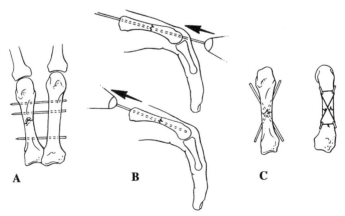

Techniques for Kirschner pin fixation of metacarpal shaft fractures. *A*, Transverse pins may be inserted percutaneously or open. *B*, Retrograde intramedullary fixation. Note that the pin is backed out so that it does not remain in the MP joint. *C*, Crossed pins *(left)* and supplemental 25-gauge stainless steel wire *(right)*. (From Green DP (ed): Operative Hand Surgery, 3rd ed. New York, Churchill Livingstone, 1993, p. 705, with permission.)

32. What are the complications of metacarpal fractures?

(1) Malunion causes dorsal angulation, which can disturb intrinsic muscle balance and produce metacarpal head prominence in the palm with pain on grasping. This complication is treated by a volar

opening wedge osteotomy and plate fixation. A rotational deformity is corrected by an osteotomy to the metacarpal base. (2) Nonunion is caused by bone loss from a gunshot wound or distraction that prevents bone approximation and healing. (3) Other complications include MCP extension contractures, intrinsic muscle contractures, pin tract infection, tendon adherence, and refracture.

33. What is a Bennett's fracture?

A Bennett's fracture is an intraarticular fracture-subluxation involving the base of the thumb metacarpal. It results in a vertical or oblique fracture through the volar beak of the metacarpal, exiting the diaphyseal-metaphyseal junction ulnarly. The strong anterior oblique ligament (volar beak ligament) stabilizes the variably sized ulnovolar fragment in anatomic position while the metacarpal fragment subluxates radially, proximally, and dorsally. The major deforming forces are the abductor pollicis longus and adductor pollicis. Supination also occurs.

34. What is the epidemiology of Bennett's fractures?

Bennett's fractures are 10 times more common in men than in women. Patients are usually in their 30s; the dominant hand is injured in 70% of cases. Most patients sustain an axial blow to the thumb with the metacarpal in some degree of flexion from a fall on an unstretched hand, striking a blow with a clenched fist, falling on a ski slope, or impact of the hand against a dashboard. Concomitant fractures are uncommon; the trapezium is most commonly involved.

35. How are Bennett's fractures treated?

Treatment requires anatomic reduction by either CRPP or ORIF and pinning or screw placement. Reduction of the fracture-dislocation is easy, but retention is difficult. Longitudinal traction is applied to the thumb metacarpal, which is radially extended and pronated with direct pressure over the fracture site. The thumb metacarpal is then stabilized by fixing it to the index metacarpal, trapezium, or both, using one or two pins—between the thumb and index metacarpals, thumb metacarpal to trapezium, thumb metacarpal to ulnovolar fragments, or any combination of the above.

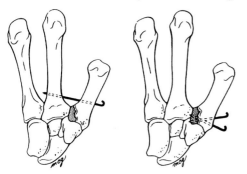

Fixation of a Bennett's fracture. *Left,* A Kirschner pin is inserted between the thumb and index metacarpals. *Right,* Pins are passed from the metacarpal shaft into the Bennett fragment. (From Green DP (ed): Operative Hand Surgery, 3rd ed. New York, Churchill Livingstone, 1993, p 749, with permission.)

36. What is a reverse Bennett's fracture?

It is an intraarticular fracture-dislocation involving the base of the little finger metacarpal. It is analogous to a Bennett's fracture of the thumb. The deforming forces are the extensor carpi ulnaris and hypothenar muscles. Anatomic reduction of the mobile carpometacarpal (CMC) joint is necessary.

37. What is a Rolando's fracture?

Rolando's fracture is an intraarticular fracture of the base of the thumb metacarpal in T, Y, or comminuted form. Treatment consists of closed or open reduction and K-wire pinning. For comminuted fractures, mold in a thumb spica cast for 3–4 weeks. A classic two-part Rolando's fracture may be reduced and interfragmentary fixation performed either with multiple K-wires or a plate. (See figure at top of next page.)

38. What role does the CMC joint of the little finger play?

The CMC joint of the little finger allows 30° of flexion and extension. Rotation allows normal cupping of the palm in grip (opposition). Inadequate reduction results in major residual functional disability with weakness of grip.

Fixation of a Rolando's fracture. *Left,* Provisional fixation is accomplished with a clamp and Kirschner pin. *Right,* The final fixation is accomplished with a T-plate (T = trapezium). (From Green DP (ed): Operative Hand Surgery, 3rd ed. New York, Churchill Livingstone, 1993, p 751, with permission.)

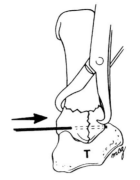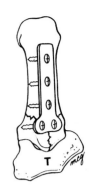

39. How are open fractures treated?

All open fractures must be cultured; patients are placed on intravenous antibiotics. Open fractures are converted to clean wounds by thorough irrigation (Hydrojet) and debridement. Fractures caused by gunshot wounds (low velocity) generally sustain minimal damage to tendons and nerves. Formal exploration of the entire bullet tract is not necessary; the entrance and exit wounds are simply cleansed. Skeletal stability is restored either primarily or as soon as possible (as in the case of extensive open injuries with multiple fractures) by simple immobilization, K-wire fixation, external fixation, or immediate bone grafting (in special cases). Severely comminuted fractures extending onto joint surfaces may discourage any form of fixation, and arthrodesis may be necessary. Soft tissue coverage may be necessary before fracture fixation or bone grafting.

40. How are fractures with segmental bone loss treated?

Fractures with segmental bone loss are treated as open fractures. Occasionally, the wound is packed open. Length and stability are maintained by K-wires or external fixation. For definitive reconstruction, the various components of the injury must be addressed. The soft tissue wound often requires flap coverage. Immediate or delayed bone reconstruction is performed with bone grafts. Nerve and tendon reconstruction and vascularized joint transfers may be necessary.

41. What is the "lag screw" technique of interfragmentary compression?

This technique provides rigid fixation and is primarily indicated for long oblique and spiral shaft fractures. It is usually indicated for fractures in which the length of the fracture line is at least twice the diameter of the bone. Lag screw fixation involves passing a screw through a gliding hole in the near fragment (nonthreaded and of wider diameter than the threads of the screw) into a smaller hole in the far fragment (tapped to the same diameter as the screw threads) which then grabs the far cortex. As the screw is tightened (lagged), the threads grip and draw the far fragment towards the near fragment, approximating the fragments and compressing the fracture. Ideally, longitudinal compressive forces are best counteracted by placing the screw 90° to the bone's long axis, and torsional stresses are best resisted by placing the screw 90° to the fracture.

BIBLIOGRAPHY

1. Green DP, Butler TE: Fractures and dislocations in the hand. In Rockwood CA, Green DP, Bucholz RW, Heckman JD (eds): Fractures in Adults. Philadelphia, Lippincott-Raven, 1996, pp 607–744.
2. Stern PS: Fractures of the metacarpals and phalanges. In Green DP (ed): Operative Hand Surgery, 3rd ed. New York, Churchill Livingstone, 1993, pp 695–758.
3. Swanson TV, Szabo RM, Anderson DD: Open hand fractures: Prognosis and classification. J Hand Surg 16A: 101–107, 1991.
4. Widgerow AD, Edinburg M, Biddulph SL: An analysis of proximal phalangeal fractures. J Hand Surg 12A: 134–139, 1987.
5. Worlock PH, Stower MJ: The incidence and pattern of hand fractures in children. J Hand Surg 11B:198–200, 1986.
6. Wray RC Jr, Glunk R: Treatment of delayed union, nonunion, and malunion of phalanges of the hand. Ann Plast Surg 22:14–18, 1989.
7. Yang SS, Gerwin M: Fractures of the hand. In Levine AM (ed): Orthopaedic Knowledge Update: Trauma. Rosemont, IL, American Academy of Orthopaedic Surgeons, 1996, pp 95–109.

91. JOINT DISLOCATIONS AND LIGAMENT INJURIES

W. Bradford Rockwell, M.D., and R. Chris Wray, Jr., M.D.

1. Explain the difference between true collateral and accessory collateral ligaments.
The thick collateral ligaments of the phalanges arise from the condyles of the proximal bone and insert on the palmar third of the distal bone and the distal lateral margin of the palmar plate. The true collateral ligament inserts distally on bone, whereas the accessory collateral ligament inserts distally on the palmar plate.

2. What soft tissue structures provide stability to the proximal interphalangeal (PIP) joint?
Soft tissue structures that form a box around the PIP joint are the collateral ligaments on either side, palmar plate, and dorsal capsule. The dorsal capsule is very thin and provides minimal stability to the joint. The collateral ligaments on the radial and ulnar sides and the palmar plate are firm structures. For dislocation to occur, at least 2 of the 3 strong structures must be disrupted.

3. How is the functional stability of a joint tested?
The stability is tested through active and passive motion. Stability during active motion suggests joint stability, although a partial ligament tear may exist. Recurrent displacement with active motion indicates major ligament disruption. The position in which displacement occurs may indicate the site of disruption. Passive motion provides the final assessment of stability. Each collateral ligament as well as the palmar plate is stressed to measure stability.

4. What are the three types of dorsal PIP dislocations?
Joint dislocations are described with respect to the distal bone in relation to the proximal bone. The three dorsal PIP dislocations are (1) subluxation with some articular surface still in contact, (2) dorsal dislocation with no articulating joint surface, indicating avulsion of the palmar plate with major bilateral split of the collateral ligaments, and (3) fracture-dislocation, which may be stable or unstable. Subluxation, dislocation, and stable fracture-dislocations are treated with closed reduction and an extension blocking splint, allowing full active motion except for the last 30° of extension. Unstable fracture-dislocations require operative repair.

5. What is the treatment for chronic PIP dorsal subluxations?
Chronic PIP dorsal subluxations may result from laxity of the PIP palmar plate or an extensor tendon imbalance, usually from a mallet deformity resulting in a swan-neck posture. If passive PIP mobilization demonstrates a distal interphalangeal (DIP) extensor lag, treatment is aimed at correcting the extensor mechanism. PIP palmar plate laxity is corrected with either palmar plate reattachment or joint tenodesis using one slip of the superficialis tendon.

6. Are dislocations of the finger DIP and thumb interphalangeal (IP) joints common?
No. These dislocations are rare and usually dorsal. The majority are treated with closed reduction and immobilization for 10–21 days before active motion is begun.

7. With an injury to another part of the hand, what anatomic difference between the metacarpophalangeal (MP) and PIP joints accounts for immobilization of MP joints in flexion and PIP joints in extension?
The metacarpal head is characterized by a cam effect in which the length of the collateral ligament attachment to the articular surface is greater with the joint flexed at least 50° than with the joint extended. The PIP joint collateral ligament possesses a uniform length. Splinting MP joints in at least 50° of flexion keeps the collateral ligaments on stretch and does not allow their shortening. PIP joint position does not affect the length of the collateral ligaments. PIP joints are splinted in extension to avoid a flexion contracture.

8. Which anatomic structures contribute to a complex or irreducible MP joint dislocation.

MP joint dislocations are most commonly dorsal and involve the index or little finger. The metacarpal head of the index finger is detached from the weak membranous portion of the palmar plate, which may become inserted between the metacarpal head and the base of the proximal phalanx. The lumbrical muscle is stretched around the radial border of the metacarpal head, and the flexor tendons are stretched around the ulnar border. The metacarpal head of the little finger is entrapped between the abductor digiti minimi and flexor digiti minimi tendons ulnarly and the lumbrical muscle and flexor tendons radially. Axial traction tightens these structures and makes reduction more difficult. MP joint flexion and axial traction may allow closed reduction.

9. Do digital carpometacarpal (CMC) dislocations occur?

The ligament configuration of the index and middle CMC joints, called the fixed unit, is highly stable. Dislocations of the digital CMC joints are uncommon. When they occur, they are usually dorsal and most commonly involve the fifth joint, followed by the the fourth. Frequently, a fifth CMC joint dislocation is accompanied by a fracture, termed *Baby Bennett's fracture-dislocation*. This fracture may be missed with only a PA radiograph and requires operative reduction and fixation.

10. What is gamekeeper's thumb?

Injury to the ulnar collateral ligament (UCL) of the thumb MP joint is common. Forced radial deviation of the thumb produces the injury, which results in trauma to the dorsal capsule, UCL, and ulnar aspect of the palmar plate. This injury is called gamekeeper's thumb or skier's thumb.

11. Describe Stener's lesion.

The UCL of the thumb MP joint has bony attachments deep to the adductor aponeurosis. In complete disruptions of the UCL from the proximal phalanx, the abductor aponeurosis may become interposed between the distal end of the UCL and the proximal phalanx, producing poor healing and persistent ligament laxity. Operative repair is required.

12. What soft tissue structure provides the most stability to the thumb CMC joint?

The saddle contour of the articular surfaces of the thumb CMC joint provides inherent intrinsic stability. The capsular thickening comprising the volar beak ligament, which passes from the trapezium to the volar beak of the thumb metacarpal, is a key structure in maintaining CMC stability.

13. Does joint subluxation occur at the thumb CMC joint?

The thumb CMC joint is also called the basal joint. Joint laxity most commonly occurs in postmenopausal women as a result of laxity of the volar beak ligament. The most common form of reconstruction uses the flexor carpi radialis (FCR) tendon as a soft tissue support for the base of the metacarpal; the rest of the tendon is interposed in the space created by excision of the trapezium.

14. What is the most common complication after joint or ligament injury?

Ligament injury requires joint immobilization and may require operative repair. Joint stiffness results and may be further worsened by intraarticular swelling and resulting fibrosis. Early joint motion minimizes postinjury stiffness, but preference must be given to joint immobilization until adequate ligament stability has developed.

BIBLIOGRAPHY

1. Abrahamsson SO, Sollerman C, Lundborg G, et al: Diagnosis of displaced ulnar collateral ligament of the metacarpophalangeal joint of the thumb. J Hand Surg 15A:457–460, 1990.
2. Dray GJ, Eaton RG: Dislocations and ligament injuries in the digits. In Green DP (ed): Operative Hand Surgery. New York, Churchill Livingstone, 1993, pp 767–798.
3. Henderson JJ, Arafa MAM: Carpometacarpal dislocation: An easily missed diagnosis. J Bone Joint Surg 69B:212–214, 1987.
4. Lubahn JD: Dorsal fracture dislocation of the proximal interphalangeal joint. Hand Clin 4:15–24, 1988.
5. Miller RJ: Dislocations and fracture dislocations of the metacarpophalangeal joint of the thumb. Hand Clin 4:45–65, 1988.
6. Vicar AJ: Proximal interphalangeal joint dislocations without fractures. Hand Clin 4:5–13, 1988.
7. Wray RC JR: Fractures and joint injuries of the hand. In McCarthy JG (ed): Plastic Surgery. Philadelphia, W.B. Saunders, 1990, pp 4593–4628.
8. Zemal NP: Metacarpal joint injuries in fingers. Hand Clin 8:745, 1992.

92. SOFT TISSUE COVERAGE OF THE HAND

Norman Weinzweig, M.D., and Jeffrey Weinzweig, M.D.

1. Which mechanisms of injury to the hand often result in significant soft tissue loss requiring reconstruction?

A plethora of destructive culprits awaits the unsuspecting hand. Examples include crush injuries, such as roller or punch press mishaps; frostbite; thermal and electrical injuries; and blast injuries. Soft tissue loss requiring reconstruction also may result from debridement for infection, excision of neoplasms, subcutaneous infiltrations of intravenous solutions, and direct injection of caustic agents.

2. What injuries present the most difficult challenges for soft tissue coverage?

Injuries involving the tactile surface of the hand with disruption of its sensory supply represent the most difficult reconstructive problems. The reconstructive goal must include restoration of sensibility if maximal function is to be achieved.

3. What are the indications for flap coverage?

A skin graft requires a suitable recipient bed, such as muscle, fascia, paratenon, or periosteum. In the absence of structures capable of revascularizing a graft, as in cases of exposed bone without periosteum or exposed tendon without paratenon, a well-vascularized flap is necessary to provide durable soft tissue coverage.

4. How is a wound prepared for flap coverage?

Pulsatile irrigation with several liters of antibiotic solution, debridement of all devitalized tissue, and eradication of infection are mandatory prior to flap coverage. Serial debridement and placement of a string of tobramycin-impregnated beads beneath a Tegaderm pouch (changed after 3–5 days) are often useful approaches in the preparation of a contaminated wound.

5. What is the significance of random and axial flaps?

In the early 1970s, Ian McGregor introduced the concept of random and axial flaps, which was a significant breakthrough in the understanding of skin vascularity. Before this time, flap size and design were largely predicated on fortuitous length-to-width ratios on a trial-and-error basis, ranging from 1:1 on the extremities to 5:1 on the face. A random pattern flap "lacks any significant bias in its vascular pattern" and "is subject to the restrictions hitherto generally accepted in flap design," whereas an axial pattern flap "has an anatomically recognized arteriovenous system running along its axis" and, therefore, "is not subject to many of the restrictions that apply to random pattern flaps."

6. Describe the venous anatomy of the upper extremity.

Three venous systems exist in the forearm: the superficial epifascial system, venae comitantes, and perforating veins. The superficial system consists of the cephalic vein, basilic vein, and communicating veins between them. The venae comitantes are paired veins that travel parallel to the radial, ulnar, anterior interosseous, and posterior interosseous arteries deep to the fascia. The perforating veins connect the superficial and deep systems. The superficial system and venae comitantes contain bicuspid valves, preventing retrograde filling. The valves in the communicating system are less constant and usually unicuspid.

7. How does blood bypass the valves in a retrograde flap?

Initially, it was thought that venous flow occurred through the bypassed valves by collateral veins in the superficial and deep systems and by crossover between the venae comitantes, which have valveless communicating branches between certain comitantes valves. However, experimental evidence casts doubt on this process as the only mechanism of retrograde flow. Recently, Timmons postulated that three processes are necessary for reverse flow to occur: (1) increased venous pressure proximal to the valve, (2) disruption of sympathetic tone, and (3) venous filling proximal and distal to the valves.

8. Can a fasciocutaneous flap be elevated from the dorsal aspect of the forearm?

Yes. A large fasciocutaneous flap—the posterior interosseous artery flap—can be elevated from the dorsal aspect of the forearm. This vessel originates from the common interosseous artery in 90% of people and the ulnar artery in 10% and usually is found 2 cm proximal to the ulnar styloid beneath the extensor indicis proprius. The posterior interosseous artery flap territory has been shown to extend from the level of the wrist to a point 4 cm below the epicondyles, although some contend that the area is limited to the distal and middle thirds of the forearm. It is useful for covering defects of the dorsal and palmar aspects of the hand and the first web space.

9. What is a distant pedicle flap? What are the indications for its use?

Distant pedicle flaps are not based on the involved extremity; donor sites include the chest, abdomen, and groin. The use of such flaps necessitates a delay period (usually 2–3 weeks) during which the pedicle flap remains attached to both the recipient and donor sites. The upper extremity is immobilized to prevent flap disruption; stiffness of the hip and upper extremity may occur in older patients as a result. After the delay, the pedicle is divided, the donor site closed, and the flap inset. The use of a distant pedicle flap is indicated when local or regional flaps are either unavailable or insufficient to provide adequate soft tissue coverage or the patient is not a candidate for free tissue transfer.

10. What is the most commonly used distant pedicle flap?

The groin flap.

11. What is the significance of the groin flap?

The groin flap, reported by Ian McGregor and Ian Jackson in 1972, was one of the first axial pattern flaps to be described. It was revolutionary because it allowed greater potential for reconstruction of difficult upper extremity wounds. It is a versatile flap with a reliable vascular supply that is capable of covering large defects of the hand and wrist and provides an excellent tissue bed for subsequent procedures such as tendon reconstruction.

12. How is a groin flap designed?

The groin flap is supplied by the superficial circumflex iliac artery (SCIA), a branch of the femoral artery, and accompanying venae comitantes. The SCIA originates 2–3 cm below the midpoint of the inguinal ligament and courses laterally parallel to the inguinal ligament until it reaches the medial border of the sartorius muscle. The flap is designed by drawing a line from the anterior superior iliac spine (ASIS) to the pubic tubercle to mark the course of the inguinal ligament. The femoral artery is palpated 2.5 cm below the ligament at the origin of the SCIA. A line is drawn laterally from this point and parallel to the inguinal ligament to mark the course of the SCIA pedicle. The flap is centered over this line; the dissection is begun laterally and extended medially to the medial border of the sartorius. The fascia over the lateral border of the sartorius is incised and reflected with the flap to ensure inclusion of the pedicle. A flap that is 10 cm wide usually allows tubing when the flap is needed for circumferential coverage of degloved digits. Donor sites up to 12 cm in width can be closed directly.

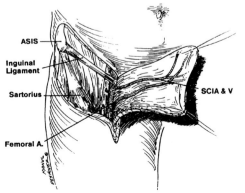

Groin flap. (From Mih AD: Pedicle flaps for coverage of the wrist and hand. Hand Clin 13:217–229, with permission.)

13. What are the disadvantages of the groin flap?
1. Dependent position of the hand during attachment and immobilization causes edema with subsequent joint stiffness
2. Difficulty with physical and occupational therapy due to immobilization of the upper extremity
3. Patient discomfort
4. Two-stage procedure

14. How are anterior chest wall and abdominal wall flaps designed?
Anterior chest wall flaps are designed on the anterolateral chest wall or the infraclavicular region. The blood supply is derived from the intercostal vessels or the thoracoepigastric system and is oriented in a transverse-to-oblique direction toward the midline. Flaps designed on the contralateral chest wall permit easier immobilization of the extremity with the elbow flexed than flaps on the ipsilateral chest wall.

Flaps elevated from the abdominal wall are called **epigastric flaps** when they are above the umbilicus and **abdominal flaps** when they are below. Epigastric flaps are useful for coverage of large defects of the distal forearm or hand. A superiorly based flap crossing the midline obtains vascular supply from both sides. The forearm is placed in a comfortable position across the lower chest and the flap is designed as needed. Most abdominal flaps are inferiorly based random flaps in which flap length is restricted to 1.5 times the width. Axial pattern abdominal flaps can be based on the superficial inferior epigastric artery (SIEA), a branch of the SCIA, as described by Shaw and Payne in 1946. These flaps vary in length from 5–18 cm and in width from 2–7 cm and can be used as tubed flaps with the base of the tube rotated through an arc of 180° to facilitate positioning of the hand. Division and inset of each of these flaps is performed at 2–3 weeks; donor site defects are covered with split-thickness skin grafts at the time of flap elevation or division.

15. What is a fillet flap?
A fillet flap is a salvage flap consisting of the vascularized soft tissue of an otherwise mutilated digit. After excision of the phalanges and tendons, the fillet flap can be used for coverage of adjacent soft tissue defects.

16. What are the indications for free tissue transfer?
Various situations preclude the use of local, regional, or distant pedicle flaps. Involvement of the hand and forearm in an injury may eliminate all potential local or regional flap donor sites. Although distant pedicle flaps, such as the groin flap, are useful for coverage of large defects, defects resulting from circumferential injuries are extremely difficult to cover with such a flap. Occasionally, defects involving the volar and dorsal aspects of the hand or more proximal circumferential defects can be covered by a combined groin and epigastric flap. However, free flaps offer far greater versatility and availability of donor sites for coverage of extensive defects. In addition, tailoring of the free flap to suit the reconstructive needs of the wound is easily accomplished because of the diversity of available flaps. Limb elevation, early mobilization, and the ability to cover even extensive circumferential defects are additional advantages to the use of free tissue transfer.

17. Which free flaps are most commonly used?
Numerous flaps are available for free tissue transfer. A flap is selected based on the particular needs of a given wound, including size, geometry, location, and function. Thin, pliable coverage for the dorsum of the hand can be provided by a temporoparietal fascia, dorsalis pedis, or radial forearm flap. Thicker coverage for a palmar or forearm defect can be provided by a scapular or lateral arm flap. Coverage of an extensive circumferential defect can be provided by a rectus abdominis, serratus anterior, or latissimus dorsi flap.

18. Which flap is commonly used as a regional pedicle flap or free flap?
The radial forearm flap.

19. How can the radial forearm flap be used as a regional pedicle flap?
The radial forearm flap is designed to include the radial artery when raised as a pedicle fasciocutaneous flap. It can be based proximally to cover defects involving the proximal forearm and elbow or distally (reversed) to cover defects involving the distal forearm, wrist, and hand.

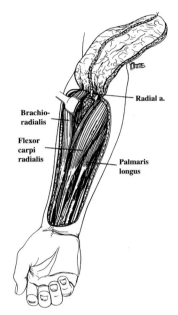

Radial forearm flap. (From Green DP (ed): Operative Hand Surgery, 3rd ed. New York, Churchill Livingstone, 1993, p 4473, with permission.)

20. How is a radial forearm flap elevated?

The course of the radial artery is mapped out with a Doppler and marked on the volar surface of the forearm. The required length of the vascular pedicle is measured, and a template of the soft tissue defect is outlined on the proximal forearm (for a reversed or distally based flap). The flap may include virtually all of the volar forearm skin, if needed (up to 14 cm by 24 cm); the donor site is then skin-grafted.

The radial artery and its two venae comitantes are invested in a layer of deep fascia known as the lateral intermuscular septum, which separates the flexor and extensor compartments of the forearm and is attached to the periosteum of the radius distal to the insertion of the pronator teres. The artery is covered proximally by the brachioradialis; it emerges distally between the brachioradialis and flexor carpi radialis to lie superficially, covered only by skin, subcutaneous tissue, and deep fascia.

Elevation of the flap is usually begun on the ulnar aspect of the flap and continued toward the radial pedicle. The antebrachial fascia is incised and elevated with the skin paddle. The flap is raised in a subfascial plane, exposing muscle bellies proximally and tendons distally, with care to preserve the paratenon for subsequent skin grafting. On the radial side of the flexor carpi radialis tendon, the dissection passes to a plane deep to the radial vessels, where it proceeds to the radial side of the pedicle. The attachment of the lateral intermuscular septum to the periosteum of the radius is divided to allow elevation of the vascular pedicle and to ensure inclusion in the flap. Division of the pedicle proximally (for a distally based reverse flap) completes the dissection.

When bone is included as an osteofasciocutaneous flap, the attachment of the lateral intermuscular septum to the periosteum of the radius must be preserved. A cuff of flexor pollicis longus muscle is left attached to the radius to ensure preservation of the periosteal vessels. A keel-shaped segment of radius, not to exceed one-third the thickness of the bone, is osteotomized and elevated with the flap.

21. What is the main contraindication to use of the radial forearm free flap?

Both proximally based and reversed (distally based) radial forearm flaps require division of the radial artery. Sacrifice of the radial artery is permissible only when sufficient perfusion of the hand by the ulnar artery has been demonstrated by a normal Allen's test. In up to 15% of hands, the ulnar artery does not perfuse the radial digits because of an incomplete superficial palmar arch or prior ulnar artery injury. Reconstruction of the radial artery with a vein graft should be performed if ischemia of the hand results.

22. Can a radial forearm pedicle flap be harvested without sacrificing the radial artery?

Elevation of a radial forearm fascial flap is possible without sacrifice of the radial artery. Weinzweig et al. described a flap based on perforators from the radial artery, which form a fascial plexus extending 1.5–7 cm from the radial styloid. It is elevated in proximal-to-distal fashion and is based on 6–10 perforators found at the distal portion of the forearm. The flap easily reaches the palmar and dorsal aspects of the hand as well as the first web space.

23. What fasciocutaneous free flap can be harvested from the lateral arm?

The lateral arm flap, described by Song and popularized by Katsaros et al., is based on the posterior radial collateral artery and encompasses the posterolateral aspect of the upper arm between the insertion of the deltoid muscle and the elbow. Advantages of this flap include (1) relatively constant anatomy; (2) relatively long pedicle (up to 6 cm); (3) thin, pliable tissue; (4) use as a neurosensory flap; (5) ease of harvest in the supine position, permitting a two-team approach; and (6) direct closure of the donor site for flaps less than 6 cm wide. The only disadvantages associated with this flap are hypoesthesia in the distribution of the posterior cutaneous nerve if it is divided or harvested and the donor site scar.

24. What is the thinnest free flap available for coverage of the dorsum of the hand?

The temporoparietal fascial flap. Described by Upton et al., this flap provides excellent coverage for defects of the hand as well as a suitable gliding surface for underlying tendons with a thin, pliable fascia that is then skin-grafted. Advantages include relative predictability of the pedicle and a concealed donor scar; disadvantages include potential injury to the frontal branch of the facial nerve during harvest and scalp alopecia.

25. What is a functional free muscle transfer?

Free tissue transfer of muscle can be performed to restore hand function when major loss of skeletal musculature in the forearm results in a significant functional deficit that cannot be sufficiently reconstructed by a simpler procedure. Reinnervation with restoration of voluntary active muscle contraction can be accomplished by suturing a motor nerve in the recipient area to the motor nerve of the transplanted muscle. Transfer of the gracilis muscle or a segment of the latissimus muscle into the flexor compartment of the forearm with suture to the flexor digitorum profundus tendons can be performed to restore active finger flexion.

26. What is a composite free flap?

Composite defects involve multiple structures such as bone, tendon, nerve, and skin. Reconstruction of such defects can be accomplished with a composite free flap that incorporates the required structures into a single unit. A defect requiring bone, tendon, sensory nerve, and skin may be reconstructed with a radial forearm flap incorporating the palmaris longus tendon, lateral antebrachial cutaneous nerve, and a segment of radius. Another choice may be the dorsalis pedis flap with incorporation of the superficial or deep peroneal nerve, long toe extensor tendons, and metatarsal bone. A third choice may be the lateral arm flap with incorporation of the posterior cutaneous nerve, triceps tendon, and a segment of humerus.

27. What are the advantages and disadvantages of composite free flaps?

Composite free flaps permit single-stage reconstruction of defects that otherwise may require two or three stages. The main disadvantages with the use of composite free flaps are donor site morbidity, flap planning and design, and technical complexity. Common sense must dictate the planning of the reconstruction and considerations to minimize donor site morbidity. In certain situations the size, geometry, or components of a particular defect are better approached by multistaged conventional procedures. An extensive soft tissue defect with a limited bone defect may be preferably managed by transfer of a skin-grafted free latissimus dorsi muscle flap and a nonvascularized iliac crest bone graft.

28. Describe the neurosensory functions of the hand.

The hand possesses a sophisticated level of sensibility with specialized neurosensory receptors on the dorsum and volar surface of the digits. Fingertips have the highest innervated density of any body surface except the tongue. Swartz has distinguished between the need for "critical sensibility" of the fingertips and "protective sensibility" of the palm and dorsum of the hand. Loss of the volar or tactile surface of the fingers requires replacement with specialized sensory cells that can be found only on the hand itself, on the toes, or on the sole of the foot—glabrous skin. Pacinian corpuscles and Meissner's corpuscles are encapsulated sensory endings found exclusively in glabrous skin. Merkel cells, which are sensory endings with expanded tips, are also found in glabrous skin. Areas of critical sensibility are covered by glabrous skin and supported by underlying pulp tissue, such as the fingertips, palm of the hand, and sole of the foot.

29. What are the indications for the use of a sensate free flap?

The hand possesses a limited amount of sensate tissue to reconstruct defects that require sophisticated innervation crucial to tactile function. It does not possess sufficient tissue to reconstruct defects greater than those that can be covered by a Littler flap or other local innervated transposition flap. Thus, larger defects often require free transfer of a sensate flap.

30. Which sensate free flaps are commonly used?

Defects of the fingers can be reconstructed using the **toe pulp neurosensory flap**, described by Buncke and Rose, which consists of glabrous skin and underlying pulp tissue from the great or second toe. Moving two-point discrimination (2PD) of the transferred pulp tissue has been reported to range from 3–12 mm. The **great toe wrap-around flap**, described by Morrison and MacLeod, is a composite flap of skin, nail, and pulp tissue, with or without the distal phalanx of the great toe. The great toe is partially degloved based on the dominant ulnar pedicle. The **first web flap,** described by May et al., uses the highly innervated tissue of the first web space of the foot. The flap is supplied by the first dorsal metatarsal artery and branches of the deep peroneal nerve and neighboring plantar digital nerves of both toes. A thin, pliable flap of glabrous skin and pulp measuring up to 12 cm × 8 cm can be harvested.

Several free fasciocutaneous flaps can be harvested to provide protective sensibility to a recipient site upon transfer. Examples include the **lateral arm flap** based on the posterior cutaneous nerve, the **radial forearm flap** based on the lateral antebrachial cutaneous nerve, and the **dorsalis pedis flap** based on the superficial peroneal nerve.

31. Does tissue expansion have a role in coverage of soft tissue defects of the hand?

In selected cases. Successful soft tissue resurfacing of defects involving the fingers, web spaces, and dorsum of the hand have been reported using seamless custom expanders in which the base of the expander is approximately the size of the defect to be corrected. Expanders also have been used to recruit tissue for congenital hand anomalies, such as syndactyly release, to avoid the use of skin grafts. Small elongated or rectangular expanders are used in such cases. Neurovascular compromise, implant extrusion, and infection may occur with the use of tissue expanders.

BIBLIOGRAPHY

1. Becker C, Gilbert A: The dorsal ulnar artery flap. In Gilbert A, Masquelet AC, Heutz VS (eds): Pedicle Flaps of the Upper Limb, 2nd ed. Boston, Little, Brown, 1992, p 129.
2. Cavanagh S, Pho RWH: The reverse radial forearm flap in the severely injured hand: An anatomical and clinical study. J Hand Surg 17B:501–503, 1992.
3. Costa H, Soutar DS: The distally-based island posterior interosseous flap. Br J Plast Surg 41:221–227, 1988.
4. Daniel RK, Terzis J, Schwarz G: Neurovascular free flaps. A preliminary report. Plast Reconstr Surg 56:13, 1975.
5. Glasson DW, Lovie MJ: The ulnar island flap in hand and forearm reconstruction. Br J Plast Surg 41:349–353, 1988.
6. Halbert CF, Wei FC: Neurosensory free flaps: Digits and hand. Hand Clin 13:251–262, 1997.
7. Katsaros J, Schusterman M, Beppu M, et al: The lateral upper arm flap: Anatomy and clinical applications. Ann Plast Surg 12:489, 1984.
8. Lister G: Free skin and composite flaps. In Green DP (ed): Operative Hand Surgery, 3rd ed. New York, Churchill Livingstone, 1993, pp 1103–1158.
9. Manktelow RT, Zuker RM, McKee NH: Functioning free muscle transplantation. J Hand Surg 9A:32, 1984.
10. McGregor IA, Jackson IT: The groin flap. Br J Plast Surg 25:3–16, 1972.
11. McGregor IA, Morgan G: Axial and random pattern flaps. Br J Plast Surg 25:3–16, 1972.
12. Mih AD: Pedicle flaps for coverage of the wrist and hand. Hand Clin 13:217–230, 1997.
13. Song R, Song Y, Yu Y, Song Y: The upper arm free flap. Clin Plast Surg 9:27, 1982.
14. Soutar DS, Tanner NSB: The radial forearm flap in the management of soft tissue injuries of the hand. Br J Plast Surg 37:18, 1984.

15. Upton J, Rogers C, Durham-Smith G, Swartz WM: Clinical applications of temporoparietal flaps in hand reconstruction. J Hand Surg 11A:475, 1986.
16. Weinzweig N, Chen L, Chen ZW: The distally-based radial forearm fasciosubcutaneous flap with preservation of the radial artery: An anatomic and clinical approach. Plast Reconstr Surg 94:675–684, 1994.
17. Wood MB: Composite free flaps to the hand. Hand Clin 13:231–238, 1997.
18. Zancolli EA, Angrigiani C: Posterior interosseous island forearm flap. J Hand Surg 13B:130–135, 1988.

93. FLEXOR TENDON INJURIES

William F. Wagner, Jr., M.D., and James W. Strickland, M.D.

1. Should acute flexor tendon lacerations be repaired primarily?

The concept that tendons can be immediately repaired in zones I and II with the expectation of restoring a favorable amount of tendon excursion has advanced from doubtful theory to general acceptance. Almost all studies have shown superior results compared with flexor tendon grafting. Advantages of primary tendon repair include the fact that the tendon is returned to its normal length, the period of disability necessitated by wound healing and later grafting is reduced, the tendency for joint stiffness is decreased, and the results of secondary lysis, when necessary, should be better.

2. What is the orientation of the flexor digitorum profundus (FDP) and flexor digitorum superficialis (FDS) tendons at the level of the proximal phalanx?

Once within the flexor sheath, the FDS tendon begins to flatten. It then splits and divides around the FDP tendon. The two slips of the FDS tendon reunite deep to the FDP tendon with one-half of the fibers decussating and the other half continuing distally on the same side. The reuniting of fibers of the FDS tendon is known as the chiasm of Camper. Beyond the chiasm, the FDS tendon splits into radial and ulnar slips, which then insert into the middle three-fifths of the middle phalanx.

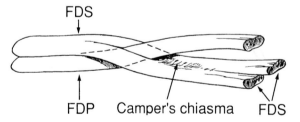

Early in the flexor sheath, the FDS tendon divides and passes around the FDP tendon. The two portions of the FDS reunite at Camper's chiasm.

3. Where does the flexor tendon sheath begin and end in the digit? Where are the various pulleys or thickened areas of the flexor sheath located?

In the fingers the flexor sheath arises at the level of the volar plate of the metacarpophalangeal (MCP) joint and ends at the proximal volar base of the distal phalanx. The flexor sheath comprises thickened areas of arcing fibers, referred to as **anular pulleys**, that alternate with thin, flexible areas of criss-crossing fibers described as **cruciate pulleys**. The first anular pulley arises from the volar plate of the MCP joint and the second anular pulley from the middle one-third of the proximal phalanx. The first cruciate pulley extends from the distal end of the second anular pulley to the proximal end of the third anular pulley, which arises primarily from the volar plate of the proximal interphalangeal (PIP) joint. The second cruciate pulley is located between the third and fourth anular pulleys, and the fourth anular pulley arises from the middle portion of the middle phalanx. The third cruciate pulley is located between the fourth and fifth anular pulleys, and the fifth anular pulley arises from the volar plate of the distal interphalangeal (DIP) plate and proximal volar base of the distal phalanx. It is not always possible to identify all of the described pulleys of the flexor sheath. (See figure at top of next page.)

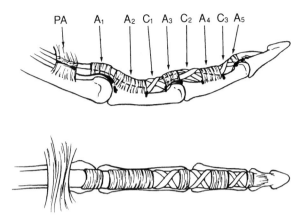

Lateral *(top)* and dorsal *(bottom)* views of the finger depict the components of the digital flexor sheath. The sturdy anular pulleys (A_1, A_2, A_3, A_4, and A_5) are important biomechanically in keeping the tendons closely applied to the phalanges. The thin, pliable cruciate pulleys (C_1, C_2, and C_3) collapse to allow full digital flexion. A recent addition is the palmar aponeurosis pulley (PA), which adds to the biomechanical efficiency of the sheath system.

4. What are the two ways in which flexor tendons receive nutrition?
Vascular injection studies have long shown the significant role of perfusion via small blood vessel networks called **vincula**, which arise from the digital arteries and ultimately connect into an intratendinous vascular network. Other studies have noted that **synovial diffusion** is the significant nutrient pathway.

5. What two areas of cellular activity contribute to flexor tendon healing?
Tendons heal by a combination of extrinsic and intrinsic cellular activity. The more intrinsic the cellular activity, the fewer the adhesions. Extrinsic cellular activity primarily relates to peripheral adhesions that are frequently associated with the tendon-healing process. Although these adhesions have been considered an essential source of repair to cells, recent studies of the intrinsic healing capacity of tendons suggest that adhesions may constitute a nonessential inflammatory response at the site of injury.

6. What is the effect of stress on healing tendons?
If the repaired flexor tendon is not stressed, the healing process may take up to 8 weeks, and repaired tendons have minimal tensile strength throughout the healing process. Stressed tendons heal faster, gain tensile strength faster, and have fewer adhesions and better excursion than unstressed tendons.

7. During what period are flexor tendons weakest after repair?
Strength usually decreases by 10–50% between 5 and 21 days after repair in unstressed tendons. It may not decrease at all in repairs subjected to early application of the appropriate amount of stress.

8. List three factors that may lead to tendon adhesion formation.
Tendon adhesion formation can be precipitated by tendon sheath injury, suture, and immobilization. Of these factors, immobilization has undergone the most extensive experimental and clinical investigation. Based on these studies, early protected mobilization to improve the mechanism by which flexor tendons heal has a sound scientific basis and is the best way of inhibiting adhesion formation. Of course, meticulous surgical technique and the underlying severity of the trauma to the tendon also affect the production of tendon adhesions.

9. What factors contribute to the strength of a repaired flexor tendon laceration?
Dorsal rather than palmar placement of core sutures for flexor tendon repairs has significant advantages in terms of strength and biomechanics. In addition, the strength of a tendon repair is roughly proportional to the number of suture strands that cross the repair site and the caliber of the suture. Increasing the number of suture strands across the repair site increases repair strength but adds to technical difficulty and increases the volume of suture material at the repair site.

10. What causes gapping at the repair site? How does it affect tendon healing?
Gapping may occur as repaired tendons begin to rupture through the suture or knot. Gapping also may occur when locking loops collapse and allow the tendon ends to pull apart. Gapping at the

repair site becomes the weakest part of the tendon, unfavorably alters tendon mechanics, and may promote adhesion formation, resulting in decreased tendon excursion.

11. How can the tendency for gapping at the repair site be decreased?

A peripheral epitendinous suture results in an increase in repair strength and a significant reduction in the tendency for gapping at the repair site. Improved strength and decreased gapping are maintained with cyclic stress. Horizontal mattress or running locked peripheral epitendinous sutures have been shown to add the greatest strength and resistance to gap formation.

12. What are the most commonly used techniques for flexor tendon repair?

Most techniques involve the use of a core suture to bridge the repair site. Many techniques now use an additional suture, but the total number of strands at the repair site is four. Our method consists of a simple two-strand core stitch that enters and exits through the tendon ends and has locking grasps on either side of the tendon. An additional palmarly placed horizontal mattress suture is inserted across the tendon ends to complete a four-strand repair. A running horizontal locked stitch is used as a peripheral epitendinous stitch to tidy the repair, increase strength, and decrease gap formation.

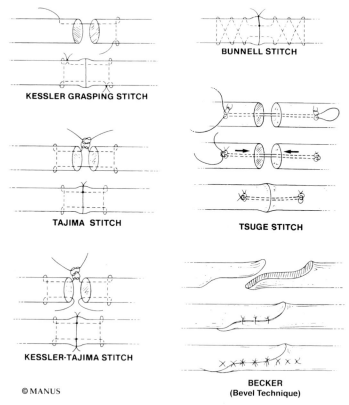

Flexor tendon repair techniques.

13. Describe the zones of flexor tendon injury.

A modification of Verdan's zone system is used by most hand surgeons in describing injuries to flexor tendon system. Zone I flexor tendon injuries occur distal to the insertion of the FDS tendon. Zone II injuries are located from the proximal edge of the fibroosseous flexor tendon canal to the insertion of the FDS. Zone III injuries occur in the area where the lumbricals arise from the FDP tendon in the mid-palm. Zone IV injuries occur within the carpal tunnel, and zone V injuries occur proximal to the carpal tunnel in the distal forearm. (See figure at top of next page.)

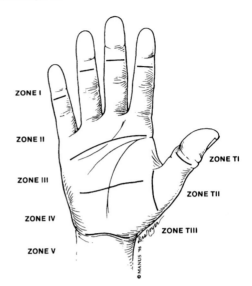

The zones of flexor tendon injuries. T = thumb zones.

14. In zone II flexor tendon laceration repairs, what area of the sheath can be opened for repair? What areas should be preserved?

In opening the intact components of the sheath, every attempt must be made to preserve the anular components, which are almost impossible to repair. Biomechanical studies have shown that the A_2 and A_4 pulleys are the most critical for adequate flexor tendon function. Tendon sutures should be performed in the cruciate synovial sheath windows, which usually can be restored after tendon suture. By acutely flexing the DIP joint and, to some extent, the PIP joint, it is possible to deliver the profundus and superficialis stumps into a cruciate window. If at least 1 cm of the distal tendons can be exposed in this manner, core sutures can be placed in the profundus tendons and two superficial slips without great difficulty. If a lesser length of distal tendon is present in the window, the next most distal cruciate synovial interval must be opened for core suture placement.

15. How does one retrieve a proximal tendon end that has retracted proximally down the tendon sheath?

Many clever tactics have been suggested to facilitate tendon capture and repositioning when the proximal ends have retracted further down the proximal sheath. One of the most commonly used methods is to pass a small catheter from the distal wound into the palm beneath the anular pulleys, where it is sutured to both tendons several centimeters proximal to the A_1 pulley. The catheter is then pulled distally and easily delivers the tendon stumps into the distal repair site. A transversely oriented needle secures the tendons for repair, and the connecting suture can be severed in the palm and the catheter withdrawn.

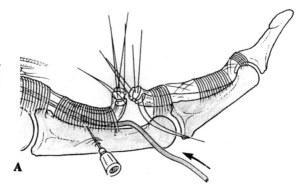

Sourmelis and McGrouther's method of retrieving flexor tendons. *A,* A 22-gauge hypodermic needle is passed transversely through the anular sheath to maintain tendon position. *(Figure continued on following page.)*

(Figure continued on following page.)

A

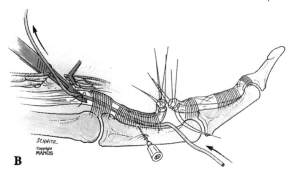

Sourmelis and McGrouther's method of retrieving flexor tendons *(continued). B,* Catheter-tendon suture is cut in palm and withdrawn.

B

16. When the proximal ends of the lacerated FDS and FDP tendons retract into the palm, how can one correctly orient these tendons when they are brought out more distally into the digit?

When the proximal tendon ends have retracted into the palm, it is extremely important to reestablish the proper anatomic relationship of the FDP and FDS tendons. The FDP must be passed back through the hiatus created by the FDS slips so that it lies palmar to Camper's chiasm and recreates the relative positioning that was present at the level of the tendon laceration. Failure to restore the correct relationship creates an impediment to unrestricted tendon gliding after repair.

17. How should zone I FDP tendon avulsion injuries be repaired?

If the distal stump is short or nonexistent, the FDP stump may be reattached by first elevating a periosteal flap from the base of the distal phalanx and then drilling an oblique hole beneath the flap to penetrate the dorsal cortex just beneath the proximal fingernail. A double-armed needle with 3-0 sutures is placed in the proximal tendon stump and passed through the bone hole. The sutures are used to pull the tendon beneath the periosteal flap and are tied over a cotton pad/button combination over the nail. If possible, the tendon attachment should be supplemented by sutures through some adjacent sheath or periosteum.

18. Describe the three main types of avulsion injuries to the profundus tendon insertion.

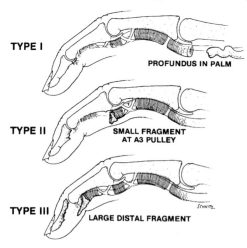

TYPE I

PROFUNDUS IN PALM

TYPE II

SMALL FRAGMENT
AT A3 PULLEY

TYPE III

LARGE DISTAL FRAGMENT

In type I injuries, the tendon retracts all the way into the palm and is held there by the lumbrical origin. In type II injuries, the tendon retracts to the level of the PIP joint. Type III injuries consist of a large bony fragment that gets caught on the A4 pulley and prevents retraction of the bony fragment beyond the distal portion of the middle phalanx.

19. How should FDP avulsions in which the diagnosis is delayed for more than several months be treated?

Late untreated patients who are asymptomatic are best left alone. For late instability of the DIP joint, fusion should be considered. A one- or two-staged flexor tendon graft can be performed in carefully selected patients, but the potential risks may outweigh the possible advantages for some patients.

20. Should partial tendon lacerations be repaired?

Most authorities agree that lacerations up to 50% of the cross-sectional area of the tendon are optimally treated without tendon repair and with early mobilization. However, if the tendon laceration is beveled, the risk of entrapment, rupture, and triggering increases significantly. In such situations, the beveled portion of the tendon can be either excised or repaired with simple sutures. The result is a tendon that allows smoother gliding through the fibroosseous sheath.

21. What are the indications for tenolysis after flexor tendon repair?

Tenolysis is indicated after repair whenever the passive range of digital joint flexion significantly exceeds the patient's ability to flex actively at the same joint. All fractures should be healed, and wounds should have reached tissue equilibrium with soft skin and subcutaneous tissues. Reaction around the scars should be minimal. In addition, joint contractures must have been overcome and a normal or near-normal passive range of digital motion achieved.

22. What is most frequent complication after early postoperative mobilization programs?

A flexion contracture at the PIP or DIP joints may develop after early postoperative mobilization. Prompt recognition of the development of contractures, modification of the motion program to permit greater extension, and judicious use of dynamic splints help to prevent or overcome such deformities before they progress too far.

23. How do ruptures occur after flexor tendon repairs? What is the treatment?

Ruptures occur almost without exception when patients have been doing so well with their rehabilitation program that they use their hands in an extremely strong manner, such as heavy lifting, well before the tendons have sufficient strength to tolerate the extremely high tensile demands of such activity. Rupture of one or both flexor tendon repairs is a significant complication. The preferred treatment is prompt reexploration and repair.

24. Is a four-strand repair augmented by some type of running locked suture strong enough to allow early active motion therapy?

Based on experimental and clinical data regarding the stress applied to digits by various degrees of active flexion, it is believed that light, active digital flexion carried out with the wrist in extension should be relatively safe for flexor tendons repaired with the four-strand technique. This goal can be incorporated into a therapy protocol by allowing light active maintenance of full composite digital flexion once the wrist is brought from flexion to extension.

25. When can strengthening exercises be initiated after flexor tendon repair and appropriate early therapy protocols?

Based on multiple studies, it is believed that repaired flexor tendons regain sufficient strength by 8 weeks to initiate strengthening exercises. The exercises are increased in a gradually progressive manner.

CONTROVERSIES

26. Should the flexor sheath be repaired after repair of the flexor tendon laceration?

For: Repairing the sheath after tendon suture has the theoretical advantages of providing a barrier for adhesion formation, restoring synovial fluid nutrition, and restoring sheath mechanics. Furthermore, repair of the sheath may decrease the coefficient of friction between the pulley and tendon during the first few millimeters of proximal excision when the repaired tendon passes under the edge of the thick anular pulleys.

Against: The sheath is often technically difficult to reestablish, and few valid clinical or experimental data substantiate that it improves the results of flexor tendon repair.

27. Should the epitendinous suture, which is used in repairing acute flexor tendon lacerations, be placed initially or after core sutures are placed?

Initially: (1) Forcible handling of the tendon is minimized; (2) enlargement of the tenorrhaphy is minimized; (3) the sutures may still be buried within the tendon; and (4) the strength of the repair is equivalent to the popular Kessler suture technique.

After: Placement of core sutures initially as part of the flexor tendon repair allows easy retrieval of the tendons from their proximal and distal sites and good approximation of the tendon ends. A running epitendinous suture can then be used to tidy the tendon ends and increase the repair strength.

BIBLIOGRAPHY

1. Strickland JW: Flexor tendon repair. Hand Clin 1:55–68, 1985.
2. Strickland JW: Results of flexor tendon surgery in zone II. Hand Clin 1:167–179, 1985.
3. Strickland JW: Opinions and preferences in flexor tendon surgery. Hand Clin 1:187–191, 1985.
4. Strickland JW: Flexor tendon surgery. Part 1: Anatomy, biomechanics, physiology, healing and adhesions. Orthop Rev 15:632–645, 1986.
5. Strickland JW: Flexor tendon surgery. Part 2: Flexor tendon repair. Orthop Rev 15:701–721, 1986.
6. Strickland JW: Flexor tendon surgery—a review. Part 1: Primary flexor tendon repair. J Hand Surg 14B:261–272, 1989.
7. Strickland JW: Flexor tendon surgery—a review. Part 2: Free tendon grafts and tenolysis. J Hand Surg 14B:368–382, 1989.
8. Strickland JW: Biologic rationale, clinical application, and results of early motion following flexor tendon repair. J Hand Ther 2:71–83, 1989.
9. Strickland JW: Flexor tendon injuries. Curr Orthop 6:98–110, 1992.
10. Strickland JW: Flexor tendon repair—Indiana method. Ind Hand Center Newslett 1(1):1–12, 1996.
11. Strickland JW: Experimental studies of the structure and function of tendon: Hand Surg Update 1:1–15, 1993.
12. Strickland JW: Flexor tendon injuries. I: Foundations of treatment. J Am Acad Orthop Surg 3:44–54, 1995.
13. Strickland JW: Flexon tendon injuries. II: Operative technique. J Am Acad Orthop Surg 3:55–62, 1995.
14. Strickland JW: The Indiana method of flexor tendon repair. Atlas Hand Clin 1:77–103, 1996.
15. Strickland JW: Tendon injuries in the upper extremity. In Dee R, Mango E, Hurst LC (eds): Principles of Orthopaedic Practice, 2nd ed. New York, McGraw-Hlll, 1997, pp 1173–1187.
16. Strickland JW: Flexor tendon repair: The Indianapolis method. In Hunter JM, Schneider LH, Mackin EJ (eds): St. Louis, Mosby, 1997, pp 353–361.
17. Strickland JW: Flexor tendon injuries. In Strickland JW (ed): The Hand: Master Techniques in Orthopaedic Surgery. Philadelphia, Lippincott-Raven, 1998, pp 473–490.
18. Strickland JW, Wagner WF: Recent advances in flexor tendon surgery. Rec Advan Orthop Surg 6:77–101, 1992.
19. Wagner WF, Carroll C, Strickland JW, et al: A biomechanical comparison of techniques of flexor tendon repair. J Hand Surg 19A:1–5, 1994.

94. EXTENSOR TENDON INJURIES

Mary Lynn Newport, M.D.

1. What are the eight zones commonly used to describe extensor tendon injuries?

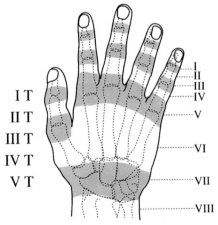

Zones I, III, V, and VII (the odd zones) overlie the joints of the hand (i.e., distal interphalangeal [DIP], proximal interphalangeal [PIP], metacarpophalangeal [MP], and carpal joints, respectively). Zones II, IV, VI, and VIII (the even zones) overlie the bones (i.e., middle phalanges, proximal phalanges, metacarpals, and distal radius/ulna, respectively).

2. The thumb is typically divided into how many extensor zones?

Five. The odd zones (I, III, and IV) overlie the joints (IP, MP, and carpal joints, respectively), and the even zones (II and IV) overlie the bones (proximal phalanx and metacarpal, respectively).

3. Do the extensor digiti minimi (EDM) and extensor indicis proprius (EIP) tendons run ulnar or radial to their respective communis tendons?

The EDM and EIP tendons usually run ulnar to the extensor digitorum communis (EDC) tendon and allow independent extension of the small and index fingers, respectively. However, significant variability of the extensor tendons to the index and small fingers, including radial EIP and EDM tendons and supernumerary tendons, has been reported in up to 19% of specimens in anatomic studies.

4. Which muscles extend the MP and IP joints? What is their innervation?

The MP joints are extended through the extrinsic EDC (as well as EIP and EDM) tendons supplied by the posterior interosseous nerve branch of the radial nerve; the IP joints are extended by the intrinsic tendons of the interossei and lumbricals supplied by the ulnar nerve. The intrinsics are able to extend the IP joints because they course dorsal to the axis of rotation for these joints.

5. Which finger and which zones are most commonly injured?

The long finger is the most frequently injured (38% of cases), followed by the index (28%), ring (18%), and thumb and small finger (10% each). Zone VI, directly over the metacarpal, is the area frequently injured. (This is also true for the thumb, in which zone IV is the area directly over the metacarpal.)

6. Which general area has the better prognosis after extensor tendon injury—the proximal (V–VIII) or the distal (I–IV) zones?

The proximal zones have a significantly better prognosis (65–75% good/excellent results) than the distal zones (0–40% good/excellent results), probably because the extensor mechanism is simpler more proximally. The extensor tendon covers only one side of bone in the proximal zones with no intricate connections except the juncturae. The more distal zones have less excursion and cover the phalanx on three sides, thereby increasing the chances of adhesion formation.

7. What are the juncturae tendinae?

Small tendinous bands that course distally from the ring finger EDC to connect with the EDC of the long and small fingers. If an EDC is lacerated in zone VI proximal to the junctura, the pull from adjacent juncturae can extend the affected finger and mask the injury.

8. What is a mallet finger or mallet deformity?

This deformity represents droop of the finger into flexion at the DIP joint with inability to extend the distal phalanx fully, if at all.

9. What causes a mallet deformity?

Almost all are secondary to acute injury of the extensor mechanism, usually from a direct blow to the tip of the finger, forcing it into flexion.

10. What are the different types of mallet fingers?

Type I is a tendinous rupture (with or without a small fleck of bone) from the distal phalanx. Type II is a tendon laceration at or proximal to the DIP joint. Type III is a deep abrasion with loss of extensor substance. Type IV includes a significant fracture of the distal phalanx.

11. How is a mallet finger treated?

Type II (lacerations) should be be sutured; some surgeons use a K-wire to hold the joint in extension. Types I and III should be treated with extension splinting consisting of a dorsal or volar alumifoam splint or a stack splint. Treatment of type IV injuries is controversial. Most experts agree that if the joint is congruous (not volarly subluxed), treatment should consist of splinting only. If the joint is volarly subluxed, many advocate reduction with percutaneous pinning. Others perform an open reduction with internal fracture fixation.

12. What is a boutonnière deformity?

A boutonnière deformity consists of a flexed position of the PIP joint and hyperextended position of the DIP joint. It is most often found in a chronic inflammatory disorder such as rheumatoid arthritis, but it may occur after an injury in an otherwise normal hand. In chronic deformity, synovitis of the PIP joint produces attenuation or destruction of the central slip insertion on the middle phalanx. The finger adopts a progressively more flexed position as the extensor pull is lost. As the finger slips more into flexion, the lateral bands of the intrinsic mechanism slide volarly, producing an ever greater flexion deformity. As they slide volarly, the tension of the intrinsics to the DIP increases, pulling the DIP joint into progressively more extension.

13. What is an acute boutonnière deformity? What biomechanical process produces it? How is it treated?

The same basic mechanism is present in an acute boutonnière, in which an injury, usually involving forced flexion of the PIP, ruptures the central slip attachment to the middle phalanx. Immediately after an acute injury, the patient usually is still able to extend the PIP joint because the lateral bands have not yet slid volarly. The patient will be tender dorsally and have pain with extension. The injured finger is most comfortable in flexion because the capsule is most capacious in this position. As a consequence, the lateral bands slide volarly, producing deformity at the PIP and DIP joints.This deformity is usually quite noticeable at around 10 days after injury. Open injuries (e.g., tendon lacerations) are directly repaired, followed by splinting of the PIP joint in full extension for 5–6 weeks. Closed injuries (e.g., avulsion) are treated by progressive splinting until extension of the PIP joint is achieved.

14. What is the currently recommended repair technique for extensor tendons?

No repair technique is completely accepted. The modified Bunnell technique has been shown to be the strongest and most biomechanically advantageous in zone VI, whereas the modified Bunnell or modified Kessler technique is best in zone IV.

15. What is the treatment protocol after extensor tendon repair?

No postoperative protocol is universally accepted. Any repair is contingent on other injuries (fractures, skin loss, flexor injury, neurovascular injury). Most surgeons have moved away from static splinting of all joints in extension to protocols that encourage tendon gliding, such as the use of an extensor outrigger with rubber bands, which allows active finger flexion and produces passive finger extension. Newer protocols encourage active finger range of motion under carefully controlled circumstances.

BIBLIOGRAPHY

1. Browne EZ Jr, Ribik CA: Early dynamic splinting for extensor tendon injuries. J Hand Surg 14A:72–76, 1989.
2. Doyle JR: Extensor tendons: Acute injuries. In Green DP, Hotchkiss RN (eds): Operative Hand Surgery, vol. 2, 3rd ed. New York, Churchill Livingstone, 1993, pp 1925–1954.
3. Gonzalez MH, Gray T, Ortinau E, Weinzweig N: The extensor tendons to the little finger: An anatomic study. J Hand Surg 20A:844–847, 1995.
4. Gonzalez MH, Weinzweig N, Kay T, Grindel S: Anatomy of the extensor tendons to the little finger. J Hand Surg 21A:988–991, 1996.
5. Kleinert HE, Verdan C: Report of the Committee on Tendon Injuries. J Hand Surg 8:794–798, 1983.
6. Newport ML, Blair WF, Steyers CM Jr: Long-term results of extensor tendon repair. J Hand Surg 15:961–966, 1990.
7. Newport ML, Pollack GR, Williams CD: Biomechanical characteristics of suture techniques in extensor zone IV. J Hand Surg 20A:650–656, 1995.
8. Newport ML, Williams CD: Biomechanical characteristics of extensor tendon suture techniques. J Hand Surg 17A:1117–1123, 1992.

95. TENDON TRANSFERS

Julie A. Melchior, M.D., and Richard I. Burton, M.D.

1. What is a tendon transfer?
The tendon of a functioning muscle is detached from its insertion and reattached to another tendon or bone to replace the function of a paralyzed muscle or injured tendon. The transferred tendon remains attached to its parent muscle with an intact neurovascular pedicle.

2. List the general principles of tendon transfers.
1. Full passive range of motion of the joints to be powered
2. Power of the donor muscle (the brachioradialis and flexor carpi ulnaris are the strongest)
3. Amplitude of the donor muscle (finger flexors have the greatest amplitude at 70 mm, wrist flexors and extensors the least at 33 mm)
4. Direction of the transfer
5. Location and nature of pulley, if needed
6. Tissue bed into which the transfer is placed
7. Selected fusions to simplify polyarticular system

3. How do you select the donor tendons?
1. List the functioning muscles.
2. List which of the functioning muscles are expendable.
3. List hand functions requiring restoration.
4. Match the second and third points.
5. Staging
6. In phase—out of phase

PERIPHERAL NERVE INJURIES

4. Which deficits in radial nerve palsy from a lesion at the midhumeral level require transfers?
1. Loss of wrist extension
2. Loss of finger extension at the metacarpophalangeal (MP) joints
3. Loss of extension and radial abduction of the thumb

5. List the standard tendon transfers for radial nerve palsy.

• Wrist extension	Pronator teres to extensor carpi radialis brevis (ECRB)
• Finger extension	Flexor carpi ulnaris (FCU) to extensor digitorum communis (EDC) (Jones)
	Flexor carpi radialis (FCR) to EDC (Starr)
	Flexor digitorum superficialis (FDS) of middle and ring fingers to EDC (Boyes)
• Thumb extension/abduction	Palmaris longus to rerouted extensor pollicis longus (EPL)

6. What area is affected by low median nerve palsy? What deficits are involved?
Low median nerve palsy affects the area distal to the innervation of the flexor pollicis longus (FPL) and flexor digitorum profundus (FDP). The following deficits are involved:
1. Loss of palmar abduction and pronation of the thumb (opposition)
2. Thenar muscles (abductor pollicis brevis [APB], opponens pollicis [OP]—variable innervation of flexor pollicis brevis [FPB] from ulnar nerve to both heads of FPB in some patients)
3. Lumbricals to index and middle fingers
4. Critical sensibility to thumb and index and middle fingers (implications of numbness for function, protection from injury, use of visual feedback after transfers)

7. **What movements are necessary for effective thumb opposition?**
Palmar abduction and pronation of the metacarpal with MP joint stability.

8. **List the standard opposition transfers.**
   • FDS of ring finger through a pulley of FCU (Bunnell)
   • Palmaris longus extended by a strip of palmar fascia to APB (Camitz)
   • Extensor indicis proprius (EIP) (Burkhalter)
   • Abductor digiti minimi (ADM) (Huber)

9. **What are the deficits in a high median nerve palsy?**
   1. Thumb opposition/critical sensibility
   2. Loss of flexion at the proximal interphalangeal (PIP) and distal interphalangeal (DIP) joints
of the index and middle fingers (FDP and all FDS)
   3. Loss of flexion at the IP joint of the thumb (FPL)

10. **List the standard tendon transfers for a high median nerve palsy.**
   • Thumb IP joint flexion: brachioradialis to FPL
   • DIP joint flexion of index and middle fingers: side-to-side tenorrhaphy of index and middle
     finger FDP tendons to ring and little finger FDP tendons
   • Conventional opposition transfer: EIP or abductor digiti quinti (ADQ) to APB

11. **What are the deficits in a low ulnar nerve palsy with preservation of the extrinsic flexors?**
   1. "Clawing" (MP hyperextension, IP flexion) of the ring and little fingers due to loss of independent MP flexion (contributes to loss of grip strength) (interossei)
   2. Loss of thumb adduction (loss of power pinch) (adductor; first dorsal interosseous; FPB, ½ or all)
   3. Loss of index finger abduction (loss of power pinch) (first dorsal interosseous)
   4. Abducted (ulnarly deviated) little finger (Wartenberg's sign) due to the ulnar deviating force
of the extensor digiti quinti (EDQ) unbalanced by loss of the third volar interosseous

12. **What are the transfers for correction of clawing?**
   • FDS of middle or ring finger, split, to radial lateral bands of middle, ring, and little fingers
     (modified Stiles-Bunnell) or to proximal phalanx (Littler)
   • ECRB extended by plantaris strips dorsally through the intermetacarpal spaces into radial lat-
     eral bands of middle, ring, and little fingers (Brand I)
   • Extensor carpi radialis longus (ECRL) extended by fascia lata strips volarly through the carpal
     tunnel into radial lateral bands of middle, ring, and little fingers (Brand II)
   • FCR + brachioradialis (BR) graft to lateral bands (Riordan)
   • EIP + EDQ to lateral bands through the intermetacarpal spaces (Bunnell-Fowler)
   • Zancolli "lasso" (FDS divided, looped through a slit in the A_2 pulley, and sutured to itself)

13. **What are the transfers for restoring thumb adduction?**
   • FDS of middle or ring finger to adductor pollicis
   • ECRB + palmaris tendon graft to adductor pollicis
   • BR/ECRL + graft between third and fourth metacarpals to adductor pollicis (Boyes)

14. **What are the transfers for restoring index finger abduction?**
   • Accessory APL + palmaris tendon graft to first dorsal interosseous (Neviaser)
   • EIP to first dorsal interosseous (Bunnell)
   • EPB to first dorsal interosseous (Bruner)
   • Many others

15. **What is the transfer to correct abduction of the little finger?**
EDQ to collateral ligament of MP joint

16. **What are the deficits in a high ulnar nerve palsy?**
   1. Less clawing of ring and small fingers (due to loss of the deforming forces of FDP of ring
and small fingers)
   2. Loss of DIP flexion of ring and little fingers

17. What are the standard tendon transfers for high ulnar nerve palsy?

1. Side-to-side tenorrhaphy of FDP of middle finger to FDP of ring and little fingers
2. Split FDS of middle finger—$\frac{1}{2}$ to ring, $\frac{1}{2}$ to small finger; radial side of A_1 or A_2 for MP flexion (to small finger, also helps to correct Wartenberg's sign)
3. Conventional tendon transfers for pinch and abducted little finger ($FDS_{middle} \pm$ graft to adductor pollicis; accessory APL + graft to first dorsal interosseous for pinch; and FDS_{ring} split volar to MP joint, then to radial lateral bands of ring and small fingers)

COMBINED NERVE PALSIES

18. In a low median/ulnar nerve palsy (the most common combined injury), what are the key deficits?

• Complete loss of palmar and volar digital sensation ("blind hand")
• Volar pulp atrophy
• Intrinsic motor loss

19. What are the recommended tendon transfers for reconstruction?

1. Thumb adduction/key pinch: ECRL + free graft between third and fourth metacarpals to abductor tubercle of thumb
2. Thumb abduction/opposition: FDS_{middle} to APB insertion through a pulley of FCU
3. Power flexion of proximal phalanx and integration of MP and IP motion (clawing): FDS_{ring}, split, to A_1/A_2 pulleys
4. Volar sensibility of thumb: free neurovascular cutaneous island flap from radial-innervated dorsum of hand (subject to debate)

20. What transfers, in addition to those for low median/ulnar nerve palsy, may be useful in a high median/ulnar nerve palsy?

1. Finger flexion: ECRL to FDP $\pm$ tenodesis of DIP joint of the middle, ring, and small fingers
2. Clawing
   • Tenodesis of all digits with free tendon graft to dorsal carpal ligament (volar to deep transverse metacarpal ligament) to extensor mechanism (dorsal aponeurosis, lateral bands)
   • Zancolli "lasso" (see question 12) using volar plate instead of A_2 pulley
3. Thumb/index (or long) pinch (tip pinch)
   • Arthrodesis of thumb MP joint
   • APL slips to first dorsal interosseous
   • EIP or EDQ to APB insertion for opposition
4. Thumb IP flexion: BR to FPL in forearm
5. Radiovolar sensibility (subject to debate)
   • Superficial radial nerve-innervated index fillet flap to palm, or
   • First dorsal metacarpal artery neurovascular island flap

CEREBRAL PALSY

21. List several common hand and upper extremity deformities seen in cerebral palsy that may benefit from tendon transfers.

• Thumb-in-palm deformity (thumb flexed, adducted)
• Thumb MP flexed, IP hyperextended *or* thumb MP hyperextended, IP flexed
• Clenched fist
• Wrist flexed, ulnar-deviated
• Forearm pronation
• Elbow flexion
The following factors also should be evaluated:
• Sensibility/cortical representation
• Fixed joint contractures vs. spasticity alone
• Adiadochokinesis (inability to perform rapid alternating movements)
• Intelligence level

• Function of opposite upper extremity
• Lower extremities and balance (need for ambulatory aids/wheelchair)
• Need for prolonged postoperative splinting and therapy to prevent recurrence

It is important to do only 1 or 2 transfers at a time; otherwise, you may overcorrect and create the opposite deformity.

22. What procedures are used to correct the thumb-in-palm deformity?
1. FPL abductoplasty (FPL to APB, fusion or tenodesis of thumb IP joint)
2. Lengthen FPL at musculotendinous junction, and transfer BR to APL
3. Flexor/pronator release
4. EPL reinforcement

23. What tendon transfers are used to correct the thumb deformities?
1. MP flexed, IP hyperextended: APL to ERB or EPL recession.
2. MP hyperextended, IP flexed: BR to APL, release adductor pollicis.
3. MP fusion is useful for both deformities and may be combined with FPL lengthening, BR to APL transfer, and release of adductor to deepen web space.

24. What transfers help to correct the clenched fist?
1. Superficialis-to-profundus transfer—most common
2. Flexor/pronator slide (release muscle origins from the medial epicondyle and proximal ulna)—less commonly done today
3. FCU or PT or BR to EDC (only after appropriate releases have been done)

25. What soft tissue procedures correct the wrist flexion/ulnar deviation, with or without pronation, seen in cerebral palsy?
1. FCU to ECRB (if primary deformity is palmar flexion) or ECRL (if primary deformity is ulnar deviation); Green procedure; with proper prolonged splinting, also helps finger contractures
2. Pronator teres tenotomy/pronator quadratus release
3. Flexor/pronator slide (rarely done)

26. If the wrist flexion, ulnar deviation, and pronation are due to a fixed bony deformity, what are the treatment options?
1. Proximal row carpectomy (preserves some wrist motion)
2. Radioulnar arthrodesis (if contracture is severe—rarely done)
3. Wrist arthrodesis (last resort or if sensory loss is profound)
Tendon transfers may still be needed for soft tissue balancing.

27. Elbow flexion contractures are common in cerebral palsy, although they do not often require surgical release. What structures would need to be released?
Biceps, brachialis, and lacertus fibrosus.

RHEUMATOID ARTHRITIS

28. What is the caput ulnae syndrome?
• Dorsal subluxation of the distal ulna, combined with supination of the carpus on the radius
• Loss of MP joint extension of the small finger due to rupture of the EDQ and EDC_{small}, followed by progressive ruptures of the EDC tendons from ulnar to radial
• Decreased active and passive forearm supination due to the distal radioulnar joint

29. After the EPL, the digital extensor tendons are the most frequently ruptured tendons in rheumatoid patients. They tend to rupture from ulnar (EDQ, $EDC_{small,ring}$) to radial ($EDC_{middle,index}$, EIP). What are the options for transfers if the EPL is intact?
1. If only EDQ, EDC_{small} are ruptured: distal end of EDQ sutured to EDC_{ring}
2. If EDQ and $EDC_{small,ring}$ are ruptured: EIP to EDC_{ring}, EDQ
3. If EDQ and $EDC_{small,ring,middle}$ are ruptured: EDC_{middle} distal end sutured to EDC_{index} plus EIP to EDC_{ring}, EDQ

4. If EIP is also ruptured: FDS_{ring} to EDQ and $EDC_{ring,middle}$
5. If all finger extensors are ruptured: FDS_{middle} to $EDC_{index,middle}$ and FDS_{ring} to $EDC_{ring,small}$

30. What are the choices for transfers if the EPL is ruptured?
1. EIP to EPL (preferred, if EIP available)
2. EDQ (if intact) to EPL
3. ECRL to EPL (least preferred)

31. What other disorders are in the differential diagnosis of extension tendon ruptures in rheumatoid patients?
• Tendon dislocation (due to attenuation of radial shroud fibers)
• MP joint dislocation (due to joint changes)
• Posterior interosseous nerve palsy

32. Flexor tendon ruptures are also seen in rheumatoid patients. Briefly discuss the major options for transfers.
1. If FPL is ruptured (Mannerfelt syndrome): FDS_{ring} to FPL or IP fusion (good choice if IP joint is already arthritic)
2. If FDP_{index} and FPL are ruptured: DIP fusion, tenodesis, or transfer FDS_{index} to FDP_{index} plus above transfers for FPL
3. IF FDS, FDP_{index}, and FPL are ruptured: distal FDP_{index} sutured to FDP_{middle} plus above for FPL
4. If FDS/P_{index} and FDS/P_{middle} are ruptured: $FDS_{middle,ring}$ to FDP_{index}, FDS_{small} to FDP
Note: If swan-neck deformities are present, try not to use FDS in transfers because it may worsen the swan-neck deformity.

QUADRIPLEGIA

33. In quadriplegic patients, elbow extension is important for transfer capabilities and to reach objects from a seated wheelchair position. How can elbow extension be reconstructed with tendon transfers?
• Deltoid to triceps with free tendon graft (Moberg)
• Biceps to triceps (Zancolli)

34. In C6 quadriplegics, the lowest functioning level is C6 and wrist extensors are functional. How can you provide useful grasp (key pinch)?
Thumb IP fusion and release of proximal thumb pulley + tenodesis of FPL to volar surface of radius (Moberg)

35. In C7 quadriplegics with elbow and wrist extension, how can you achieve pinch?
• Divide FDS_{ring} and transfer to APB; then use BR/ECRL to proximal end of FDS_{ring}.
• BR to EDC, EPL + FDS lasso to correct MP joint hyperextension + thumb MP volar capsulodesis + thumb CMC fusion (or APL tenodesis) + PT to FPL and ECRL to FDP (House's two-stage reconstruction).

36. List the priorities of reconstruction of function in quadriplegia.
1. Elbow extension
2. Simple hand mechanics by selected small joint fusions (i.e., thumb)
3. Reestablish effective key pinch (rather than opposition)
4. Reestablish active finger flexion (with passive tenodesis for digital extension)
5. In lower lesions, if active digital flexion and extension are restored, intrinsic function is reestablished by dorsally routed tenodesis

BRACHIAL PLEXUS

37. What are the most common types of brachial plexus injury?
• C5–C6 (upper trunk; Erb-Duchenne palsy)
• C8–T1 (lower trunk; Klumpke's palsy)
• C5–T1 (complete plexus)

38. For a patient with C5–C6 (upper trunk) palsy, what muscles are deficient? What transfers are useful?

1. Shoulder weakness of abduction/external rotation
   - Glenohumeral arthrodesis
   - L'Episcopo transfer (latissimus dorsi, teres major to posterolateral humeral head with or without anterior capsule and subscapularis release
2. Elbow flexion
   - Free innervated muscle flaps, using musculocutaneous nerve to multiple intercostal nerves
   - Pectoralis major to biceps (Clark)
   - Latissimus dorsi to biceps
   - Triceps to biceps
   - Steindler flexoplasty (transfer origin of flexor/pronator muscles to 5 cm proximal on humerus)

39. For a patient with C8–T1 (lower trunk) injury, what muscles are deficient? What transfers are useful?

The intrinsics are deficient as well as FCU and $FDP_{ring,small}$.
- Finger flexion: BR to FPL, ECRL to FDP
- Opposition: EIP to APB, ECU + tendon graft through intermetacarpal spaces to lateral bands

ARTHRODESES

40. What are the primary purposes for arthrodesis in patients with a nerve palsy, cerebral palsy, or rheumatoid arthritis?

To provide stabilization, to simplify a polyarticular system, and to provide motor power now available for transfer

41. To facilitate thumb/index tip pinch and to provide proximal thumb abduction stability in combined nerve palsies, cerebral palsy, and quadriplegia, what arthrodeses may be used?
- Thumb MP joint arthrodesis
- Thumb IP joint arthrodesis
- Index PIP, DIP joint arthrodeses

42. In combined nerve injuries, wrist stability is often a problem. What arthrodesis is useful?

Radiocarpal arthrodesis, which also makes extensor tendons available for transfer in a combined median/ulnar palsy.

43. If an adducted thumb cannot be stabilized by transfers (as in cerebral palsy, quadriplegia, and combined median/ulnar injury), what bony procedure may be helpful?

Thumb CMC fusion.

44. In an upper trunk brachial plexus palsy, shoulder weakness and/or instability may be seen. What procedure apart from tendon transfer may be useful?

Glenohumeral arthrodesis.

BIBLIOGRAPHY

1. Brand PW: Tendon transfer reconstructions for radial, ulnar, median and combined paralyses: Principles and Techniques. In Brand PW, Hollister A (eds): Clinical Mechanics of the Hand, 2nd ed. St. Louis, Mosby, 1993, pp 208–248.
2. Burton RI: The arthritic hand. In Evarts CM (ed): Surgery of the Musculoskeletal System. New York, Churchill Livingstone, 1990, pp 1087–1158.
3. Green DP, Burkhalter WE, Omer GE, et al: Nerve reconstruction. In Operative Hand Surgery, 3rd ed. New York, Churchill Livingstone, 1993, pp 1401–1531.
4. Jones NF: Tendon transfers for reconstruction of the hand and wrist. In Russel RC (ed): Instructional Courses in Plastic and Reconstructive Surgery. St. Louis, Mosby, 1992.
5. Littler JW: In Converse JM (ed): Reconstructive Plastic Surgery. Philadelphia, W.B. Saunders, 1977, pp 3103–3151, 3166–3214, 3266– 3305.

6. Littler JW: Tendon transfers and arthrodesis in combined median and ulnar nerve paralysis. J Bone Joint Surg 31A:225–234, 1949.
7. Moberg EA: Upper limb surgical rehabilitation in tetraplegia. In Evarts CM (ed): Surgery of the Musculoskeletal System. New York, Churchill Livingstone, 1990, pp 915–941.
8. Ramselaar JM: Tendon Transfers to Restore Opposition of the Thumb. Leiden, H.E. Stenfert Kroese N.V., 1970.
9. Smith RJ: Tendon Transfers of the Hand and Forearm. Boston, Little, Brown, 1987.

96. PROBLEMS INVOLVING THE PERIONYCHIUM

Duffield Ashmead, IV, M.D.

1. Describe fingernail anatomy and fingernail production.

The nail is a plate of flattened cells layered together and adherent to each other. The **nailbed** is composed of the **germinal matrix** (intermediate nail), which produces 90% of nail plate volume; the **sterile matrix** (ventral nail), which contributes additional substance that is largely responsible for nail adherence; and the **roof of the nail fold** (dorsal nail), which is responsible for the smooth, shiny surface of the nail plate. The sterile matrix is closely associated with the periosteum of the distal phalanx. The germinal matrix is immediately adjacent to the extensor tendon insertion. Distal phalangeal injuries are frequently associated with nail bed disruption.

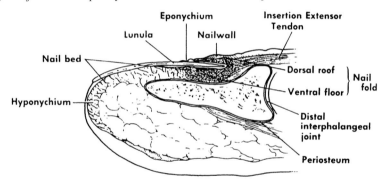

The anatomy of the nail bed in sagittal section. (From Zook EG, Brown RB: The perionychium. In Green DP (ed): Operative Hand Surgery, 3rd ed. New York, Churchill Livingstone, 1993, p 1284, with permission.)

2. What function does the fingernail serve?

In all likelihood, the fingernail evolved for scratching and self-defense as well as protecting the fingertip. In addition, it serves more delicate functions. By providing counterforce to the finger pulp, it increases the sensitivity of the fingertip; two-point discrimination widens if the nail plate is removed. Nails also assist in picking up fine or thin objects.

3. Describe the surrounding structures and their importance.

The **hyponychium**, or area immediately under the fingernail at its cut edge, is a keratinous plug that lines the juncture of the overhanging nail plate, the distal margin of sterile matrix, and the fingertip skin. It is heavily populated with lymphocytes and polymorphonuclear leukocytes as a barrier to subungual infection. The **perionychium** is the skin at the nail margin, folded over its proximal and lateral edges. It is a site of frequent, minor trauma and occasional infection.

4. What is the lunula?

The lunula is the whitish area of the most proximal nail. Attributed to differences in nail adherence and light reflection, it corresponds to the area beyond which cell nuclei within the nail plate have degenerated.

5. Describe several common nail changes that are manifestations of systemic disease.

Clubbing. This exaggerated curvature of the nail plate may be congenital but is classically described in association with pulmonary, bowel, or liver disease.

Onycholysis. Premature separation of the nail plates is seen with thyrotoxicosis and psoriasis. Psoriasis often leads to associated pitting and ridging of the nail plate.

Chromonychia. Changes in nail color may be seen in renal failure. They also may reflect drug effects.

6. Describe several nail changes associated with trauma.

Premature nail plate separation may reflect transverse scarring of the sterile matrix, frequently seen after fingertip crush injuries.

Longitudinal splitting of the nail plate may be due to scar adhesions from the nail roof to the nail floor (synechia).

Longitudinal grooving may reflect disturbances of the nail fold due to adjacent tumors or underlying skeletal change with secondary distortion.

Nail spikes or remnants frequently complicate traumatic fingertip amputations. Residua of germinal or sterile matrix continue to produce small volumes of nail plate, which grow over several months. Ultimately they may prove a source of pain or secondary infection, necessitating excision.

Beaking is a nail deformity caused by inadequate support of the distal sterile matrix. It is usually seen after distal fingertip amputations with loss of phalangeal tuft or healing of distal open wounds by secondary intention. As a result of the process of wound contracture, sterile matrix is drawn volar across the distal tip.

7. What are the usual patterns of infection associated with the fingernail?

Acute paronychia. Infection (usually staphylococcal) of the nail margin (perionychium) usually responds to direct drainage, marsupialization, or partial nail plate removal.

Chronic paronychia. Typically seen in patients whose hands are frequently wet (e.g., dishwashers). Maceration appears to lower defenses against local bacterial or fungal colonization. The condition often leads to nail plate deformity and onycholysis. It may respond to local or systemic antibiotics and antifungals with or without limited drainage. Complete nail plate removal is sometimes necessary.

Onychomycosis. Chronic fungal infestation of the perionychium and nail plate may be associated with dramatic discoloration of the nail as well as thickening and onycholysis. Although treatment with systemic antifungals such as griseofulvin has been advocated, simple nail plate removal and use of a topical antifungal as the nail regrows may be equally successful without the risks of systemic drug toxicity.

8. What is the significance of a subungual hematoma?

Crush injuries to the fingertip are extremely common. Development of a subungual hematoma invariably reflects nailbed injury with or without an associated fracture of the distal phalanx. Radiographs are almost always indicated. Even small subungual hematomas may be quite painful and should be decompressed. Classic techniques of trepanation include the use of a hot paperclip or battery-powered cautery, although drilling through the nail plate with a large-bore needle is also an option. More significant hematomas (> 50%) imply more extensive nailbed injury and should be explored by nail plate removal. In addition to providing complete decompression, nail plate removal allows nailbed repair. Most practitioners advocate the use of fine, absorbable suture (e.g,. 6.0 cat gut). The nail plate (or a substitute) is then replaced to splint the repair and stent the nail fold to prevent synechiae.

9. Discuss common benign periungual tumors.

Mucous cysts are small ganglia arising from the distal interphalangeal (DIP) joint, usually in association with a small osteophyte(s). As they encroach on the perionychium either deep or superficial to the germinal matrix, splitting or deep grooving may be seen in the nail plate. Larger cysts are associated with significant attenuation of the overlying skin and occasionally may drain spontaneously. Mucous cysts are usually treated by excision, taking care to address the associated osteophyte.

Glomus tumors (tumors of the glomus body) are frequently subungual. Although often extremely small (1–2 mm), they are characteristically painful, exquisitely tender, and highly sensitive to cold. The diagnosis is often empirical. Resection may require transungual exposure or elevation of the nailbed from a lateral approach.

Pyogenic granulomas represent an exuberant excess of granulation tissue in response to relatively minor trauma. They are frequently encountered in the perionychium. Most respond to curettage and chemical or electrical cautery of the base.

10. What is the differential diagnosis for pigmented subungual lesions?
The most common pigmented subungual lesion is **posttraumatic hemorrhage**, although the patient frequently reports no history of injury. These lesions usually "grow out" with the nail plate and can be identified by scoring the overlying plate and observing for several weeks.

Benign nevi occasionally present in a subungual location.

Subungual melanoma is potentially serious and often diagnosed late. The threshold for nail plate removal and incisional biopsy of a suspicious lesion should be low.

11. What is the significance of pigment deposition within the nail plate? What is Hutchinson's sign?
Benign pigment streaks in the nail plate (melanonychia striata longitudinalis) are extremely common in black patients and often occur spontaneously, particularly with advancing age. Similar streaking of pigment in the nail plate may reflect the presence of a benign subungual (germinal matrix) nevus. Broader streaks of variegated color and streaks with cuticular pigmentation (Hutchinson's sign) should raise suspicion of a subungual melanoma.

BIBLIOGRAPHY
1. Fleegler E, Zienowicz RJ: Tumors of the perionychium. Hand Clin 6:113–134, 1990.
2. Guy RJ: The etiologies and mechanisms of nail bed injuries. Hand Clin 6:9–20, 1990.
3. Keyser JJ, Littler JW, Eaton RG: Surgical treatment of infections and lesions. Hand Clin 6:137–154, 1990.
4. Van Beek AL, Kassan MA, Adson MH, Dale V: Management of acute fingernail injuries. Hand Clin 6:23–36, 1990.
5. Zook EG: Anatomy and physiology of the perionychium. Hand Clin 6:1–8, 1990.
6. Zook EG, Brown RE: The perionychium. In Green DP (ed): Operative Hand Surgery, 3rd ed. New York, Churchill Livingstone, 1993, pp 1283–1314.
7. Zook EG, Van Beek AL, Russell RC, Beatty ME: Anatomy and physiology of the perionychium: A review of the literature and anatomic study. J Hand Surg 5:528–536, 1980.

97. FINGERTIP INJURIES

Richard J. Zienowicz, M.D.

1. Which is the most frequently injured finger?
The long (middle) finger. Fingertips are the most frequently injured part of the hand, and the long finger is most vulnerable because it is the last to be withdrawn from a machine or car door.

2. Where is the greatest quantity of dermal lymphatics in the human body?
The hyponychium. Teleologically it make sense to protect the parts of the body (fingers and toes) most frequently in contact with potential disease-causing organisms.

3. What is the anatomic significance of the lunula?
The lunula represents the transition zone of the proximal germinal matrix and distal sterile matrix of the nailbed. The cells at this point become pycnotic (lose their nuclei).

4. What is the clinical significance of the lunula?
The lunula visibly demarcates the germinal matrix even without the nail plate intact, unless it is heavily contused. If sufficient turgid soft tissue support can be restored (i.e., thick thenar flap), the possibility of preservation of the tip and a reasonable, albeit shorter, nail can be anticipated.

5. What are the treatment goals for fingertip injuries?

All treatment decisions involve a FAT compromise (function, appearance, and time). In general, the hand surgeon must endeavor (1) to preserve length and sensibility, (2) to prevent joint contracture and symptomatic neuroma, (3) to encourage early return of function, and (4) to honor aesthetic considerations of the patient when feasible.

6. Do most injuries involving primarily skin loss from the fingertip heal better with skin grafts?

Usually not. Good results after conservative treatment (healing by secondary intention) are the rule; in several studies both cosmesis and sensibility were superior compared with skin grafting.

7. If the nail has been destroyed, why not just shorten the digit to the level of the distal interphalangeal joint?

The profundus tendon attaches to the base of the distal phalanx. Shortening results in profound loss of strength because the insertion of the tendon is discarded.

8. Describe the lumbrical-plus finger.

The lumbrical-plus finger may arise after amputation of the distal phalanx or unrepaired laceration of the profundus tendon. Loss of its distal insertion allows the profundus tendon to migrate proximally, along with the lumbrical muscle attached to it in zone IV of the palm. When a lumbrical contracts, ordinarily it pulls the profundus tendon in a distal direction and the lateral band in a proximal direction, resulting in extension of the proximal (PIP) and distal interphalangeal (DIP) joints and flexion of the metaphalangeal (MP) joint. When flexion is attempted in the lumbrical-plus finger, paradoxical extension occurs as the proximally migrated profundus tendon pulls the lumbrical proximally, forcing the IP joints into extension via the lateral band.

9. Why not preserve the profundus function and pad the stump by suturing it to the extensor tendon?

In most cases, this procedure would result in the **quadriga syndrome**, which Verdan named after the Roman charioteers who had to control the reins to four horses. Tendon balance is upset by relatively minor changes in length. Verdan described the inability to achieve full composite flexion (i.e., clenched fist) if the profundus tendon of one finger is pulled to greater-than-normal resting length. The effect is simulated by holding the long or ring finger in extension while attempting to make a fist with the others.

10. Which local flap is most suitable for reconstruction of multiple fingertip injuries on the same hand?

The cross-finger flap uses tissue from the dorsum of the middle phalanx but can be designed with equal versatility and reliability from the proximal phalanx or palmar or axial surfaces. This technique allows concurrent repair of 3 or sometimes even 4 adjacent fingertip injuries.

11. What vital structure is susceptible to injury during elevation of a thenar flap?

The radial digital sensory nerve to the thumb, which courses along the surface of the flexor pollicis brevis muscle.

12. Some authors have worried about permanent joint contractures after thenar flap use and cautioned against this technique in older patients. Is such concern warranted?

The thenar flap requires 10–14 days of immobilization with the PIP joint in flexion. In a careful review of 150 cases, Melone and Beasley found only 6 patients who demonstrated stiffness, usually with less than 15° of extension loss. Thirty-one patients were over 50 years of age, and only one had persistent stiffness.

13. Neglect of what key technical element in direct closure of a digital amputation typically results in a persistently painful finger?

Failure to resect a sufficient length of each digital nerve to avoid neuroma formation in the prehensile surface area.

14. Anesthesia for fingertip injuries is usually accomplished by digital block. What measures can significantly decrease the pain associated with local injection?

The first step is to choose the dorsal web spaces, where pain and pressure receptor distribution is proportionately far less than in palmar skin. A small-gauge needle (25 G or less) disturbs fewer receptors. The pain of injection has been shown to be related primarily to the acidic pH of the injectate (plain xylocaine ~ 3.3–5.5). Addition of sodium bicarbonate (44 mEq/L) to xylocaine in a 1:9 ratio (i.e., 1 cc bicarbonate to 9 cc xylocaine) raises the pH to approximately normal tissue range (7.35–7.45); lowers the pKa; and results in quicker initiation of the block and shorter duration of action. This procedure can be supplemented with straight local injection and/or bupivacaine to extend the duration of anesthesia. Avoid mixing bicarbonate with marcaine because it will cause milky precipitation. Lastly, a slow injection avoids excessive pressure receptor activation until the anesthetic effect has begun.

15. What is glabrous skin?

Glabrous skin is devoid of pilosebaceous units and generally heals with less scarring. The best location for obtaining glabrous skin for use on hand and fingertip injuries is the ulnar aspect of the hypothenar eminence.

16. Are there any tricks to obtaining a graft of uniform thickness?

The Pitkin technique used to obtain skin grafts from difficult donor sites is ideal for the hypothenar region. Xylocaine with epinephrine is injected subcutaneously to raise a wheal in the shape of the intended graft (drawn with a marking pen). A long blade (Weck or Goulian) is necessary except for small grafts, which may be taken with a no. 10 or 20 blade. The best instrument for this area is a Davol dermatome, which looks like an electric toothbrush (Stanley Simon, a general surgeon, designed it in his basement workshop). The Davol dermatome allows harvest of a nearly full-thickness graft that will contract minimally yet leave an inconspicuous donor site.

17. Describe the terminal vascular anatomy of the finger.

The two digital arteries form an anastomotic arch near the terminal insertion of the profundus tendon. The arch then gives off two smaller collateral arteries and one larger (< 0.7-mm diameter) artery, all of which remain contiguous distally with the dorsal network of much smaller caliber. Lateroungual veins are too narrow for microsurgical anastomosis. Suitable veins for anastomosis are present on the palmar pulp surface immediately beneath the skin.

18. What is the cap technique?

Using the robust periosteal circulation of the distal phalanx, Rose described a technique of limited removal of proximal soft tissue, including nailbed, and replacement of amputated distal parts usually not suitable for replantation over this bone. His technique improved survival of composite tip grafts.

19. Do neurovascular island flaps eventually integrate sensorally with their new site after transfer?

In only 20–40% of adults but more frequently in children.

20. Aside from local flaps, what other techniques may be used to correct soft tissue losses to the fingertip?

Composite grafts from the toe distal phalanges provide like tissue with minimal donor morbidity and deformity. Distant flaps from the groin, abdomen, chest, and elsewhere are occasionally used, especially when involvement of multiple digits makes local donor sites unusable or impractical. Free tissue transfer of toes, either complete or partial, is an excellent choice for distal phalangeal reconstruction of the thumb because it results in optimal functional and aesthetic restoration.

21. Cold intolerance after fingertip injury is common. When does it resolve?

Probably never. Previous teaching that cold intolerance was a transient phenomenon has been challenged lately by many surgeons' reports of longstanding persistent symptoms that may become more tolerable but nevertheless remain bothersome.

22. How is sensibility affected after advancement flap reconstruction of the fingertip?

The typical V-Y flaps provide near normal (5–7 mm) two-point discrimination, whereas the Moberg and other axial refinements of this flap can restore normal sensation (≤ 5 mm).

23. Flaps are composite tissues intended to replace missing soft tissues (and occasionally muscle, bone, or cartilage) with similar components. Their common denominator, when successful, is patency of arterial inflow and venous outflow. Associate the following flaps with their respective anatomic descriptions.

    1. Axial flap   2. Random flap   3. Island flap   4. Pedicle flap

    A ( ) Perfusion derived exclusively through the subdermal plexus of vessels.

    B ( ) Arteriovenous connection; "leash" of blood vessels supplies flap.

    C ( ) Harvested from an area with a known arteriovenous blood supply while remaining connected by skin and subcutaneous tissue to its donor site.

    D ( ) In all respects identical to axial pattern flap, but skin and soft tissue attachments are divided, leaving the flap attached only to its dominant blood vessels.

    Answers: A (2), B (4), C (1), D (3)

24. Choose the descriptive name or eponym for the following flaps:

    A ( ) V-Y advancement flap with unilateral or bilateral applications

    B ( ) Heterodigital random pattern flap, optionally providing sensation

    C ( ) Axial advancement flap most appropriate for thumb

    D ( ) Heterodigital neurovascular island flap that leaves insensate donor site

    E ( ) Axial dorsal flap with hetero- and homodigital applications

    F ( ) Versatile island flap based on the first dorsal metacarpal artery (first described by Foucher)

    G ( ) Random-pattern, palmar-based flap with myriad configurations

    H ( ) Palmar advancement flap best suited for dorsal oblique amputations

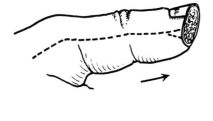

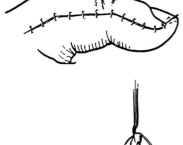

FIGURE 1.   Moberg volar advancement flap. Midlateral incisions are made on the radial and ulnar sides of the thumb, and the volar flap is elevated. The MP and IP joints are flexed at a 30–40° angle, and the flap is advanced. (From Tsuge K: Comprehensive Atlas of Hand Surgery. Chicago, Year Book, 1989, p 84, © Nankodo, Tokyo, 1984, with permission.)

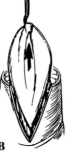
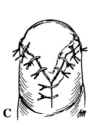

FIGURE 2.   Atasoy-Kleinert volar V-Y advancement flap. *A*, Flap design. *B*, Flap elevation and advancement. *C*, Inset. (From Green DP (ed): Operative Hand Surgery, vol. 1, 3rd ed. New York, Churchill Livingstone, 1993, p 56, with permission.)

A   B   C

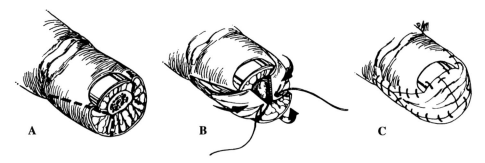

FIGURE 3.   Kutler lateral V-Y advancement flap. *A,* Flap design. *B,* Flap elevation and advancement. *C,* Inset. (From Green DP (ed): Operative Hand Surgery, vol. 1, 3rd ed. New York, Churchill Livingstone, 1993, p 56, with permission.)

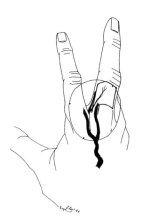

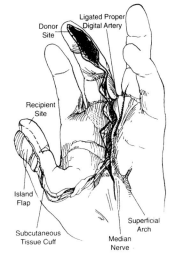

FIGURE 5 *(right).*   Littler flap. The flap is elevated based on the ulnar neurovascular pedicle and passed through a tunnel to the thumb defect. The donor site is closed with a full-thickness skin graft. (From Coleman DA, Valnicek SM: Neurovascular island flaps. In Blair WF (ed): Techniques in Hand Surgery. Baltimore, Williams & Wilkins, 1996, p 62, with permission.)

FIGURE 4 *(above).*   Flag flap. The reliability of the flap is improved when at least one cutaneous vein and a dorsal digital artery are included in the staff of the flag. (From Foucher G, Khouri RK: Digital reconstruction with island flaps. Clin Plast Surg 24:17, 1997, with permission.)

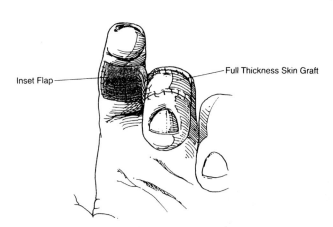

FIGURE 6.   Cross-finger flap. This flap is typically elevated from the dorsum of a middle phalanx for coverage of a volar defect on an adjacent digit or the thumb. The donor site is closed with a skin graft. (From Calkins ER, Smith DJ: The cross-finger flap. In Blair WF (ed): Techniques in Hand Surgery. Baltimore, Williams & Wilkins, 1996, p 49, with permission.)

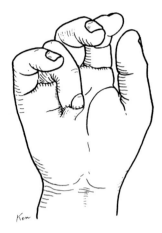

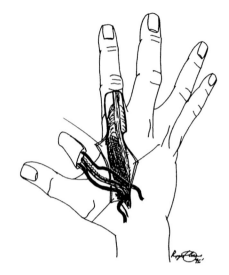

FIGURE 7. Thenar flap. (From Tsuge K: Comprehensive Atlas of Hand Surgery. Chicago, Year Book, 1989, p 82, © Nankodo, Tokyo, 1984, with permission.)

Answers (figure number in parentheses): A (3), B (6), C (1), D (5), E (4), F (8), G (7), H (2)

FIGURE 8. Kite flap. This flap is raised from the dorsum of the proximal phalanx of the index finger and transferred to the thumb. Superficial branches of the radial nerve that innervate the skin island are included in the neurovascular pedicle. (From Foucher G, Khouri RK: Digital reconstruction with island flaps. Clin Plast Surg 24:21, 1997, with permission.)

BIBLIOGRAPHY

1. Cronin TD: The cross finger flap: A new method of repair. Am Surg 17:419–425, 1951.
2. Henderson HP, Campbell Reid DA: Long term follow-up of neurovascular island flaps. Hand 12:113–122, 1980.
3. Lister GD: Skin flaps. In Green DP: Operative Hand Surgery, vol. 2, 3rd ed. New York, Churchill Livingstone, 1993, p 1741.
4. Littler JW: Neurovascular skin island transfer in reconstructive hand surgery. Transactions of the Scandinavian International Congress of the Society of Plastic Surgeons, 1960, pp 175–179.
5. Louis DS. Amputations. In Green DP: Operative Hand Surgery, vol. 1, 3rd ed. New York, Churchill Livingstone, 1993, p 53.
6. Russell RC: Fingertip injuries. Plast Surg 7:4477, 1990.
7. Russell RC, Casas LA: Management of fingertip injuries. Clin Plast Surg 16:3, 1989.
8. Zook EG: The perionychium: Anatomy, physiology, and care of injuries. Clin Plast Surg 8:21–31, 1981.

98. INFECTIONS OF THE HAND

Norman Weinzweig, M.D., and Mark H. Gonzalez, M.D.

1. Who was Allen B. Kanavel?

Allen B. Kanavel, Professor of Surgery at Northwestern University Medical School in Chicago, wrote the classic treatise, *Infections of the Hand*, in 1912 during the preantibiotic area, expounding many basic principles in hand surgery. His work served as an invaluable guide to the surgical treatment of acute and chronic suppurative processes of the fingers, hand, and forearm, including the pathways of spread of infection and placement of surgical incisions. He also promulgated the fascial-space concept.

2. What was the mortality rate associated with hand infections in the preantibiotic era?

Acute lymphangitis caused by streptococcal infections of the hand was associated with significant morbidity and mortality in the preantibiotic area. Mortality rates as high as 28% were cited in the literature. After the introduction of antibiotics, streptococcal species were found to be exquisitely sensitive to penicillin.

3. What is the most common hand infection?
Paronychia.

4. What is the most common pathogen responsible for hand infections?
Staphylococcus aureus.

5. What is the etiopathogenesis of felons?
Felons arise when a penetrating wound contaminates the fat pad of the distal phalanx, producing a closed-space abscess. The abscess is associated with progressive tenderness and throbbing pain. A vicious cycle of inflammation, congestion, venous compromise, necrosis, and abscess formation is initiated. The abscess generally points in the path of least resistance, the site of maximal tenderness. Spontaneous decompression may occur with skin necrosis. If the skin is unyielding, felons may result in osteomyelitis, tenosynovitis, or septic arthritis.

6. What are the possible consequences of untreated or inappropriately treated felons?
- Painful, unstable, insensate, unaesthetic scars
- Acute flexor tenosynovitis
- Septic arthritis
- Osteomyelitis
- Deep space infection
- Amputation

7. What are the different types of incisions for drainage of felons?
- Fishmouth
- J or hockey stick
- Through-and-through
- Volar transverse
- Midvolar longitudinal
- Unilateral high midlateral

8. Describe the advantages and disadvantages of the above incisions.
Various incisions have been described for the treatment of felons. The fishmouth or alligator mouth incision is mentioned only to be condemned; it often results in a painful, unstable scar. The J or hockey stick and through-and-through incisions are similar to the fishmouth incision. The volar transverse incision may injure the terminal digital nerve branches at the level of the trifurcation. Popular incisions for the treatment of felons include the traditional unilateral high midlateral incision and the less-known but equally acceptable midvolar longitudinal incision. The midvolar longitudinal incision must *not* be carried proximal to the distal interphalangeal joint crease to avoid problems with contracture. This incision avoids the potential problems with a high midlateral incision when the abscess points volarly, predisposing to necrosis of the intervening skin bridge.

9. What are the advantages of the midvolar longitudinal incision?
- Most direct approach: drain an abscess where it points
- Most efficient drainage
- Minimizes injury to digital nerves
- Least amount of scarring
- Maintains stability of soft tissue pad

10. What complications may follow treatment of felons?
- Slough of the bridge of normal skin between the incision and central necrosis (high midlateral)
- Anesthesia with blind digit tips after cutting terminal digital nerve branches (transverse volar)
- Pain due to neuroma formation or cicatricial entrapment of nerve endings (transverse volar)
- Unstable pulp due to division of fibrous septae (fishmouth)
- Unsightly scars

11. What is the clinical presentation of herpetic whitlow?
This infection is common in health care workers, such as dentists and respiratory therapists, who are exposed to the herpes simplex virus. The incubation period is 2–14 days. It is characterized by throbbing pain, swelling, and erythema in the affected finger. Vesicles of clear fluid often coalesce to form ulcers over 10–14 days.

12. Is herpetic whitlow an aseptic felon?
Herpetic whitlow is often described as an aseptic felon. This is a misnomer because herpetic whitlow is a *cutaneous* disease and therefore does *not* involve the deep pulp space.

13. How is herpetic whitlow treated?

Herpetic whitlow is treated conservatively. The infection runs a self-limited course and usually resolves spontaneously within 3 weeks with normal healing. Herpes infections may be prolonged in immunocompromised patients and patients with secondary bacterial infection. The treatment of herpes infections of the hand should be conservative with analgesics and elevation to reduce pain and swelling. Incision and drainage are to be avoided unless a secondary bacterial abscess develops. Antiviral agents such as acyclovir or foscarnet may be used in immunocompromised patients with a refractory herpetic infection.

14. Is surgical drainage ever indicated for the treatment of herpetic whitlow?

No. Incision and drainage may lead to devastating complications involving the entire distal phalanx with bacterial superinfection and even ascending encephalitis that results in death. The only possible role for surgery is segmental nail removal for relief of pain over the involved portion of the nailbed.

15. What are acute paronychia?

Acute paronychia are infections of the soft tissue fold around the fingernail (nail fold). They involve disruption of the seal between the proximal nail fold and the nail plate and provide a portal of entry for bacteria.

16. What is a "run-around" infection?

Continuity of the paronychial tissue with the eponychial tissue overlying the tissue of the nail may result in extension of the infection to involve both the eponychium and paronychium. A run-around abscess usually involves the entire nail fold, spreading under the nail sulcus to the opposite side; it is most commonly seen in young children and cases of neglected paronychia. Most often, gram-positive cocci such as staphylococci and streptococci are the culprits. In children, the infection has an increased distribution of anaerobic and mixed bacterial flora.

17. How are acute paronychia treated?

Early in their course, acute paronychia occasionally can be treated by soaks, hand elevation, splintage, and antibiotics. Once the nail fold is elevated by accumulation of pus, drainage should be performed. First the involved finger is soaked in warm suds water for 15–30 minutes to loosen the nail fold; a Freer elevator is then used to tease gently the eponychial fold in the area of pus accumulation and thus facilitate drainage. One-fourth-inch plain gauze is loosely packed in the wound, the hand is splinted and elevated, and antibiotics are given. Often, no anesthetic (digital nerve block) is necessary. In rare cases, it is necessary to incise the eponychial fold longitudinally, as described by some surgeons.

18. What are chronic paronychia?

Chronic paronychia demonstrate an indurated and rounded cuticle as a result of recurring episodes of increased inflammation, drainage, and eventual thickening and longitudinal grooving of the nail plate. They are most often seen in middle-aged women as a result of prolonged occlusion of the nail fold in the presence of *Candida albicans* (cultured in 95% of cases). Mechanical separation of the undersurface of the cuticle from the upper layer of the nail plate may be due to trauma, manicure, prolonged immersion in water (dishwashers), fungal invasion of the subcuticular area, retained foreign body, and necrotic nail.

19. How are chronic paronychia similar to acute paronychia?

Chronic paronychia are a completely distinct entity from acute paronychia with no similarities except involvement of the nail fold.

20. How are chronic paronychia treated?

Chronic paronychia are far more difficult and frustrating to eradicate than the acute form. Nonoperative treatment is universally unsuccessful. Surgical procedures include marsupialization of the eponychium, as described by Keyser and Eaton in 1976, and total onychiectomy (nail plate removal) and application of antifungal-steroid ointment to the nailbed (3% Bio-form in Mycolog), as described in Kilgore and Graham in 1977.

21. How many cardinal signs did Kanavel originally describe?
Kanavel originally described only three cardinal signs. Although he mentioned in his treatise that "the whole of the finger is uniformly swollen," this observation was not a cardinal sign.

22. What are Kanavel's four cardinal signs of flexor tenosynovitis?
1. Exquisite tenderness that affects the entire tendon sheath and is limited to the sheath
2. Intense pain with passive extension of the finger, most marked at the proximal end
3. Semiflexed finger
4. Fusiform or symmetric swelling of the entire finger

23. How is acute flexor tenosynovitis treated?
Acute flexor tenosynovitis is treated by tendon sheath irrigation. The patient is taken to the operating room, and either the open or closed approach is used.

24. What are the open and closed approaches to tendon sheath irrigation for acute flexor tenosynovitis?
The **closed approach** to tendon sheath irrigation involves limited incisions for drainage of the involved tendon sheath. Placement of the incisions varies, but they are usually located distal to the A_4/A_5 pulley at the level of the distal interphalangeal (DIP) joint and just proximal to the A_1 pulley at the level of the distal palmar crease. Vigorous intraoperative irrigation of the tendon sheath is key to the treatment of this hand emergency. Although some surgeons prefer 10% antibiotic solutions for irrigation, the mechanical action of the irrigant appears to be more important than the nature of the irrigant. Many surgeons set up an irrigating system postoperatively, with 2 catheters situated proximal and distal to the ends of the flexor sheath, but it is most likely that intraoperative irrigation plays the critical role in treating the tenosynovitis. The closed approach allows primary wound healing with less scarring, less risk of desiccation and tendon necrosis, shorter hospitalization (< 72 hours), active flexion and extension exercises within 48–72 hours, rapid and complete functional recovery with minimal morbidity usually within 7–10 days, greater patient compliance with less pain on exercise, and a smaller primary wound.
The **open approach**, which uses midaxial or volar zig-zag incisions, exposes delicate structures to infection with subsequent fibrosis and loss of function. Other problems include increased risk of tendon necrosis, greater scarring, and significant morbidity. The open approach essentially involves filleting the volar aspect of the involved finger with direct drainage of any purulent material. Treatment may require secondary procedures and prolonged hospitalization and rehabilitation and yield a less desirable functional result.

25. How is gonococcal flexor tenosynovitis treated?
Gonococcal flexor tenosynovitis most commonly arises by hematogenous spread from a genitourinary focus. It is often the only manifestation of disseminated gonorrhea. The clinical picture is acute flexor tenosynovitis. Treatment is by closed sheath irrigation and intravenous penicillin G, 1 million U every 4 hours, or a third-generation cephalosporin. Good functional recovery is the rule.

26. Which pathogens are most commonly responsible for acute flexor tenosynovitis?
Most cultures are sterile because of the initiation of antibiotic therapy before culture. The most common pathogens are gram-positive cocci.

27. What are the complications of untreated or inappropriately treated acute flexor tenosynovitis?
- Skin necrosis
- Tendon adhesions
- Tendon necrosis and rupture
- Joint ankylosis
- Septic arthritis
- Osteomyelitis
- Deep space abscess
- Amputation

28. What are the fascial spaces in the hand?
The fascial spaces are potential spaces located throughout the hand that swell after implantation of bacteria, such as by penetrating injuries.

29. Name the fascial spaces of the hand.

- Thenar space
- Middle palmar space
- Hypothenar space
- Subfascial web space in the palm and interdigital area ("collar button")
- Dorsal subaponeurotic space
- Dorsal subcutaneous space
- Radial bursa
- Ulna bursa
- Parona's space

30. Why are the fascial spaces pertinent to hand infections?

Pus from an infection in the flexor tendon sheath of the ring or middle finger may rupture into the middle palmar space. Similarly, pus from an infection in the index flexor tendon sheath may rupture into the thenar space. Infection in the hypothenar space is rarely described. The dorsal subcutaneous space is a large potential space overlying the entire dorsum of the hand and may contain large volumes of pus. The dorsal subaponeurotic space lies deep to the aponeurosis of the extensor tendons.

31. What is a "collar-button" abscess?

A collar-button abscess is an infection of the subfascial palmar space, which is contiguous with the dorsal subcutaneous space between the fingers. The subfascial palmar space and the dorsal subcutaneous space are the two most superficial of the deep spaces in the hand. Collar-button abscesses begin as blisters, which become infected with intracutaneous and subcutaneous pus in the palm. Tethering of the skin to the palmar fascia makes it difficult for a subcutaneous infection in this area to track superficially beneath the space or between the skin and fascia. Consequently, instead of spreading peripherally, the abscess extends dorsally to the palmar fascia. Contiguity with the dorsal subcutaneous tissues causes a great deal of dorsal swelling with abduction of the fingers because of purulence between the digits palmarly and dorsally. Treatment requires incision and drainage of the subcutaneous blister with excision of the palmar fascia. Exposure of the superficial dorsal extension allows complete unroofing of the subfascial infection. Great care must be taken to identify the bifurcation of the digital arteries to the adjacent sides of the fingers. Local wound care and early motion usually result in full functional recovery.

32. What are the causes of dorsal hand swelling?

(1) Lymphatic drainage to the dorsum of the hand from either palmar or dorsal infection sites, (2) dorsal subcutaneous abscess, and (3) dorsal subaponeurotic abscess.

33. Describe the treatment of a dorsal hand abscess.

The dorsal subaponeurotic space in the hand is a potential space that usually becomes secondarily infected from a local penetration injury. It is often difficult to differentiate this infection from a dorsal subcutaneous abscess. The problem should be approached as the worst case scenario—a subaponeurotic infection. Two linear incisions should be made on the dorsum of the hand, one over the second metacarpal and one between the fourth and fifth metacarpal. This technique permits differentiation of the infection, drainage, and satisfactory coverage of the tendons. A dorsal midline incision in the case of a subaponeurotic abscess may result in extensor tendon loss due to desiccation, infection, and ischemia. Early motion is mandatory after drainage and should involve all three digital joints plus the wrist joint to maintain extensor tendon gliding.

34. What are the boundaries of the thenar space?

Dorsal: musculature of the adductor pollicis

Volar: fascia overlying adductor pollicis

Radial: fusion of adductor pollicis and adductor fascia at their insertion into the proximal phalanx of the thumb

Ulnar: midpalmar space or oblique septum extending from the palmar fascia to the volar ridge of the third metacarpal

The thenar space is contiguous with the flexor tendons of the index finger. It is exposed to local penetrating injury.

35. What is the position of the thumb in thenar space infections?

The thumb is held in marked abduction because this maneuver reduces pressure within the abscess cavity. Progressive infection within the thenar space usually tracks dorsally over the adductor pollicis and first dorsal interosseous muscles. This progression produces a dumbbell effect with extension of the abscess from its origin deep to the flexor tendons of the index finger over the adductor pollicis and first dorsal interosseous to its site of presentation superficial to the first dorsal interosseous.

36. What incisions are used for drainage of thenar space abscesses?

Adequate drainage of a thenar space infection must permit exposure to the dumbbell abscess with care to protect the digital nerve and artery to the radial aspect of the index finger as well as the nerve and volar blood supply to the thumb (ulnar digital nerve and princeps pollicis artery or only the ulnar digital artery to the thumb). The recommended incisions are perpendicular to the web space approximately 1 cm proximal to the thenar crease and extend proximally on the dorsum or palm toward the convergence of the index and thumb metacarpals. The fascia overlying the adductor muscle and first dorsal interosseous can be excised widely. Incisions parallel to the web space either volarly or dorsally result in a contracture web space between the thumb and index finger.

37. What are the boundaries of the midpalmar space?

Midpalmar space infections are located ulnar to the oblique septum. They may result from either indirect inoculation by a penetrating injury or rupture of flexor tenosynovitis involving the middle or ring fingers. They occur less commonly than thenar space infections, probably because of the relatively protective nature of the midpalmar space compared with the dorsum of the thumb-index web. Flexor tenosynovitis involving the little finger tracks proximally through the ulna bursa and does not enter the midpalmar space. Infection results in dorsal swelling (as in a thenar abscess). It is the only infection resulting in loss of palmar concavity. The infection is located deep (dorsal) to the flexor tendons and volar to the metacarpals.

38. What incisions are used for drainage of a midpalmar space abscess?

An oblique or transverse palmar incision should allow wide exposure of the palmar fascia with identification and protection of the neurovascular bundles of the adjacent fingers as well as the deep palmar arch and ulnar motor nerve.

39. What structures are connected to form a "horseshoe" abscess?

The sheath of the flexor pollicis communicates with the radial bursa. Likewise, the sheath of the little finger communicates with the ulnar bursae. The two bursae communicate with the deep space just superficial to the pronator quadratus, termed Parona's space. An infection of the tendon sheath of the thumb or little finger may progress through Parona's space into the other side, forming a horseshoe abscess.

40. What factors lead to the development of osteomyelitis after a human bite?

Delayed treatment, inadequate initial debridement, and initial suturing of the wound.

41. What organisms are encountered in a human bite infection? What is appropriate initial antibiotic therapy?

The organisms are microbes commonly found on the skin or in the mouth. Examples include gram-positive aerobic organisms (*Staphylococcus aureus, Staphylococcus epidermidis, Streptococcus* species) and anaerobes (*Peptococcus* species, *Peptostreptococcus* species, *Bacteroides* species, and *Eikenella corrodens*, a facultative anaerobe). Antibiotic coverage must cover gram-positive and anaerobic organisms. A first-generation cephalosporin in combination with penicillin or ampicillin in combination with clavulonic acid fosters adequate coverage. In penicillin-sensitive patients, clindamycin may be used, but *E. corrodens* is resistant to clindamycin and an additional antibiotic may be added based on culture and sensitivity.

42. What organisms are associated with wounds contaminated with river or sea water? What antibiotic therapy is appropriate?

Vibrio vulnificus occurs in coastal and brackish water and commonly infects cuts acquired while cleaning or shelling crabs. The organism is sensitive to tetracycline and chloramphenicol. *Mycobacterium marinum* infection, termed "swimming pool granuloma," is a cutaneous infection acquired in fresh water. Appropriate antibiotics are rifampin and ethambutol or trimethoprim-sulfamethoxazole. *Aeromonas hydrophila* is also commonly found in fresh water and may infect open cuts in swimmers. Appropriate antibiotics are ciprofloxacin, trimethoprim-sulfamethoxazole, and tetracycline.

43. What factors predispose to the development of necrotizing fasciitis? What are the etiologic organisms? Describe the pathologic process.

Necrotizing fasciitis is most frequently seen in intravenous drug abusers, diabetics, and alcoholics. The organisms most frequently noted are beta-hemolytic streptococci and mixed aerobic-anaerobic organisms. The infection causes liquefaction necrosis of the fascia with selective spread along fascial planes. Involvement of the skin and muscle occurs at later stages with bullae formation, skin slough, and myonecrosis.

44. What organisms are frequently seen in dog and cat bites?

Dog bites: *S. aureus, Streptococcus viridans, Pasteurella multocida,* and *Bacteroides* species. Cat bites: *P. multocida.*

45. Describe the clinical presentation of sporotrichosis in the upper extremity. How is it treated?

Sporotrichosis is a chronic granulomatous infection caused by the saprophytic fungus *Sporothrix schenckii*. After inoculation through a skin abrasion or thorn puncture, a local ulceration develops. The disease then spreads through the lymphatic channels with red, hard nodules and ulcerations along the path of lymphatic spread in the arm. On rare occasions, the disease presents with inflammatory arthritis of the joints of the hand or wrist. Treatment is a long course of oral potassium iodide. Refractory disease and extracutaneous disease respond to intravenous amphotericin B.

46. What factors predispose to the development of gas gangrene? How is it treated?

Gas gangrene is caused by *Clostridium* species or other gas-forming organisms. The condition is frequently seen in grossly contaminated wounds with crushed or anoxic tissue. Suturing of a contaminated and inadequately debrided wound also may predispose to this condition. Treatment requires emergent debridement and appropriate antibiotics.

47. What organisms are frequently cultured from abscesses due to intravenous drug abuse?

The cultured organisms are common skin or oral flora. Saliva contamination is common because of the practice of licking needles. The drugs are not sterile and also may harbor organisms. The most commonly cultured organisms are streptococci, *S. aureus, E. corrodens,* and *Bacteroides* species. Antibiotic coverage must include gram-positive organisms and anaerobes. A combination of cephalosporin and penicillin or ampicillin and clavulonic acid provides adequate initial coverage pending culture results.

48. In diabetic hand infections, what factors correlate with an increased risk of amputation?

The risk factors are infections involving structures below the subcutaneous tissue, concomitant renal failure, and infections with gram-negative, anaerobic, or polymicrobial organisms.

BIBLIOGRAPHY

1. Bolton H, Fowler P, Jepson R: Natural history and treatment of pulp space infection and osteomyelitis of the distal phalanx. J Bone Joint Surg 31B:499, 1949.
2. Brown P, Kinman PB: Gas gangrene in a metropolitan community. J Bone Joint Surg 56A:1445–1451, 1974.
3. Gonzalez MH, Papierski P, Hall RF Jr: Osteomyelitis of the hand after a human bite. J Hand Surg 18A:520–522, 1993.
4. Gonzalez MH, Kay T, Weinzweig N, et al: Necrotizing fasciitis of the upper extremity. J Hand Surg 21A:689–692, 1996.
5. Gonzalez MH, Garst J, Nourbash P, et al: Abscesses of the upper extremity from drug abuse by injection. J Hand Surg 18A:868–870, 1993.
6. Gonzalez MH, Bochar S, Novotny J, et al: Upper extremity infections in patients with diabetes mellitus. J Hand Surg (in press).
7. Freeland AE, Burkhalter WE, Mann RJ: Functional treatment of acute suppurative digital tenosynovitis. Orthop Trans 5:113–114, 1981.
8. Kanavel A: Infections of the Hand. Philadelphia, Lea & Febiger, 1912.
9. Keyser J, Eaton RG: Surgical cure of chronic paronychia by eponychial marsupialization. Plast Reconstr Surg 58:66, 1976.
10. Kilgore E, Brown L, Newmeyer W, et al: Treatment of felons. Am J Surg 130:195, 1975.
11. Mann RJ (ed): Hand infections. Hand Clin 5(4), 1989 [entire issue].
12. Mann RJ: Infections of the Hand. Philadelphia, Lea & Febiger, 1988.
13. Nevaiser RJ: Closed tendon sheath irrigation for pyogenic flexor tenosynovitis. J Hand Surg 3:462–466, 1978.
14. Polayes I, Arons M: The treatment of herpetic whitlow—a new surgical concept. Plast Reconstr Surg 65:815, 1980.
15. Stone O, Mullins J: Chronic paronychia. Arch Dermatol 86:324, 1962.

99. REPLANTATION AND REVASCULARIZATION

Rudolf F. Buntic, M.D., and Harry J. Buncke, M.D.

1. What is the goal of replantation surgery?

The goal of replantation surgery is successful restoration of function. Revascularization of an amputated part does not necessarily mean success. If the revascularized part has no useful function, or interferes with normal activity, proceeding with replantation must be questioned. The surgeon needs to decide whether the patient will best be served by replantation or completing the amputation. Multiple factors, such as the nature of the affected part(s), other injuries, mechanism of injury, age, work status, and motivation of the patient, influence the decision.

2. What important factors affect outcome in extremity replants?

Multiple factors affect outcome in replantation. Certainly patient age and general health are among them. Factors specific to the amputation and not related to general health include the following:

1. Level and complexity of the injury. The more distal the injury, the greater the chance for success. An exception is distal replants beyond the trifurcation and distal interphalangeal (DIP) joints, in which establishing circulation may be more difficult.
2. Ischemia time. The longer the ischemia, especially warm ischemia, the worse the prognosis.
3. Upper extremity replants tend to do better than lower extremity replants.
4. Sharp injuries tend to do better than crushing or avulsion injuries.
5. Multiple-level injuries do not do as well as single-level injuries.

3. What are the indications for replantation?

Each patient needs to be evaluated on an individual basis, taking into account all of the patient's history and needs. The following factors are strong indications for replantation: (1) multiple finger amputations, (2) thumb amputations, (3) hand amputations at the palm or wrist, and (4) pediatric amputations. The following factors are less absolute indications and are considered controversial by some: (1) loss of a single digit, excluding the thumb, and (2) ring avulsion injuries. However, in appropriately selected cases with motivated patients, results can be excellent.

4. What are the contraindications to replantation?

(1) Upper extremity amputation proximal to the midforearm with ischemia time longer than 6 hours, (2) concomitant life-threatening injuries, (3) multiple-level injuries, (4) severe crush or avulsion, (5) extreme contamination, (6) systemic illness or surgical history precluding replantation, and (7) self-mutilation cases and psychotic patients.

5. Is an operating microscope required to perform a replant?

Although some surgeons report success with loupe magnification when performing free flaps, this is not the case for replantation, especially in digital replantation, in which the vessels can be quite small. A good microscope is essential for adequate visualization and precise technique. Digital replants, especially in children, often have vessel diameters less than 1 mm. Loupe magnification is usually used to examine and dissect the amputated part in preparation for vessel and nerve repair.

6. What closing pressure in a microvascular clamp may result in intimal injury?

Clamp-closing pressures > 30 gm tend to cause intimal damage. The clamp size is not as relevant as closing pressures. Precise atraumatic technique is essential to minimize the risk of thrombosis.

7. Describe the operative sequence in finger or hand replantation.

Bone shortening and osteosynthesis are usually performed first. Shortening of bone facilitates tension-free anastomosis. Arterial repair or flexor tendon repair is usually done next. Nerve repair can be performed after artery repair. The hand can then be turned over, and the extensor tendon repair is performed. A dorsal vein is repaired next. The skin is then closed. Sometimes skin grafting is necessary to complete the closure. Of course, circumstances are variable, and this order may be changed to suit the particular circumstances of an amputation. A skin graft for an open wound, even if placed over an anastomosis, is safer than a tight closure.

8. In what situation is bone fixation postponed?

Usually bony alignment and fixation are performed first, because the procedure can be quite traumatic and disrupt vessel, nerve, and tendon repairs. However, in proximal injuries in which muscle ischemia is a factor, a temporary vascular shunt can be performed first to perfuse the part. With a large part susceptible to warm ischemia, immediate perfusion with a temporary synthetic tube in the artery returns ischemia time to zero. Toxic metabolites that collect in the ischemic part are washed out. The part and proximal structures can then be dissected without the urgency of ongoing ischemia. Bone fixation can be done while shunting continues, or the shunting can be temporarily stopped.

9. What is the treatment for arterial insufficiency after replantation?

If a finger turns white after successful revascularization, inflow usually has been interrupted. Signs are a pale digit that has poor capillary refill and does not bleed if stuck with a needle. These signs may indicate vasospasm, extrinsic pressure on the vessel, or clotting. Vasospasm can be avoided by maintaining a warm environment, administering analgesics, and possibly performing regional blocks. The dressing may be too tight and should be removed or replaced as a first step. Another cause of ischemia may be pressure on the artery from swelling, tight closure, or hematoma. A few key sutures that may cause tension can be removed. If this strategy fails, operative exploration and repair are indicated if the part is believed to be salvageable.

10. Why do most replants fail?

Venous insufficiency is usually responsible for replant failure because venous structures are the most difficult to repair.

11. How many arteries need to be repaired to revascularize a finger successfully?

Usually only one artery repair needs to be performed. In patients with distal obstruction or an unrecognized distal artery injury, a second artery may need to be repaired.

12. How many veins need to be repaired?

One vein can be enough to establish adequate venous drainage. Some surgeons advocate 2 or 3 venous repairs, but this approach is time-consuming and may not be feasible in very distal amputations or in small children.

13. What is the treatment for venous insufficiency?

A finger that turns blue and lacks venous drainage will fail just as miserably as one without arterial inflow. Capillary refill is immediate, and the part often swells. Bleeding from the digit is usually quite dark, indicating poor oxygenation. Removing the dressing and, possibly, several sutures should be considered first. The nail can be removed and the nailbed scrubbed and soaked with heparin sponges to allow continuous bleeding of the finger. Leeches also may be used. Leeches secrete a powerful anticoagulant, hirudin, that results in bleeding of the bite site for several hours after the leech has filled its stomach and fallen off. The continuous oozing of blood from the replanted part allows inflow and outflow to continue until neovascularization occurs and blood can drain via capillaries. Because leeching can result in significant blood loss over time, blood counts need to be done at least daily. The possibility of blood transfusion should be discussed with the patient beforehand.

14. How do you sacrifice a leech after it has been used?

Leeches are used only once and then sacrificed. They cannot be reused. Sacrificing can usually be performed by placing the leech in pure rubbing alcohol.

15. What kind of infection is associated with leeches?

Leeches are colonized with *Aeromonas hydrophila*, which may cause serious soft tissue infections in replants. For this reason all patients who undergo leech treatment should be covered for *A. hydrophila* with prophylactic cefotaxamine or ciprofloxacin.

16. Which vessels are used in ear replantation?

Ear replantation can be one of the most difficult challenges for a microsurgeon. Commonly the injury is an avulsion type with a crush component. Motor vehicle accidents and human bites are frequent causes. Good vessels can be difficult to find, and venous congestion is common postoperatively. Branches from the superficial temporal vessels or posterior auricular vessels can be used if present. However, because ear injuries usually have a crush avulsion component, these vessels are often too severely damaged for microsurgical repair. The superficial temporal vessels can be used directly, with or without vein grafting. The disadvantage is the loss of a pedicle for the temporoparietal fascia flap if it is required later.

17. Which vessels are used in scalp replantation?

Despite reports of scalp replantation with a single artery and vein, multiple arterial and venous anastomoses are usually performed to provide adequate flow for the scalp. Vein grafting is often required. Any arteries or veins that are present are candidates, including the supraorbital, temporal, postauricular, and occipital vessels.

18. A man presents to the emergency department with a four-finger saw amputation. The thumb was not amputated. The fingers are replantable. The small and long fingers are easy to identify, but the index and ring fingers are difficult to distinguish because they are the same length. How do you tell them apart?

The index finger does not usually have hair on the dorsal midphalangeal skin, whereas the ring finger does. In the long term, this may not be important. But the patient certainly may be able to tell the difference later and wonder why you put his fingers back on the wrong way.

19. What methods are used to monitor replants?

Early recognition of circulatory compromise in a replanted part is essential if salvage is to be achieved. Many types of monitoring systems have been reported with variable results. The ideal system provides continuous and accurate information in a noninvasive fashion. To date, the ideal system has not been created. Clinical evaluation of the replanted part by experienced physicians and nurses is the best method of monitoring. Color, capillary refill, temperature, and edema should be evaluated. Other more objective methods are also used. Quantitative fluorimetry has proved successful as an objective form of measuring perfusion. Other methods, such as surface temperature recordings and Doppler measurements, also have been described.

20. Should isolated ulnar artery or radial artery injuries be repaired if hand perfusion is judged to be good?

Isolated repairs of ulnar and radial arteries have previously had poor results. Patency has improved with microvascular technique. Single-vessel patency rates without vein grafting have been reported at 100% in one series, as measured by Doppler ultrasound imaging. Evidence of cold intolerance after radial artery sacrifice argues for primary repair of damaged radial or ulnar arteries.

21. What is heterotopic replantation?

Heterotopic replantation implies replacing an amputated part in a different area from the area in which it originated. With multiple amputations, for instance, a crushed thumb may be replaced with a less injured digit, or a digit may be moved to an ulnar position to improve grip. With bilateral upper or lower extremity amputations, one limb may be replanted on the opposite side to maintain length or function. In major multiple trauma cases, an amputated part may be stored in a distant uninjured area to be retransplanted later when the recipient area and the patient are stabilized. It is conceivable that a critical part may be stored in a surrogate host who is temporarily immunosuppressed while the injured victim is treated and stabilized.

CONTROVERSY

22. What type of anticoagulation is required after replantation?

Thrombosis of small vessels continues to be a problem after a microsurgical repair. To decrease failure rates, multiple pharmacologic agents have been used in the laboratory and clinically to prevent thrombosis. No one regimen has proved to be most successful. Daily aspirin is commonly used as a suppressor of platelet aggregation. Often low-molecular-weight dextran is added, usually just before the micro-vascular clamps are removed. It is normally used for approximately 5 days postoperatively. Dextran is believed to have both antiplatelet and antifibrin properties. It also appears to act as a volume expander. Heparin binds to antithrombin III and inactivates thrombin and other enzymes in the clotting cascade. As with other anticoagulants, administration of heparin can increase the hematoma and bleeding rate. It is commonly used as a vessel irrigant before anastomosis and systemically when postoperative thrombosis develops. If heparin is used systemically, rare patients may require short-term Coumadin treatment.

BIBLIOGRAPHY

1. Buncke HJ (ed): Microsurgery: Transplantation-Replantation. An Atlas Text. Philadelphia, Lea & Febiger, 1991.
2. Davies DM: A world survey of anticoagulation practice in clinical microvascular surgery. Br J Plast Surg 35:96, 1982.
3. Partington MT, Lineweaver WC, O'Hara M, et al: Unrecognized injuries in patients referred for emergency microsurgery. J Trauma 34:238, 1993.
4. Rothkopf DM, Chy B, Gonzalez F, et al: Radial and ulnar artery repairs: Assessing patency rates with color Doppler ultrasonographic imaging. J Hand Surg 18A:626, 1993.

100. THUMB RECONSTRUCTION

Donald R. Laub, Jr., M.D., and Vincent R. Hentz, M.D.

1. What methods are available for thumb reconstruction?
The available surgical methods are osteoplastic reconstruction, finger pollicization (usually of the index finger), and microsurgical toe transfer. Prosthetic replacement is also a consideration.

2. In the era of microsurgery, why even consider prosthetics?
The patient may not be a surgical candidate. A prosthesis may lengthen and make useful a shortened digital stump; it also may give a more esthetic appearance to the hand. Even after successful hand reconstruction, the patient may request an esthetic prosthesis for "going out on Sunday."

3. Is the child with a congenitally missing part an "amputee"?
No. It is a mistake to think of a child with congenital hand differences as an amputee. Children with congenital hand anomalies view themselves as normal, and the vast majority function well by using their own techniques. They are disabled only in comparison with others. To imagine what it would be like to have their deformity, we imagine an amputation.

4. Should you fit a prosthesis on a child?
If the child has a functional pinch, no. The prosthesis will be more of an encumbrance. Children with congenitally absent thumbs usually develop a pinch between the index and long finger.

5. What is the treatment of choice for aplastic and severely hypoplastic thumbs?
Pollicization of the index finger.

6. Why not a toe-to-thumb transfer?
Usually absence of a thumb is part of a more significant longitudinal deficiency with lack of recipient structures. Even in cases of hypoplasia, if the child has a functioning pinch between the index and middle fingers, existing function should be enhanced by pollicization rather than replaced.

7. How is the index finger pollicized?
The digit is shortened by removing almost all of the metacarpal, save the metacarpal head, which assumes the function of the trapezium. The finger is dissected as an island flap on the flexor and extensor tendons, the two neurovascular pedicles, and dorsal veins and nerves. The finger is pronated 140–160° and fixated into the correct axis of the thumb. Hyperextension of the index metacarpophalangeal (MCP) joint is prevented by fixing the metacarpal head in palmar rotation.

8. Why is the metacarpal head palmarly rotated?

The MCP joint of the index finger is a condylar joint that can be hyperextended some 45°, whereas the carpometacarpal (CMC) joint of the thumb is a saddle joint that circumducts but resists hyperextension. Therefore, to allow the transposed index finger to generate the forceful pinch needed, it is fixed with the joint extended to full passive range. The palmar capsule and volar plate then resist further hyperextension.

9. Which muscles of the index finger assume the function of which muscles of the thumb?

Index finger muscle	Thumb muscle
First dorsal interosseous	Abductor pollicis brevis
First palmar interosseous	Adductor pollicis
Extensor digitorum to the index	Abductor pollicis longus
Extensor indicis proprius	Extensor pollicis longus

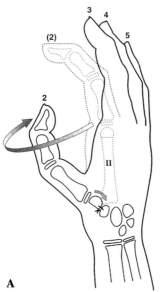 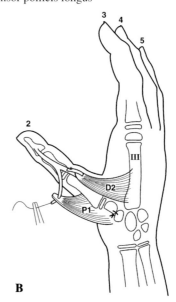

A, Pollicization of index finger, with shortening and pronation of the index ray and hyperextension of the MCP joint. B, The index interosseous muscles are used to supply function of thenar muscles.

10. How is hypoplasia of the thumb classified?

Blauth described five types of hypoplasia of the thumb:

Type I	Minimal shortening or narrowing
Type II	Narrow first web space
	Intrinsic thenar muscle hypoplasia
	MCP joint instability
Type IIIA	Narrow first web space
	Intrinsic thenar muscle hypoplasia
	MCP joint instability
	Extrinsic tendon abnormalities
	Metacarpal hypoplasia with stable CMC joint
Type IIIB	Same as type IIIA with unstable CMC joint
Type IV	Rudimentary phalanges
	Thumb attached by skin bridge
Type V	Aplastic thumb

11. When should reconstruction of a hypoplastic thumb be attempted?

Types II and IIIA are candidates for reconstruction. Types IIIB, IV, and V are best served by index finger pollicization.

12. What techniques can be used for less severe hypoplasia of the thumb?

- Deepening of the first web space by transposition flaps
- Stabilization of the MCP joint
- Correction of extrinsic tendon abnormalities
- Opponensplasty, usually with the abductor digiti minimi (Huber technique)

13. What is osteoplastic reconstruction?

It is a multistage reconstructive technique that employs bone grafting or lengthening osteotomies, covered with skin flaps, on the remaining thumb stump to add length and to provide opposition. No joints are reconstructed. Sensation can be provided in the form of a neurovascular island flap, transferred from a finger (the usual donor is the ulnar side of the middle or ring). Most experts believe that microvascular toe transfer provides a better reconstruction with more similar tissue and joints for partial amputation of the thumb.

14. Does loss of the first toe cause gait disturbance?

Gait studies show shifting of weight distribution away from the first metatarsal head, but if the metatarsal head is preserved, the disturbance in gait is minimal.

15. What is the vascular pedicle of the transferred first toe?

The first dorsal intermetatarsal artery, which arises in most cases from the dorsalis pedis artery but occasionally from the deep plantar system. The origin may be determined at the time of operation. If the deep system is dominant, a reversed vein graft extension may be needed. The more important question concerns the recipient blood vessels in the hand. In patients with any degree of injury to the hand, an arteriogram should be obtained to determine the residual vascular anatomy.

16. Can parts of toes be used?

Yes. Neurovascular island flaps can be used to provide innervated pulp to the oppositional surfaces. This technique is especially useful in the multiply traumatized hand, to which traditional neurovascular island flap techniques would add further debility. There have been reports of transferring vascularized joints from the foot to the thumb in severe isolated joint trauma.

17. When is pollicization preferable to toe transfer for reconstruction of a traumatically amputated thumb?

When the metacarpal is completely absent. There is no way to reconstruct an adequate basilar joint with a toe.

CONTROVERSY

18. Which toe is preferred for thumb reconstruction?

1. **The great toe**. In the United States, generally the great toe is preferred because it provides a stronger and more stable thumb for a pincer grip. The great toe is more like the thumb in appearance, although a bit broader. The transplanted toe atrophies and thins after time, and usually the difference is apparent only in side-by-side comparison.

2. **The second toe.** In Asian cultures in which Zori-type sandals are worn, the loss of a first web space in the foot is a disability; therefore, the second toe is preferred. Women who wear open-toe footwear also may find loss of the great toe disturbing. In addition, the second toe can provide greater metatarsal length for transfer, so in cases in which less than one-third of the first metacarpal remains, the second toe is preferred.

BIBLIOGRAPHY

1. Buck-Gramcko D: Pollicization. In Blair WF: Techniques in Hand Surgery. Baltimore, Williams & Wilkins, 1996.
2. Buncke HJ: Great toe transplantation and digital reconstruction by second-toe transplantation. In Buncke HJ: Microsurgery: Transplantation–Replantation. Philadelphia, Lea & Febiger, 1991.
3. Pillet J, Mackin EJ: Aesthetic hand prosthesis: Its psychological and functional potential. In Hunter IM, Schneider LH, Mackin EJ, Callahan AD (eds): Rehabilitation of the Hand, 3rd ed. St. Louis, Mosby, 1990.
4. Wei FC, el-Gammal TA: Toe-to-hand transfer. Current concepts, techniques and research. Clin Plast Surg 23:103, 1996.

101. THE MUTILATED HAND

Jeffrey Weinzweig, M.D., and Norman Weinzweig, M.D.

1. What is a mutilated hand?

A mutilated hand results from a complex injury with composite tissue loss and significant functional compromise (usually impaired prehension) and often requires bone, soft tissue, and microneurovascular reconstruction. Without surgical intervention, a mutilated hand remains virtually functionless. Even with surgical intervention, the hand usually functions in an assist fashion. In addition to the loss of function, patients often complain of intractable pain and psychological stress.

2. What is prehension?

The functional hand possesses prehension—the ability to oppose the fingers to grip or grasp. According to Tubiana, "prehension is a complex function of the hand that gives it mechanical precision combined with a standard sensory pattern."

3. What are the main objectives in the treatment of a mutilated hand?

The main goals in management of a mutilated hand are restoration of form and function. Ideally, the injured parts are restored to their pretraumatic state. Although replantation of sharply severed parts may approach the ideal from an aesthetic point of view, function rarely can be restored to the preinjury level.

4. Outline a treatment plan for the management of mutilating injuries of the hand.

1. Initial assessment must include:
   - Accurate history, including age, handedness, occupation, avocations, mechanism of injury, time of injury, general health
   - Physical examination, including evaluation of perfusion, motor and sensory function, contamination, severity of tissue damage, and other life-threatening injuries
   - Radiographs of the hand and any amputated part
   - Angiography, when indicated
2. Tetanus prophylaxis
3. Broad-spectrum intravenous antibiotics
4. High-pressure jet lavage and aggressive debridement of devitalized tissues (except in electrical burns)
5. Reduction and immobilization of fractures and dislocations
6. Revascularization of ischemic tissues
7. Immediate or delayed reconstruction of nerve, tendon, bone, and soft tissue
8. Early wound closure by skin grafts and/or flaps
9. Secondary procedures such as pollicization and toe-to-thumb transfer
10. Postreconstruction physical rehabilitation (Uninjured or minimally injured structures must be appropriately splinted or undergo occupational therapy to avoid stiffness or instability, especially when other parts of the hand are absent or functionless.)

5. How are mutilating injuries of the hand classified?

Because mutilated hands assume a myriad of forms, they should be precisely described. The goals of a classification system should be (1) accurate description of any mutilating injury, (2) user-friendliness, (3) progression of injury complexity, and (4) facilitation of communication between clinicians. Furthermore, a classification system should ideally (5) direct treatment, (6) predict functional outcome, and (7) allow derivation of a staging system based on functional outcome. This system should allow the examining surgeon to describe accurately and reproducibly any mutilating injury of the hand.

Several classifications of mutilating hand injuries exist in the literature; unfortunately, injuries are grouped arbitrarily according to the part of the hand predominantly involved. Reid's classification groups mutilating injuries into six categories: dorsal injuries, palmar injuries, radial hemiamputations, ulnar hemiamputations, distal amputations, and degloving injuries. The modified Pulvertaft classification groups mutilating injuries into five categories: radial, ulnar, central, transverse, and other. Wei's classification groups mutilating injuries into two categories: type I (all fingers are amputated proximal to the proximal interphalangeal joint but the thumb is intact) and type II (at least 3 fingers are amputated proximal to the proximal interphalangeal joint, and the thumb is amputated proximal to the interphalangeal joint so that opposition is impossible).

6. What is the "tic-tac-toe" classification system for mutilating injuries of the hand?

A devascularized hand with radial hemiamputation and ulnar degloving cannot be accurately described by any of the classifications discussed above. Because a mutilated hand may have sustained several different types of complex injuries, a comprehensive classification must incorporate the degree and precise location of soft tissue and/or bony destruction and vascular integrity, in addition to the predominantly involved part of the hand. Recently we devised a classification system for mutilating injuries of the hand that categorizes them into seven types and three subtypes with subscript notation to indicate vascular status:

TIC-TAC-TOE CLASSIFICATION SYSTEM

Injury types	Injury subtypes
I. Dorsal mutilation	A. Soft tissue loss
II. Palmar mutilation	B. Bony loss
III. Ulnar mutilation	C. Combined tissue loss
IV. Radial mutilation	
V. Transverse amputation	**Vascular status** (subscript)
VI. Degloving injury	0. Vascularity intact
VII. Combined injury	1. Devascularization

The hand is then systematically divided into nine numerical zones in tic-tac-toe fashion with radial, central, and ulnar columns and proximal, central, and distal row). The "tic-tac-toe" classification system allows the examining surgeon to describe precisely any mutilating injury of the hand. It permits accurate assessment of each hand injury by assignment of the appropriate classification type, subtype, vascular status, and zone involvement in a user-friendly and practical fashion.

"Tic-tac-toe" classification zones. (From Weinzweig J, Weinzweig N: The "Tac-Tac-Toe" classification system for mutilating injuries of the hand. Plast Reconstr Surg 100:1200–1211, 1997, p 1210, with permission.)

7. What are dorsal mutilation injuries (type I)?

Dorsal mutilation injuries involve the dorsal skin, extensor tendons, and bones. The tactile surface (palmar skin) of the hand is preserved. Vascularization is intact. Type I injuries are usually the least severe of the mutilating injuries but often require soft tissue coverage of the dorsum of the hand and immediate or staged extensor tendon repairs and/or reconstructions. The most common mechanism is crush-avulsion, in which the loose, mobile dorsal soft tissue is avulsed along with the extensor tendons. Occasionally, bony injury may be associated with a crush component. In both cases, volar tissues such as the flexor tendons, neurovascular structures, and tactile soft tissue, are preserved, thus minimizing functional losses. Functional outcome is relatively favorable and directly related to the extent of bony injury and the need for prolonged immobilization.

8. What are palmar mutilation injuries (type II)?

Palmar mutilation injuries involve the palmar skin (tactile surface), flexor tendons, and bones. They often involve the radial and ulnar arteries, deep and superficial palmar arches, and common and proper digital arteries with possible devascularization of one or more fingers. The median and ulnar nerves and common and proper digital nerves also may be involved. Type II injuries are generally more severe and complex than dorsal injuries. They disrupt the tactile surface of the hand, often necessitating resurfacing with regional or distant flaps. In addition, they may require open or closed reduction and internal fixation of fractures and/or flexor tendon repair with or without staged reconstruction. Neurovascular compromise to one or more fingers is occasionally seen.

9. What are ulnar mutilation injuries (type III)?

Ulnar mutilation injuries involve loss of the ulnar digits, destruction of the ulnar column (phalanges, metacarpals and/or carpus), and interference with grasp or power grip mechanisms. Type III injuries involve bone, tendon, soft tissue, and neurovascular structures along the ulnar aspect of the hand, resulting in significant functional disability due to interference with grip mechanisms. An objective of reconstructive surgery is to maintain the breadth of the hand.

10. What are radial mutilation injuries (type IV)?

Radial mutilation injuries involve loss of the thumb, destruction of the radial column, and loss of opposition or pinch mechanisms. Type IV injuries are serious and may involve total or subtotal loss of the thumb and thenar musculature. Without restoration, they result in severe disability with loss of 50% or more of total hand function. Damage to the remainder of the hand plays a role in the choice of reconstructive options, such as pollicization of the index finger or remnants of other injured fingers, osteoplasty, or toe-to-thumb transfer. When replantation or revascularization is successful, functional results are generally good, depending on the status of the remainder of the hand.

11. What are transverse amputations (type V)?

Transverse amputations result in loss of the hand or digits at different levels with corresponding functional losses. Restoration of functional pinch depends on the level of loss. Amputations distal to the metacarpophalangeal (MCP) joint level may result in a phalangeal hand, whereas amputations proximal to the MCP joint level may result in a metacarpal hand (see below). Complete hand amputation also may occur. Type V injuries occur at or proximal to the MCP joint of the fingers and involve at least three fingers, with possible involvement of the thumb. They often result in significant functional losses, depending on the success of replantation or revascularization of the amputated part(s), including the fingers as a metacarpal unit and possibly the thumb. Involvement of the thumb adds the component of radial mutilation to the equation, making this a combined injury (type VII, see below).

Successful replantation and revascularization at the transmetacarpal level generally result in fair-to-poor functional results, even with guillotine-type amputations. The main reason is probably ischemic insult to the interosseous and lumbrical muscles as a result of direct muscle injury or interruption of the delicate blood supply to these tiny muscles. The zone of injury is often extensive, with destruction of the intrinsic muscles, flexor and extensor tendons, MCP joints, and neurovascular structures. Multiple reconstructive procedures are required in staged fashion. Bilateral mutilations present a special circumstance with respect to functional outcome.

Complete hand replantations have a better prognosis than transmetacarpal replantations. The flexor tendons are injured in zone 5, and the intrinsic muscles of the hand are spared.

12. What is a metacarpal hand?

A metacarpal hand is a hand that has lost its prehensile ability due to amputation of all fingers with or without amputation of the thumb. Functional restoration can be achieved by various microvascular toe transfer techniques. The choice of procedure depends on the level of amputation of the fingers and the functional status of the thumb. Based on their extensive experience with metacarpal hands reconstructed with toe-to-hand transfers, Wei et al. described a classification system that served as a guide to their treatment philosophy. They identified two major types of metacarpal hand based on whether the thumb is injured.

13. What is the Krukenberg procedure?

Originally described by Krukenberg in 1917, this operation was mainly used in Germany during World War I. The forearm is fashioned into an active pincer with the arms covered by inner- vated sensate soft tissue. It is indicated in cases of congenital or traumatic amputations of the hand. In unilateral amputations, a prosthesis is preferred except in patients whose occupation demands sensibility of both upper limbs. However, when both hands have been amputated, the Krukenberg operation is cited as the best approach, performed either bilaterally or unilaterally with a prosthesis on the other side. It helps bilateral amputees to regain total independence. A sensate pincer is espe- cially necessary in blind patients. This operation is particularly indicated when both hands and both eyes have been damaged.

14. What are degloving injuries (type VI)?

Degloving injuries involve circumferential loss of innervated skin and tactile surface(s) of the hand. They are often associated with nerve, vessel, or tendon avulsion. Degloving injuries are seri- ous injuries usually caused by avulsion of soft tissue by a roller-type mechanism. No local inner- vated skin is available to resurface important tactile areas of the hand. Soft tissue coverage occasionally can be achieved by harvesting a skin graft from the degloved part. Often, a groin flap or emergency free flap is required. Reconstruction is especially difficult for simultaneous provision of skin on both aspects of the hand.

15. What are combination injuries (type VII)?

Type VII injuries usually involve a combination of types I–VI as well as other injuries that do not fit the more rigid definitions of injury types. Type VII injuries are usually the most severe, often caused by extreme forces such as punch presses and thermal or electrical burns.

16. What is an emergency free flap?

Based on Godina's work with early microsurgical reconstruction of complex trauma to the limb, Lister and Scheker defined the emergency free flap as one performed after primary debridement or within 24 hours of surgery, and reported a success rate of 93.5% (29/31 flaps). More recently, Ninkovic et al. reported their experience in 29 patients who underwent 27 emergency free flaps and 3 emergency toe-to-hand transfers without flap failure, infections, or wound-healing complications. Long-term follow-up demonstrates successful functional and aesthetic results with reduced rates of free flap failure, postoperative infection, and secondary operative procedures as well as reduced hos- pital stay and medical costs.

17. What is spare parts surgery?

Amputated parts that are not suitable for replantation can be salvaged for use as possible donors, such as pliable dorsal skin for coverage, nailbed for split- or full-thickness nailbed grafts, tendons for interpolated grafts, pulley reconstruction, or soft tissue arthroplasty, nerve grafts from nonre- plantable digits, or bone grafts to bridge bony defects. Mutilating injuries usually demonstrate dev- astating involvement of bone and soft tissue structures; one has to carefully examine the remaining extremity and amputated parts in an attempt to maximize function. Every amputated part should be considered a possible spare part before it is discarded.

18. What is ectopic parts surgery?

Ectopic parts surgery involves transfer of an amputated part to a different location where it may serve a more useful function. Short stumps of fingers (index, middle, or ring) with little function can often be pollicized to provide a useful and sensate thumb reconstruction. In addition, an amputated part may be banked ectopically in a more favorable location until the site from which it came is ready for anatomic replantation.

19. When is amputation indicated?

Realistic assessment of potential function may indicate that the revascularized part will be insensate, painful, immobile, or nonfunctional with possible decreased function of the adjacent normal digits. Amputation is not failure; instead, it often serves a patient better than multiple complex operations that restore little function.

20. What is the role of prostheses in the management of the mutilated hand?

Cable-operated or myeloelectric prostheses help to restore useful function to an otherwise functionless hand.

BIBLIOGRAPHY

1. Adani R, Castagnetti C, Landi A: Degloving injuries of the hand and fingers. Clin Orthop Rel Res 314:19–25, 1995.
2. Brown HC, Williams HB, Woodhouse FM: Principles of salvage in mutilating hand injuries. J Trauma 8:318, 1968.
3. Godina M: Early microsurgical reconstruction of complex trauma of the extremities. Plast Reconstr Surg 78:285, 1986.
4. Harris GD, Nagle DJ, Bell JL: Mutilating injuries. In Jupiter JB (ed): Flynn's Hand Surgery. Baltimore: Williams & Wilkins, 1991, pp 103–114.
5. Joshi BB: Sensory flaps for the degloved mutilated hand. Hand 6:247, 1974.
6. Kleinman WB, Dustman JA: Preservation of function following complete degloving injuries to the hand: Use of simultaneous groin flap, random abdominal flap, and partial-thickness skin graft. J Hand Surg 6A:82, 1981.
7. Lister G, Scheker L: Emergency free flaps to the upper extremity. J Hand Surg 13A:22, 1988.
8. Midgler RD, Entin MA: Management of mutilating injuries of the hand. Clin Plast Surg 3:99, 1976.
9. Nicolle FV, Woodhouse FM: Restoration of sensory function in severe degloving injuries of the hand. J Bone Joint Surg 48A:1511, 1966.
10. Ninkovic M, Deetjen H, Ohler K, Anderl H: Emergency free tissue transfer for severe upper extremity injuries. J Hand Surg 20B:53–58, 1995.
11. Pribaz JJ, Pelham FR: Upper extremity reconstruction using spare parts. Prob Plast Reconstr Surg 3:373–390, 1993.
12. Reid DAC, Tubiana R: Mutilating Injuries of the Hand. Edinburgh, Churchill Livingstone, 1984.
13. Scheker LR: Salvage of a Mutilated Hand. In Cohen M (ed): Mastery of Plastic Surgery. Boston, Little, Brown, 1994, pp 1658–1681.
14. Sundine M, Scheker LR: A comparison of immediate and staged reconstruction of the dorsum of the hand. J Hand Surg 21B:216, 1996.
15. Tsai T-M, Jupiter JB, Wolff TW, Atasoy E: Reconstruction of severe transmetacarpal mutilating hand injuries by combined second and third toe transfer. J Hand Surg 6:319–328, 1981.
16. Tubiana R: Prehension in the Mutilated Hand. In Reid DAC and Tubiana R (eds): Mutilating Injuries of the Hand. Edinburgh, Churchill Livingstone, 1984, p 61.
17. Tubiana R, Stack HG, Hakstian RW: Restoration of prehension after severe mutilations of the hand. J Bone Joint Surg 48B:455, 1966.
18. Tubiana R: Reconstruction after traumatic mutilations of the hand. Injury 2:127, 1970.
19. Wei F-C, El-Gammal TA, Lin C-H, et al: Metacarpal hand: Classification and guidelines for microsurgical reconstruction with toe transfers. Plast Reconstr Surg 99:122–128, 1997.
20. Weinzweig N, Chen L, Chen Z-W: Pollicization in the severely injured hand by transposition of middle and ring finger remnants. Ann Plast Surg 34:523–529, 1995.
21. Weinzweig N, Sharzer L, Starker I. Replantation and revascularization at the transmetacarpal level: Long-term functional results. J Hand Surg 21A:1, 1996.
22. Weinzweig, N, Starker I, Sharzer LA, Fleegler EJ: Vascular supply to the lumbrical and interosseous muscles. Plast Reconstr Surg 99:785-790, 1997.
23. Weinzweig J, Weinzweig N: The "Tic-Tac-Toe" classification system for mutilating injuries of the hand. Plast Reconstr Surg 100:1200–1211, 1997.

102. PERIPHERAL NERVE INJURIES

Rahul K. Nath, M.D., and Susan E. Mackinnon, M.D.

1. Describe the functional anatomy of peripheral nerves.
Peripheral nerves are basically composed of four components:

1. **Neurons**, the primary functional units of peripheral nerve, are composed of cell bodies and axons. The cell bodies of motor axons are found in the anterior horn area of the spinal cord, and sensory cell bodies are found in the dorsal root ganglia of the spinal cord.

2. **Connective tissues** of the nerve are arranged in three layers: endoneurial connective tissue, which is found around individual axons; perineurial tissue, which surrounds fascicles; and epineurial tissue, which runs between fascicles and around the outside of the nerve and constitutes the main support structure of the nerve itself.

3. **Schwann cells** supply myelin for efficient electrical nerve conduction. In addition, they appear to influence maturation and resting metabolism of axons.

4. **End-organs**, including the motor endplates, sensory receptors, and autonomic receptors, transduce electrical activity into function.

Motor recovery appears to become refractory to reinnervation after about 1 year of denervation. Sensory recovery has been described up to 20 years after initial denervation. Autonomic function after denervation has not been well-studied.

2. How are nerve injures classified? What is the clinical importance of classification?
Seddon's original classification, proposed in 1943, described three types of nerve injury:

1. **Neurapraxia** involves a local conduction block at a discrete area along the course of the nerve; subsequent wallerian degeneration does not occur.

2. Axonal damage is the basis of **axonotmesis**; wallerian degeneration occurs distal to the site of injury.

3. Transection of a peripheral nerve constitutes **neurotmesis**.

Sunderland expanded Seddon's classification with grades of nerve injury from I–V. Mackinnon described a mixed injury that she called a grade VI injury. The Sunderland classification describes injury to peripheral nerves in relation to axon and connective tissue anatomy. Clinical prognosis is proportional to the level of injury.

Classification of Nerve Injury

DEGREE OF INJURY	TINEL SIGN/ PROGRESSES DISTALLY	RECOVERY PATTERN	RATE OF RECOVERY	SURGICAL PROCEDURE
I. Neurapraxia	No Tinel sign	Complete	Fast (days to 12 wk)	None
II. Axonotmesis	+/+	Complete	Slow (1 in/mo)	None
III.	+/+	Great variation*	Slow (1 in/mo)	None or neurolysis†
IV. Neuroma in continuity	+/–	None	No recovery	Nerve repair or nerve graft
V. Neurotmesis	+/–	None	No recovery graft	Nerve repair or nerve graft
VI. Combination of grades I–V and normal	Varies by fascicle, depending on injury	Varies by fascicle	Varies by fascicle	Varies by fascicle

* Recovery is at least as good as nerve repair but varies from excellent to poor, depending on the degree of endoneurial scarring and the amount of sensory and motor axonal misdirection within the injured fascicle.
† If injury localizes at a known anatomic site of nerve compression, nerve decompression may enhance recovery.

3. What is meant by wallerian degeneration?

The distal segment in a complete nerve injury undergoes a series of degenerative changes collectively known as wallerian degeneration. In 1850 Waller described the gross changes of turbidity or coagulation seen even at the distalmost end of the neural tube after nerve transection. This ground-glass appearance represents the remnants of degenerated myelin and axonal material after loss of axonal continuity. The initial breakdown products of the axon and myelin are phagocytosed by macrophages and Schwann cells. Eventually, the space originally occupied by myelinated axons is filled with columns of Schwann cell nuclei and their basement membranes.

4. What are the bands of Büngner?

The collapsed columns of Schwann cells filling the distal segment of a complete nerve injury have a characteristic bandlike appearance under electron microscopy; these columns are known as the bands of Büngner.

5. Does the number of nerve fibers in the distal nerve stump equal the number of proximal stump axons successfully crossing the repair or graft site?

No. Axons affected by a complete injury develop numerous growth cones or sprouts from each injured axon that attempt to connect with the distal stump. Therefore, each injured proximal axon is responsible for the production of numerous distal growth cones that by electron microscopy resemble small normal axons surrounded by an intact or fragmentary basal membrane.

6. Do regenerating axonal growth cones grow through the lumens of the original endoneurial tubes vacated by distal axons during wallerian degeneration?

Sometimes. In Sunderland grade II injuries, which are characterized by axonal discontinuity in the presence of endoneurial integrity, regeneration occurs through the original endoneurial tubes to the target organ. Thus grade II injuries have excellent outcomes. In grade III and higher injuries, in which endoneurial disruption is accompanied by axonal discontinuity, growth cones preferentially attach to molecules such as laminin and extend along basal laminar tissue. Because Schwann cells within the bands of Bungner are associated with large amounts of basal lamina, growth cones tend to advance along these structures rather than through the lumens of the collapsed collagen-based endoneurial tubes.

The affinity that growth cones exhibit for Schwann cell basal lamina has suggested the use of artificial sources of basal lamina as scaffolding for nerve regeneration. Experiments with freeze-dried skeletal muscle grafts (a rich source of basal lamina) have been partially successful in allowing nerve regeneration across short nerve defects.

7. What is Tinel's sign?

Percussion over the site of a nerve injury or nerve repair elicits a tingling or electric shocklike sensation in the distribution of the injured nerve. This sensation represents the leading edge of nerve regeneration. An advancing Tinel's sign after nerve repair implies successful nerve regeneration toward the target organ. A Tinel's sign that does not advance with time may be due to extraepineurial growth cones that have become misdirected outside the epineurial boundary at the level of the nerve repair. Although sensory in nature, Tinel's sign is also found in regenerating motor nerve, probably because of the presence of proprioceptive afferent fibers within all motor nerves.

8. How fast do nerves regenerate?

As a general rule, regenerating nerves advance at the rate of about 1 mm/day or 1 inch/month. However, several clinical studies based on advancing Tinel's sign after nerve repair have given a rate of recovery up to 2 mm/day.

9. If nerves regenerate at the rate of 1 inch/month and the hand is about 30 inches from the axilla, does this mean that a complete ulnar nerve injury at the level of the axilla will take $2\frac{1}{2}$ years to restore sensibility to the ulnar two fingers in the hand?

Yes. The time course of nerve regeneration is relatively predictable, based on the distance from the most proximal extent of injury to the end-organ supplied by the nerve.

10. In the same situation as question 9, will the ulnar-innervated hand intrinsic muscles regain function 2½ years after injury?

No. Like most voluntary skeletal muscle that becomes denervated and unlike sensory receptors, the intrinsic muscles of the hand become functionally refractory to reinnervation after a finite period. The absolute time is not known, but with muscle reinnervation the sooner the reconstruction the better. In closed injury, reconstruction should be performed 3 months after injury if recovery is not forthcoming. With open nerve injuries, repair should be performed as soon as clinically feasible. Intrinsic muscles in the hand do not regain function after an injury in the axilla because the prolonged denervation time precludes recovery of motor function.

11. Do all proximal motor nerve injuries result in permanent loss of function?

No. Excellent recovery is possible across long distances under certain circumstances. Early primary repair of sharp transections that maintain motor and sensory topography by excellent coaptation along anatomic landmarks on the epineurium results in good recovery of function. Similarly, because of enhanced nerve regenerative capacity and possibly greater central plasticity, nerve repairs in children tend to have good outcomes even with long nerve grafts. Protective sensibility and improved muscle function are possible after long nerve grafts when meticulous microtechnique is used and sensory/motor topography is correct.

12. What are nerve transfers? How are they designed?

It is possible to provide motor inflow to motor nerves close to the target muscle by using motor nerve donors; this is the concept of nerve transfer. Nerve transfers are designed by selecting donor nerves that supply nonessential muscles or muscles with redundant fiber innervation and that hopefully are synergistic with the recipient nerve. An example is transfer of the medial pectoral nerve branches to the musculocutaneous nerve for biceps recovery; many other transfers are possible for both motor and sensory reconstruction.

13. How long should you wait before operating on nerve injuries?

In general, nerve injuries associated with open wounds require immediate exploration. The classic case is a sharp laceration causing nerve injury that can be repaired primarily. However, one exception to this general rule is a gunshot wound, which, although open, causes injury by indirect heat and shock effects. Such injuries more closely resemble closed or blunt trauma, which initially should be managed expectantly. In closed or blunt injury, the clinical course is watched closely. If complete recovery is not present within 6 weeks, nerve conduction and electromyographic studies are obtained for baseline evaluation. The clinical course is followed for about 12 weeks, and repeat electrical studies are obtained. An improving clinical course at 12 weeks or electrical evidence of reinnervation suggests continuation of conservative therapy. Failure to progress clinically and electrically suggests that operative intervention with intraoperative electrical testing is indicated. The exact surgical procedure varies from neurolysis to nerve grafting or nerve transfer, depending on the grade of the injury and the distance of the injury from the end-organ.

14. What is the best way to treat peripheral nerve injuries resulting in segmental loss of continuity?

Many different solutions have been proposed for the problem of nerve gaps. However, the use of autogenous nerve grafts harvested from appropriate donor sites is the gold standard for reconstruction of nerve defects. Experimental evidence suggests that vein grafts and artificial conduits can successfully bridge cutaneous nerve defects up to 3 cm in length; longer gaps are not effectively reconstructed with vein or other conduits. Nerve grafts can restore function after reconstruction of defects even longer than 15 cm. However, the success rate of nerve grafting is inversely proportional to the length of graft required. In massive loss of nerve segments, transplanted nerves can be used for grafting. This technique is especially useful in children, in whom the amount of autogenous nerve available for grafting may be limited. Harvested donor nerves are preserved in cold University of Wisconsin solution for 7 days before transplantation to reduce antigenicity. Recipients and donors must be blood-type compatible, but HLA compatibility is not necessary. Immunosuppression with steroids and cyclosporin A is required until there is evidence of regeneration across the graft into native distal nerve, at which point immunosuppression is stopped. Clinical success with this management in a small series of patients has been good.

15. What is the best method for surgical nerve repair?

Surgical repair of nerve injuries is best performed with a few interrupted 9-0 or 10-0 Nylon stitches through the epineurium. Other techniques, including fibrin glue and laser energy for epineurial coaptation, have been investigated. However, fibrin glue carries a risk of transmission of bloodborne diseases, and lasers produce heat that damages neural tissue and also results in unacceptably decreased tensile strength at the repair site. The gold standard remains microsuture applied under microscope control. Attempts at fascicular and grouped fascicular repair have shown no advantage over simple epineurial repair.

16. Which nerves innervate the hand?

The median, ulnar, and radial nerves.

17. Describe clinical tests for nerve function in the hand.

A simple and comprehensive way to diagnose nerve injuries in the upper extremity is to test three functions of each nerve: extrinsic motor function, intrinsic motor function, and sensibility in autonomous areas.

Clinical Tests for Nerve Function

FUNCTION	RADIAL NERVE	MEDIAN NERVE	ULNAR NERVE
Extrinsic motor	Wrist extension	Profundus index finger	Profundus small finger
Intrinsic motor	None	Abductor pollicis brevis	First dorsal interosseous
Sensory	Dorsal first web space	Pulp of index finger	Pulp of small finger

18. What is a Martin-Gruber anastomosis? Why is it important in nerve injury of the hand?

Ten to twenty percent of patients have an anatomic connection between the median and ulnar nerves high in the forearm. In 60% of these connections median nerve fibers travel to the ulnar nerve to innervate "median" muscles in the hand. About 35% send median nerve fibers to the ulnar nerve to innervate "ulnar" muscles in the hand. Five percent of Martin-Gruber anastomoses involve ulnar nerve fibers that go to the median nerve. Martin-Gruber anastomoses are important in understanding certain clinical patterns in high injury to the ulnar nerve. For example, a complete injury to the ulnar nerve, if it occurs above a Martin-Gruber anastomosis, may present with numbness in the ulnar nerve distribution of the hand but intact function of hand intrinsic muscles.

19. What is the difference between neurotropism and neurotrophism?

Neurotropism refers to the selective guidance of nerve regeneration toward target organs by hypothetical factors produced by the target itself. The implication is that muscle and sensory targets are able to promote differential functional regeneration of nerves after a period of denervation. No strong experimental evidence supports the concept of motor/sensory specificity. However, tissue specificity does exist (i.e., nerve-to-nerve connections preferentially occur vs. nerve to other tissue), and fascicular specificity is also likely.

Neurotrophism defines influences that promote maturation and nutrition of regenerating axons. Many growth factors, extracellular matrix components, and hormones are important to successful nerve regeneration.

CONTROVERSY

20. Can you deliver functional axons to an injured nerve by suturing it to the side of an uninjured nerve (i.e., an end-to-side nerve repair)?

Sometimes. Animal experiments indicate that some fibers will grow from an intact nerve into another nerve end sutured to the side of the uninjured donor nerve. Retrograde staining for sensory fibers has indeed shown small amounts of stain uptake at the level of the dorsal root ganglion of the intact nerve. The functional importance of this finding is unknown, but probably it does not have great significance. When retrograde tracers are used in motor nerves with end-to side repair, no evidence of tracer at the level of the anterior horn cells has been found. Therefore, provision of motor function with this approach cannot be expected. Nevertheless, there is a growing interest in end-to-side nerve repair because of its theoretical usefulness in high nerve injuries.

BIBLIOGRAPHY

1. Brandt KE, Mackinnon SE: A technique for maximizing biceps recovery in brachial plexus reconstruction. J Hand Surg 18A:726–733, 1993.
2. Clark D: Jules Tinel and Tinel's sign. Clin Plast Surg 10:627–628, 1983.
3. Mackinnon SE: New directions in peripheral nerve surgery. Ann Plast Surg 22:257–273, 1989.
4. Mackinnon SE, Dellon AL: Surgery of the Peripheral Nerve. New York, Thieme, 1988.
5. Mackinnon SE: Nerve allotransplantation following severe tibial nerve injury. J Neurosurg 84:671–676, 1996.
6. Nath RK, Mackinnon SE, Jensen JN, Parks WC: Spatial pattern of type I collagen expression in injured peripheral nerve. J Neurosurg 86:866–870, 1997.
7. Nath RK, Mackinnon SE, Shenaq SM: New nerve transfers following peripheral nerve injuries. Oper Techn Plast Reconstr Surg 4:2–11, 1997.
8. Seddon H: Surgical disorders of the peripheral nerve. New York, Churchill Livingstone, 1975.
9. Sunderland S: The intraneural topography of the radial, median and ulnar nerves. Brain 68:243–249, 1945.
10. Sunderland S: Nerves and Nerve Injuries. Edinburgh, Churchill Livingstone, 1978.

103. NERVE COMPRESSION SYNDROMES

A. Lee Dellon, M.D.

1. Name the peripheral nerve compressed in carpal tunnel syndrome, cubital tunnel syndrome, radial tunnel syndrome, supinator syndrome, pronator syndrome, and Guyon's canal syndrome.

The median nerve is compressed in the carpal tunnel. The more proximal median nerve compression syndromes are called either anterior interosseous nerve syndrome (associated with weakness in the flexor pollicis longus and profundus to the index and middle finger) or pronator syndrome (associated with little motor involvement but numbness in the median-innervated fingers). The ulnar nerve is compressed at the wrist in Guyon's canal (the ulnar tunnel) and in the postcondylar groove at the elbow (cubital tunnel syndrome). Proximal ulnar nerve compression is associated with numbness over the ulnar dorsum of the hand and weakness of the profundus to the little finger and the ulnar wrist flexor. The entire radial nerve is compressed in the radial tunnel syndrome, whereas its motor branch is compressed beneath the supinator muscle and its sensory branch is compressed beneath the fascia in the distal third of the forearm.

2. Name the peripheral nerve compressed in tarsal tunnel syndrome, fibular tunnel syndrome, and anterior tarsal tunnel syndrome.

The common peroneal nerve, a branch of the sciatic nerve, can be compressed beneath the peroneal longus muscle at the fibular head. The deep peroneal nerve is compressed in the anterior tarsal tunnel syndrome beneath the inferior extensor retinaculum. The posterior tibial nerve is compressed beneath the flexor retinaculum in the tarsal tunnel, whereas the medial and lateral plantar and calcaneal nerves have their own separate tunnels immediately distal to the tarsal tunnel.

3. Name the peripheral nerve compressed in thoracic outlet syndrome.

There is no nerve in the thoracic outlet. The thoracic outlet is the diaphragm. The thoracic inlet contains the brachial plexus, which may become compressed beneath or between the scalene muscles or between congenital anomalies that are related to the clavicle, first rib, subclavian artery and vein, pleural fascia, or a cervical rib.

4. What area of sensibility is abnormal with pronator syndrome but not with carpal tunnel syndrome?

The thenar eminence. It is innervated by the palmar cutaneous branch of the median nerve, which arises about 5–7 cm proximal to the wrist.

5. What chronic nerve compression occurs between the metatarsal heads?

Morton's neuroma. Morton, who described the symptom complex related to this anatomic area in 1875, believed that there was a true injury to the nerve. Histopathology clearly demonstrates that this swelling in the common plantar digital nerve is due to chronic compression. Perhaps the treatment of Morton's neuroma will change from excision of the nerve to division of the intermetatarsal ligament.

6. What nerve compressions cause symptoms related to sleep?

1. **Carpal tunnel syndrome** causes the patient to awaken from sleep because the flexor muscle group, which is stronger than the extensor group, brings the wrist into flexion, placing pressure on the median nerve. Night awakening is almost always part of the history, unless the patient is an extremely heavy sleeper and awakens with the whole hand feeling numb.

2. **Tarsal tunnel syndrome** causes the patient to have trouble falling asleep. Typically the arch or metatarsal head region (the ball of the foot) or the toes will tingle or burn because the fluid that has built up during the day's activities causes a relative increase in pressure on the posterior tibial nerve.

3. **Ulnar nerve compression** in the cubital tunnel worsens when the patient sleeps with the elbow flexed and may contribute to the whole hand complaints that the patient experiences by morning.

7. What nerve compression causes pain?

Usually chronic nerve compression does not cause pain. Pain is due to acute nerve compression and is a sign that the nerve is dying. Acute compression may become superimposed on chronic compression.

8. What nerve compression causes weakness and clumsiness?

Ulnar nerve compression at the elbow. Carpal tunnel syndrome does not cause weakness, even of pinch, until the compression is severe and associated with thenar muscle atrophy. Carpal tunnel syndrome is not associated with clumsy dropping of objects until it is so severe that no two-point discrimination remains.

9. What nerve compression gives the feeling that the leg is "giving out"?

Compression of the common peroneal nerve at the fibular head. The muscles innervated by this nerve control ankle extension and eversion, and weakness of these muscles creates the sensation of loss of control of the foot.

10. What common injury antedates a common peroneal nerve compression?

An inversion sprain of the ankle. Because the common peroneal nerve innervates the muscles at the fibular head, the nerve is relatively fixed in this location. With an inversion sprain, the peroneal branches that cross the ankle are stretched, causing the proximal stretch/traction injury.

11. What are the symptoms of compression of the lateral femoral cutaneous nerve?

Numbness over the anterolateral thigh and buttock is the most common. Knee aching or pain and hip pain are also common complaints.

12. What common incidents may antedate development of meralgia paresthetica?

Motor vehicle injury when a seat belt is worn, harvest of an iliac crest bone graft, wearing a girdle, diabetes, and lower abdominal surgeries, including hernia repair and hysterectomy, may cause compression of the lateral femoral cutaneous nerve. In about one-third of cadavers, this nerve crosses from within the pelvis to the thigh by going *through*, not under, the inguinal ligament, and in about 4% of cadavers a branch crosses superficial to the iliac crest.

13. What is Tinel's sign?

Jules Tinel was a prisoner during World War I. Kaplan's translation of Tinel's French paper appears in Spinner's book about peripheral nerve injury. Tinel's "tingling" or "buzzing" sign was noted to be present when the site of nerve injury was tapped with the examiner's finger. In prisoners in whom nerve function was regained, tapping along the course of the nerve produced a tingling site that travelled distally. A positive Tinel sign, therefore, is traditionally a sign of neural regeneration. When Phalen popularized the carpal tunnel syndrome, he described a positive Tinel sign over the median nerve at the wrist. Tinel's sign has become almost synonymous with a tingling that radiates distally along the distribution of a nerve at the site at which the nerve is compressed.

14. Is Tinel's sign always positive in patients with nerve compression?

Nerve compression induces pathophysiologic changes that ultimately cause axonal degeneration. Early in the course of nerve compression, when ischemia is localized, the Tinel sign is negative. It also may be negative late in the course of nerve compression, when axons have died and no further regeneration is occurring.

15. What is the value of provocative tests in the diagnosis of nerve compression?

The symptoms of numbness and tingling are produced by ischemia. If the nerve is put under increased pressure by certain physical examination maneuvers, symptoms may be elicited.

16. Describe the provocative tests for compression of the median, ulnar, and radial nerves.

Phalen described wrist flexion as the provocative sign for median nerve compression at the wrist. McMurty described pressure over the median nerve in the proximal forearm for the pronator syndrome. Resisted forearm pronation, resisted elbow flexion, and resisted middle or ring finger superficialis function also may elicit symptoms of pronator syndrome. Wartenberg described hyperpronation of the forearm to elicit the dorsoradial burning characteristic of radial sensory compression. Elbow flexion causes ulnar nerve compression in the cubital tunnel.

17. How do you distinguish de Quervain's tenosynovitis from radial sensory nerve compression?

The Finkelstein test (pain with ulnar deviation of the wrist when the thumb is adducted and flexed) is positive for both conditions. Pain with resisted thumb extension and abduction, when the wrist is motionless, is present with tendinitis of the first dorsal extensor compartment but absent with nerve compression. Tenderness over the radial styloid is also present with tendinitis but not with nerve compression. Decreased sensation to touch and a positive Tinel's sign are present with nerve compression but not with tendinitis.

18. How do you distinguish tennis elbow from radial tunnel syndrome?

Tennis elbow is due to inflammation of the extensors of the wrist and the fingers at their origin from the lateral humeral epicondyle. Swelling and tenderness are found at the site of inflammation. Pain with resisted radial wrist extension or resisted extension of all fingers suggests tennis elbow. Tenderness to palpation about 1 cm anterior or volar to the lateral humeral condyle suggests radial nerve compression. The radial nerve may become compressed by the fibrous edge of the extensor carpi radialis, which inserts into the base of the third metacarpal. Pain referred to the elbow region with resisted middle finger extension is a sign of radial tunnel syndrome.

19. What are the earliest physical findings of nerve compression?

Patients with reversible ischemic changes have symptoms without signs. The earliest signs of nerve compression are related to the larger-diameter nerve fibers. Compression decreases oxygen tension, and the larger-diameter fibers, which are related to motor function and perception of touch/vibration, are affected before the smaller-diameter fibers, which are related to perception of temperature and pain. Therefore, manual muscle testing detects weakness, or the muscle can be measured for pinch and grasp. Testing of the touch fibers detects sensory changes. The qualitatively altered perception of vibration stimulated with a tuning fork is the earliest and easiest sign to detect. Quantitation of cutaneous vibratory threshold or cutaneous pressure threshold changes gives the best documentation (quantitative sensory testing).

20. What physical findings correlate with advanced nerve compression?

With sufficient duration even a small degree of pressure results in nerve compression that may manifest with axonal loss. For motor fibers, axonal loss results in atrophy or wasting of the appropriate muscles. For sensory fibers, it results in a decrease and ultimately a loss of two-point discrimination.

21. With computer-assisted quantitative sensory testing of pressure threshold, what is the first measurable change in chronic nerve compression?

The pressure required to discriminate one-point static from two-point static touch.

22. What are the earliest signs of recovery from decompression of a peripheral nerve?

The relief of numbness and tingling often occurs first, but in patients with axonal loss, degeneration may be accompanied by the pain of neural regeneration. Quantitative sensory testing documents recovery in the following order: recovery of perception of low-frequency vibration before higher-frequency vibration (it is easier to reinnervate the Meissner corpuscles than the Pacinian corpuscles) and recovery of moving two-point discrimination before static two-point discrimination (it is easier to reinnervate the Meissner corpuscles than the Merkel-cell neurite complexes). With computer-assisted sensory testing, the order of recovery is (1) one-point moving touch, (2) one-point static touch, (3) moving two-point discrimination, and (4) static two-point discrimination. Muscle strength recovers at a variable rate, determined by the distance of the muscle from the site of compression and the amount of weakness and degree of rehabilitation. Muscle wasting may never recover.

23. What is electrodiagnostic testing?

The function of the peripheral nerve can be tested electrically. Such testing is traditionally done by neurologists or physiatrists, but sometimes is done by therapists. The peripheral nerve is electrically stimulated, usually transcutaneously, and the reading is recorded at a different site. By such techniques the conduction velocity, latency, and amplitude can be determined. For muscles, electromyography can be done, usually with a percutaneous needle. Denervation of the muscle can be detected.

24. Do patients like electrodiagnostic testing?

No. It is invasive. It is painful. It is expensive ($500–1500). Most patients will not have it repeated.

25. What does an abnormal latency or amplitude mean?

The conduction velocity of the peripheral nerve is related to the thickness of the axon and myelin. Traditional electrodiagnostic testing evaluates only the large-diameter fibers and thus cannot detect problems with nerves transmitting information about temperature or pain perception. A decrease in latency or conduction velocity means that the myelination is decreased or thin. This is the first change associated with chronic nerve compression. The amplitude is related to the number of nerve fibers present. A decrease in amplitude means a loss of nerve fibers.

26. If electrodiagnostic testing is still abnormal after carpal tunnel decompression, should the patient undergo repeat surgery?

After decompression of a peripheral nerve, electrodiagnostic testing may never return a normal result. Regenerating nerves do not remyelinate completely.

27. Why should you stage the degree of compression of a peripheral nerve?

With any disease or medical condition, the treatment is determined by how advanced the disease is.

28. How is nerve compression staged?

The earliest stage of compression is associated with reversible ischemic block and perhaps symptoms of numbness and tingling but no signs. Thus the earliest stage involves a **minimal degree** of nerve compression. With longer duration of compression, the nerve develops endoneural edema, perineural thickening, and an increase in interfascicular epineurium. Changes can be provoked by pressure or physical examination maneuvers, and the patient shows changes in cutaneous vibratory or cutaneous pressure threshold and measurable weakness. This stage involves a **moderate degree** of compression. Sufficient duration of pressure results in axonal loss with wallerian degeneration, a decrease in two-point discrimination, and muscle atrophy. This stage involves a **severe degree** of compression.

29. How does treatment of a nerve compression vary with staging?

For a **minimal degree** of compression, the treatment consists of alteration of daytime and probably work activities, splinting or postural changes, and nonsteroidal antiinflammatory medications. Patients with associated medical conditions should be returned to the primary care physician to ensure treatment. For a **moderate degree** of compression, all of the treatments for minimal compression should be tried for at least 3 months. Then further intervention may be required. For sites of compression with no known synovial collections, such as the carpal tunnel, a cortisone injection may be tried. Additional changes in activities of daily living or working conditions, such as time off from work, may be tried. If the moderate degree of compression persists and the patient does not wish to continue with treatment, surgical decompression of the nerve should be considered. For a **severe degree** of compression, surgical decompression of the nerve should be considered; other treatments are not likely to be effective.

30. Does the result of electrodiagnostic testing influence the treatment of nerve compression?
If the results of electrodiagnostic testing demonstrate muscle denervation or the absence of electrical activity in a peripheral nerve, the degree of nerve compression should be considered severe, and surgical decompression should be the primary treatment. Any other electrical testing result simply demonstrates the presence of nerve compression; the degree of compression can be determined clinically. Nonoperative treatment should be offered to the patient.

31. When is internal neurolysis indicated for the treatment of chronic nerve compression?
Although much has been written about this subject, Mackinnon et al. performed the best study, which was prospective and randomized. They found no advantage to doing internal neurolysis at the time of simple decompression for carpal tunnel release. The randomization was done preoperatively and not based on intraoperative findings. In addition, all patients had "routine" carpal tunnel syndrome; therefore the results of that study cannot be applied to patients with recurrent carpal tunnel syndrome or an underlying neuropathy.

32. How long should a patient be splinted after a nerve decompression?
The shorter time the better—usually about 1 week. If the nerve is prevented from moving for more than 1 week, collagen deposition and fibrin cause adherence to the nerve postoperatively and set up the conditions for recurrence or failure.

33. What is the best surgical technique for ulnar nerve decompression at the elbow?
Five surgical options are currently used throughout the world: simple decompression, anterior subcutaneous transposition, medial epicondylectomy, anterior intramuscular transposition, and submuscular transposition. For a minimal degree of nerve compression, each of these procedures gives a high percentage of excellent results. For a severe degree of nerve compression, each has at least a 25% failure or recurrence rate. One technique for submuscular transposition, which uses a musculofascial Z-lengthening procedure, appears to give the highest percentage of excellent results and the lowest recurrence rates, presumably because the ulnar nerve rests in a location with no new pressures on it.

34. What nonoperative treatment should be considered for radial tunnel syndrome in the patient with coexisting tennis elbow?
The counterforce brace commonly used to reduce the force delivered to the lateral humeral epicondyle can directly decompress the radial nerve in the radial tunnel. Many patients with a diagnosis of recurrent or resistant tennis elbow have a coexisting radial tunnel syndrome. Before operating on the radial tunnel, try the counterforce brace.

35. What is the most common avoidable complication of nerve decompression?
Injury to a nearby cutaneous nerve. For example, the most common cause of postoperative pain after carpal tunnel surgery is a neuroma of the palmar cutaneous branch of the median nerve. Similarly, for cubital tunnel surgery the most common cause of postoperative pain is injury to the medial antebrachial cutaneous nerve. For tarsal tunnel decompression, it is injury to a posterior branch of the saphenous nerve.

CONTROVERSIES

36. Should every patient suspected of having a nerve compression undergo electrodiagnostic testing?
Electrodiagnostic testing is truly objective and gives information about a patient who is uncooperative, malingering, or comatose; it is the only technique to evaluate the presence of a myopathy. Although electrodiagnostic testing is highly specific, it is not highly sensitive. In many patients suspected clinically of having a nerve compression electrodiagnostic testing is interpreted as "normal." The physician evaluating the patient for nerve compression usually can be certain of the diagnosis from the history and physical examination and initiate therapy without electrodiagnostic testing. The cost of testing is often more than the cost of the nonoperative and operative treatment. Another issue is the legal liability faced by the surgeon who operates on a patient with a "normal" electrodiagnostic test. Quantitative sensory testing is noninvasive, nonpainful, and less expensive (often less than $300). It may be more sensitive than electrodiagnostic testing, but it is less specific. If you suspect

coexisting cervical or lumbar disc disease or peripheral neuropathy or if the patient has undergone previous surgery, it is prudent to obtain electrodiagnostic testing.

37. What are the advantages and disadvantages of endoscopic carpal tunnel decompression?
The advantages are one or two short incisions, a little less postoperative pain, and perhaps a return to work 2 days earlier. The disadvantages relate to inability to do other required surgery, the occasional need to convert to an open procedure or to reoperate using an open technique, the increased risk of injury to the median nerve or its branches, and the increased risk to adjacent blood vessels. Typically, the endoscopic technique requires a longer operative time, an endoscope, and extra training by the surgeon. It is, therefore, not at all clear that well-informed patients, considering the risks and potential benefits, will choose endoscopic carpal tunnel release.

BIBLIOGRAPHY

1. Dellon AL: Tinel or not Tinel. J Hand Surg 9B:216, 1984.
2. Dellon AL: Treatment of Morton's neuroma as a nerve compression: The role for neurolysis. Am Podiatr Med Assoc 82:399–402, 1992.
3. Dellon AL: Somatosensory Testing and Rehabilitation. Bethesda, MD, American Occupational Therapy Association, 1997.
4. Dellon AL, Change E, Coert JH, Campbell K: Intraneural ulnar pressure changes related to operative techniques for cubital tunnel decompression. J Hand Surg 19A:817–830, 1994.
5. Dellon AL, Keller KM: Computer-assisted sensorimotor testing in patients with carpal and cubital tunnel syndromes. Ann Plast Surg 38:493–502, 1997.
6. Dellon ES, Aszman OC, Dellon AL: Lateral femoral cutaneous nerve and its susceptibility to compression and injury. Plast Reconstr Surg 100:600–604, 1997.
7. Dellon ES, Keller KM, Moratz B, Dellon AL: Validation of cutaneous pressure threshold measurements for the evaluation of hand function. Ann Plast Surg 38:485–492, 1997.
8. Mackinnon SE, Dellon AL: Surgery of the Peripheral Nerve. New York, Thieme, 1988.
9. Mackinnon SE, McCabe S, Murray JF, et al: Internal neurolysis fails to improve the results of primary carpal tunnel decompression. J Hand Surg 16A:211–218, 1991.
10. Nahabedian M, Dellon AL: Meralgia paresthetica: Etiology, diagnosis and outcome of surgical management. Ann Plast Surg 35:590–594, 1995.
11. Nath R, Mackinnon SE, Weeks PM: Ulnar nerve transection as a complication of two-portal endoscopic carpal tunnel release: A case report. J Hand Surg 18A:896–898, 1993.
12. Nouhan R, Kleinert JM: Ulnar nerve decompression by transposing the nerve and Z-lengthening the flexor-pronator mass: Clinical outcome. J Hand Surg 22A:127–131, 1997.
13. Novak CB, Lee GW, Mackinnon SE, Lay L: Provocative testing for cubital tunnel syndrome. J Hand Surg 19A:817–820, 1994.
14. Spinner M: Injuries to the Major Branches of Peripheral Nerves of the Forearm, 2nd ed. Philadelphia, W.B. Saunders, 1978.

104. BRACHIAL PLEXUS

Mark H. Gonzalez, M.D.

1. Which nerve roots supply the brachial plexus?
The brachial plexus is most frequently supplied by the fifth through eighth cervical (C) and first thoracic (T) nerve roots (see figure at top of next page).

2. What is a prefixed plexus? A postfixed plexus?
A prefixed plexus has a contribution from the fourth cervical nerve root, and a postfixed plexus has a contribution from the second thoracic nerve root.

3. Which nerves form the trunks of the brachial plexus?
Most frequently, the upper trunk is formed by the C5 and C6 nerve roots, the middle trunk is formed by the C7 nerve root, and the lower trunk is formed by the C8 and T1 nerve roots.

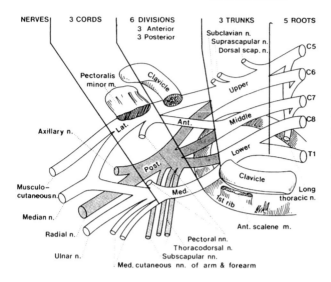

The brachial plexus. (From Lister GL: The brachial plexus. In Lister GL: The Hand. Edinburgh, Churchill Livingstone, 1993, pp 243–246, with permission.)

4. Which nerves form the cords of the brachial plexus?

Each trunk divides into an anterior and posterior division. The anterior divisions of the upper and middle trunks unite to form the lateral cord, the anterior division of the lower trunk forms the medial cord, and the posterior divisions of the three trunks form the posterior cord.

5. How are the peripheral nerves formed in the brachial plexus?

The musculocutaneous nerve arises from the lateral cord and the ulnar nerve from the medial cord. The median nerve is formed by contributions of the medial and lateral cords. The radial, axillary, and thoracodorsal nerves arise from the posterior cord.

6. What is the common mechanism of closed brachial plexus injury in adults?

Downward (caudal) traction to the shoulder usually causes upper trunk injuries. Traction to the abducted arm (cephalad) causes lower trunk injuries, and front-to-back force applied to the shoulder has been associated with an isolated C7 injury. Anterior dislocation of the shoulder and proximal humerus fracture have been associated with suprascapular and axillary nerve injury.

7. What are the common clinical patterns of closed brachial plexus injury in adults?

Proximal injuries of the brachial plexus are termed supraclavicular injuries, and distal injuries are termed infraclavicular injuries. The most common patterns of supraclavicular injury are Erb's palsy and whole plexus injury. Erb's palsy involves damage to the C5 and C6 nerve roots. Supraspinatus, infraspinatus, deltoid, brachialis, and biceps function is lost. Clinically the arm is internally rotated and adducted, and the elbow is extended. The C7 nerve root also may be damaged, causing loss or weakness of elbow, wrist, and finger extension. The whole plexus injury causes complete or nearly complete loss of arm function (flail arm). Isolated involvement of the C8 and T1 nerve roots (Klumpke's paralysis) is extremely uncommon and shows loss of hand function with sparing of the elbow and shoulder. Infraclavicular injuries commonly show loss of shoulder abduction and flexion but also may be associated with loss of hand, wrist, and elbow function.

8. What are the indications for an arteriogram after an injury to the brachial plexus?

1. Penetrating trauma to the region of the brachial plexus
2. Abnormal pulses associated with blunt or penetrating trauma
3. A normal initial exam followed by subsequent brachial plexus neurologic deficit that may be due to an expanding hematoma.

The risk of arterial injury after brachial plexus injury is 10%, and some authors recommend arteriography for all brachial plexus injuries.

9. **What is the significance of a preganglionic and postganglionic lesion of the brachial plexus?**

A preganglionic lesion of the nerve root is within the intervertebral foramen proximal to the sensory root ganglion and is also termed a root avulsion. A postganglionic lesion is distal to the sensory root ganglion. Preganglionic lesions are not reconstructable by nerve graft, and regeneration is not possible. A postganglionic lesion can be grafted and has regenerative potential.

10. **What is Horner's syndrome? What is its significance?**

Horner's syndrome consists of ptosis (drooping eyelid), miosis (small pupil), and enopthalmos (sunken eyeball) on the same side of the face. It is also associated with anhidrosis (absence of sweat secretion) of the affected side of the face. The presence of Horner's syndrome implies interruption of the sympathetic fibers to the face that arise in the cervicothoracic ganglion. This interruption is due to a proximal lesion to the C8 and T1 roots that is frequently preganglionic.

11. **What is the histamine triple response?**

Histamine is injected into the skin, and the triple response is vasodilation followed by a wheal and flair. The response is an axonal reflex involving the sympathetic ganglion and dorsal root ganglion. Skin denervation with an intact triple response implies a preganglionic lesion.

12. **How can a preganglionic and postganglionic lesion be differentiated?**

Preganglionic lesions are associated with Horner's syndrome; transverse process fractures of the cervical spine; denervation of the serratus, rhomboids, or supraspinatus; an intact histamine response; paralysis of the hemidiaphragm; and absence of any return in the distribution of a nerve root. They are also associated with nerve root avulsion. The presence of intact sensory nerve conduction with absent somatosensory evoked potential also implies a preganglionic lesion. Traumatic meningocoeles on myelogram and proximal nerve lesions on MRI suggest a preganglionic lesion. Surgical exploration is required to determine the level of a nerve root lesion with certainty.

13. **What is the indication for neurolysis of the brachial plexus?**

Neurolysis removes scar surrounding intact nerve fibers. Posttraumatic scarring of the brachial plexus can arrest nerve regeneration or cause loss of regenerated function. In this setting, neurolysis is indicated to release scar that surrounds functioning fascicles and to determine which fascicles are discontinuous and require grafting. Intraoperative nerve stimulation may be useful in identifying and protecting intact fascicles.

14. **What is the indication for nerve grafting of the brachial plexus?**

Postganglionic lesions with loss of fascicular continuity are reconstructed by nerve grafts. A sharp laceration to the brachial plexus can be sutured primarily, but most traction injuries require grafting because of scarring and an ensuing gap. The sural nerve is the most common donor nerve.

15. **What is the indication for neurotization of the brachial plexus? What nerves can be used?**

Neurotization is used for nerve root avulsions that are not reconstructable by nerve grafting. A functioning nerve is used to provide nerve fibers for the distal stump of an avulsed nerve root. The anastomosis can be made directly or with an interposed nerve graft. The intercostal nerves, spinal accessory nerve, cervical plexus, medial pectoral nerve, and contralateral C7 nerve root have been used as donors.

16. **Describe the optimal timing of exploration of an adult traction injury of the brachial plexus.**

Surgery must be performed before 6 months after injury to maximize nerve regeneration. Many surgeons advise surgery after several weeks or months for severe injuries with no evidence of any return.

17. **What causes obstetric palsy?**

Obstetric palsy is believed to be due to a traumatic lesion at birth. Two situations may predispose to obstetric palsy. Large infants with cephalic presentation and shoulder dystocia are at risk during delivery, as are small infants born with a breech presentation. Obstetric palsy may occur after a seemingly normal delivery and has been documented even after a cesarean section.

18. **What are the indications and timing for exploration of obstetric palsy?**

The absence of any return of biceps or deltoid function by 3 months of age is a strong indication for brachial plexus exploration. Other criteria include the absence of elbow flexion/extension, wrist extension, or thumb/finger extension by 9 months of age. Most surgeons recommend exploration before 6–9 months of age.

19. What symptoms are associated with thoracic outlet syndrome?

Neurologic symptoms are most commonly associated with thoracic outlet syndrome. Burning pain involving the shoulder occurs with radiation into the inner arm and the hand. Tingling and numbness of the C8 and T1 nerve root distribution, including the ulnar two fingers, are common. Weakness and wasting of the intrinsic hand muscles, including the thenar eminence, are less common. Vascular changes of the arm and hand are infrequent but may cause venous congestion, cold intolerance, color changes. and cold sensitivity.

20. What is the anatomy of the thoracic outlet?

The thoracic outlet is a triangular space bounded anteriorly by the scalenus anticus, posteriorly by the scalenus medius, and inferiorly by the first rib. The brachial plexus and subclavian artery pass through the outlet.

21. What is the cause of thoracic outlet syndrome?

Any structure that narrows the thoracic outlet may cause thoracic outlet syndrome. A cervical rib, fibrous bands, or a mass effect (tumor) may cause nerve compression. Postural changes such as the military brace position or stooped shoulders also may contribute to the development of thoracic outlet syndrome.

22. What is the Roos test?

The patient is seated with the arms abducted 90° and the elbows flexed 90°. The patient is asked to open and close the hands repeatedly for 3 minutes. The patient with thoracic outlet syndrome experiences an exacerbation of symptoms and is unable to complete the test.

23. What is the treatment of thoracic outlet syndrome?

The initial therapy of thoracic outlet syndrome is conservative, including physical therapy, weight loss when appropriate, and avoidance of conditions that exacerbate the condition, such as carrying heavy weights on the shoulder. Therapy involves postural exercises. Refractory symptoms may be amenable to surgical therapy. The thoracic outlet may be decompressed through a supraclavicular or axillary approach. The supraclavicular approach allows release of fibrous bands and the scalene muscles. The first rib or a cervical rib can be excised through an axillary approach.

24. What is Parsonage Turner syndrome? What is the recommended treatment?

Parsonage Turner syndrome is also called neuralgic amyotrophy and acute brachial neuritis. Acute pain involving the shoulder with radiation into the arm is the initial symptom with subsequent partial or complete paralysis of the arm. The paralysis is a lower motor neuron type with flaccidity. Surgical intervention is not recommended; most patients regain complete function.

BIBLIOGRAPHY

1. Boome RS (ed): The Brachial Plexus. New York, Churchill Livingstone, 1997.
2. Gallen J, Wiss D, Cantelmo N, Menzoin J: Traumatic pseudoaneurysm of the axillary artery: Report of three cases and literature review. J Trauma 24:350–354, 1984.
3. Gilbert A, Whitaker I: Obstetrical brachial plexus lesions. J Hand Surg 16B:489–491,1991.
4. Leffert RD: Brachial Plexus Injuries. New York, Churchill Livingstone, 1985.
5. Lister GL: The Hand. Edinburgh, Churchill Livingstone, 1993.
6. Michelow BJ, Clarke HM, Curtis CG et al: The natural history of obstetrical brachial palsy. Plast Reconstr Surg 93:675–681, 1994.
7. Millesi H: Brachial plexus injury in adults: Operative repair. In Gelberman RH (ed): Operative Nerve Repair and Reconstruction. Philadelphia, W.B. Saunders, 1991, pp 1285–1301.
8. Roos DB: New concepts of thoracic outlet syndrome that explain etiology, symptoms, diagnosis, and treatment. Vasc Surg 13:313–321, 1974.
9. Sturm J, Perry J: Brachial plexus injuries from blunt trauma—a harbinger of vascular and thoracic injury. Ann Emerg Med 16:404–406, 1987.
10. Waters PM: Obstetrical brachial plexus palsy injuries: Evaluation and management. J Am Acad Orthop Surg 5:205–214, 1997.

105. RHEUMATOID ARTHRITIS

Nabil A. Barakat, M.D., and W. P. Andrew Lee, M.D.

1. What is the normal presentation of rheumatoid arthritis (RA)?

RA is a systemic, chronic inflammatory disease involving the synovial tissues of both joints and tendons. It typically presents in the third and fourth decades of life as symmetric involvement of multiple joints. It has a variable course, including remissions and exacerbations. The diagnosis depends on clinical symptoms and criteria. The cause is likely to be multifactorial, with some evidence of genetic predisposition.

2. What is the pathophysiology of RA?

The precise cause is unknown but is thought to be an autoimmune reaction to an unknown agent within the synovial tissue. IgG and IgM are thought to interact with the antigen to form autoantibody-antigen complexes that cause synovial infiltration with leukocytes. The leukocytes release inflammatory mediators that cause the synovitis. The IgG and IgM autoantibodies are also termed rheumatoid factors (RFs) and are present in more than 70% of affected patients, making them RF-positive.

3. What are the radiographic features of RA?

A uniform joint space narrowing is noted as well as characteristic erosions without the subchondral sclerosis that is prominent in osteoarthritis. Osteophytes are usually not seen, although osteoporosis and soft tissue swelling are often present.

4. What are the clinical features of RA?

Symmetric joint swelling and pain, along with decreased range of motion, are often noted. Untreated, the condition leads to deformity of the joints and subsequent loss of function. Similarly, inflammation of the tendons leads to localized areas of tenderness that move with excursions of the affected tendon. The synovial proliferation may lead to tendon ruptures and subsequent loss of function. Triggering and various nerve compressions are also noted subsequent to the inflammation. Muscle wasting secondary to all of the above may result. Extraarticular manifestations include eye, lung, heart, blood vessel, muscle, and neurologic signs as well as associated autoimmune diseases.

5. What is the caput ulnae syndrome?

The caput ulnae syndrome includes dorsal dislocation of the distal ulna, supination of the carpus, and volar subluxation of the extensor carpi ulnaris. The syndrome is thought to result form the synovitis that stretches the ulnar triangular fibrocartilage complex. It is seen in up to one-third of patients and causes weakness and pain that are aggravated by forearm rotation. Examination of the wrist reveals prominence of the distal ulna with supination of the carpus on the forearm. This finding sets the stage for attrition ruptures of the extensor tendons.

6. What are the causes of tendon ruptures in RA?

Both extensor and flexor tendon ruptures occur in RA. They are thought to be secondary to attrition of the tendons against a bony prominence. On the **extensor side**, the extensor digitorum communis tendon ruptures from ulnar styloid abrasion (Vaughan-Jackson lesion), whereas the extensor pollicis longus is abraded by Lister's tubercle. On the **flexor side**, the flexor pollicis longus is the most commonly ruptured flexor tendon from attrition against the scaphoid bone (Mannerfelt lesion). Flexor tendon ruptures also result from direct invasion by inflammatory infiltrate as well as ischemic necrosis from proliferation of the synovium.

7. What is the differential diagnosis of an extensor tendon rupture leading to lack of metacarpophalangeal (MP) joint extension?

Lack of MP joint extension is usually due to extensor rupture. Other causes include MP joint dislocation, fixed MP joint flexion contracture, and extensor subluxation at the MP joint. Extensor paralysis due to posterior interosseous nerve compression from elbow synovitis also has been reported.

8. How is RA treated medically?

Nonsteroidal antiinflammatory drugs (NSAIDs) and corticosteroids are the first line of treatment. Second-line drugs include azathioprine, gold compounds, and hydrochloroquinone. Local steroid injections occasionally give transient relief of symptoms, as do joint protection and splinting.

9. What are the principles of treatment in rheumatoid hand and wrist surgery?

First and foremost, deformity without pain or functional loss is not an indication for surgery. Many grossly abnormal-appearing hands are painless and have no functional loss. The entire patient should be assessed, including both upper and lower extremities as well as the spine. Functional loss and effects on activities of daily living should be assessed specifically.

10. What are the four objectives of surgical treatment of rheumatoid hand deformity?

1. To relieve pain and its debilitating effects.
2. To improve and restore useful function, most importantly for activities of daily living.
3. To prevent ongoing destruction.
4. To correct cosmetic deformity. Remember: deformity without pain or functional loss is not an indication for surgery.

11. What three general categories of surgical procedures are performed on the rheumatoid hand and wrist?

Nearly all surgical procedures for RA may be categorized as preventive, reconstructive, or salvage surgeries. Preventive surgeries include synovectomies and tenosynovectomies. Reconstructive surgeries include soft tissue reconstruction, such as tendon rebalancing, arthroplasties, and tendon transfers. Salvage surgeries include different types of joint arthrodesis.

12. What is the surgical sequence in rheumatoid patients?

Lower extremity joints should be addressed first, and a proximal joint should be addressed before a distal joint (e.g., elbow before wrist or hand, wrist before MP or proximal interphalangeal [PIP] joints). The painful joint should be approached first with uncomplicated procedures that have the best outcome.

13. What are the indications for an extensor tenosynovectomy?

Significant dorsal swelling persistent after 6 months of medical treatment is thought by most experts to be an indication for extensor tenosynovectomy. The Darrach procedure, in which the ulnar head is excised, is sometimes added to help prevent tendon rupture. Similarly, repositioning of the volarly dislocated extensor carpi ulnaris (ECU) together with a tendon transfer (typically the extensor carpi radialis longus [ECRL]) is also indicated in later stages of the disease.

14. What is the preferred treatment of extensor ruptures?

In the case of a single rupture of the extensor to the little finger, the distal stump is sutured to the neighboring extensor tendon to the ring finger. Double ruptures of the extensors of the little and ring fingers may be treated in a similar fashion, or an extensor indicis proprius (EIP) tendon transfer may be performed. Rupture of three or sometimes four extensor tendons is treated by transfer of the flexor digitorum superficialis (FDS) of the middle finger to the extensor side. Rupture of the extensor pollicis longus (EPL) is usually treated by transfer of the EIP.

15. What are the indications for wrist arthrodesis?

Pain, loss of function, and wrist deformity, along with radiographic findings of extensive carpal destruction and collapse, are the typical indications for an arthrodesis. Wrist synovectomy is indicated in patients with minimal bony destruction. Wrist arthroplasty using different silicone implants has fallen out of favor because of multiple complications, although metal prostheses are used at some centers.

16. What are the indications for MP joint arthroplasty?

The indications are pain, loss of function, and ulnar drift, along with radiographic evidence of advanced destruction of the joint. Absence of pain with a functional hand is a contraindication to surgical treatment. MP joint arthroplasty with silicone implants has enjoyed relative success in comparison with wrist arthroplasties. On the other hand, MP joint arthrodesis is usually avoided in view of the significant limitation that it imposes on motion.

17. What are the common finger deformities in the rheumatoid hand?

A swan-neck deformity with hyperextension of the PIP joint and flexion of the distal interphalangeal (DIP) joint and the boutonnière deformity with hyperextension of the DIP joint and flexion of the PIP joint are often noted. Both deformities are secondary to imbalances in the extensor mechanism caused by the synovitis within the joint spaces.

18. What is the surgical approach to correction of the swan-neck deformity?

The treatment depends on the mobility of the PIP joint. If the PIP joint is flexible in all positions, DIP arthrodesis or a sublimis sling is indicated. If PIP joint flexion is limited, intrinsic release, PIP joint manipulation, or lateral band mobilization is indicated. A stiff PIP joint with radiographic evidence of advanced intraarticular changes requires either PIP joint fusion or arthroplasty. PIP joint arthroplasty in the setting of RA has generally met with poor long-term results.

19. What is the mechanism leading to the boutonnière deformity?

Inflammation within the PIP joint is thought to stretch the extensor mechanism, causing the lateral bands to displace volarly and become fixed. They thus act as flexors of the PIP joint and become the sole extensors of the DIP joint, leading to hyperextension of the DIP joint. Surgical correction of boutonnière deformity is often associated with limited functional improvement and a high recurrence rate. Soft tissue correction is indicated only if passive extension of the PIP joint is possible and the joint is preserved. Plication or reinsertion of the central tendon and relocation of the lateral bands dorsally may be performed. If the PIP joint cannot be extended passively or if it is painful, an arthrodesis of this joint is indicated.

20. What are the indications for thumb fusions in RA?

Fusions of MP or IP joints of the thumb are excellent operations, addressing pain, functional deformity, and cosmesis of the joints. The stability and overall function of the hand is often improved after such procedures despite the lack of motion at the involved joint.

BIBLIOGRAPHY

1. Friedman R: Rheumatoid arthritis. Sel Read Plast Surg 7(35):9–17, 1995.
2. Feldon P, Millender L, Nalebuff E: Rheumatoid arthritis in the hand and wrist. In Green D: Operative Hand Surgery, 3rd ed. New York, Churchill Livingstone, 1993.
3. O'Brien E: Surgical principles and planning for the rheumatoid hand and wrist. Clin Plast Surg 23:407–420, 1996.
4. Towheed T, Anastassiades T: Rheumatoid hand: Practical approach to assessment and management. Can Fam Physician 40:1303–1309, 1994.

106. SMALL JOINT ARTHRODESIS AND ARTHROPLASTY

Alan Rosen, M.D., and Andrew J. Weiland, M.D.

SMALL JOINT ARTHRODESIS

1. List the indications for small joint arthrodesis.

The general indications for arthrodesis of any joint pertain to the hand: (1) pain; (2) instability; (3) joint destruction; (4) deformity resulting from trauma, osteoarthritis, or rheumatoid-type conditions; and (5) loss of muscle or tendon function across the joint. Failure of prior procedures aimed at maintaining motion, such as implant arthroplasty, are also an indication for arthrodesis as a salvage procedure. More specific indications for small joint arthrodesis in the hand include (1) painful posttraumatic arthrosis or deformity; (2) fixed contractures after burns; (3) rheumatoid arthritis; (4) severe infection unresponsive to pharmacologic therapy; (5) Dupuytren's contracture with fixed deformity; (6) nerve palsy leading to instability that impedes function; (7) chronic mallet finger deformity unresponsive to conservative treatment; and (8) as a salvage procedure after failed arthroplasty or tendon reconstruction for deformity such as boutonnière or mallet finger.

2. Should all chronic mallet deformities be fused?

No. Studies have shown that even chronic mallet finger deformities may respond to treatment with 8 weeks of distal interphalangeal (DIP) joint splinting. Patient preference also should be taken into account. Many patients would rather live with a 10–15° extensor lag than undergo surgery to fuse the joint. However, if a significant secondary hyperextension deformity develops at the proximal interphalangeal (PIP) joint, arthrodesis of the DIP joint may be indicated to preserve PIP joint function.

3. Describe the ideal position for fusion of the metaphalangeal (MP), PIP, and DIP joints of the index, middle, ring, and little fingers.

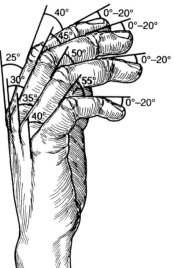

In general, finger MP joints should be cascaded from a radial to ulnar direction, beginning with 25° of flexion in the index finger and adding 5° for each finger as one progresses ulnarward. The PIP joints also should be cascaded from a radial to ulnar direction, beginning with 40° of flexion in the index finger and adding 5° for each finger as one progresses ulnarward. The DIP joints should be fused in 0° of flexion. (*Note:* The editor prefers DIP joint fusion in slight flexion of 20°). No rotation, ulnar deviation, or radial deviation from the normal anatomic position should be allowed in joints undergoing fusion. An exception to this rule is the DIP joint of the index and middle fingers, for which 5–10° of supination may be useful in achieving pulp-to-pulp pinch with the thumb.

(From Brockman R, Weiland AJ: Small joint arthrodesis. In Green DP (ed): Operative Hand Surgery, 3rd ed. New York, Churchill Livingstone, 1993, p 100, with permission.)

4. What is the ideal position for fusion of the MP and IP joints of the thumb?

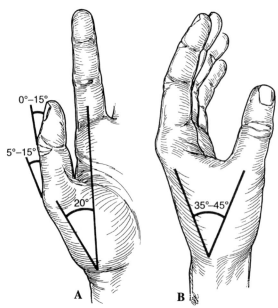

Ideal position for arthrodesis in the thumb. *A*, The MP joint is flexed 5–15° with approximately 10° of pronation to facilitate pulp-to-pulp pinch with the fingers. The IP joint is also fused in slight flexion (0–15°). *B*, If the CMC joint needs to be fused (very unusual), it should be placed in 35–45° of palmar abduction and 20° of radial extension. (From Brockman R, Weiland AJ: Small joint arthrodesis. In Green DP (ed): Operative Hand Surgery, 3rd ed. New York, Churchill Livingstone, 1993, p 101, with permission.)

5. A stiff finger is less cumbersome if it is slightly shorter. True or false?

This statement is true for the index, middle, ring, and little fingers. In the thumb, which is involved in nearly all hand activities, maximal length should be obtained to allow functions such as pinch and opposition.

6. What general principles need to be followed to obtain a successful fusion?

Many techniques have been described for fixation of small joint arthrodeses, each with its own proponents and applications. However, no matter what technique is used, several general principles need to be followed: (1) avoid interposition of any soft tissues between bony surfaces; (2) remove all cartilage from the joint surfaces; (3) surface preparation should result in good cancellous-to-cancellous bone contact; (4) the bony surfaces must be held securely together by either internal or external fixation; and (5) the position of fusion should be as close as possible to the position of function.

7. What internal fixation techniques are available for small joint arthrodesis?

Several techniques are available. Internal fixation techniques include (1) Kirschner wires, which may be trimmed at the bone surface and left in situ or protruding from the bone so that they can be removed once the fusion has set; (2) interosseous wiring; (3) tension band wiring; (4) lag screw fixation; (5) plate fixation; and (6) bioabsorbable rods and pin, the clinical use of which is still in its infancy.

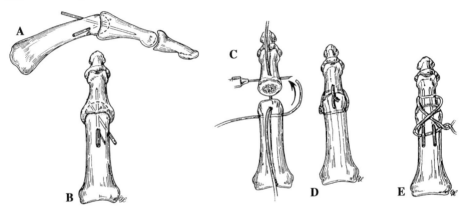

Internal fixation techniques for small joint arthrodesis. *A* and *B*, Kirschner wiring. *C* and *D*, Interosseous wiring. *E*, Tension band wiring. *F*, Lag screw fixation. (From Brockman R, Weiland AJ: Small joint arthrodesis. In Green DP (ed): Operative Hand Surgery, 3rd ed. New York, Churchill Livingstone, 1993, p 104, with permission.)

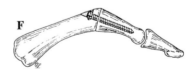

8. Discuss the indications for external fixation.

External fixation is not generally used for uncomplicated phalangeal and metacarpal joint arthrodesis. The limited indications for external fixation include (1) open joint injuries with severe bone and articular surface loss; (2) septic arthritis or osteomyelitis with joint destruction; and (3) failed prior arthrodesis by other methods.

9. Is bone grafting necessary for small joint fusions?

Bone grafts are not usually necessary to obtain successful digital joint arthrodeses. They may be useful in patients with significant bone loss due to trauma; failed arthroplasty; failed arthrodesis; infection; or the arthritis mutilans form of rheumatoid arthritis with severe bone loss.

10. Is small joint arthrodesis performed in children with open physes?

Yes. Indications for arthrodesis of digital joints in children with open physes are rare, but the procedure may be indicated in cases involving congenital problems or cerebral palsy.

11. It is possible to perform a digital fusion in children without interfering with digital growth. True or false?

True. The articular cartilage is carefully shaved off, avoiding damage to the ossification center and the physeal (growth) plate. The prepared articular surfaces are then reduced into the desired position of fusion and held in place with Kirschner wires until fusion has occurred.

12. What are the most common complications of small joint arthrodesis?

Arthrodesis of the small joints is not a fail-safe operation. Numerous complications may occur, including (1) nonunion; (2) malunion; (3) pin tract infection; (4) cold intolerance; and (5) vascular insufficiency, which is seen most often after arthrodesis for a fixed flexion deformity (restoration of digital length may place the neurovascular bundles under excessive stretch).

SMALL JOINT ARTHROPLASTY

13. What are the indications for arthroplasty vs. arthrodesis?

In deciding whether to perform arthroplasty or arthrodesis in the hand, the adjacent joints must be taken into account. Fusion of contiguous joints is usually not recommended because it severely curtails range of motion of the affected digit. As a general rule, arthrodesis provides power and stability, whereas arthroplasty provides range of motion. Arthroplasty is more commonly indicated proximally (for example, at the metacarpophalangeal [MCP] joints of the index, middle, ring, and little fingers), whereas arthrodesis is more commonly performed distally (at the DIP joints). Joints that require stability for specific functions such as pinch—for example, the PIP joint of the index finger and the MCP joint of the thumb—are more amenable to fusion.

14. Discuss the common indications for arthroplasty in the small joints of the hand.

Rheumatoid arthritis and related collagen diseases such as psoriatic arthritis and systemic lupus erythematosus are among the most common disease processes that lead to joint destruction requiring arthroplasty. Arthroplasty also may be indicated for degenerative or posttraumatic disease. Therefore, the two major indications for arthroplasty in general are (1) pain and deformity secondary to arthritis and (2) stiffness due to loss of joint surface or joint incongruity.

15. What are the primary contraindications to arthroplasty?

Ongoing infection is an absolute contraindication for any type of implant arthroplasty. Loss of active range of motion across a joint due to damage or paralysis of the flexor or extensor tendons is also a primary contraindication.

16. Name the structures necessary for a stable arthroplasty.

Sufficient bone stock should be present to allow for a stable arthroplasty. In addition, it is necessary to obtain reasonable stability of the joint by restoration or preservation of the capsule and surrounding ligamentous structures. Functional flexor and extensor tendons to provide active range of motion across the joint are also required. If restoration of joint stability is doubtful, arthrodesis is a better option.

17. Describe the different types of arthroplasty.

1. Resection arthroplasty, in which the diseased articular surfaces are resected and soft tissue is interposed between the two bones.

2. Silicone elastomer arthroplasty, in which the distal end of the proximal bone and the proximal end of the distal bone are resected and a flexible silicone spacer is interposed between the two. (See figure on p. 543.)

3. Cemented arthroplasty, which involves placement of a prosthesis composed of two articulating components, usually made of a combination of metal (titanium or cobalt chrome) and ultra-high-molecular-weight polyethylene (UHMWP).

4. Hemiarthroplasty, in which only one of the joint surfaces is replaced, usually by a silicone or titanium implant. (See figure on p. 544.)

5. Allograft joint replacement.

6. Vascularized whole joint transfer.

The last two procedures have limited application and indications (e.g., traumatic loss of several fingers or injury to an essential joint in a child).

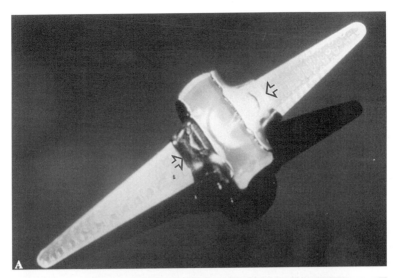

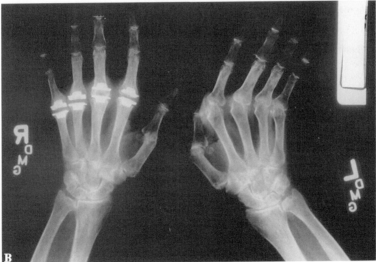

Hinged silicone prosthesis with grommets (arrow). *A*, Prosthesis before implantation. *B*, Radiograph of implanted prostheses at the metacarpophalangeal joints of the index, middle, ring, and little fingers on the right hand.

18. What is perichondral arthroplasty?

Perichondral anthroplasty was first described in Europe during the 1970s. Chondral grafts are harvested from the costal cartilages and sutured over the resurfaced ends of adjacent bones of the affected joint. When only cartilage is used, the procedure fails as a result of cartilage necrosis. When an osseous base with overlying cartilage is used, satisfactory results have been reported, but only in a small series of patients.

19. Discuss the common complications of silicone implants.

The most common complications associated with the use of silicone implants are prosthetic fracture, dislocation, and formation of silicone-induced particulate synovitis with osteolysis and cyst formation. The use of a new high-performance (HP) elastomer and circumferential grommets has reportedly decreased the incidence of fracture in hinged implants. However, HP elastomer (especially when used in areas of heavy loading such as the carpus) has been associated with a higher incidence of silicone-induced particulate synovitis, which curtails the indications for its use.

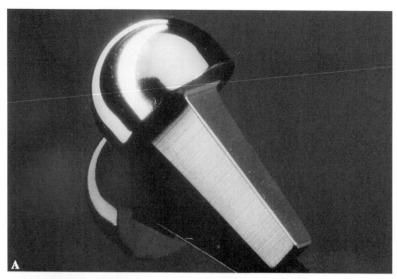

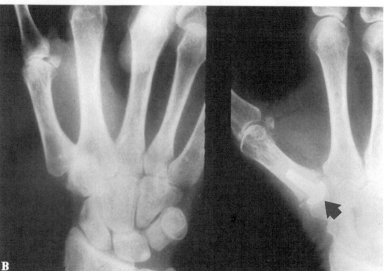

Convex condylar titanium implant. *A,* Prosthesis before implantation. *B,* Radiograph of a thumb with car-pometacarpal arthritis before *(left)* and after *(right)* implantation of the prosthesis *(arrow).*

20. What are the early and late complications of small joint arthroplasty?

The common complications of small joint arthroplasty are essentially the same as the complications of arthroplasties in general. Early complications include (1) wound breakdown, (2) infection, (3) prosthetic dislocation, and (4) nerve injury. Late complications include (1) loss of motion, (2) recurrent deformity, (3) prosthetic loosening, and (4) prosthetic fracture.

BIBLIOGRAPHY

1. Brockman R, Weiland AJ: Small joint arthrodesis.In Green DP (ed): Operative Hand Surgery, 3rd ed. New York, Churchill Livingstone, 1993, pp 99–111.
2. Beckenbaugh RD, Linscheid RL: Arthroplasty in the hand and wrist. In Green DP (ed): Operative Hand Surgery, 3rd ed. New York, Churchill Livingstone, 1993, pp 143–188.
3. Gould JS: Arthroplasty of the metacarpophalangeal and interphalangeal joints of the digits and thumb. In Peimer CA (ed): Surgery of the Hand and Upper Extremity. New York, McGraw-Hill, 1996, pp 1677–1689.

4. Hanel DP: Reconstruction of finger deformities. In Hand Surgery Update. Rosemont, IL, American Society for Surgery of the Hand, 1996, pp 33–44.
5. Thompson JS: Small joint arthrodeses. In Peimer CA (ed): Surgery of the Hand and Upper Extremity. New York, McGraw-Hill, 1996, pp 973–997.
6. Weiland AJ: Small joint arthrodesis and bony defect reconstruction. In McCarthy JG (ed): Plastic Surgery, vol 7: The Hand. Philadelphia, W.B. Saunders, 1990, pp 4671–4694.
7. Wright PE: Arthritic hand. In Crenshaw AH (ed): Campbell's Operative Orthopaedics, 8th ed, vol 3. St. Louis, Mosby, 1992, pp 3301–3339.

107. CONGENITAL ANOMALIES

Joseph Upton, M.D., and Benjamin J. Childers, M.D.

1. At what age of development does the limb bud appear? When are digital rays evident?

Streeter divided human embryonic development into 23 stages. Limb development and differentiation are rapid processes occurring between the third and eighth postovulatory weeks. The limb bud, called Wolff's crest, is well defined at day 30. It is a ventral swelling mesoderm covered by a thick layer of ectoderm, called the apical ectodermal ridge (AER). By day 41 digital rays are present, and by day 48 joint interzones are evident histologically. Usually by the time the expectant mother is sure that she is pregnant, most of the upper limb differentiation has been completed.

2. What does syndactyly mean? Is it the most common congenital anomaly?

Syndactyly (Greek: *syn* = together, *dactyly* = finger) is commonly used to describe webbed digits and is the second most common congenital anomaly. The most common are duplications, particularly preaxial or thumb duplications in the Asian population and postaxial or ulnar duplications in African American and Native American populations. The incidence of duplications varies according to the population but overall occurs in 3.8–12.0/1000 live births.

3. What type of correction is best for syndactyly?

No one repair is absolutely best. Over 60 methods have been described in the literature, and most use the same basic surgical principles. The surgeon must be comfortable with a few repairs that she or he learns to do well and not experiment with each case.

4. What are the principles of syndactyly correction?

1. Use of full-thickness flaps for commissure reconstruction
2. Zig-zag incisions on the palmar surface
3. Use of full-thickness skin grafts
4. Equal division of flaps between each partner digit
5. Meticulous, atraumatic technique
6. Adequate postoperative immobilization
7. Staged release of the radial and ulnar sides of a digit. Release of both sides during one procedure may compromise the vascular supply to the digit.

In operating on young children, it is also important to work under general anesthesia and to use a pneumatic tourniquet and absorbable 6-0 or 5-0 chromic suture material.

5. What are the most common problems after syndactyly correction?

Infection, graft or flap maceration, and graft loss are almost always related to the child's activity and/or inadequate immobilization. Surgeons with children of their own do not hesitate to protect operated limbs in a long arm cast extending well proximal to the elbow flexed at 90°. Single residents without children do not always appreciate the problems that most parents encounter with controlling active young children. Early problems also may occur after children wet their casts or dressings in bathtubs or swimming pools.

Long-term problems include recurrence of the webbing or "web creep," which is related to scar contracture at the base of the commissure or along the incision lines. Zig-zag incisions are intended to reduce this potential contracture. Skin grafts are often hyperpigmented and, if harvested within the hair-bearing escutcheon, may become hirsute during adolescence. Inadequate correction of the first web release may be obtained with tight contractures, which can be widened only with additional soft tissue.

6. What is the most important web space in the hand?
The thumb-index or first web space is unquestionably the most important. Of all techniques described for correction of congenital hand anomalies, release of the first web space is the most significant functionally and aesthetically. In a pure analysis, a "basic hand" has three components: a mobile digit or thumb on the radial side, a first web space, and a post or digit on the opposite side of the hand.

7. What is the best method for surgical release of the first web space?
The surgeon must learn to use one or two methods well. For minimal-to-moderate contractures, the four-flap Z-plasty provides the greatest release and maintains the best concavity between the thumb and index MP joints. A single Z-plasty and the five-flap Z-plasty, also called the "jumping man," are good alternatives. Many varieties of dorsal rotational flaps from the thumb or index metacarpal regions have been described with the use of skin grafts. These techniques are not preferred because they leave a conspicuous skin graft in a visible position of the hand. These local flaps are indicated in complex problems such as the Apert hand.

For severe contractures soft tissue is often needed. Free tissue transfers in infants or young children are often quite cumbersome and technically difficult. Distally based forearm (radial artery or dorsal interosseous artery) fasciocutaneous flaps have been described for children with arthrogryposis, windblown hands, and hypolastic thumbs with tight contractures, and are advised for experienced surgeons.

8. What contributes to thumb-index contracture?
Tight skin is the most obvious etiology, but tight investing fascias of the first dorsal interosseous and adductor pollicis muscles almost always are found and must be excised. Often a tight band is present between the two muscles. Occasionally, a tight thumb carpometacarpal (CMC) joint may be found; it is usually suspected on physical examination.

9. How is syndactyly clinically classified?
The level of webbing between digits is **complete** if it extends to the fingertip and **incomplete** with a more proximal termination. A **simple** syndactyly refers to soft tissue connections between adjacent digits, whereas **complex** refers to bone or cartilaginous unions. **Complicated** refers to abnormal duplicated skeletal parts within the interdigital space. The most common pattern is bilateral simple, incomplete syndactyly of the long and ring fingers. Many such patients have a simple syndactyly involving toes 2 and 3 on one or both feet.

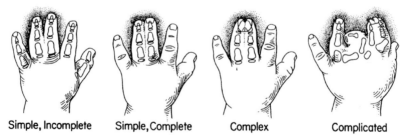

Simple, Incomplete   Simple, Complete   Complex   Complicated

Classification of syndactyly. (From Upton J: Congenital anomalies of the hand and forearm. In McCarthy JG, May J, Littler JW (eds): Plastic Surgery. Philadelphia, W.B. Saunders, 1990, p 5280, with permission.)

10. Do children need more surgery after syndactyly repair?
There is always a chance that contractures will require future correction. The literature cites a secondary operation rate of about 10%. The incidence is much higher in complex and complicated cases and cases with postoperative complications. There is a direct relationship between carefully planned and executed surgery and a low complication rate. Children and adults with central complex polysyndactyly invariably need secondary corrections. This variety is the most difficult to treat.

11. Geneticists and pediatricians use the terms *malformation, deformation,* **and** *disruption.* **What do they mean?**

The dysmorphology approach to congenital anomalies divides defects into one of three sequences, which are defined as problems that lead to a cascade of events:

1. In a **malformation** sequence poor formation of tissue within the fetus initiates the chain of defects, which may range from minimal to severe. All gradations of radial dysplasia, ranging from absence of the thenar muscles to complete absence of the radius resulting in the club hand posture, are examples. Occurrence rate is in the 5% range. Radial dysplasias also are associated with malformation in other organ systems, such as the VATERR association (vertebral anomalies, anal atresia, tracheoesophageal fistula, renal anomalies, and radial dysplasia) and Holt-Oram syndrome (radial dysplasia and congenital heart disease).

2. The **deformation** sequence involves no intrinsic problem with the fetus or embryo; instead, abnormal external mechanical or structural forces cause secondary distortion or deformation. Tethering or constriction of limb parts by anular bands in the constriction ring syndrome is a prime example. The occurrence rate is very low.

3. In the **disruption** sequence the normal fetus or embryo is subjected to tissue breakdown or injury, which may be vascular, infectious, mechanical, or metabolic in origin. The hand deformities associated with maternal ingestion of thalidomide or alcohol are good examples.

Often the patient's problem cannot be explained by a single initiating factor. When the cause of a defect is unknown, the term **malformation** is preferred. Multiple defects are usually referred to as a **malformation syndrome.**

12. What is the relative incidence of congenital hand duplications? How are they clinically classified?

Duplications are the most common anomalies in all large series. They are classified by their position within the hand as preaxial (radial), central and postaxial (ulnar). In the U.S. duplication is most prevalent among African-Americans, who have an extremely dominant inheritance pattern with a frequency of 1 in 300 live births and a predilection for the postaxial border of the hand. In contrast, Caucasians and Asians primarily have preaxial duplication at a rate of 1 in 3000 live births. (See question 2.)

Preaxial thumb duplications are classified into six categories by the level of the duplications. Type II at the interphalangeal (IP) joint and type IV at the metaphalangeal (MP) joint are the most common. The more proximal varieties, type V at the thumb metacarpal level and type VI at the CMC joint level, are uncommon. Additional designations are made if there is an extra phalanx (delta phalanx) or a triphalangeal partner (type VII). Triphalangeal thumbs are unusual and well beyond the experience of most residents.

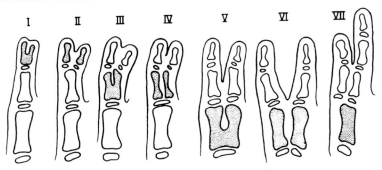

Classification of thumb duplications based on the level of duplication. Type VII describes the triphalangeal thumb. (From Upton J: Congenital anomalies. In Jurkiewicz M, Krizek TJ, Mathes SJ, Ariyan S (eds): Plastic Surgery: Principles and Practice. St. Louis, Mosby, 1990, p 573, with permission.)

Central duplications are unusual and account for less than 10% of all duplications; they have no systematic clinical classification system. Because central duplications are often associated with webbing, the term **synpolydactyly** is used.

Postaxial duplications of the fifth ray are divided into three categories. Type I is characterized by a soft tissue nubbin with a skin bridge. Skeletal connections are present in type II, and a complete duplication of the entire ray is seen in type III. Most cases are type I.

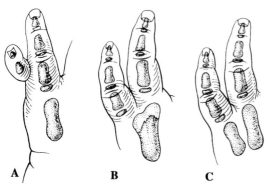

Classification of polydactyly (postaxial) demonstrates digits with *(A)* no skeletal attachment (type I), *(B)* skeletal connections (type II), and *(C)* complete duplication of the entire ray, including the metacarpal bone (type III). (From Upton J: Congenital anomalies of the hand and forearm. In McCarthy JG, May J, Littler JW (eds): Plastic Surgery. Philadelphia, W.B. Saunders, 1990, p 5345, with permission.)

A   B   C

13. Is any special work-up needed in newborns with a duplication?
In most cases, no. Thumb duplications may have a positive inheritance pattern and are common in Caucasian and Asian populations, whereas fifth finger duplications are extremely common in Afro-Americans and Native American populations. When the opposite is seen, a work-up is in order. Over 30 syndromes are associated with postaxial duplications, primarily in non–Afro-American populations. Conversely, an Afro-American with thumb duplication and negative family history may have a syndrome such as fetal alcohol syndrome. Referral to a geneticist is in order.

14. How do you treat a newborn in the nursery with a type I floppy nubbin attached to the fifth finger?
Pediatricians like to "tie them off" with a suture. Type I duplications with large skin bridges often do not fall off. Many such children present to the dermatologist 8 years later with a bump at the site of duplication, which is misdiagnosed as a wart. The "wart" does not respond to application of a triple acid ointment or solution. This lump is a cartilaginous remnant or scar. Simple excision and closure with one or two sutures under local anesthesia in the newborn nursery is a more appropriate option.

15. Which side of a thumb duplication should be preserved?
The correct answer depends on which thumb has the better parts. In most patients the radial of the two partners is the more hypoplastic and is ablated. In some more proximal type V and type VI varieties at the metacarpal level, the distal portion of the ulnar partner is transposed on top of the proximal portion of the radial partner.

16. What are the basic principles of thumb duplication correction?
1. Create the best possible thumb by using the best parts of each partner.
2. Preserve an intact ulnar collateral ligament at the MP joint level.
3. Reattach all thenar intrinsic muscles.
4. Release a tight thumb index web space (Four-flap Z-plasty is most commonly used.)
5. Preserve as much mobility as possible and preferably have motion at at least two of the three (CMC, MP, IP) joints.

17. What do you tell parents after a thumb duplication correction? Will the thumb be normal?
No. Most large series are incomplete and do not include critical long-term outcomes. What you see initially is what you get later. The reconstructed thumbs are usually smaller and less mobile than the normal side. Thenar muscles, especially the abductor pollicis brevis and flexor pollicis brevis, may be weak. Metacarpophalangeal joint instability or stiffness may occur after a collateral ligament reconstruction. A bulge on the radial side of the metacarpal in a type IV thumb represents a bifid metacarpal head that was not excised. The proximal type V and VI thumbs are never normal postoperatively, do not have normal intrinsic muscles, have short metacarpals, and commonly have inadequate extrinsic extensor and flexor tendon excursion.

18. What are the genetics and incidence of the constriction ring syndrome (CRS)?

There is no positive inheritance in CRS. The incidence is less than 10% in large reported series of congenital hand malformations. The cause is related to an in utero deformation in which strands of the inner layer of the chorionic sac detach and wrap around parts of the fetus, usually fingers and toes. There are many examples of monozygotic twins with only one partner affected.

19. What anatomic features distinguish CRS from other congenital anomalies of the upper limb?

The anatomy proximal to the level of deformation or in utero injury is completely normal. For this reason, toe transfers for thumb and digital reconstruction are much more predictable. Unfortunately, many severely affected children have no toes to transfer.

20. What other terms have been used to describe CRS?

Many terms have been used to describe the clinical features seen in CRS:

Acrosyndactyly refers to digits joined together at the tips and creating the appearance of a peak (Greek: *acro* = peak).

Anular band is a ring around a body part; **constriction ring** is the preferred term to describe the same phenomenon.

Fenestrated syndactyly refers to the sinuses at the base of the webbed digits. At the time of ischemic insult caused by the constricting band, the separation of the digit via programmed cell death has started. Although the webbing recurs as a result of the distal inflammatory process, the separation may persist and presents as a dorsal-to-palmar epithelial-lined sinus that can be easily probed. The actual level of the sinuses is always distal to the level of the normal commissure.

Placental bands and **amniotic bands** refer to the strands that wrap around body parts. At birth, desiccated strands wrapped around digits represent the loose strands of the chorionic sac that have separated and become entangled around fingers, toes, and other body parts.

Congenital amputations refer to transverse loss of tissue or failure of formation. They are commonly seen in CRS but are not exclusive to it.

This condition has been around for a long time and has been confused in past and recent literature. The term **constriction ring syndrome** has been adopted by the American Society for Surgery of the Hand (ASSH) and the International Federation of Societies of Surgery of the Hand (IFSSH).

21. What is a constriction ring or anular (ring) band?

The constricting ring acts as a tourniquet around the developing digit, toe, or other body part and results in a soft tissue depression beneath the skin. The ring may be superficial or deep, extending into the periosteum; it may extend completely or partially around the circumference of the part. Most digital rings are deep dorsally and extend only partially around the palmar surface. However, this explanation does not account for the frequent association of cleft lip/palate and club feet with CRS. The clefts are often wide lateral clefts that result in a monstrous clinical appearance. It has been postulated that wide bands or aprons of partially separated sac obstruct the fusion of the lateral lip with the prolabial segment.

22. How is CRS treated?

In the past, surgeons performed simple Z-plasties that did nothing more than leave the mark of the infamous cowboy Zorro on operated hands. After excision of the scarred constriction ring it is necessary to advance flaps of fat and fascial tissue across the depression to correct the contour deformity. Straight-line dorsal incisions are preferred to Z-plasties; they are conveniently placed along the less visible sides of the digit.

23. Why are transverse absences associated with CRS ideal for toe-to-thumb transfers?

CRS is the only congenital anomaly in which the anatomy proximal to the level of complete or partial loss is completely normal. In other conditions, intrinsic and extrinsic muscle and neural and vascular anatomy may be anomalous.

24. What does symphalangism mean? What are the more common clinical presentations?

Symphalangism (Greek: *sym* = together, *phalanx* = bone) refers to phalanges that are fused because of a failure of segmentation or incomplete segmentation with cavitation. More than 15 clinical conditions are associated with these stiff, often short and slender digits. The most important clinical sign is the lack of a flexion crease. There are three general categories of symphalangism:

1. **True symphalangism** demonstrates digits of normal length, positive inheritance, fusion of one or more digits, PIP involvement (common), and long, slender fingers.

2. **Symbrachydactyly** demonstrates all variations of short digits with and without varying degrees of webbing. Formerly many affected hands were classified as atypical cleft hands. DIP and PIP joints are commonly fused.

3. **Syndromic symphalangism** is most commonly seen in the Apert and Poland syndromes. In both the central three rays are most commonly involved. Some degree of digital fusion may be seen in the other acrocephalosyndactyly (ACS) syndromes. In neither of these conditions are the MP joints involved.

25. How is symphalangism treated?
The stiff fingers will always be stiff. Angulation and especially rotation should be corrected early in life without damage to growth centers.

26. In what position should PIP joints be fused?
Index finger, 10°; middle finger, 25–30°; ring finger, 40°; and small finger, 45–50°.

27. How can IP joints be reconstructed?
Many methods have been tried; none is satisfactory. Examples include:
- Silicone caps and spacers
- Silicone implants with stems into the medullary canals
- Perichondrial resurfacing
- Incision of early cartilage bridges followed by early motion
- Osteointegrated implants (this technique has promise for the future)
- Microvascular second-toe joint transfer

All of these reconstructions have their advantages and disadvantages. In children it is preferable to use autogenous materials to avoid the secondary disadvantages of incompatible biomaterials. Perichondrial resurfacing at the MP and PIP levels results in fibrocartilage and stiff joints. Early release and continued motion result in floppy digits that ultimately become stiff. Osteointegrated concepts have not yet been used in children but may have promise. Microvascular defects are labor-intensive and biologically make the most sense. The balance of the thin intrinsic and extrinsic extensor mechanism is never maintained.

28. What is the difference between clinodactyly and camptodactyly?
Clinodactyly (Greek: *clino* = deviated, *dactylos* = digit) refers to a digit or thumb that is deviated in a radioulnar or mediolateral direction. An inward (radial) deviation of the fifth digit is most commonly seen and in fact is so often associated with various other types of congenital hand anomalies that it represents "background noise" and gives no specific indication of one condition over another.

Camptodactyly (Greek: *campto* = bent, *dactylos* = digit) refers to a flexion deformity of a digit or thumb in an anteroposterior plane. This deformity also commonly involves the PIP joint of the fifth finger and is seen in two distinct age groups: infants and adolescent girls.

29. What is the main anatomic problem in camptodactyly?
As the digit develops in the fetus or infant or as it continues to grow in the young child and adolescent, the balance of flexion and extension forces at each joint is quite precise. More than 20 abnormal origins and particularly insertions of the intrinsic and extrinsic muscle tendon units within the hand have been described. The most common variations involve abnormal distal insertions of the lumbrical and interosseous muscles within the digits, particularly on the ulnar side of the hand. Tight joint capsules, collateral ligaments, joint contractures, abnormal articulating surfaces, and proliferative fibrous bands (fibrous substrata) within the digit are more likely secondary and are not the primary forces causing camptodactyly.

30. What are the radiologic signs of congenital camptodactyly?
A true lateral radiograph of the digit gives an indication about the duration of congenital camptodactyly. Digits that have been flexed at the PIP joints for longer periods show the following:
1. Flattening of the dorsal condylar surface of the proximal phalanx
2. Widened base of the middle phalanx

3. Flattening of the palmar surface of the condyle
4. Indentation within the surface of the middle phalanx
5. Narrowed joint space

The most important determining factor in joint formation is motion. A joint that is not moved early in life will not have a rounded condyle and will demonstrate a flat articular surface.

31. What are the indications for joint release in camptodactyly?

Most joint contractures are treated successfully with stretching and splinting. Few require surgical release. Contractures of 15–50° usually have favorable outcomes. Adults and adolescents with longstanding contractures > 70° of flexion are best treated with arthrodesis. The results of soft tissue releases are inversely proportional to the severity of the contracture. Often initial tight contractures can be improved with conscientious stretching but may need surgery later in childhood to obtain full correction. Surgery may be difficult and must be followed by a strict stretching and night-splinting regimen.

32. What is the differential diagnosis of bilateral flexion deformities of the thumb?

Trigger thumbs due to flexor tenosynovitis are the most common cause. Newborns and infants may demonstrate congenital absence of the extrinsic extensor (EPL), a condition in which the thumb is adducted into the palm (commonly called "clasped thumb"). Congenital camptodactyly does not involve the thumb but should be considered with any flexion deformity of a digit. More generalized musculoskeletal conditions, such as arthrogryposis and Freeman-Sheldon syndrome, also must be considered.

33. When should a trigger thumb be released surgically?

In children under 18 months of age spontaneous resolution *may* be seen within 6 months. After 2 years of age children with persistent locking develop compensatory hyperextension of the MP joint as the palmar plate is stretched. This hyperextension may not correct itself with growth after the trigger is corrected. No additional surgery is indicated unless functional problems are present. Forget about approaching a young child with a needle for a steroid injection in your office. This method will not work. Percutaneous needle releases have been described in older patients but have little place in the treatment of young children, in whom surgical division of the A_1 pulley is indicated.

34. What is the worst complication of a trigger release?

The radial digital nerve to the thumb is easily severed with blind cutting in a proximal direction.

35. What conditions should be considered in a child born with gross enlargement of a digit?

Macrodactyly (Greek: *makros* = large, *dactylos* = digit) and **gigantism** have been used to describe enlarged digits and thumbs. Gigantism is preferred by some because it encompasses enlargement of both soft tissues and skeletal elements. The clinician should consider:

1. Neurofibromatosis (NF)
2. Nerve territory-oriented lipofibromatosis not associated with NF
3. Multiple hereditary exostosis
4. Proteus syndrome with hyperostotic lesions and overgrowth of phalanges
5. Vascular malformations, particularly venous, lymphatic, and mixed venous-lymphatic
6. Hemihypertrophy of the limb

These unusual conditions should be referred to the pediatric hand specialist.

36. What is the work-up for macrodactyly?

These conditions are rare. Common sense dictates that the clinician obtain radiographs, complete a thorough physical examination, and then hit the books. NF is suspected on clinical examination and has specific criteria. Biopsies are rarely necessary. Genetic analysis is available. Vascular anomalies are distinguished by MRI. Bone tumors often require biopsy. Hemihypertrophy is the most difficult and is often a diagnosis by exclusion. In this condition there is a high incidence of adrenal masses, which must be detected by ultrasound. No one other than the pediatric hand specialist has a detailed working knowledge of all of these conditions. It is helpful to contact someone locally or nationally with experience in treatment of each particular condition.

37. What is the difference between hemangioma and vascular malformation?

During the past 10 years knowledge has increased exponentially. Mulliken made the most significant contribution with his classification, which makes a clearcut distinction between the two on biologic grounds. **Hemangiomas** are vascular birthmarks that appear shortly after birth, undergo a period of rapid growth and proliferation, and spontaneously involute by age 7–9 years. The endothelial cells actively proliferate and create new vascular channels during the growth phase. The mechanism for involution is unknown. **Vascular malformations** are biologically quiescent lesions. They result from defective embryogenesis, are present at birth or recognized shortly after birth, and do not undergo a biphasic growth cycle like hemangiomas. The endothelial cells do not actively proliferate. Malformations are subgrouped according to cell types into capillary, venous, lymphatic, mixed venous-lymphatic, and arterial malformations. Arterial malformations include arteriovenous fistulas (AVFs) with active shunting between the arterial and venous sides of the circulation.

38. Outline the five types of hypoplastic thumbs.

Type 1: hypoplastic thumb with all joints present; median nerve-innervated intrinsic muscles present but hypoplastic; joints stable; function normal.

Type 2: thumb skeleton more hypoplastic; joints intact with some collateral ligament instability at the MP level; greater hypoplasia of median nerve-innervated intrinsic muscles; first web space often deficient.

Type 3: thumb phalanges present but much smaller; increased collateral ligament instability at the MP level; thenar intrinsic muscles small and weak; ulnar intrinsic muscles hypoplastic; extrinsic muscles hypoplastic; first web space very tight. **Type 3A:** metacarpal intact but small; intact CMC joint. **Type 3B:** metacarpal incomplete; no CMC joint.

Type 4: thumb and all of its components highly deficient; no skeletal connection to the rest of the hand; skin bridge only, constituting a floating thumb or "pouce floutant."

Type 5: aplasia.

39. What are the possible options for reconstruction of type 3B thumbs?

The options are (1) staged osteoplastic reconstruction and (2) excision of the thumb and index pollicization. The second option is preferred by most pediatric hand specialists. Staged reconstruction involves (1) provision of skeletal continuity with a standard bone graft or a microvascular second toe transfer, (2) creation of an adequate web space, and (3) tendon transfers to provide palmar abduction of the first ray as well as MP and IP flexion and extension.

40. What are the long-term functional limitations of a well-performed pollicization procedure?

Such thumbs are never normal. Grip and pinch maneuvers involving the thumb are always deficient. Results fall into two basic groups: (1) complete or partial radius deficiency and (2) normal radius and preoperative range of motion. The second group has predictably better outcomes because extrinsic flexor and extensor muscles as well as intrinsic muscles to the index ray are normal. A stiff index finger preoperatively will become a very stiff thumb.

41. Describe the hand in patients with Apert syndrome.

Apert syndrome (acrocephalosyndactyly) is common only in craniofacial clinics. It occurs in more than 1 of 45,000 live births. Both hands have anantiomorphic (mirror image) deformities:

- Short radially deviated thumb (radial clinodactyly)
- Deficient first web space
- Complete, complex syndactyly involving the central three rays
- Simple, complete syndactyly between the ring and fifth rays

Three specific types of hand configurations have been described with varying degrees of severity. Additional skeletal anomalies include carpal coalitions, a ring-fifth metacarpal synostosis, symphalangism between the proximal and middle phalanges, and varying degrees of conjoined nails. The hands are subclassified into three separate groups depending on the severity of skeletal coalition.

42. What is Poland syndrome?

In 1849 Alfred Poland, a student dissector in gross anatomy, described a cadaver with chest wall anomalies associated with a hypoplastic webbed hand. The illustration made by a friend did not include the hand, but the head, neck, and thorax were depicted in detail. A century after this description appeared in the Guy's Hospital Reports, Clarkson, the hospital hand surgeon, found the hand that had been preserved in the hospital museum, redescribed the condition, and introduced the term Poland syndrome. The hand surgeon's definition includes (1) absence of the sternal head of the pectoralis major muscle (the clavicular head is usually present), (2) hypoplastic hand, and (3) brachysyndactyly (short, webbed fingers). We have further described the hand anomalies as affecting primarily the central three rays of the hand. The four variations of severity range from least affected (hypoplastic but present index, long, and ring digits) to the hand with no digits or thumb.

43. How is the chest wall reconstructed in children with Poland syndrome?

Nothing is usually done in children. In adolescents conspicuous deformities can be reconstructed with correction of the pectus carinatum (pigeon breast) or pectus excavatum (caved-in chest) deformities, followed by a latissimus dorsi muscle transfer to recreate the missing pectoralis major muscle.

44. What is the most persistent request of girls with Poland syndrome?

Girls request breast reconstruction, which is different from a simple augmentation or reconstruction after mastectomy. Expansion and overexpansion must be completed before final implant placement because the integument, including the areola, is often highly deficient. Subpectoral implants are preferred, but this muscle is either deficient or absent. Latissimus transfer with submuscular implants is then performed. It is wise to wait until adulthood before doing a transverse rectus abdominis muscle (TRAM) or free tissue transfer reconstruction.

45. A child is born with impending gangrene of portions of one or both forearms. What condition does the child have? What type of work-up is indicated?

This rare and often catastrophic condition, called **cutis aplasia congenita**, probably results from mechanical impingement or pressure on the upper limbs. Usually the forearms are caught between the head or trunk and the pelvic brim. The condition is often associated with multiple births. Mothers often give a history of lack of movement for one or more days before delivery. Routine work-up, including blood tests and radiographs, is normal. This condition can be viewed as an in utero Volkman's contracture.

46. What is Holt-Oram syndrome?

In the late 1950s two pediatricians, working independently in the United States and England, described the association between congenital *hand anomalies* and *congenital heart defects*. The cardiac anomalies vary greatly, but the hand malformations consist primarily of some form of radial dysplasia. If a surgeon has the opportunity to examine a large number of infants with congenital heart defects, he or she will find many cases of minimal radial dysplasias, such as hypoplastic thenar intrinsic muscles. Children with radial club hand or thumb hypoplasia or absence are not difficult to diagnose.

47. What single operation is most beneficial for patients with a congenital hand anomaly?

Release of the first (thumb-index) web space. For mild-to-moderate deficiencies we prefer the four-flap Z-plasty and for tight, constricted web spaces the distally based radial forearm flap or dorsal interosseous flap. Dorsal sliding flaps are not preferred because of the unsightly, hyperpigmented skin grafts in the donor region. However, they are popular in both orthopedic and plastic surgical literature because of the mobility of the dorsal skin and the technical ease of the procedure.

48. Describe the hand in a child with Freeman-Sheldon syndrome.

The "whistling face" syndrome presents with characteristic hand and facial anomalies. The hands are often narrow with prominent ulnar drift. Incomplete, simple syndactyly and varying degrees of PIP camptodactyly are often present. The first web space is usually tight. The descriptive term "windblown hand" is often applied. Many other musculoskeletal anomalies, such as scoliosis, hip dysplasia, and radial head dislocation, may be present. These children are not retarded mentally.

49. A child presents with a swollen hand and forearm and an associated neck mass diagnosed as a "cystic hygroma." What is the underlying pathophysiology?

Cystic hygroma describes a lymphatic malformation in the head and neck region. The upper limb as well as mediastinum also may be involved. In the hand and forearm the interconnecting lymphatic channels may be much smaller. The size of the limb may be quite large, grotesque on occasion. Besides the symptoms related to bulk and increased weight, many children develop high fevers related to episodic beta streptococcal infections, which usually originate in the cutaneous vesicles often found in lymphatic lesions. Skeletal enlargement may be present but is not a hallmark of these macrodactylies, which are difficult to treat. Staged aggressive debulking is the treatment of choice once conservative measures and compression garments have failed.

50. What is the difference between a typical and atypical cleft hand?

They are completely different. A **typical cleft** hand has the following characteristics: bilaterality, positive inheritance, foot involvement, V-shaped cleft, and syndactyly (common). A portion or all of the middle ray is commonly missing. It is often called simply a cleft hand. The **atypical cleft** refers to a unilateral anomaly that is nonfamilial and has a U-shaped cleft with no foot involvement. Small nubbins often represent rudimentary digits. This condition often has been called "lobster claw hand." After much discussion at various international meetings, the committees for the study of congenital anomalies of the hand recommend that "atypical cleft hand" be officially classified as symbrachydactyly.

51. Describe the upper limb in a child with severe arthrogryposis multiplex congenita.

Arthrogryposis, a syndrome of unknown etiology, is always present at birth and manifests with persistent joint contractures. It is classified into **myopathic** and **neurogenic** forms. The bottom line is that the muscles do not function. The upper limb appearance is unmistakable. The shoulders are thin and held in adduction and internal rotation. The elbows are extended, and the forearms are usually held in a semiflexed pronated position. Some elbow passive range of motion may be present. In severe cases the wrist is held in flexion and ulnar deviation, and the thumb is tightly adducted into the palm. The digits are flexed and ulnarly deviated at the MP joints. The skin may be atrophied and waxy. Skin dimples dorsally and flexion creases on the palmar surfaces signify mobile joint spaces. The lower extremities are more frequently involved than the upper.

BIBLIOGRAPHY

1. Dobyns JH, Wood VE, Bayne LG: Congenital. In Green DP (ed): Operative Hand Surgery, vol. 1, 3rd ed. New York, Churchill Livingstone, 1993, pp 251–549.
2. Flatt AE: The Care of Congenital Hand Anomalies. St. Louis, Quality Medical Publishing, 1994.
3. Lister G: Congenital. In Lister G (ed): The Hand, 3rd ed. New York, Churchill Livingstone, 1993, pp 459–512.
4. Mulliken JB, Young AE: Vascular Birthmarks: Hemangiomas and Malformations. Philadelphia, W.B. Saunders, 1988.
5. Upton J: Congenital anomalies of the hand and forearm. In McCarthy JG, May J, Littler JW (eds): Plastic Surgery, vol. 8. Philadelphia, W.B. Saunders, 1990, pp 5213–5398.

108. DUPUYTREN'S DISEASE

Robert M. McFarlane, M.D., F.R.C.S.(C), and Douglas C. Ross, M.D., F.R.C.S.(C)

1. What is the cause of Dupuytren's disease (DD)?

DD is a familial disease and until recently was considered to be a genetic disease due to a single dominant gene of variable penetrance. The cause is probably multifactorial, involving more than one gene as well as environmental factors.

2. What diseases are associated with DD?

1. **Diabetes mellitus.** About 5% of people with DD are diabetic (type I or II). The frequency of DD in diabetic patients increases with age and duration of diabetes. For instance, at 20 years' duration, 67% of diabetic patients have DD, although the disease is mild and rarely requires treatment. Patients also have a type of finger joint contracture called limited joint mobility, which prevents them from fully extending the fingers. The explanation for the association between DD and diabetes is unknown.

2. **Seizure disorders.** The incidence of epilepsy is 1.5% in the general population and 3.0% in people with DD. There are two conflicting explanations: (1) genetic linkage and (2) the theory that DD is caused by long-term barbiturate medication.

3. **Chronic alcoholism.** The prevalence of DD varies, but severe alcoholics often have severe DD. Despite frequent statements to the contrary, DD is not due to liver disease. The association is related to the volume of alcohol consumed and the age of the patient. There also may be a genetic predisposition.

3. Is DD related to work or injury?

Despite many attempts to answer this question, no study is conclusive. Patients often attribute their disease to some work pattern, whether they are manual or sedentary workers. Some studies report an increase of DD in heavy manual workers, whereas several others have found no greater incidence. Recent reports suggest an association with vibration injury, but the figures are not significant. The association of DD with acute injury is a separate problem. Several reports, most of which are anecdotal and involve one or two cases, relate the onset of DD to a fracture, penetrating wound, or laceration of the hand. The suggested causes are swelling and immobilization in a genetically predisposed person.

4. What are the risk factors for developing DD?

Because DD is a familial disease, the chance that a child will develop DD depends on the clinical features possessed by the parent, which were described by Hueston as "diathesis factors." The presence of one or more of these factors increases the chance that other members of the family may develop DD:

1. Positive history in first- or second-degree relative
2. Presence of ectopic deposits—Dupuytren's tissue that appears beyond the palmar surface of the hand. The usual sites are knuckle pads over the dorsum of the PIP joints, plantar fibromatosis, and penile fibromatosis (Peyronie's disease).
3. Early age of onset of disease (before 40 years)
4. Presence of severe bilateral disease, especially involving the radial side of the hand

The examiner should determine the presence or absence of each factor in every patient. Diathesis factors are not only of prognostic value; they are also essential in planning treatment.

5. Does the diseased tissue exhibit specific patterns?

Yes. The diseased fascia is not laid down haphazardly but in certain components of the normal palmar fascia:

1. The pretendinous bands of the palmar aponeurosis become the pretendinous cords (normal fascia is bandlike, whereas diseased fascia is cordlike).
2. The natatory ligament becomes the natatory cord.
3. The termination of the transverse fibers of the palmar aponeurosis attach to the skin at the metaphalangeal (MP) joint of the thumb. In the fingers, the subcutaneous tissue between the neurovascular bundles becomes the central cord; the spiral, lateral, and retrovascular bands also become cords.

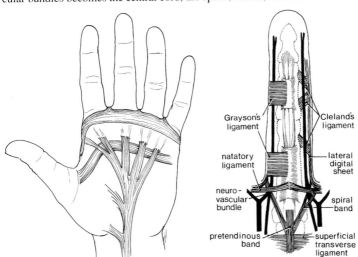

Grayson's ligament
Cleland's ligament
natatory ligament
lateral digital sheet
neuro-vascular bundle
spiral band
pretendinous band
superficial transverse ligament

The normal parts of the palmar (*left*) and digital (*right*) fascia that become diseased.

6. Which fascia causes the various flexion contractures in the hand?

1. MP joint contracture is caused only by the pretendinous cord, which attaches to the skin and tendon sheath distal to the MP joint.

2. The proximal interphalangeal (PIP) joint is contracted most often by the central cord, followed, in descending order, by the spiral cord and lateral cord. All three cords attach to the base of the middle phalanx and may be involved alone or together.

3. Contracture of the distal interphalangeal (DIP) joint is uncommon. It is caused by the retrovascular and, to some extent, the lateral cord because both cords attach to the distal phalanx.

4. The natatory cord contracts the web space from side to side and prevents the fingers from separating.

5. The MP joint of the thumb is contracted by the pretendinous cord but usually by no more than 30° because the cord is not well developed. The disabling deformity of the thumb is an adduction contracture caused by the natatory cord and termination of the transverse fibers of the palmar aponeurosis.

7. By what mechanism is the neurovascular bundle displaced?

An understanding of the mechanism is important to avoid digital nerve injury during surgery. The spiral cord passes deep to the neurovascular bundle to reach the side of the finger. It then passes superficial to the bundle to reach the base of the middle phalanx, where it attaches. In other words, it spirals around the neurovascular bundle. As the spiral cord shortens, the bundle is drawn toward the midline of the finger, where it may be cut inadvertently.

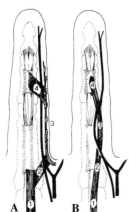

The components of the spiral cord *(A)* and the mechanism by which the neurovascular bundle is displaced toward the midline of the finger *(B)*. 1 - pretendinous band, 2 = spiral band, 3 = lateral digital sheet, 4 = Grayson's ligament.

8. To which group of diseases does DD belong? How are they classified?

DD is one of the fibromatoses, a group of nonmetastasizing tumors that tend to invade locally and to recur after surgical excision. According to Allen (1977) and Enziger and Weiss (1983), they are classified as follows:

Infantile—11 types
Adult

I. Superficial (fascial): Dupuytren's disease
   1. Palmar fibromatosis
   2. Knuckle pads
   3. Plantar fibromatosis
   4. Penile fibromatosis

II. Deep (musculoaponeurotic): desmoid tumors
   1. Extraabdominal
   2. Abdominal
   3. Intraabdominal: pelvic, mesenteric, Gardner's syndrome

9. What are the histologic features of the nodules of DD?

The clinically apparent nodule is composed of a number of smaller nodules that are nonencapsulated but surrounded by connective tissue and collagen bundles. The predominant cell is the fibroblast. Early in the disease the cells are spindle-shaped perivascular fibroblasts. Later, when contracture is apparent, the cells are more closely packed and collagen production is evident. Ultrastructurally, the predominant cell is the myofibroblast, which contains myofibrils (actomyosin) in the cytoplasm; cell-to-cell attachments are also apparent. The nuclei have deep indentations that indicate contracture. Special stains show many new blood vessels. In the late stages of the disease, the nodules disappear, and the few cells in the cords are inactive fibroblasts or fibrocytes.

10. What is the role of the myofibroblast?

Because of its electronmicroscopic appearance, contractile properties in tissue culture, and the presence of alpha-smooth muscle actin in the cytoplasm, the myofibroblast is assumed to have a contractile function as well as the ability to produce collagen. As new collagen is produced, the tissue is shortened by action of the myofibroblast. The result is joint contracture.

11. What is different about the collagen of normal fascia and Dupuytren's tissue?

Almost all of the collagen in normal fascia is type 1, whereas about 25% of the collagen in Dupuytren's specimens is type 3.

12. Where are nodules usually located?

Nodules are usually just distal or just proximal to the distal crease of the palm, in line with the ring and/or small finger. They also appear at the base of the small finger and the MP crease of the thumb. However, they may occur anywhere on the volar surface of the palm or digits.

13. What clinical features and other conditions should be considered in the differential diagnosis of DD?

The location of the nodule is almost diagnostic. It is firm and adherent to skin. It does not move with finger flexion or extension, and the skin over the proximal segment of the finger will blanch on hyperextension of the MP joint. Examine the other hand for nodules, the dorsum of the fingers for knuckle pads, and the feet for plantar nodules. All of these findings are signs of DD.

Other lumps should be easily differentiated. A **ganglion** at the base of the finger is small, spherical, mobile, and tender to palpation. An **inclusion cyst** or **benign tumor** is mobile and not adherent to the skin. **Epithelioid sarcoma** is a rare condition that mimics the nodule of DD. If the diagnosis is in doubt, a biopsy is indicated after further consultation. PIP joint contractures are commonly misdiagnosed as DD. **Camptodactyly** is usually noted by the age of 12 years in one or both small fingers. No nodules or cords are present, although the skin on the ulnar side of the proximal segment of the finger becomes tight with PIP extension. The PIP joint contracture may be fixed or passively correctable. In some cases of **trigger finger**, the patient cannot correct the PIP joint flexion. Prior triggering and pain should rule out DD. Other flexion contractures that can be differentiated by the absence of nodules are the lack of PIP joint extension often seen in diabetic patients, called **limited joint mobility**, and contractures due to **trauma** or **arthritis**. **Finger contractures in the elderly** simulate DD. All fingers are involved and flexed at both MP and PIP joints. The flexor tendons in the palm are prominent, and the contractures are not correctable. Finally, nodular thickening in the palm is a feature of **reflex sympathetic dystrophy**. The nodules are neither as discrete nor as large as DD nodules, but they are often diagnosed as DD. Histologically they are fibrosis rather than fibromatosis.

14. Is there a role for nonoperative treatment?

Yes, but at present it is limited. The only modality that has persisted over the years is steroid injections into the nodule. Ketchum believes that repeated injections will relieve pain and delay or sometimes stop the progress of the disease. He also advocates steroid injections for painful knuckle pads and plantar nodules. To date, attempts to weaken or disrupt contracted cords with collagenolytic agents, various drugs, stretching, ultrasound, and x-rays have not been successful. Future efforts are likely to include interferon and substances that affect growth factors.

15. What are the indications for operative treatment?

There are no absolute or urgent indications for surgery, but 30° of flexion contraction at the MP or PIP joint is a nuisance and indicates the extent of disease and the likelihood of progression. Many patients are seen soon after they notice a nodule in the palm, because it is painful or they are concerned that it may be malignant. An explanation of the nature of DD usually allays their concern. If the pain persists, one or two steroid injections may help. Excision of a nodule is not satisfactory because the thickening of the fascia and the scarring of the operation may worsen the condition. If it is necessary to excise a nodule for diagnosis or pain, a generous excision of the surrounding fascia is advised.

16. What are the goals of surgery?

The goals are different at each joint. At the MP joint the surgeon should be able to completely correct the contracture regardless of its severity and assure the patient that the contracture will not recur. At the PIP joint the surgeon should forewarn the patient that joint contracture may not be fully corrected. The residual contracture may be as much as 40°, depending on the severity of the original contracture. There is also the likelihood that the residual contracture will worsen.

17. What are the options in designing an operation for DD?

By considering the three following steps separately, the operation can be individualized:

1. **Skin incision.** Exposure may be longitudinal (linear, zig-zag, lazy S) or transverse. If a single ray is involved, a longitudinal incision from the proximal palm to beyond the diseased fascia in the finger permits exposure of both the fascia and the neurovascular bundles. If the disease is more widespread in the palm, a transverse incision provides good exposure. Separate longitudinal incisions may be made in the involved fingers to join the palmar incision if necessary.

2. **Management of the diseased fascia.** The diseased fascia may be incised (fasciotomy) or excised locally or widely (regional or extensive fasciectomy). Subcutaneous or open fasciotomy has been advocated for old and debilitated patients, but it is an incomplete operation that either fails to correct the contracture or results in temporary improvement. A more definitive operation is a regional fasciectomy in which only the diseased fascia is removed. It is the usual procedure in the palm to correct MP joint contracture. However, because as many as four cords may be involved in a PIP joint contracture, a more extensive operation is often required in the finger. The diseased as well as the potentially diseased tissue is excised by extensive fasciectomy.

3. **Treatment of the wound.** The wound may be sutured, left open, or skin-grafted. Usually the wound is closed in both palm and finger procedures. In the finger, longitudinal incisions are lengthened and appropriately oriented by the use of Z-plasty. Closure of a transverse wound in the palm creates a dead space where the fascia was excised, and a hematoma is likely. A hematoma can be avoided to some extent by suction drainage, but a more reliable method is to leave the wound open and let it heal by second intention (McCash technique). Healing requires 4–6 weeks, depending on the width of the wound. This procedure is contrary to surgical principles, but it is a justifiable exception.

18. What is the rationale for using skin grafts? What are the indications?

Hueston made the empirical observation that Dupuytren's tissue does not grow under a full-thickness skin graft. Therefore, full-thickness skin grafts are recommended for patients in whom recurrence is likely, including (1) patients with an increased diathesis, (2) patients with recurrent PIP joint contracture, and (3) patients with primary, severe PIP joint contracture. The procedure is called a dermofasciectomy. The diseased fascia is excised, after which areas of skin are excised, usually near the PIP joint, and the defects are covered by full-thickness skin grafts.

19. What is the difference between extension and recurrence?

Extension refers to postoperative appearance of disease in an area of the hand not involved in the surgery. Recurrence refers to the postoperative appearance of disease in the area of previous surgery. If follow-up is long enough (10–20 years), virtually all patients have one or both. However, no more than 10–15% will have enough joint contracture to justify reoperation.

20. What are the complications of surgery?

1. During surgery, division of digital arteries and nerves and inadequate excision of fascia are often due to poor planning of incisions, inadequate hemostasis, and failure to use magnification.

2. Hematoma, skin necrosis, and infection usually occur in sequence and are due to inappropriate undermining of skin and lack of hemostasis.

3. Joint stiffness is due primarily to the above complications and is worsened by inappropriate splinting and therapy.

4. Reflex sympathetic dystrophy is usually idiopathic, but statistically it occurs more frequently after an extensive operation or after one of the above complications. It occurs after 3% of operations in men and 7% of operations in women.

5. Uncorrected or early recurrent joint contracture (seen more frequently at the PIP joint) is due to inadequate fascial excision.

21. How are patients managed postoperatively?

The affected fingers are usually splinted in extension in the operating room. The surgeon is responsible for wound care, but ideally a therapist should see the patient within the first week to begin exercises and to fashion an appropriate splint. Splinting techniques vary, depending on whether surgical release involved the MP or PIP joint or whether an open palm technique was used. MP joint contractures do not require splinting if full extension is maintained with therapy alone. However, with an open palm procedure, the MP joint should be splinted in extension until the wound is closed. PIP joints require 6 weeks of full-time splinting and at least 3 months of nighttime splinting to prevent flexion contractures secondary to scar tissue.

BIBLIOGRAPHY

1. Baird KS, Alwin WH, Crossan JF, Wojciak B: T-cell mediated response in Dupuytren's disease. Lancet 341:1622–1623, 1993.
2. Berger A, Delbruck A, Brenner P, Hinzmann R (eds): Dupuytren's Disease: Pathobiochemistry and Clinical Management. New York, Springer-Verlag, 1994.
2a. Burge P, Hoy G, Regan P, Milne R: Smoking, alcohol, and the risk of Dupuytren's contracture. J Bone Joint Surg 79B(2):206–210, 1997.
3. Chiu HF, McFarlane RM: Pathogenesis of Dupuytren's contracture: A correlative clinical-pathological study. J Hand Surg 3:1–10, 1978.
4. Darby I, Skalli O, Gabbiani G: Alpha-smooth muscle actin is transiently expressed by myofibroblasts during experimental wound healing. Lab Invest 63:21–29, 1990.
5. Gabbiani G, Majno G: Dupuytren's contracture: Fibroblast contraction? An ultrastructural study. Am J Pathol 66:131–146, 1972.
6. Hueston JT: Dermofasciectomy for Dupuytren's disease. Bull Hosp Joint Dis 44:224–232, 1984.
7. McCash CR: The open palm technique in Dupuytren's contracture. Br J Plast Surg 17:271–280, 1964.
8. McFarlane RM: Dupuytren's disease. In Georgiade GS, Riefkohl R, Levin LS (eds): Plastic, Maxillofacial and Reconstructive Surgery. Baltimore, Williams & Wilkins, 1996, pp 1038–1045.
9. McFarlane RM: Patterns of the diseased fascia in the fingers in Dupuytren's contracture. Plast Reconstr Surg 54:31–44, 1974.
10. McFarlane RM, McGrouther DA, Flint MH (eds): Dupuytren's Disease. New York, Churchill Livingstone, 1990.
11. Wurster-Hill DH, Brown F, Park JP, Gibson SH: Cytogenetic studies in Dupuytren's contracture. Am J Hum Genet 43:285–292, 1988.

109. STENOSING TENOSYNOVITIS

Richard J. Wassermann, M.D., M.P.H., and Daniel P. Greenwald, M.D.

1. Describe the two basic categories of tenosynovitis.

The nonspecific inflammatory group is most closely associated with overuse or repetitive trauma syndromes and contains the subset of stenosing tenosynovitis. The second major category has an infectious etiology and may be suppurative or nonsuppurative.

2. The dominant hand is more commonly involved in flexor and extensor tenosynovitis. True or false?

True. The dominant hand is more commonly involved in cases of tenosynovitis, giving credence to the overuse/repetitive trauma theory of etiology. Tenosynovitis affects females more than males, which may highlight hormonal and anatomic differences as well as the arthritides as causes.

3. What conditions or physiologic states are associated with stenosing tenosynovitis?

Rheumatoid arthritis, osteoarthritis, pregnancy, diabetes, hypothyroidism, end-stage renal disease.

4. Trigger digits in adults are most commonly a result of what condition?

A nonspecific process resulting in the proliferation of flexor tenosynovium, which restricts entry to the fibroosseous canal at the level of the A_1 pulley.

5. What other causes should be considered in the differential diagnosis of digital triggering?

Foreign body, ganglion of the tendon sheath (sesamoid ganglion), fibromas, giant cell tumors of the tendon sheath, onchronotic pigment, chondrometaplasia, true locking of the metacarpophalangeal joint, de Quervain's tenosynovitis, flexor tendon restriction at the second anular pulley (A_2), and partial flexor tendon laceration.

6. What are the options for treatment of stenosing flexor tenosynovitis?

Although the injection of aqueous steroid into the tendon sheath at the level of the A_1 pulley remains the mainstay of initial treatment, percutaneous release in the office has yielded excellent long-term results. Patel et al. studied 225 percutaneous releases with and without steroid injection. They reported relief of triggering and pain in an average of 8 weeks for 89% of the group treated with percutaneous release alone, and 96% of patients were symptom-free in an average of 6 weeks in the percutaneous release and steroid group. Turowski et al. demonstrated a 97% cure rate for operative release and reported no major complications. They recommend the open approach for patients seeking quick and definitive relief. Only open surgical release is recommended for treatment of the congenital trigger digit.

7. What is the common presentation of congenital flexor tenosynovitis?

A painless digit flexed in a fixed position in an infant or child constitutes the most common clinical scenario. Most patients present after 6 months of age. The thumb is most commonly involved, and approximately 25% of cases are bilateral. Females are more frequently affected than males. Most cases are sporadic and nonfamilial, although several cases have been observed in twins. Abnormal sesamoid bones and inherent tendon abnormalities have been suggested as causative factors. The powerful grasping reflex and the tendency for infants to hyperflex the thumb interphalangeal joint also may be contributing factors.

8. In patients with constant triggering on active range of motion of the middle finger, how do you grade the severity of stenosing tenosynovitis in the digits? How do you calculate total hand, upper extremity, and total person impairment?

Stenosing tenosynovitis is graded as mild, moderate, or severe. The following table correlates the clinical findings with percent of digit impairment.

Grade	Clinical Findings	% Digital Impairment
Mild	Inconstant triggering on active range of motion	20
Moderate	Constant triggering on active range of motion	40
Severe	Constant triggering on passive range of motion	60

Adapted from Swanson AB, Mays JD, Yamauci Y: A rheumatoid evaluation record for the upper extremity. Surg Clin North Am 48:1003–1013, 1968.

This value is then multiplied by the contribution of each from the following table.

Units and Joints	Unit	% Impairment		
		Hand	Upper Extremity	Whole Person
Entire hand		100	90	54
Thumb	100	40	36	22
Carpometacarpal joint	75	30	27	16
Metaphalangeal joint	10	4	4	2
Interphalangeal joint	15	6	5	3
Index and middle fingers				
Entire digit	100	20	18	11
Metaphalangeal joint	100	20	18	11
Proximal interphalangeal joint	80	16	14	8
Distal interphalangeal joint	45	9	8	5
Ring and little fingers				
Entire digit	100	10	9	5
Metaphalangeal joint	100	10	9	5
Proximal interphalangeal joint	80	8	7	4
Distal interphalangeal joint	45	4	4	2

Adapted from Swanson AB, deGroot Swanson G: Principles and methods of impairment evaluation of the hand and upper extremity. In Guides to the Evaluation of Permanent Impairment, 4th ed. Chicago, American Medical Association, 1994.

The calculation is performed as follows: $0.4 \times 11 = 4.4\%$ whole body impairment, $0.4 \times 18 = 7.2\%$ upper extremity impairment, and $0.4 \times 20 = 5\%$ hand impairment. This disability falls under the musculotendinous category of impairments. It is the physician's responsibility to provide a medical evaluation of impairment, not a rating of disability.

9. How can tenosynovitis of the first dorsal compartment, also known as de Quervain's disease, be distinguished from arthritis of the first carpometacarpal (CMC) joint?
Physical examination reveals a positive grind test, abduction test, and adduction test in the case of CMC arthritis compared with localized tenderness over the first dorsal compartment and a positive Finkelstein's test in the case of de Quervain's disease. Radiographic examination reveals destruction of the articular surface of the first CMC joint and possible subluxation in the case of CMC arthritis; patients with de Quervain's disease usually have normal radiographs.

10. Can CMC arthritis and de Quervain's disease coexist?
Yes. They are two separate entities that have the same high incidence in middle-aged women.

11. Normal radiographs usually exclude a diagnosis of CMC arthritis. What other diagnoses can be excluded by normal radiographic examination?
Scaphoid fracture, radiocarpal arthritis, and intercarpal arthritis.

12. Name the contents of the six synovial lined compartments that course beneath the dorsal carpal ligament.

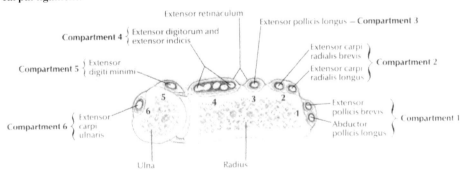

Compartments beneath the dorsal carpal ligament. (From Netter FH: Atlas of Human Anatomy. Ciba Pharmaceuticals Division, Ciba-Geigy Corporation, 1989, with permission.)

13. The first dorsal compartment is composed of a single sheath containing two tendons and demonstrates minimal anatomic variation. True or false?
False. The first dorsal compartment is the site of numerous variations in tendon structure and organization. In 20–30% of reported cases, the compartment is divided into two tunnels, one ulnar for the extensor pollicis brevis (EPB) and one more radial for one or more slips of the abductor pollicis longus (APL). A third deep tunnel containing an anomalous tendon has also been reported. The EPB is absent in 5–7% of the population. Inadequate identification and release of all slips of the APL is a common cause for failed operative management. Failure to identify and release the separate tunnel of the EPB, when present, also results in unsuccessful treatment.

14. During operative release of first dorsal compartment, how can the separate tendon of the EPB be specifically identified?
Passive extension of the thumb metaphalangeal (MP) joint isolates the EPB tendon.

15. What is intersection syndrome? How can it be differentiated from first dorsal compartment tenosynovitis?
The basic pathology is a nonspecific tenosynovitis of the second dorsal compartment. It is frequently associated with repetitive trauma at the wrist. It was previously thought to result from friction between the APL and EPB muscle bellies and those of the second the dorsal compartment. Physical

examination reveals tenderness, swelling, and, in severe cases, crepitus 4 cm proximal to the wrist joint where the two compartments cross.

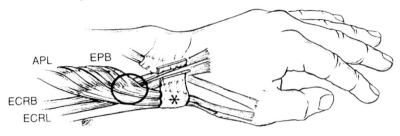

The circled area shows where the extensor pollicis brevis (EPB) and abductor pollicis longus (APL) cross the common radial wrist extensors. The location of the first dorsal compartment where de Quervain's disease occurs is indicated with a star. The second dorsal compartment has been released in the manner recommended for treatment of intersection syndrome. ECRB = extensor carpi radialis brevis; ECRL = extensor carpi radialis longus. (From Froimson AI: Tenosynovitis and tennis elbow. In Green DP (ed): Operative Surgery of the Hand. New York, Churchill Livingstone, 1993, p 1193, with permission.)

16. Tenderness, swelling, and crepitus at the level of Lister's tubercle on physical examination lead to a diagnosis of which less common tenosynovitis that requires early operative treatment?

Tenosynovitis of the third dorsal compartment often leads to rupture of the extensor pollicis longus tendon. The tenosynovitis may be caused by a distal radius fracture (despite anatomic reduction), rheumatoid disease, and, rarely, overuse (the classic drummer boy palsy).

17. List the other common examples of stenosing tenosynovitis. How are they treated?

Stenosing tenosynovitis also may involve the following tendons: flexor carpi radialis, extensor carpi ulnaris, extensor indicis proprius, and extensor digiti minimi. The mainstays of treatment are injection of water-soluble steroid, nonsteroidal antiinflammatory drugs, rest, and splinting.

BIBLIOGRAPHY

1. Froimson AF: Tenosynovitis and tennis elbow. In Green DP (ed): Operative Hand Surgery. New York, Churchill Livingstone, 1993, pp 1989–2000.
2. Patel MR, Moradia VJ: Percutaneous release of trigger digit with and without cortisone injection. J Hand Surg 22A:150–155, 1997.
3. Savage RC: Tenosynovial disorders of the hand and wrist. In McCarthy JG (ed): Plastic Surgery. Philadelphia, W.B. Saunders, 1990, pp 4725–4742.
4. Steenwercky A, De Smet L, Fabry G: Congenital trigger digit. J Hand Surg 21A:909–911, 1996.
5. Swanson AB, de Groot Swanson G, Goran-Hagert C: Evaluation of impairment of hand function. In Hunter JN, Schnieder LH, Mackin EJ (eds): Tendon and Nerve Surgery in the Hand. St. Louis, Mosby, 1997, pp 617–670.
6. Turowski GA, Zdankiewicz PD, Thomson JG: The results of surgical treatment of trigger finger. J Hand Surg 22A:145–149, 1997.

110. TUMORS

Earl J. Fleegler, M.D.

1. What is a tumor?

Although tumor means "swelling," the word usually refers to a new growth or proliferation of cells at an increased rate, possibly with other abnormalities in relation to the surrounding normal cells.

2. How do you evaluate a patient with a spontaneously developing ulnar claw hand without sensory defect?

A careful history may yield information about underlying neurologic disease, trauma, or a previous malignancy, such as lymphoma. Malignant proliferation about the ulnar nerve (in this case, probably distal to the division into sensory motor branches in the hand) would explain the findings. If standard radiographic evaluation fails to help, MRI can define space-occupying lesions and identify occult ganglia or other conditions (e.g., atypical acid fast infections, lymphoma, or even a primary neoplasm).

3. Is the approach to an upper extremity mass different from the approach to a mass elsewhere?

No. Masses in any anatomic location require careful evaluation. Because the nonneoplastic ganglion is the most common mass found in the hand and wrist, serious tumors are too often considered to be cysts. However, there are differences based on anatomy. Early tumors can hide within the complex anatomy of the hand. One must understand the local lymphatic anatomy, including the epitrochlear and axillary lymph node groups, to evaluate the tumors fully. Certain tumors, such as squamous cell carcinomas involving the perionychium, subungual melanoma, and epithelioid sarcoma, can be insidious. Often they are not associated with symptoms or signs in their early development. Melanomas and epithelioid sarcoma are especially dangerous.

4. All malignant tumors of the upper extremity are sarcomas. True or false?

False. In addition to malignant tumors of the musculoskeletal system (sarcomas), there are large numbers of benign and malignant neoplasms of all of the tissue of the upper extremity, including carcinomas (both epithelial and glandular in origin).

5. Are epithelioid sarcomas the most common malignant tumor of the upper extremity?

No. Overall, squamous cell carcinomas are probably the most common malignant tumors of the upper extremity.

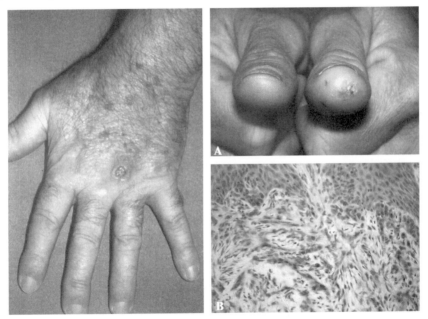

Left, Ulcerated mass on the dorsum of the hand of a middle-aged man. This lesion was a biopsy-proven squamous cell carcinoma. Note the surrounding actinic changes. *Right,* Epithelioid sarcoma. *A,* Enlargement and ulceration of the distal phalanx of the thumb, which was indurated on examination. *B,* Histology demonstrates an epithelioid pattern in association with spindle cells consistent with an epithelioid sarcoma.

6. Do even small masses in the hand require a preoperative MRI?

Use of expensive studies, such as MRI, requires careful consideration. The typical ganglion can be diagnosed clinically, especially when transillumination or aspiration is carried out. However, the physician can still be led to a misdiagnosis. The MRI is important in diagnosing occult masses deep within the hand. Masses that are not clearly benign cysts or other benign, nonaggressive lesions require diagnostic studies that provide information about their nature and extent. Sometimes this information can be obtained from less expensive studies, such as ultrasound evaluation. Early in their development, even serious malignancies are small masses.

7. List the most common causes of a lump in the hand.
Actinic keratoses, ganglion, giant cell tumor of the tendon sheath, inclusion cyst.

8. Of the following tumors of the upper extremity, which is least likely to metastasize via lymphatics: squamous cell carcinoma, basal cell carcinoma, epithelioid sarcoma, malignant fibrous histiocytoma, synovial sarcoma, rhabdomyosarcoma, or clear cell sarcoma?
Basal cell carcinoma. All of the other tumors certainly may metastasize via lymphatics, but it is extremely rare for basal cell carcinoma to do so.

9. Which of the tumors listed in question 8 is most likely to be encountered in children?
Rhabdomyosarcoma—the most common soft tissue sarcoma of childhood.

10. What association do the following have in common: epidermodysplasia verruciformis, human papilloma virus, osteomyelitic draining sinuses, excessive sun, radiation exposure, and immunosuppression?
Squamous cell carcinoma develops in association with all of these conditions.

11. After frozen section confirmation of adequate margins of excision around a malignant tumor specimen, what should the surgeon do next?
Attempt to eliminate tumor cell deposits from the site by copiously irrigating the site and changing everything that is contaminated by tumor cells and will come in contact with the area, including gloves, gowns, instruments, and drapes.

12. Is brown/black pigmentation of the eponychial fold diagnostic of melanoma?
Although not always diagnostic of melanoma, pigmentation of the eponychial fold—Hutchinson's sign—requires investigation to evaluate the possibility of melanoma.

13. What is the importance of Clark's levels and Breslow's measurements?
Both help to assess aggressiveness of the lesion, provide insight into treatment modalities, and are helpful in outcome studies.

14. How do you stage a patient with a malignant tumor?
Staging, according to the American Joint Committee, depends on tumor size and extension (T), lymph node involvement (N), metastasis (M), and grade of tumor (G). Enneking developed a similarly useful, somewhat simpler system. T is defined by whether the tumor is confined within an anatomic compartment (T_1) or extends through a compartment (T_2). G_1 refers to low-grade and G_2 to high-grade lesions. Enneking does not use nodal involvement as a separate classification, considering that nodal involvement is similar, with regard to outcome, to presence of metastatic disease (M). A stage I sarcoma corresponds to a low-grade sarcoma without metastatic disease. A high-grade lesion without metastasis is designated stage II; stage III indicates metastatic disease for either grade.

15. Who should biopsy a mass in the hand—the dermatologist, primary care physician, general surgeon, orthopedist, plastic surgeon, or hand surgeon?
The physician who is both qualified and prepared to carry out definitive surgery.

16. How do you evaluate a roughened, subungual mass?
If the lesion has typical characteristics of a wart and is treated with one of the modalities for warts (e.g., freezing) but recurs or persists, biopsy should be considered. Such lesions, especially in older patients, may represent a subungual squamous cell sarcoma. Radiographic evaluation of the area should be completed before biopsy.

17. What should you know about a patient presenting with a pigmented linear streak involving the nail area?
One should know whether the patient has a history of trauma producing a subungual hematoma, whether the patient is taking any medications that may predispose to pigmented lesions, and the race

of the patient. Benign pigmented streaks, especially in older patients, are not unusual in African-American patients. Whether the lesion started as a small line and increased in size may be of importance. However, considerable clinical judgment is required in this situation, and biopsy is frequently warranted.

18. What findings are suspicious in relation to a pigmented skin lesion?

Size greater than 6 mm, variation in color, change to an irregular margin, alteration of normal skin markings (such as obliteration of skin creases), and ulceration. Of course, certain melanomas (e.g., amelanotic) may not exhibit pigmentation.

19. During carpal tunnel release an unusual, moderately firm thickening is encountered within the synovial tissue. What is the approach to this finding?

Among other etiologies, one must consider neoplasia. Because the surgeon does not know the extent of the lesion (staging) or the diagnosis and does not have permission for definitive treatment, incisional biopsy is recommended. The operation is concluded after carpal tunnel release. Additional work-up is completed as necessary. If the lesion proves to be a serious neoplasm, appropriate additional work-up, consultations, and discussions with the patient are carried out before definitive treatment.

20. In preparation for biopsying a mass in the hand, do you exsanguinate the hand?

No. Stripping blood from the area of the tumor with the pressure of a tourniquet may increase the risk of tumor cells entering the lymphatics.

21. A 65-year-old man complains of a small ulcerated area on the dorsum of the hand. What is the differential diagnosis and approach?

A careful history is taken to assess a possible traumatic vs. infectious cause. Regional nodes should be assessed. A common cause of such lesions in a sun-exposed area is squamous cell carcinoma. After radiographic evaluation of the area as well as the chest, incisional biopsy can confirm the diagnosis and direct definitive treatment, which includes excision of the lesion with a histologically normal margin of tissue. In more advanced cases, regional lymph node dissection also may be required.

22. The patient described in question 21 is found to have a firm, slightly moveable ipsilateral axillary mass. What surgical treatment do you recommend?

With squamous cell carcinoma, once the remainder of the work-up is found to be negative, axillary lymphadenectomy is recommended along with treatment of the primary tumor.

23. What are the treatment options for a 14-year-old girl with a primary rhabdomyosarcoma of the hand and Enneking stage III involvement?

The patient should be treated in conjunction with an oncologist. Modalities of treatment include control of the primary tumor site by surgery or irradiation as well as systemic chemotherapy.

24. What treatment options would you recommend for a 50-year-old man with an Enneking stage IIb synovial sarcoma of the antecubital area?

Staging studies, including MRI, a metastatic work-up (including CT scan of the lungs), and consultation with an oncologist and radiation therapist are recommended. Many centers recommend wide excision with adequate margins of normal tissue along with consideration of irradiation.

25. What is the most common benign skeletal tumor in the hand?

Enchondromas are the most common primary tumor found in the bones of the hand.

26. A 30-year-old woman presents with a history of pain in the distal phalanx of her middle finger, and a ridged fingernail extends proximally to the eponychial area, where a reddish-blue, slightly elevated area about 3 mm in diameter is noted. The area is tender. What is the most likely diagnosis? How would you treat the patient?

After a careful history and physical examination, a radiograph should be taken. The radiograph may demonstrate a small area of underlying bony damage. A glomus tumor is first in the differential diagnosis. Surgical treatment requires complete excision of the lesion and pathologic evaluation.

27. What is an osteoid osteoma?

An osteoid osteoma is a benign lesion producing a core (nidus) in the bone and the surrounding reactive area. It is frequently associated with pain in young patients. Routine radiographs may confirm the diagnosis. Treatment includes excision and curettage.

28. If the pathologic diagnosis of a small mass that you "shelled out" of the index-middle finger web area is synovial sarcoma, what is the major treatment problem?

Because you dissected in the marginal-reactive zone, you probably left scattered, multiple deposits of tumor in different planes.

29. A 70-year-old, otherwise healthy man complains of feeling a mass in the area of an incision scar after release of the carpal tunnel and simultaneous excision of a small nodule from the ring-little finger area. The nodule was found to be a sweat gland carcinoma. Findings are compatible with a mass in the old carpal tunnel incision. What is the probable cause of this mass?

Growth of a deposit of sweat gland carcinoma.

BIBLIOGRAPHY

1. Bednar MS, McCormack RR Jr, Glasser D, Weiland J: Osteoid sarcoma of the upper extremity. J Hand Surg 18A:1019–1028, 1993.
2. Belinkie SA, Swartz WB, Zitelli JA: Invasive squamous cell carcinoma of the carpus: Malignant transformation of epidermis dysplasia verruciformis. J Hand Surg 11A:273–275, 1986.
3. Bogumill GP, Fleegler EJ (eds): Tumors of the Hand and Upper Limb. Edinburgh, Churchill Livingstone, 1993.
4. Bray PW, Bell RS, Bowen CVA, et al: Limb salvage surgery and adjunct radiotherapy for soft tissue sarcomas of the forearm and hand. J Hand Surg 22A:495–503, 1997.
5. Enzinger FM, Weiss SW: Soft Tissue Tumors, 2nd ed. St. Louis, Mosby, 1988.
6. Fleegler EJ: Skin tumors. In Green DP (ed): Operative Hand Surgery, 3rd ed. New York, Churchill Livingstone, 1993, pp 2173–2196.
7. Mulligan RM: Introduction to the pathology of cancer. In Nealon TF Jr (ed): Management of the Patient with Cancer. Philadelphia, W.B. Saunders, 1965, pp 11–37.

111. REFLEX SYMPATHETIC DYSTROPHY

Rahul K. Nath, M.D., and Susan E. Mackinnon, M.D.

1. Describe the functional anatomy of the sympathetic nervous system.

Sympathetic nerve fibers originate in the hypothalamus. Somatic sympathetic axons descend through the posterior columns of the spinal cord and synapse at the level of spinal sympathetic chain ganglia. Postsynaptic fibers travel to end-organs intimately associated with coterminous blood vessels. Peripheral terminals release norepinephrine, which acts on $alpha_1$, $beta_1$, and $beta_2$ receptors. $Alpha_2$ receptors on the sympathetic end terminals prevent release of norepinephrine. $Alpha_1$ receptors are responsible for vasoconstriction of peripheral blood vessels in the normal setting.

2. The sympathetic nervous system has "fight or flight" functions. What is their relevance to pain?

The exact mechanism for sympathetic involvement in chronic pain is not known. The presumed anatomic basis for sympathetically maintained pain syndrome (SMPS) is the formation of abnormal short circuits between nociceptive and mechanoreceptor afferents and sympathetic fiber efferents at the level of the spinal cord. The mechanism by which abnormal short circuits develop is obscure, but tissue trauma apparently leads to inappropriate release of terminal norepinephrine that in some way causes the pain and tissue changes seen in the clinical setting.

3. Does experimental evidence suggest the involvement of sympathetic nerves in some chronic pain syndromes?

Yes. Electrical stimulation of sympathetic nerves in patients with clinical signs of SMPS results in exacerbation of pain. Similar stimulation of sympathetic fibers in patients who are undergoing sympathectomy for vascular disease does not produce pain. Other studies have shown that injection of norepinephrine into the skin of normal patients does not cause pain but that norepinephrine injection into the skin of postsympathectomy patients recapitulates the pain present before sympathectomy. Animal studies support these clinical data.

4. What is RSD? What is CRPS? What is the difference between them?

Reflex sympathetic dystrophy (RSD) is a clinical pain syndrome with sympathetic manifestations that classically occur after minor trauma to an extremity. Three criteria are basic to the definition: (1) diffuse pain in an area not corresponding to the distribution of a peripheral nerve; (2) diminished function of the affected area and stiffness of involved joints; and (3) characteristic skin and soft tissue changes, ranging from swelling, rubor, hyperhidrosis, and warmth in early stages to atrophy, stiffness, and coldness as the syndrome progresses. Vasomotor instability is usually present. These signs are consistent with sympathetic overactivity, implying involvement of the sympathetic nervous system in the pathogenesis of the syndrome. Three classic stages are described, corresponding to the physical changes accompanying progression of the disease from acute inflammatory onset (stage I, early) through dystrophy (stage II, intermediate) to atrophy or disuse stiffness (stage III, late).

Recently, many pain investigators have suggested that the term RSD should be replaced by a term more descriptive of the characteristic features of the syndrome. The International Pain Nomenclature Group has proposed the term **complex regional pain syndromes (CRPS)**. Patients are subdivided into two categories: (1) sympathetically maintained pain syndromes (SMPS) and (2) sympathetically independent pain syndromes (SIPS), depending on the presence or absence of abnormal sympathetic discharge. Therefore, CRPS encompasses the concept that pain becomes chronic because of maintaining factors, which may be sympathetic or nonsympathetic. The idea of regionality also is emphasized. The intent of the change in nomenclature is to address the prevalent overdiagnosis of sympathetically maintained pain by emphasizing the concept that nonsympathetically mediated pain is much more common.

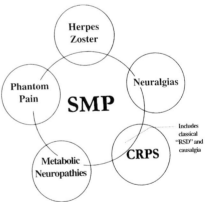

Venn diagram of several painful conditions and sympathetically maintained pain (SMP). Note that only a small percentage of patients with chronic regional pain syndrome (CRPS) have a sympathetic component to their pain. (Modified from Stanton-Hicks M, Janig W, Hassenbusch S, et al: Reflex sympathetic dystrophy: Changing concepts and taxonomy. Pain 63:127–133, 1995.)

5. Is SMPS the same as RSD?

Not exactly. SMPS is subdivided into type 1 and type 2. Type 1 SMPS describes cases previously labeled RSD—that is, sympathetically maintained pain with various initiating factors other than the special situation of nerve injury. Type 2 SMPS describes patients whose pain syndrome is specifically initiated by a nerve injury of any type; type 2 was previously classified as causalgia.

6. What is (or was) causalgia?

The word *causalgia* derives from the Greek for *burning pain*. Silas Weir Mitchell described the syndrome of chronic burning pain after gunshot wounds during the American Civil War. Such wounds were found to have nerve injury as a common factor, and the associated chronic pain syndrome with sympathetic manifestations eventually became known as causalgia. It now is referred to as SMPS type 2.

7. CRPS consists of SMPS and SIPS. What is the incidence of each?

The actual incidence of CRPS is unknown and probably cannot be determined. However, the proportion between SMPS and SIPS can be estimated based on the personal experience of pain specialists who see these problems on a daily basis. Some groups place the percentage of SMPS at only 10% of CRPS. This figure cannot be proved but reflects the concept that nonspecialists who manage patients with pain vastly overdiagnose sympathetically maintained pain.

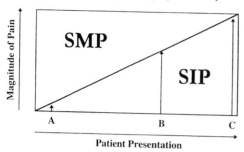

Patient Presentation

Relative contribution of SMP and SIP to total pain experienced by the patient. *A* represents a patient with primarily SMP-related pain, and *C* represents a patient with no sympathetic component. *B* represents an intermediate mix. Most patients with CRPS are closer to *C*. Sympatholytic procedures are most efficacious in patients resembling patient *A*. (Modified from Stanton-Hicks M, Janig W, Hassenbusch S, et al: Reflex sympathetic dystrophy: Changing concepts and taxonomy. Pain 63:127–133, 1995.)

8. Why is sympathetically maintained pain overdiagnosed?

Probably because patients with chronic pain have complex problems that defy easy categorization. It is well known that pain with a sympathetic overlay is often resistant to treatment, and diagnosing patients with sympathetically maintained pain categorizes them as difficult to manage. Therefore, management failures can be rationalized.

9. How can you diagnose sympathetically maintained pain accurately?

A given patient's pain syndrome may have components of both sympathetic and nonsympathetic pain. A structured, logical approach using objective diagnostic criteria improves the chances of managing the pain syndrome correctly. One approach is first to define the proportion of pain caused by sympathetic activity and then to look for the nonsympathetic maintaining causes, if any. Four aspects of the diagnostic protocol are important:

1. **Clinical features** associated with the pain syndrome are noted and signs of increased sympathetic tone are looked for.

2. **Cold testing.** Patients with sympathetically maintained pain are hypersensitive to minor cold stimulation as with an ice cube or ethyl chloride.

3. **Temporary sympatholysis** by blockade of alpha1 adrenergic receptors blocks the component of pain resulting from abnormal sympathetic connections. Alpha-adrenergic blockade protocols using intravenous phentolamine and including placebo testing have been worked out. Patients grade their pain on an analog scale while receiving phentolamine or placebo. The proportion of pain reduction that occurs during phentolamine flow but not during placebo administration represents pain related to abnormal sympathetic connections.

4. **Triple-phase bone scanning.** The delayed phase of testing reveals diffuse periarticular radionuclide uptake in cases of sympathetically maintained pain. This test has shown greater than 95% sensitivity and specificity when correlated with strong clinical signs of sympathetic overactivity in chronic pain syndromes.

After correlating clinical and objective findings, a rational diagnosis can be formulated and the patient treated accordingly.

10. Does CRPS occur only in the extremities?

The definition of CRPS includes regionality as an important diagnostic feature of the pain syndrome. Regionality can extend to many body areas, including the head and neck, chest, breast, and penis. Both SMPS and SIPS may occur in these regions. Diagnosis and management are similar regardless of the region.

11. What inciting events may cause sympathetically maintained pain?

Classically, minor blunt trauma to an extremity is identified as the causative event on retrospective review. However, many other possible agents have been proposed, including ischemia, myocardial infarction, psychological trauma, nerve compression, surgery, and viral disease. In one large series, no cause was identified in 10% of patients.

12. What are the principles of management of SMPS?

Early diagnosis before the onset of permanent soft tissue changes is important. Aggressive physical therapy to prevent disuse stiffness is crucial. In addition to these ancillary measures, active treatments are designed and implemented based on anatomic and pharmacologic principles. However, truly permanent relief of all pain and associated symptoms is unusual.

The first principle of management after diagnosis of SMPS is to define and treat any underlying causes of the pain, such as nerve compression. If this is not possible, sympatholysis or interruption of the sympathetic effector pathway is considered. Several possible levels of intervention in the sympathetic pathway are possible. Medical therapy targets the alpha$_1$ receptor via intravenous phentolamine (primarily for diagnosis) and bretylium (for treatment). Phenoxybenzamine is orally efficacious but unfortunately limited by side effects. Interruption of sympathetic flow at the level of the ganglion is possible as a temporary (blockade with local anesthetic injection) or permanent treatment (transection of the sympathetic chain).

13. How effective are the treatments for sympathetically maintained pain?

The answer is not clear. A review of the literature about ganglion blockade, intravenous sympathetic blockade, and surgical sympathectomy from 1945–1994 reveals serious methodologic flaws in all reports. Double-blinded, randomized, prospective studies were done only in three reports, and none of the reports stated a mean length of follow-up. However, if trends are studied, surgical sympathectomy appears to be more effective than intravenous sympathetic blockade, which in turn appear to provide better relief than ganglion blockade.

14. If surgical sympathectomy has the highest efficacy, why is it not used for every patient?

Surgical sympathectomy is designed to interrupt permanently the anatomic continuity of the sympathetic chain at the level of the sympathetic ganglion. In upper extremity pain the upper thoracic chain (stellate ganglion) is transected, whereas in lower extremity pain the lumbar chain is interrupted. The procedures can be done in an open fashion or, recently, through an endoscope, which may result in lower surgical morbidity. Although endoscopic techniques are effective and safe, they are still surgical procedures and should not be undertaken lightly. In addition, the physiologic consequence of sympathetic loss to an extremity must be accepted: erythema, warmth, anhidrosis, and frequent temperature lability. Because of these morbidities, surgical sympathectomy is indicated only in severe, intractable cases of SMPS. In such cases, however, early surgical intervention often slows progression of the disease and affords symptomatic relief. Recurrent pain after unilateral surgical sympathectomy may be treated by bilateral sympathectomy or application of dorsal column spinal electrostimulation.

CONTROVERSY

15. Are certain people more prone to developing SMPS?

When time has passed and the pain has not been treated adequately, it is clear that psychological factors become more important in the clinical syndrome. Depression is common, and personality disorders are often seen. The controversy arises in trying to attach prior significance to personality traits in patients who manifest SMPS. According to one school of thought, patients with a certain personality profile are more prone to develop SMPS after minor inciting events, including psychological trauma. Advocates of this theory believe that SMPS is best managed by psychotherapy and claim reversal of physical characteristics of SMPS with this treatment. This theory is not widely accepted, and diagnosis of patients is not based on objective criteria and testing.

BIBLIOGRAPHY

1. Amadio PC, Mackinnon SE, Merritt WE, et al: Reflex sympathetic dystrophy syndrome: Consensus report of an ad hoc committee of the American Association of Hand Surgery on the definition of reflex sympathetic dystrophy syndrome. Plast Reconstr Surg 87:371–375, 1991.
2. Campbell JN, Meyer RA, Raja SN: Is nociceptor activation by alpha-1 adrenoreceptors the culprit in sympathetically maintained pain? Am Pain Soc J 1:3–8, 1992.
3. Kumar K, Nath RK, Toth C: Spinal cord stimulation is effective in the management of reflex sympathetic dystrophy. Neurosurgery 40:503–509, 1997.
4. Mackinnon SE, Dellon AL: Painful sequelae of peripheral nerve injury. In Mackinnon SE, Dellon AL (eds): Surgery of the Peripheral Nerve. New York, Thieme, 1988, pp 492–504.

6. Nath RK, Mackinnon SE: Reflex sympathetic dystrophy. Clin Plast Surg 23:435–446, 1996.
7. Ochoa JL, Verdugo RJ: Reflex sympathetic dystrophy: A common clinical avenue for somatoform expression.
    Neurol Clin 13:351–363, 1995.
8. Stanton-Hicks M, Janig W, Hassenbuch S, et al: Reflex sympathetic dystrophy: Changing concepts and taxon-
    omy. Pain 63:127–133, 1995.

112. REHABILITATION OF THE INJURED HAND

Lois Carlson, O.T.R./L., C.H.T., and Lynn Breglio, P.T., C.H.T.

1. What are the physiologic effects of early motion programs after tendon repair?
Experimental studies have demonstrated that early motion favors intrinsic vs. extrinsic healing.
Positive results of early motion after tendon repair include improved tendon excursion, increased
tensile strength, and decreased edema and joint stiffness.

2. Describe early passive mobilization after flexor tendon repair in the hand.
This technique mobilizes the repaired tendon using passive flexion and limited active or passive
extension. The repair is immobilized using a forearm-based dorsal block splint, which limits extension of the wrist and metacarpophalangeal (MP) joints. Current therapy protocols are based on one or
both of the following approaches:

1. **Kleinert traction.** Rubber band traction provides passive flexion and allows active extension
to the limits of the splint. The traction is secured distally to the fingernail using a nail hook and attached proximally to the forearm portion of the splint. Use of a palmar pulley increases flexion at the
distal interphalangeal joint.

2. **Duran method.** The repaired tendon is mobilized using isolated passive extension of proximal interphalangeal (PIP) and distal interphalangeal (DIP) joints. The protocol is based on the need
for 3–5 mm of tendon excursion to prevent adhesions.

Active motion is generally started by 3–6 weeks. Progression of treatment for individual patients varies with the level of scar formation and demonstrated active motion.

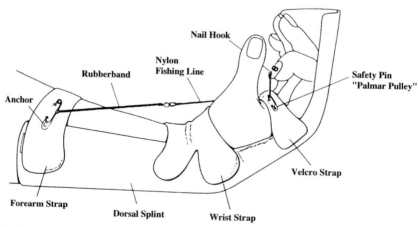

Modification of Kleinert dynamic traction splint using palmar pulley. (From Chow JA, Thomes LJ, Dovelle S, et
al: Controlled motion rehabilitation after flexor tendon repair and grafting. J Bone Joint Surg 70B:591–595,
1988, with permission.)

3. When are early active mobilization protocols used after flexor tendon repair?
Early active mobilization may be used if the repair is sufficiently strong to withstand early motion,
if the patient is reliable, and if the protocol is guided by an experienced therapist. The repaired tendon

is still protected using splinting, and elements of passive mobilization are generally incorporated into the rehabilitation program. The active part of the program may involve gentle active muscle contraction in a limited range or use of a "place-and-hold" technique. A method popularized by Strickland and Cannon includes use of a tenodesis splint (hinged wrist splint limiting wrist extension and MP extension) combined with "place-and-hold" exercises.

4. Describe early passive mobilization protocols used for extensor tendons in zones V, VI, and VII.

Early passive mobilization protocols use a reverse Kleinert approach. The splint maintains the wrist in approximately 45° of extension, with dynamic traction positioning the MP (and interphalangeal) joints in 0° of extension. Active flexion in the splint is allowed to a predetermined level, depending on the protocol and the quality of the repair. Evans recommends splinting initially to provide MP flexion equal to approximately 30° for the index and middle and 40° for the ring and little fingers to achieve 5 mm of passive tendon glide for adhesion prevention.

5. What is the SAM protocol for zone III and IV extensor tendon repairs?

The SAM (short arc motion) protocol, developed by Evans, is an example of an early active motion protocol for zone III and IV extensor tendon repairs. Early active motion is initiated for the repaired tendon, using volar static splints as templates. The patient flexes and extends the joints, using minimal active muscle tendon tension (MAMTT). During exercise, the wrist is positioned in 30° of flexion and the MP joint at neutral to slight flexion. The interphalangeal (IP) joints are maintained in an extension splint between exercises.

1. The patient actively flexes to 30° at the PIP joint and 20–25° at the DIP joint. If no extensor lag develops after 2 weeks, flexion is gradually increased by 10° each week over the next several weeks.

2. With the PIP joint positioned in extension, the patient actively flexes and extends the DIP joint. Full flexion is allowed unless the lateral bands have been repaired, in which case flexion is limited to 30–35°.

6. What are flexor tendon gliding exercises?

Tendon gliding exercises are used to obtain maximal total and differential flexor tendon glide: flexor digitorum superficialis (FDS), straight fist; flexor digitorum profundus (FDP), full fist; and hook (or claw) position, maximal differential glide.

7. Describe splinting after MP implant arthroplasty.

The patient is splinted with the MP joints in the position of extension and neutral to slight radial deviation. Two splints are commonly used:

1. **Dynamic splint.** This splint is used during the day to maintain joint alignment, assist extension, and provide controlled flexion for 3–4 weeks after surgery. The splint helps to train the capsule to be adequately loose in the flexion/extension plane and relatively tight in the mediolateral plane. Active and passive flexion exercises are done initially within the splint. Components of the splint also may include a supinator strap to the index, and taping the little finger to the ring finger to provide a flexor assist; a thumb outrigger may be needed to avoid excessive radial deviation force.

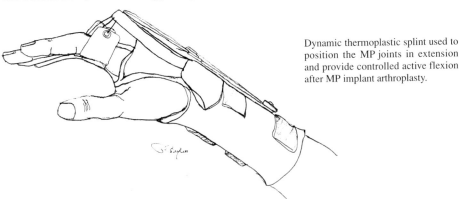

Dynamic thermoplastic splint used to position the MP joints in extension and provide controlled active flexion after MP implant arthroplasty.

2. **Static splint.** A volar splint is fabricated with the wrist in 15–20° of extension and MP joints at 0° extension and 0–10° radial deviation. Thermoplastic or soft materials may be used to position the fingers. The splint is worn at night for up to 3 months or longer as needed.

Additional splinting for flexion also may be required, including splints to block IP flexion during MP flexion exercise and dynamic splinting, most commonly for the little finger.

8. Name three possible long-term postoperative complications of MP implant arthroplasty.

1. Loss of flexion or extension. In general, the goal is to achieve 0° extension and 70° flexion. According to Swanson, flexion of index and middle fingers is less critical and should be limited to 45–60° of flexion for stability.
2. Ulnar drift
3. Fracture/dislocation of implant

9. Describe examples of joint protection techniques for patients with arthritis.

These techniques minimize stress to joints during daily activities and are appropriate for patients with arthritis in general as well as for patients who have undergone surgery such as implant arthroplasty. Examples include: (1) use of larger, stronger joints; (2) three-point pinch (preferable to lateral pinch); (3) avoidance of deforming forces, such as twisting and ulnar deviation; and (4) balance of work and rest.

10. What factors must be evaluated to determine the cause of limited passive motion?

Restricted motion may be due to soft tissue and/or joint restrictions. In evaluating limited flexion at the PIP joint, for example, the following factors should be considered:

1. **Extrinsic extensor tightness.** Flexion is affected by the position of the MP joint; flexion is decreased if the MP joint is flexed.
2. **Intrinsic extensor tightness.** Flexion is affected by the position of the MP joint; flexion is decreased if the MP joint is extended (intrinsic stretch position).
3. **Joint restrictions.** Flexion is unaffected by the position of the MP joint.

11. When is it appropriate to initiate active motion after an intraarticular fracture of the PIP joint?

The initiation of active motion depends on the stability of the fracture. Early active motion is possible if rigid fixation is achieved with protective splinting between exercise sessions. If less rigid fixation is used, active motion generally may be started at 3 weeks, and passive motion at 6 weeks.

12. What important principles must be followed in planning a treatment program after limited wrist arthrodesis to correct wrist instability?

Rehabilitation must be guided by the need for a stable, pain-free wrist with functional mobility. Keys to successful management after surgery include adequate immobilization, early active motion of uninvolved joints, a focus on regaining finger and thumb motion as soon as possible, and allowing the wrist to adapt gradually to its new kinematics through active exercise and use.

13. Why should a patient be referred for hand therapy after a nerve injury?

1. Before regeneration it is important to prevent deformity and improve function through the use of splinting and to educate the patient about methods of compensation for loss of sensibility and autonomic function.
2. During regeneration, goals of therapy may include sensory desensitization and reeducation, muscle reeducation and strengthening, and restoration of functional patterns of use.

14. What are the potential deformities and splinting needs for radial nerve injuries?

The major problem is wrist drop from loss of wrist extensors (radial wrist extensors are spared with posterior interosseous nerve injury). Finger extension and thumb extension/radial abduction are also affected. Splinting options include wrist extension (dynamic or static), with or without finger and thumb outriggers to provide dynamic extension force, and the tenodesis splint, as described by Colditz (static outrigger from forearm-based splint to the proximal phalanges reproduces tenodesis effect).

15. For ulnar nerve injuries?

Ulnar nerve injuries may be high (affecting one-half of the flexor digitorum profundus [FDP], flexor carpi ulnaris [FCU], and ulnar intrinsics) or low (affecting the adductor pollicis, one half of the flexor pollicis brevis [FPB], interossei, one-half of the lumbricals, abductor digiti minimi [ADM], flexor digiti minimi [FDM], and opponens digiti minimi [ODM]). The major deformity at both levels is claw deformity, caused by loss of all intrinsics to the ring and little fingers. The claw gets worse as a high ulnar palsy improves (increased flexion by the FDP). A splint that prevents MP hyperextension allows substitution by the long extensors to extend the IP joints. The simplest design is a figure-of-eight splint molded to the patient with thermoplastic material, which allows full flexion and permits functional use.

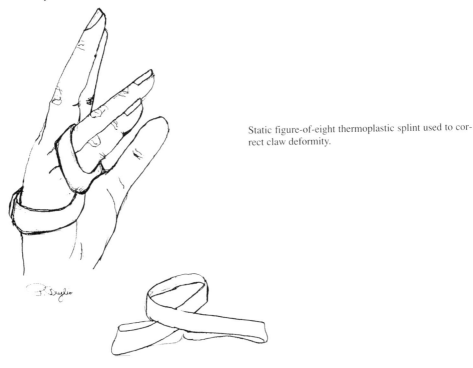

Static figure-of-eight thermoplastic splint used to correct claw deformity.

16. For median nerve injuries?

Median nerve injuries may be high (affecting all forearm flexor/pronator muscles except one half of the FDP and FCU), or low (affecting one-half of the lumbricals, opponens pollicis [OP], abductor pollicis brevis [APB], and one-half of the flexor pollicis brevis [FPB]). The major deformity requiring splinting at both levels is "ape hand" or loss of opposition. An opposition splint places the thumb in the corrected position to prevent deformity and improve function.

17. What readily available tests are used for determining early changes in sensibility due to nerve compression?

Semmes-Weinstein monofilaments and vibrometry (threshold tests) have been shown to be more sensitive than innervation density tests such as two-point testing in identifying early changes due to nerve compression.

18. What are the most common postural faults noted in patients with thoracic outlet syndrome (TOS) that can be improved with therapy?

Rounded shoulders with a forward head posture; tight pectoral muscles (major and minor), with weak middle and lower trapezius muscles secondary to the slumped position; and tight neck flexors and scalenes with overstretched levator scapulae and upper trapezius muscles, which cause the forward head position.

19. Describe the benefits of hand therapy for patients with carpal tunnel syndrome or other forms of cumulative trauma.

Splinting is appropriate for relative rest. Splints should be used judiciously to avoid problems such as disuse or development of abnormal compensatory patterns. Night splinting is recommended for carpal tunnel syndrome to prevent wrist flexion during sleep and median nerve compression. **Exercises** include active nerve and tendon gliding, stretching of overused tight muscles, and strengthening of opposing weak muscles, as indicated from evaluation. **Postural assessment and training** focus on the areas of malalignment, muscle tightness, or weakness. **Work-related evaluation and modification** should address factors related to repetition, force, and posture, including the work station, work style assessment, and work requirements (e.g., production incentives and breaks). Finally, **biofeedback training and relaxation** may be used to relax muscle groups typically used in a state of sustained contraction.

20. What are upper limb tension tests?

Upper limb tension tests assess neural tension in the upper extremity by bringing the patient through sequential motions designed to place the neural tissues on stretch. A positive test reproduces the patient's symptoms and/or demonstrates resistance or limitations in movement. Test results are assessed in reference to expected normal responses. Butler describes four basic tests for the upper extremity, with different movement patterns for the median, radial and ulnar nerves.

21. What general principle can be used to activate a muscle after tendon transfer?

The patient is instructed to perform the original function of the transferred muscle or to combine the original function with the new function. For example, after an opponensplasty using the ring FDS, the thumb is opposed to the tip of the ring finger.

22. Should the burned hand be splinted in the functional position?

No. The burned hand should be placed in the antideformity position, depending on the size and location of the burn. The position of antideformity is 15–20° of wrist extension, 60–70° of flexion at the MP joints, and full extension at the IP joints, with the thumb in palmar abduction.

23. Name three methods to prevent hypertrophic scarring after a burn to the hand.

1. Compression, which includes Jobst garments, Isotoner gloves, and Tubigrip. In addition, inserts under compression garments or in conjunction with splints may be made using elastomer, other silicone-based products, or padding materials.
2. Silicone gel pads
3. Massage

24. Describe examples of splints used after surgery for Dupuytren's contracture.

Splinting to maintain extension is critical after surgery. Depending on the extent of involvement, options include:
- Thermoplastic extension pan splint for extension of all fingers
- Joint spring splint for extension of all joints of one finger
- Joint jack splint for PIP extension

Serial casting may be used to increase extension at the PIP joint if it remains unresponsive to other forms of splinting.

25. What are tests of maximal voluntary effort?

As part of functional testing or a formal functional capacities evaluation, a battery of tests is used to determine whether a patient is giving maximal effort. Such testing may be necessary to help validate findings in patients who have the potential for secondary gain from their disability.

Static strength tests are performed using the Jamar dynamometer and Baltimore Therapeutic Equipment (BTE) Work Simulator (passing scores based on coefficients of variation of 10–15% or less as well as correlation of grip test results), position of dynamometer handle test (skewed bell-shaped curve is anticipated with maximal effort), and the rapid exchange test using the dynamometer (increased speed of performance results in decreased ability to control force at submaximal level).

26. What are some of the advantages and disadvantages of whirlpool treatment vs. direct application of heat, such as a hot pack or paraffin bath?

The whirlpool can be a modality of heat or neutrality because of the adjustability of temperature, thus not compromising vascularity or damaging insensitive parts. In addition, it may be used with chemical additives to decrease bacterial count in a small open wound, and the turbulence may assist in tissue debridement. The buoyancy of the water allows the patient to exercise during treatment. The primary disadvantage of whirlpool treatments is that the extremity is placed in a position of dependency, potentially increasing edema.

Paraffin and hot packs have the advantage of being able to position the hand in elevation and place the hand in a position of stretch. In addition, the oil in the paraffin provides lubrication to dry tissues. When used for treatment of the hand, paraffin and hot packs can provide vigorous heating, which increases tissue extensibility, and are useful adjuncts before exercise or splinting of the stiff hand.

27. How can edema be measured in the hand?

Edema can be evaluated using circumferential measurements and/or a volumeter (measures total volume of the hand using water displacement). Values are then compared with the unaffected side as well as sequentially over time for the involved hand.

28. Name a modality that may be prescribed for edema reduction.

High-voltage galvanic stimulation used for 10–20 minutes is a beneficial adjunct to other edema reduction methods, such as exercise, massage, compression, and elevation. The electrodes are placed surrounding the edematous tissue, with interrupted current sufficient to produce a rhythmic muscular contraction and relaxation of the affected area. The intensity is increased based on patient tolerance. A distinct advantage of this modality is its ability to be used under water, eliminating the need to strap the electrodes in place.

29. Define categories of splints used to gain joint motion.

1. **Serial static casts or splints** provide a static force at end range. This method is based on the principle that tissue lengthens and grows in response to gentle constant tension at the end of its elastic limit. Changes are made as gains in motion are achieved by remolding or refabricating the cast or splint. This type of splinting is most effective in more chronic joint contractures or joints with a hard end feel that require steady, gentle pressure over a prolonged period. Additional benefits include total contact and even pressure distribution, which assist in reduction of edema and increase wearing tolerance. Unfortunately, this type of splinting may not be removable.

2. **Static progressive splints** apply a steady, nonelastic force that can be progressed during each splinting session to accommodate improvements in motion. This type of splinting has the advantage of being removable and allows reciprocal splinting into flexion and extension if required.

3. **Dynamic splints** provide a dynamic force (for example, from a rubber band or spring) and are most effective with joints that have a soft end feel.

CONTROVERSY

30. Describe a course of treatment for reflex sympathetic dystrophy (RSD).

There is lack of consensus about almost everything related to RSD, including its definition, etiology, and most effective treatment approach. The authors' approach focuses on use of specific active loading exercises. Other approaches use gentle exercise as well as a wide array of other modalities, with or without sympathetic blocks.

Stress loading is defined as active, sustained exercise requiring forceful use of the entire extremity with minimal motion of painful joints. Clinically, two simple exercises actively load the affected arm—scrubbing and carrying. The stress-loading program follows basic principles of exercise physiology. The body adapts in response to demand. Exercise places a demand on the neural, vascular, and sensorimotor systems, all of which may play a role in initiating and/or perpetuating RSD. An overload is needed to achieve a training effect. Exercise must be of sufficient intensity, duration and frequency to achieve this training effect. Theoretically, training may be due to the effect of stress-loading exercise on central processing abnormalities and neurovascular control mechanisms.

Keys to the success of the program include maximal load, compliance, structure and emotional support, and separation of treatment of RSD vs. fibrosis. Passive exercise, splinting, and other forms of therapy are used only after the RSD is under control. During the acute stage, symptoms generally resolve within days or weeks. If the patient is first seen during the dystrophic stage, the time required for resolution of RSD is generally longer, and treatment of fibrosis will inevitably be required through conservative measures. If treatment begins in the atrophic stage, motion gains with stress loading may be minimal, although improvement in function and a decrease in pain can still be achieved. Surgical intervention may include capsuloplasty of the MP joints, check rein release (PIP joints), and intrinsic release.

BIBLIOGRAPHY

1. Bell-Krotoski JA, Figarola JH: Biomechanics of soft-tissue growth and remodeling with plaster casting. J Hand Ther 8:131–137, 1995.
2. Butler DS: Mobilisation of the Nervous System. New York, Churchill Livingstone, 1991.
3. Carlson LK, Watson, HK: Treatment of reflex sympathetic dystrophy using the stress loading program. J Hand Ther 1:149–154, 1988.
4. Chow JA, Thomes LJ, Dovelle S, et al: Controlled motion rehabilitation after flexor tendon repair and grafting. J Bone Joint Surg 70B:591–595, 1988.
5. Evans RB: Immediate active short arc motion following extensor tendon repair. Hand Clin 11:483–512, 1995.
6. Hunter JM, Mackin EJ, Callahan AD (eds): Rehabilitation of the Hand: Surgery and Therapy. St. Louis, Mosby, 1995.
7. King JW, Berryhill BH: Assessing maximum effort in upper-extremity functional testing. Work 1(3):65–76, 1991.
8. Michlovitz SL (ed): Thermal Agents in Rehabilitation. Philadelphia, F.A. Davis, 1996.
9. Sanders MJ: Management of Cumulative Trauma Disorders. Boston, Butterworth-Heinemann, 1997.
10. Wehbe MA (ed): Early Motion in Hand and Wrist Surgery. Hand Clin 12(1): 1996.

XII. The Wrist

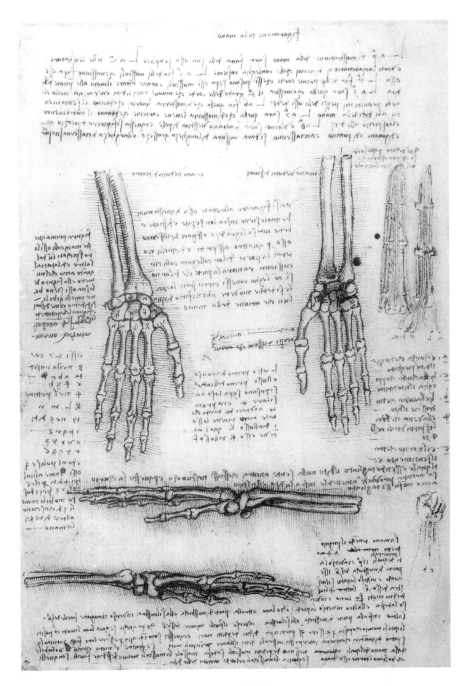

The Bones of the Hand and Wrist
Leonardo da Vinci
ca. 1510–1511
Pen and ink with wash over traces of black chalk
The Royal Library at Windsor Castle, Windsor
The Royal Collection
© 1998 Her Majesty Queen Elizabeth II

113. ANATOMY OF THE WRIST

Richard A. Berger, M.D., Ph.D.

1. What is the normal blood supply pattern of the scaphoid? The capitate? The lunate? The hamate?

The **scaphoid** receives its blood supply through small branches, primarily from the radial artery, that enter the bone through two channels. The distal pole is supplied by the palmar scaphoid branch, which enters the scaphoid through the palmar cortex. The dorsal scaphoid branch enters the scaphoid along the dorsal ridge of the scaphoid near the waist region. No consistent nutrient vessels enter the scaphoid proximally, and internally the nutrient vessels do not anastomose. Because the proximal pole is supplied solely by vessels entering distally and coursing proximally, the proximal pole is at particularly high risk of avascular necrosis with fractures proximal to the waist of the scaphoid.

The **capitate** is supplied by multiple nutrient vessels entering the palmar and dorsal cortices of the body of the capitate. Because there are no soft tissue attachments proximal to the neck, the head of the capitate depends on retrograde flow from the more distal nutrient vessels and is vulnerable to avascular necrosis in the case of a fracture through the neck.

The **lunate** has consistent nutrient vessels entering through the palmar and dorsal cortices, although there may be some dominance of the palmar nutrient vessels. The intraosseous anastomosis patterns have been described as forming X, Y, and I patterns.

The **hamate** has three general areas of nutrient vessel penetration: dorsal cortex, palmar cortex, and hamulus. The dorsal and palmar vessels have been shown to anastomose in approximately 50% of specimens. The pole of the hamate is without direct soft tissue attachments and therefore relies on retrograde flow from the more distal palmar and dorsal nutrient vessels. Thus the pole is at risk of avascular necrosis (although it is rare) in the event of a fracture. The hamulus typically has a rich blood supply but rarely anastomoses with the vessels entering the body of the hamate. This pattern may contribute to the nonunion rate in fractures of the hamulus.

2. What is the normal percentage of force or load transmission through the ulnocarpal joint?

Under normal conditions, approximately 20% of the entire longitudinal force or load is transmitted through the ulnocarpal articulation; the remaining 80% is transmitted through the radiocarpal articulation. Factors that increase ulnocarpal load transmission include wrist ulnar deviation, positive ulnar variance, and pronation of the forearm.

3. Describe the ligaments that interconnect the bones of the proximal carpal row.

The ligaments that connect the bones of the proximal carpal row are the **scapholunate** and **lunotriquetral interosseous** ligaments. They are similar to each other in that both are C-shaped, connecting the palmar, proximal, and dorsal regions but leaving the distal surfaces of the joints without direct ligamentous connections. This pattern explains why in a normal midcarpal arthrogram contrast material passes proximally into the clefts of the scapholunate and lunotriquetral joints. A normal radiocarpal arthrogram shows no passage of contrast material into the scapholunate and lunotriquetral joint clefts because of the intact scapholunate and lunotriquetral interosseous ligaments. In both ligaments, the palmar and dorsal regions are composed of true ligaments with collagen fascicles, blood vessels, and nerves, whereas the proximal regions are composed of fibrocartilage without blood vessels, nerves, or distinct collagen fascicle orientations. The differences between the two ligaments are limited primarily to the relative thickness of the dorsal and palmar regions and to the merging of the radioscapholunate ligament with the scapholunate interosseous ligament between the palmar and proximal regions. The dorsal region of the scapholunate ligament and the palmar region of the lunotriquetral ligament are the thickest, whereas the palmar region of the scapholunate interosseous ligament and the dorsal region of the lunotriquetral ligament are the thinnest.

4. How much of the proximal surface of the lunate normally articulates with the distal articular surface of the radius in the neutral wrist position?

Under normal circumstances, in a frontal radiographic projection at least 50% of the proximal articular surface of the lunate articulates with the lunate fossa; the average is 60%. If less than 50% of the proximal articular surface of the lunate articulates with the lunate fossa of the radius, ulnar translocation of the lunate is diagnosed. Generally, this translocation results from substantial disruption of the long and short radiolunate ligaments. In posteroanterior (PA) radiographs, substantial information also can be gained about the position and orientation of the lunate, simply by identifying the shape of the lunate. If the outline of the lunate is quadrangular, the lunate is dorsiflexed. If triangular in shape, the lunate is palmarflexed.

5. What are the normal radiolunate and scapholunate angles as measured on a lateral radiograph?

Before attempting to determine intercarpal or radiocarpal angles, it is imperative to ensure that a standardized quality lateral radiograph of the wrist is obtained. The ulnar margin of the wrist is placed on the x-ray cassette with the shoulder adducted to the side, the elbow flexed 90°, and the forearm positioned in neutral rotation. The wrist is positioned in neutral extension, whereby the axis of the third metacarpal is within 10° of the axis of the diaphysis of the radius. Confirmation of a true lateral radiograph of the wrist can be made by identifying the palmar cortices of the scaphoid tubercle, the body of the capitate, and the pisiform. If the palmar cortex of the pisiform falls between the palmar cortices of the scaphoid tubercle and the body of the capitate, the wrist has been positioned within 5° of a true lateral projection and is within acceptable limits. If the palmar cortex of the pisiform is seen palmar to the scaphoid tubercle, the forearm is in supination; conversely, if the palmar cortex of the pisiform is dorsal to the palmar cortex of the capitate body, the forearm is pronated.

The axis of the radius is defined by bisecting the diaphysis in two locations and connecting the bisection points. The axis of the scaphoid can be determined in several manners. First, the midpoint of the proximal and distal articular surfaces can be estimated, and a line can be drawn between the two points. Second, a tangent to the palmar cortex of the waist of the scaphoid can be drawn. The axis of the lunate is best determined by drawing a cord between the distalmost tips of the palmar and dorsal horns of the lunate. A perpendicular to this cord defines the axis of the lunate.

Under normal circumstances, the radiolunate angle should measure ± 10°. A positive angle indicates dorsiflexion of the lunate, and any value greater than +10° is labeled as dorsiflexion intercalated segment instability (DISI). A negative angle indicates palmarflexion of the lunate, and any value less than –10° is labeled as volarflexion intercalated segment instability (VISI). The normal scapholunate angle is 46°, but it has a rather wide range of variance from 30°–60°. A scapholunate angle greater than 70° indicates carpal instability. In a recent study of intra- and interobserver variability in making such measurements, it was determined that an overall estimated error of measurement averaged 7.4°.

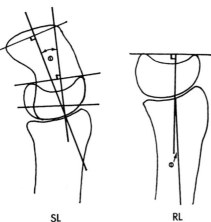

SL RL

Lines for determining scapholunate angle (SL) and radiolunate angle (RL).

6. How does the relative length of the radius and ulna, termed ulnar variance, change with forearm rotation?

The axis of rotation of the forearm passes through the radial head proximally and the ulnar head distally. The obliquity of orientation of this axis changes the orientation of the radius and ulna during pronation and supination, whereby the two bones are relatively parallel in supination and essentially crossed in pronation. This "crossing" generates a relative change in the distal projections of the two bones, whereby the radius projects less distally in forearm pronation. This change has implications in determining ulnar variance, which is a radiographic measurement of the relative lengths of the radius and ulna. This determination must be made with a PA radiograph taken with the forearm in neutral rotation. A pronated forearm may give the impression of positive ulnar variance (ulna projecting more distally than the radius), and supination may give the impression of a negative ulnar variance (ulna projecting less distally than the radius). Neutral forearm rotation is best assured by taking the radiograph with the hand and wrist placed flat on the x-ray cassette with no wrist deviation, the shoulder in 90° abduction, and the elbow in 90° flexion.

7. The proximal carpal row moves in what general motion during wrist radial and ulnar deviation? During wrist flexion and extension?

Although there are measurable motions among the scaphoid, lunate, and triquetrum, the proximal row bones move, in general, in the same overall direction as the wrist. During wrist flexion and extension the proximal row bones also move synchronously with the distal row bones in flexion and extension, respectively. During wrist radial deviation the proximal row bones move primarily in flexion, whereas during wrist ulnar deviation the proximal row bones move primarily in extension. A simplified method to remember these motion patterns is to realize that the proximal row bones move in the same *flexion* direction during *wrist flexion and radial deviation* and in the same *extension* direction during *wrist extension and ulnar deviation*.

8. Why is the radioscapholunate ligament no longer believed to be a significant mechanical stabilizer of the scaphoid and lunate?

The radioscapholunate ligament was postulated early to behave as an important stabilizer of the scaphoid and lunate, based largely on its position and orientation. It is located between the long and short radiolunate ligaments and appears to pierce the palmar radiocarpal joint capsule. It is grossly oriented vertically and appears to attach to the proximal surfaces of the scaphoid and lunate. There have even been isolated reports of disruption of this ligament associated with scapholunate dissociation.

Recent studies, however, have defined the histology of the radioscapholunate ligament and have shown that it is highly atypical, composed of a large number of blood vessels and nerve fibers, with a minimal content of poorly organized collagen that is covered by a thick layer of synovial tissue. Furthermore, it has been demonstrated that the radioscapholunate ligament is a termination of an anastomosis of the anterior interosseous artery and palmar radial arch of the radial artery and branches from the anterior interosseous nerve. Finally, material property studies have shown that the radioscapholunate ligament fails at significantly lower load levels and has a much higher strain level than contiguous ligaments. Therefore, the radioscapholunate ligament behaves more as a mesocapsule than a ligament and should not be considered a stabilizing structure of the wrist.

9. What are the normal anteroposterior and lateral intrascaphoid angles?

The normal posteroanterior intrascaphoid angle is less than 35°, and the normal lateral intrascaphoid angle is less than 35°. Patients with scaphoid malunions or nonunions with an intrascaphoid angle > 45° are considered at statistically increased risk for development of degenerative changes and show radiographic signs of carpal collapse. It has been found that either trispiral tomograms or computed axial tomograms may enhance the ability to measure these angles. The method used for determining the intrascaphoid angle in either plane measures the angle of intersection of perpendiculars drawn from the cords of the proximal and distal articular surface curves. (See figure at top of next page.)

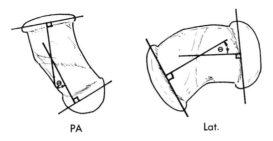

PA   Lat.

Lines for determining posteroanterior (PA) and lateral intrascaphoid angles.

10. Describe the normal arterial blood supply of the distal radius.

Recent descriptions of the arterial blood supply of the radius have prompted the use of vascularized pedicled bone grafts in the treatment of scaphoid nonunions, avascular necrosis of the scaphoid proximal pole, and Kienböck's disease. The nutrient blood vessels entering the distal radius have a consistent pattern that makes identification and isolation relatively easy.

The longitudinally oriented vessels arise from the radial artery, ulnar artery, or posterior division of the anterior interosseous artery. Three major transverse arches interconnect the longitudinal vessels, which are named from proximal to distal: dorsal supraretinacular arch (found on the extensor retinaculum), dorsal radiocarpal arch, and dorsal intercarpal arch (both found in the joint capsule proper).

There are two distinct types of nutrient vessels: supraretinacular (between the extensor compartments) and compartmental (within the extensor compartments). The supraretinacular vessels (SRA) are numbered to reflect the compartments between which they are found; the compartmental vessels (ECA) are numbered according to the compartment within which they are found.

The identified nutrient vessels are, beginning radially, 1,2 SRA; 2,3 SRA; and 4 ECA. A consistent vessel found within the fifth extensor compartment is called the 5 ECA, but it has no direct penetration into the radius; rather, it is useful as a retrograde conduit to extend the length of a 4 ECA graft pedicled to the dorsal radiocarpal or intercarpal arches, through the proximal anastomosis of the 4 ECA, 5 ECA, and posterior division of the anterior interosseous artery.

Dorsal view of carpal region illustrating the arterial blood supply. The supraretinacular arteries are found between the first and second extensor compartments (1,2 sra) and between the second and third extensor compartments (2,3 sra). Arteries are consistently found within the fourth (4 eca) and fifth (5 eca) extensor compartments. ra = radial artery, ia = posterior division of anterior interosseous artery, dsra = dorsal supraretinacular arch, drca = dorsal radiocarpal arch, dica = dorsal intercarpal arch, R = radius, U = ulna, S = scaphoid L = lunate, C = capitate.

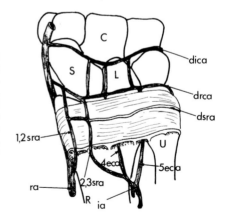

11. Name the four principal ligaments of the first carpometacarpal joint.

On the palmar surface of the joint is the anterior oblique ligament, also called the "beak ligament." Near the ulnar extreme of the joint is the ulnar collateral ligament. Dorsally, the ulnar half of the joint is covered by the posterior oblique ligament, whereas the radial half is covered by the dorsoradial ligament. There are no true ligament fibers near the radial extent of the joint, deep to the abductor pollicis longus tendon. The base of the first metacarpal is stabilized to the base of the second metacarpal by the intermetacarpal ligament, which is extracapsular and not considered a proper carpometacarpal joint ligament.

12. Describe the anatomy of the triangular fibrocartilage complex.

The triangular fibrocartilage complex is based around the triangle-shaped articular disc, which is interposed between the ulnar head and carpal bones. This articular disc is composed of fibrocartilage; its base is attached to the radius along the distal edge of the sigmoid notch. Along the dorsal margin of the articular disc is the dorsal radioulnar ligament, which connects the dorsal aspect of the sigmoid notch of the radius to the styloid process of the ulna. Extending from the dorsal radioulnar ligament in a distal direction are fibers called the extensor carpi ulnaris tendon subsheath, which variably extends to the base of the fifth metacarpal. Along the palmar edge of the articular disc is the palmar radioulnar ligament, which connects the palmar edge of the sigmoid notch to the area at the base of the ulnar styloid process, called the fovea. Emanating from the palmar radioulnar ligament are the ulnolunate and ulnotriquetral ligaments. Near the ulnar apex of the articular disc is a depression called the prestyloid recess, which is generally filled with synovial villi and variably communicates with the tip of the ulnar styloid process. Between the ulnar attachments of the dorsal and palmar radioulnar ligaments is a region of small blood vessels called the ligamentum subcruentum. The meniscus homologue is the edge of the articular disc distal to the prestyloid recess, which in selected coronal sections resembles the profile of a knee meniscus.

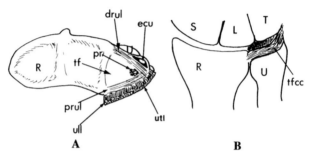

Transverse *(A)* and dorsal *(B)* views of the triangular fibrocartilage complex (tfcc). R = radius, U = ulna, S = scaphoid, L = lunate, T = triquetrum, tf =triangular fibrocartilage, pr = prestyloid recess, drul = dorsal radioulnar ligament, ecu = ecu subsheath, prul = palmar radioulnar ligament, ull = ulnolunate ligament, utl = ulnotriquetral ligament.

13. Where is the center of rotation of the wrist?

The center of rotation of the wrist is somewhat controversial because of the complex compound motion of all of the carpal bones. If taken as a unit, the wrist movements have been labeled as dorsiflexion (extension), palmarflexion (flexion), radial deviation (abduction), ulnar deviation (adduction), axial rotation (pronation/supination), and circumduction. Any combination of these motions is possible, but the classic axes of rotation of the wrist have been identified as the flexion-extension axis and radial-ulnar deviation axis. Kinematic studies have identified the head of the capitate as the anatomic location at which these axes intersect the wrist. A functional axis, called the "dart-throw" axis, also passes through the capitate but represents the motion created by throwing a dart from wrist extension and radial deviation to flexion and ulnar deviation. It is important to recognize that the axes of rotation are mere approximations and that each individual carpal bone is considered a rigid body, displaying its own kinematics, which, when summed with the remaining carpal bones, creates the overall motion that we perceive as wrist motion.

14. The midcarpal joint normally communicates with which carpometacarpal joints?

The midcarpal joint is in direct communication with the second, third, fourth, and fifth carpometacarpal joints. Only the first carpometacarpal joint is isolated from the midcarpal joint.

15. Is it normal for the radiocarpal joint to communicate with the pisotriquetral joint? With the distal radioulnar joint?

It is estimated that in 90% of normal adults the radiocarpal joint communicates with the pisotriquetral joint, as evidenced by arthrography. It is considered abnormal for the radiocarpal joint to communicate with the distal radioulnar joint, although such communications do not necessarily imply mechanical instability. Such communications, usually identified with arthrography, imply a defect in the triangular fibrocartilage complex, particularly the articular disc, which normally isolates the two joints from communication. Degenerative changes may occur in the central aspect of the articular disc as early as the third decade and increase in incidence with increasing age thereafter.

16. Are there any normal direct tendinous insertions to any of the carpal bones?

Only the pisiform has a tendinous attachment under normal circumstances, serving as the insertion of the flexor carpi ulnaris tendon. There have been reports of anomalous insertions of the abductor pollicis longus and flexor carpi radialis tendons into the trapezium. The abductor and flexor pollicis brevis originate from the trapezium, whereas the abductor and flexor digiti minimi originate from the pisiform. The origin of the opponens digiti minimi from the hook of the hamate is variable.

17. Is there normally substantial motion between the bones of the distal carpal row?

Kinematic studies, which define motions without reference to force, have demonstrated negligible motion between the bones of the distal row because of the heavy investment of interconnecting ligaments. Between each bone are strong, transversely oriented palmar and dorsal interosseous ligaments. In addition, deep interosseous ligaments connect the trapezoid to the capitate and the capitate to the hamate. Disruptions of these ligaments result from high-energy trauma, typically with substantial additional soft tissue disruption, and are termed axial instabilities.

18. Is it normally possible for the lunate to articulate with the hamate?

Viegas has demonstrated two broad categories of architecture of the distal surface of the lunate. The type I lunate, which occurs in 66% of normal wrists, has no appreciable articulation with the hamate. Rather, the distal surface of the lunate articulates solely with the head of the capitate. The type II lunate, which occurs in the remaining 33% of normal wrists, has a distinct sagittal ridge with an ulnar-sided fossa for articulation with the proximal surface of the hamate. Type II lunates have a distinct predilection to develop degenerative changes in the hamate fossa as well as accompanying degenerative changes on the proximal surface of the hamate.

19. Describe the dorsal capsular ligaments of the wrist.

The dorsal capsule of the wrist is reinforced with two major ligaments, the dorsal radiocarpal and dorsal intercarpal ligaments. In the regions between the two ligaments, the joint capsule is devoid of ligament tissue. The dorsal intercarpal (DIC) ligament connects the trapezoid and scaphoid with the triquetrum, whereas the dorsal radiocarpal (DRC) ligament connects the radius, lunate, and triquetrum. The DIC and DRC ligaments share an insertion on the dorsal cortex of the triquetrum. Proximally, the dorsal radioulnar (DRU) ligament originates adjacent to the radial attachment of the DRC but is not considered a wrist ligament per se. The anatomic arrangement of the dorsal ligaments has been put to use by introducing a fiber-splitting capsulotomy, based on their orientation. This concept promises several advantages, including minimizing scar and stiffness, enhancing visualization and accuracy in orientation, and maintaining stability when it is necessary to enter the wrist from the dorsal side. The DIC and DRC ligaments can be safely bisected, creating a radially based flap that can be extended even further by dividing the radiocarpal joint capsule from the radius to the level of the radial styloid process. This exposes the radial two-thirds of the radiocarpal joint and virtually the entire midcarpal joint. To expose the ulnar one-third of the ulnocarpal joint, the DRC ligament can be bisected and connected to a capsular incision paralleling the fifth extensor compartment creating a proximally based flap.

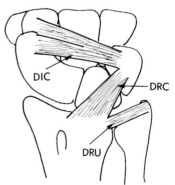

Dorsal view of the wrist illustrating the dorsal capsule ligaments. DRU=dorsal radioulnar ligament, DRC=dorsal radiocarpal ligament, DIC=dorsal intercarpal ligament.

20. What is carpal height ratio? How is it determined?

Carpal height refers to the longitudinal length of the carpus from the distal articular surface of the radius to the distal articular surface of the capitate. It is a useful concept clinically because malrotation of the proximal carpal row bones, from problems such as rheumatoid arthritis, scapholunate dissociation, and scaphoid nonunions, may result in shortening of the carpal height. Detection of such shortening helps to classify the severity of the wrist abnormality. The problem with carpal height as a dimensional measure lies in the variability of wrist sizes, presumably proportionate to the size of the individual. In an attempt to bypass this variability, the concept of **carpal height ratio** nondimensionalizes the carpal height. In the classic method, the length of the carpus is defined along the projected axis of the third metacarpal, measured from the base of the third metacarpal to the point at which the projected third metacarpal axis intersects the distal surface of the radius. This measurement is then divided by the length of the third metacarpal, also defined along the axis of the third metacarpal. The normal values for the carpal height ratio are 0.054 ± 0.03. This measurement must be made from a standard PA radiograph with the wrist in a neutral position and the entire length of the third metacarpal visible.

Because the third metacarpal is not consistently imaged on standard wrist radiographs, an alternate method for determining the carpal height ratio was developed. The denominator is the greatest length of the capitate, as determined from a standard PA radiograph. The carpal height measurement is made in the same manner as the standard carpal height ratio. Using the alternate method, the normal range of the revised carpal height ratio is 1.57 ± 0.05.

BIBLIOGRAPHY

1. Amadio PC, Berquist TH, Smith DK, et al: Scaphoid malunion. J Hand Surg 14A:679–687, 1989.
2. Berger RA, Crowninshield RD, Flatt AE: The three-dimensional rotational behaviors of the carpal bones. Clin Orthop 167:303–310, 1982.
3. Berger RA, Kauer JMG, Landsmeer JMF: The radioscapholunate ligament: A gross anatomic and histologic study of fetal and adult wrists. J Hand Surg 16A:350–355, 1991.
4. Berger RA: The gross and histologic anatomy of the scapholunate interosseous ligament. J Hand Surg 21A:170–178, 1996.
5. Berger RA, Bishop AT, Bettinger PC: A new dorsal capsulotomy for the surgical exposure of the wrist. Ann Plast Surg 35:54–59, 1995.
6. Cooney WP, Linscheid RL, Dobyns JH (eds): The Wrist: Diagnosis and Operative Treatment. St. Louis, Mosby, 1998.
7. Gelberman RH, Bauman TD, Menon J: The vascularity of the lunate bone and Kienböck's disease. J Hand Surg 5:272–278, 1980.
8. Gelberman RH, Menon J: The vascularity of the scaphoid bone. J Hand Surg 5:508–513, 1980.
9. Jiranek WA, Ruby LK, Millender LB, et al: Long-term results after Russe bone-grafting: The effect of malunion of the scaphoid. J Bone Joint Surg 74A:1217–1228, 1992.
10. Linscheid RL, Dobyns JH, Beabout JW, Bryan RS: Traumatic instability of the wrist: Diagnosis, classification and pathomechanics. J Bone Joint Surg 54A:1612–1632, 1972.
11. Nattrass GR, King GJ, McMurtry RY, Brant RF: An alternative method for determination of the carpal height ratio. J Bone Joint Surg 76A:88–94, 1994.
12. Palmer AK, Werner FW: The triangular fibrocartilage complex of the wrist: Anatomy and function. J Hand Surg 6:153–161, 1981.
13. Palmer AK, Werner FW: Biomechanics of the distal radioulnar joint. Clin Orthop 187:26–34, 1984.
14. Panagis JS, Gelberman RH, Taleisnik J, Baumgaertner M: The arterial anatomy of the human carpus. Part II: The intraosseous vascularity. J Hand Surg 8:375–382, 1983.
15. Sheetz KK, Bishop AT, Berger RA: The arterial blood supply of the distal radius and ulna and its potential use in vascularized pedicled bone grafts. J Hand Surg 20A:902–914, 1995.
16. Tountas CP, Bergman RA: Anatomic Variations of the Upper Extremity. New York, Churchill Livingstone, 1993.
17. Viegas SF, Wagner K, Patterson RM, Patterson R: Medial (hamate) facet of the lunate. J Hand Surg 15A:564–571, 1990.
18. Youm Y, McMurtry RY, Flatt AE, Gillespie TE: Kinematics of the wrist. I: An experimental study of radioulnar deviation and flexion-extension. J Bone Joint Surg 60A:423–431, 1978.

114. PHYSICAL EXAMINATION OF THE WRIST

Jeffrey Weinzweig, M.D., and H. Kirk Watson, M.D.

1. What constitutes the first part of every thorough physical examination?

A thorough history. Information about the patient's age, handedness, chief complaint, occupation, avocational activities, previous wrist injury or surgery, exact onset of symptoms and their relationship to specific activities, frequency and duration of postactivity ache, factors that exacerbate or improve symptoms, subjective loss of wrist motion, current work status, and, certainly, worker's compensation status complement findings noted during the physical examination and aid in deriving a diagnosis.

2. Is it necessary to assess the range of motion of the wrist?

Absolutely. Every examination should begin with an evaluation of passive and active range of motion of both wrists. With the patient's elbows resting on the exam table, an assessment of flexion and extension is performed. Any loss of passive motion compared with the contralateral, asymptomatic wrist is usually a sign of underlying carpal pathology. A bilateral assessment of pronation and supination is made with the examiner's hands rotating the patient's wrists from the midforearm level. Full forced pronosupination without pain eliminates the distal radioulnar joint (DRUJ) and triangular fibrocartilage complex (TFCC) as potential sources of the patient's symptoms. Degenerative joint disease (DJD) or dislocation of the DRUJ or a substantial tear of the TFCC results in pain and diminished pronosupination.

RADIAL WRIST EXAMINATION

3. Which carpal bone is involved in more than 95% of all cases of degenerative joint disease of the wrist?

The scaphoid. Periscaphoid arthritic changes involve the scapholunate advanced collapse (SLAC) pattern in 57%, the triscaphe (scaphotrapeziotrapezoid) joint in 27%, and a combination of these in 14%. The scaphoid is also involved in the etiopathogenesis of over 90% of all ganglia.

4. Which aspect of the wrist, radial or ulnar, is involved in the majority of carpal pathology?

The majority of carpal pathology involves the radial aspect of the wrist. Although ulnar wrist pain often presents a more complex diagnostic problem than radial wrist pathology, fortunately it is less common in the typical practice.

5. How many maneuvers does the radial wrist exam include? Name them.

The examination of the radial wrist consists of five maneuvers:

1. Dorsal wrist syndrome (DWS) test
2. Finger extension test (FET)
3. Articular/nonarticular (ANA) test
4. Scaphotrapeziotrapezoid (STT) test
5. Scaphoid shift maneuver (SSM)

None of these maneuvers is necessarily diagnostic by itself, nor is it intended to be. However, a diagnosis usually can be derived by assimilating the entire picture of wrist mechanics and pathomechanics with the history, symptoms, and appropriate radiographic examination.

6. Which maneuver directly examines the scapholunate (SL) joint?

The DWS test. Identification of the SL joint is facilitated by following the course of the third metacarpal proximally until the examiner's thumb falls into a recess that lies over the capitate. The SL articulation is readily palpable just proximal between the extensor carpi radialis brevis and the extensors of the fourth compartment. A normal joint produces no pain with palpation. SL dissociation, Kienböck's disease, dorsal wrist syndrome (i.e., SL joint overloading with wrist pain secondary to SL ligamentous synovitis and/or tear preceding evidence of rotary subluxation of the scaphoid), or other pathology involving the SL or radiolunate joints or the lunate itself elicits pain with direct palpation.

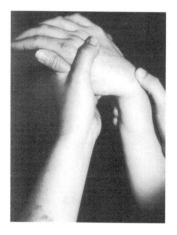

Dorsal wrist syndrome (DWS) of the scapholunate (SL) joint. Identification of the SL joint is facilitated by following the course of the third metacarpal proximally until the examiner's thumb falls into a recess. The SL articulation is readily palpable between the carpi radialis brevis and the extensors of the fourth compartment. (From Watson HK, Weinzweig J: Physical examination of the wrist. Hand Clin 13:20, 1997, with permission.)

7. Which maneuver indirectly examines the wrist with exceptional sensitivity?

The FET. The increased mechanical advantage on carpal loading during the FET produces a reliable indicator of carpal pathology. With the patient's wrist held passively in flexion, the examiner resists active finger extension. In patients with significant periscaphoid inflammatory change, radiocarpal or midcarpal instability, symptomatic rotary subluxation of the scaphoid, or Kienböck's disease, the combined radiocarpal loading and pressure of the extensor tendons cause considerable discomfort. In our experience, such patients always demonstrate a positive FET. The FET has become a highly reliable indicator of problems at the SL joint. Full-power finger extension against resistance (i.e., a negative FET) eliminates the common dorsal wrist syndrome diagnosis as well as rotary subluxation of the scaphoid, Kienböck's disease, and SLAC wrist.

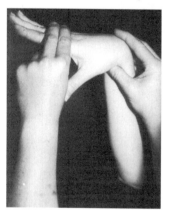

Finger extension test (FET). With the patient's wrist held passively in flexion, the examiner resists active finger extension. (From Watson HK, Weinzweig J: Physical examination of the wrist. Hand Clin 13:24, 1997, with permission.)

8. Which maneuver specifically assesses synovitis of the scaphoid?

The ANA maneuver. The proximal pole of the scaphoid articulates with the radius as the radiocarpal joint. The articular surface of the proximal scaphoid continues distally toward a junctional point along the radial aspect, where the surface changes from articular to nonarticular. With the wrist in radial deviation, the ANA junction is obscured by the radial styloid. With the wrist in ulnar deviation, the ANA junction is easily palpated just distal to the radial styloid. The ANA maneuver is performed with the examiner's index finger firmly palpating the radial aspect of the patient's wrist just distal to the radial styloid with the wrist initially in radial deviation. Pressure is maintained as the patient's wrist is brought into ulnar deviation with the examiner's other hand. The normal asymptomatic wrist demonstrates mild-to-moderate tenderness and discomfort at the ANA junction with direct palpation in almost every person. However, the patient with periscaphoid synovitis, scaphoid instability, or SLAC changes at the styloid experiences severe pain with this maneuver. For purposes of comparison, it is necessary to perform the maneuver bilaterally.

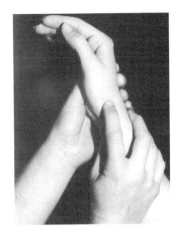

Articular/nonarticular (ANA) junction of the scaphoid. With the wrist in ulnar deviation, the ANA junction is easily palpated just distal to the radial styloid. The ANA maneuver is performed with the examiner's index finger firmly palpating the radial aspect of the patient's wrist just distal to the radial styloid with the wrist initially in radial deviation. Pressure is maintained as the patient's wrist is brought into ulnar deviation with the examiner's other hand. (From Watson HK, Weinzweig J: Physical examination of the wrist. Hand Clin 13:19, 1997, with permission.)

9. Which maneuver directly assesses the STT joint?

The STT test. Identification of the STT or triscaphe joint is facilitated by following the course of the second metacarpal proximally until the examiner's thumb falls into a recess. That recess is the triscaphe joint. A normal joint produces no pain with palpation. Triscaphe synovitis, degenerative disease, or other pathology involving the joint or scaphoid elicits pain with direct palpation.

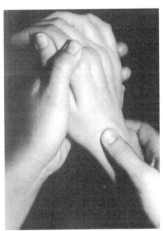

Scaphotrapeziotrapezoid (STT) or triscaphe joint. Identification of the triscaphe joint is facilitated by following the course of the second metacarpal proximally until the examiner's thumb falls into a recess, just ulnar to the anatomic snuffbox. (From Watson HK, Weinzweig J: Physical examination of the wrist. Hand Clin 13:20, 1997, with permission.)

10. Which maneuver assesses the pathomechanics of the scaphoid?

The SSM, which provides qualitative assessment of scaphoid stability and periscaphoid synovitis compared with the contralateral asymptomatic wrist. We do not refer to the SSM as a "test" or to the findings of increased pain or ligamentous laxity as a "positive scaphoid shift." Instead, laxity or discomfort with the SSM does not necessarily indicate pathology; however, asymmetric laxity that reproduces the patient's characteristic pain is indicative of pathology. This exam, therefore, is meaningful only when performed bilaterally.

11. How is the scaphoid shift maneuver performed?

With the patient's forearm slightly pronated, the examiner grasps the patient's wrist from the radial side with the examiner's same-sided hand (e.g., the examiner's right hand is used to examine the patient's right hand) and places the thumb on the palmar prominence of the patient's scaphoid while wrapping the fingers around the patient's distal radius. This position enables the thumb to push on the scaphoid with counterpressure provided by the fingers. The examiner's other hand grasps the patient's hand at the metacarpal level to control wrist position. Starting in ulnar deviation and slight extension, the wrist is moved radially and slightly flexed with constant thumb pressure on the scaphoid.

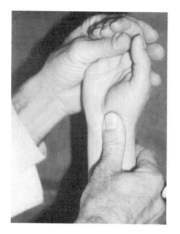

Scaphoid shift maneuver (SSM). The examiner grasps the patient's wrist from the radial side and places the thumb on the palmar prominence of the patient's scaphoid while wrapping the fingers around the patient's distal radius. This position enables the thumb to push on the scaphoid with counterpressure provided by the fingers. The examiner's other hand grasps the patient's hand at the metacarpal level to control wrist position. Starting in ulnar deviation and slight extension, the wrist is moved radially and slightly flexed with constant thumb pressure on the scaphoid. (From Watson HK, Weinzweig J: Physical examination of the wrist. Hand Clin 13:21, 1997, with permission.)

12. Explain the biomechanical mechanism of the scaphoid shift maneuver.

When the wrist is in ulnar deviation, the scaphoid axis is extended and lies nearly in line with the long axis of the forearm. As the wrist deviates radially and flexes, the scaphoid also flexes and rotates to an orientation more nearly perpendicular to the forearm, and its distal pole becomes prominent on the palmar side of the wrist. The examiner's thumb pressure opposes this normal rotation and creates a subluxation stress, causing the scaphoid to shift dorsally in relation to the other bones of the carpus. This scaphoid shift may be subtle or dramatic. In patients with rigid periscaphoid ligamentous support, only minimal shift is tolerated before the scaphoid continues to rotate normally, pushing the examiner's thumb out of the way. In patients with ligamentous laxity, the combined stresses of thumb pressure and normal motion of adjacent carpus may be sufficient to force the scaphoid out of its elliptical fossa and onto the dorsal rim of the radius. As thumb pressure is withdrawn, the scaphoid returns abruptly to its normal position, sometimes with a resounding thunk.

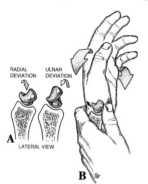

Mechanism of scaphoid shift. *A,* Relationship of the scaphoid and radius as seen in a lateral view. In ulnar deviation the scaphoid dorsiflexes, and its long axis lies nearly in line with the axis of the radius. In radial deviation the scaphoid volar flexes; its long axis lies nearly perpendicular to the axis of the wrist, and its distal pole becomes prominent on the palmar side of the wrist. *B,* During the scaphoid shift maneuver, the examiner's thumb prevents the normal palmar tilt of the scaphoid. (From Watson HK, Weinzweig J: Intercarpal arthrodesis. In Green DP (ed): Operative Hand Surgery, 4th ed. New York, Churchill Livingstone, in press, with permission.)

13. What is the clinical significance of the scaphoid shift maneuver?

The scaphoid may shift smoothly and painlessly or with a gritty sensation or clicking, accompanied by pain. Grittiness suggests chondromalacia or loss of articular cartilage, and clicking may indicate bony change sufficient to produce impingement. Pain is a significant finding, especially when it reproduces the patient's symptoms. Pain associated with unilateral hypermobility of the scaphoid is virtually diagnostic of rotary subluxation. A less well-localized pain associated with normal or decreased mobility is encountered in patients with periscaphoid arthritis, whether of triscaphe or SLAC pattern.

14. What percentage of normal asymptomatic people have an abnormal scaphoid shift?

Of 1000 normal asymptomatic people, 209 demonstrated a unilateral abnormal scaphoid shift maneuver with hypermobility of the scaphoid and/or pain. This finding, which represents 21% of examined people and 10% of examined wrists, stresses the importance of performing the maneuver bilaterally.

ULNAR WRIST PAIN

15. How do you examine a patient with ulnar wrist pain?

Ulnar wrist pain is a complex problem requiring a keen understanding of both intraarticular and extraarticular anatomy of the region. Distinguishing between abnormalities involving the distal radioulnar joint (DRUJ), triangular fibrocartilage complex (TFCC), and ulnar carpus necessitates discerning soft tissue problems from bony ones. Each region of the ulnar wrist must be systematically addressed during a thorough physical examination.

16. How can you rule out pathology involving the DRUJ?

An abnormality of the DRUJ, such as degenerative disease or subluxation, should be immediately suspected on the basis of decreased or painful pronosupination. With the patient's hand in full ulnar deviation, significant pain elicited by pressing on the ulnar head by the examiner's thumb is suggestive of DRUJ pathology. Pain produced during pronosupination while the ulnar head is pressed volarward and the pisiform pressed dorsally is often indicative of an ulnar impingement or impaction syndrome.

17. How can you diagnose a TFCC injury or tear on physical exam?

The diagnosis of a TFCC tear or injury is by exclusion. It is difficult, if not impossible, to confirm the diagnosis on the basis of physical examination alone. Other more common causes of ulnar wrist pain, such as DJD and carpal instability, must first be excluded. Examination may demonstrate loss of forearm pronosupination and wrist motion, tenderness over the TFCC dorsally, and a palpable and/or audible click with forearm rotation or radioulnar deviation of the wrist. Suspicion of TFCC pathology requires evaluation by three-compartment wrist arthrography. The presence of a radiocarpal-DRUJ arthrographic communication is pathognomonic of a TFCC perforation. However, perforations are common and do not necessarily indicate pathology.

18. What is the ulnar snuffbox?

The ulnar snuffbox is the depression palpated immediately beyond the ulnar styloid. This space is circumscribed by the ECU and FCU tendons, which run posteriorly and anteriorly, respectively, over the ulna at the wrist. In radial deviation, the floor of the depression is formed by the triquetrum; in ulnar deviation, the floor is formed by the joint between the triquetrum and hamate.

19. What is the lunotriquetral (LT) compression test?

The LT compression test directs load across the LT joint along an ulnoradial axis by palpating within the ulnar snuffbox. Direct pressure in this area elicits pain from a patient with LT joint instability, synovitis, degenerative disease, or partial synchondrosis.

20. What are ballottement tests? How can they assess LT instability?

Ballottement tests, or shear tests, demonstrate joint instability by exerting pressure in opposite directions on adjacent carpal bones. Instability of the LT joint can be demonstrated by **Reagan's test**. The examiner's thumb is used to apply pressure on the patient's lunate dorsally while the examiner's index finger applies pressure on the triquetrum volarly. **Masquelet's test** is another ballottement test of the LT joint in which the examiner uses both hands to apply shear force across the articulation. The examiner's thumbs are used to apply dorsal pressure to the lunate and triquetrum while counterpressure is applied to these bones volarly by the examiner's index fingers.

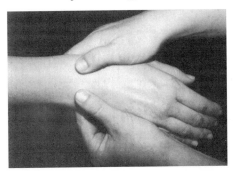

Masquelet's test of lunotriquetral (LT) instability. The examiner uses both hands to apply shear force across the LT joint. The examiner's thumbs are used to apply dorsal pressure to the lunate and triquetrum while counterpressure is applied to these bones volarly by the examiner's index fingers. (From Watson HK, Weinzweig J: Physical examination of the wrist. Hand Clin 13:25, 1997, with permission.)

21. What is TILT? How can it be diagnosed?

A new etiology for ulnar wrist pain that specifically involves the triquetrum has recently been described. The triad of localized triquetral pain along the proximal ulnar slope of the bone, a history of a hyperflexion injury, and normal radiographs is diagnostic of TILT—triquetral impingement ligament tear. The mechanism of TILT involves a cuff of fibrous tissue that has become detached from the ulnar sling mechanism and chronically impinges on the triquetrum, resulting in synovitis, bony eburnation, and pain. Point tenderness can be appreciated by palpating the ulnar aspect of the triquetrum just distal to the ulnar styloid.

RADIOCARPAL AND MIDCARPAL JOINTS

22. How can instability of the radiocarpal or midcarpal joint be evaluated?

The **anteroposterior drawer test** can be used to evaluate instability of either the radiocarpal or midcarpal joints. One of the examiner's hands holds the patient's hand by the metacarpals to apply axial traction while the other hand stabilizes the patient's forearm. While traction is maintained, anteroposterior force is applied and a drawer is elicited first at the radiocarpal and then at the midcarpal joint.

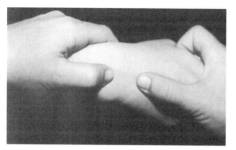

The anteroposterior drawer test of radiocarpal or midcarpal instability. One of the examiner's hands holds the patient's hand by the metacarpals to apply axial traction while the other hand stabilizes the patient's forearm. While maintaining traction, anteroposterior force is applied and a drawer is elicited at the radiocarpal and the midcarpal joint. (From Watson HK, Weinzweig J: Physical examination of the wrist. Hand Clin 13:27, 1997, with permission.)

23. What is the pivot shift test?

The pivot shift test of the midcarpal joint consists of supinating and volar subluxing the distal row of the carpus. With the patient's elbow at 90°, the hand is placed in a fully supinated position while the distal forearm is held firmly. The wrist is maintained in a neutral position while the hand is moved into full radial deviation. The ulnar side of the carpus is forced into further supination and a volar subluxed position. At this point, the hand is moved from radial to full ulnar deviation. Midcarpal instability secondary to excessive ligamentous laxity or rupture allows the capitate to sublux volarly from the lunocapitate fossa during this maneuver.

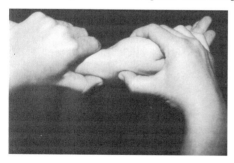

The pivot shift test of midcarpal instability. This maneuver consists of supinating and subluxing volarly the distal row of the carpus. With the patient's elbow at 90°, the hand is placed in a fully supinated position while the distal forearm is held firmly. The wrist is maintained in a neutral position while the hand is moved into full radial deviation. The ulnar side of the carpus is forced into further supination and a volarly subluxed position. (From Watson HK, Weinzweig J: Physical examination of the wrist. Hand Clin 13:27, 1997, with permission.)

CARPOMETACARPAL JOINT

24. Do all five carpometacarpal (CMC) joints demonstrate equal motion?

Absolutely not. The CMC joints link the digital rays with the carpus. The normal hand has no clinically detectable mobility at the second and third CMC joints and only several degrees of motion at the fourth CMC joint, which are functionally negligible. The fifth CMC joint has approximately 20° of motion, which permit functional adaptation to the transverse arch of the palm.

25. Which is the most important of the CMC joints?

The first CMC (trapeziometacarpal) joint is functionally the most important joint of the thumb ray because it allows movement of the entire column of the thumb. Movements of this joint are quite complex, involving multiplanar motion that includes anteposition, retroposition, adduction, and abduction.

26. Degenerative joint disease most commonly involves which CMC joint?

Although degenerative disease may involve any of the five CMC joints secondary to arthritis or trauma, the first CMC joint of the thumb is most commonly involved.

27. What three tests are used to examine the first CMC joint?

1. **Grind test.** The examiner places the thumb and index finger of one hand on either side of the patient's CMC joint. While the metacarpal is held with the examiner's other hand, the CMC joint is axially loaded. The examiner's first hand then moves the metacarpal base laterally in several directions. Symptoms are exacerbated, grating and chondromalacia are palpated, and the quality of cartilage is determined.

2. **Adduction test.** The examiner's thumb is placed on the midportion of the patient's first metacarpal while the fingers are placed along the length of the fifth metacarpal. The first and fifth metacarpals are then passively adducted toward each other with gentle pressure.

3. **Abduction test.** The patient's hand is positioned flat with the palm facing upward. The examiner's index and middle fingers are placed on the volar aspect of the phalanges or metacarpal of the patient's thumb as the thumb metacarpal is passively abducted into the plane of the finger metacarpals.

28. What is the carpal boss?

The carpal boss represents a partial or complete coalition or synchondrosis of the second and third CMC joints. This anomaly is usually asymptomatic but may result in pain secondary to localized degenerative arthritis.

29. How can you diagnose a carpal boss on examination?

Examination involves malalignment of the second and third metacarpals. The examiner grasps the heads of these bones with the thumb and index fingers of each hand and simultaneously shifts one metacarpal head volarly and the other dorsally. Pain with this maneuver is highly suggestive of a carpal boss.

EXTRAARTICULAR CAUSES OF WRIST PAIN

30. What is Finkelstein's test?

Stenosing tenosynovitis of the first dorsal compartment, also known as de Quervain's disease, is a common cause of wrist and hand pain, involving the abductor pollicis longus (APL) and extensor pollicis brevis (EPB) sheaths at the radial styloid process. The findings of local tenderness and moderate swelling of the extensor retinaculum of the wrist over the first dorsal compartment and a positive Finkelstein's test confirm the diagnosis. This test is performed by having the patient grasp his or her own thumb within the ipsilateral palm. Moderate-to-severe pain is elicited as the patient's wrist is brought from radial deviation into extreme ulnar deviation.

31. What is a "wet leather" sign?

Crepitus with tendon movement, suggestive of an inflammation-induced change in the synovium or synovitis, is known as a wet leather sign.

32. How can you evaluate a problem involving the sheath of the ECU?

The ECU sheath extends from the ECU groove on the ulnar head to the dorsal base of the fifth metacarpal. Conditions such as ECU synovitis or tendinitis, subluxation, stenosis, and partial rupture result in pain on direct palpation of the tendon at the level of, or just distal to, the ulnar head with the wrist in ulnar deviation.

33. How can you diagnose a fracture or degenerative disease of the pisiform?

Pisiform fractures are uncommon, representing approximately 1% of all carpal bone fractures. Diagnosis is often overlooked because roughly 50% of all pisiform fractures are associated with more severe upper extremity injuries. In addition, pisiform fractures are missed because they are difficult to see on routine radiographs of the wrist. Subpisiform degenerative joint disease, usually secondary to delayed diagnosis of pisiform fractures or untreated injuries, is another infrequent etiology of ulnar wrist pain. Examination of the pisiform is performed quite easily by loading the subpisiform joint laterally as with the thumb CMC joint.

34. How can you diagnose an injury or fracture of the hook of the hamate?

Pain secondary to an acute fracture or nonunion of the hook of the hamate may be an elusive cause of wrist pain. Examination of the hook of the hamate is performed by deep palpation over the tip of the hamular process in the palm by the examiner's thumb and by pressure on the dorsal ulnar aspect of the same bone with the examiner's index and middle fingers. The hook is easily located by first placing one's thumb on the volar pisiform. Movement approximately 2 cm along a line connecting the pisiform to the head of the second metacarpal (45° angle) locates the hamular process.

35. How can you diagnose flexor carpi radialis (FCR) tendinitis?

FCR tendinitis, often seen in laborers who perform repetitive wrist motions, may cause pain over the flexor aspect of the wrist. On examination, pain is elicited by palpating over the osteofibrous FCR tunnel, which begins approximately 3 cm proximal to the wrist and extends to the main insertion of the FCR on the base of the second metacarpal. In our experience, the region of greatest acute tenderness is an area less than 1 cm in diameter centered where the FCR tendon enters the trapezium tunnel at the level of the wrist crease. Pain usually increases with resisted wrist flexion and resisted radial deviation of the wrist.

36. What is intersection syndrome? How can it be diagnosed on examination?

Pain and swelling of the muscle bellies of the APL and EPB in the area where they cross the common radial wrist extensors are characteristic of intersection syndrome. This area is approximately 4 cm proximal to the radiocarpal joint. With severe cases, swelling, redness, and crepitus may be found. Examination of the region with gentle palpation elicits marked tenderness. Tenosynovitis of the second dorsal compartment is the cause of this disorder, which occurs less commonly than de Quervain's disease and must be differentiated from it.

37. What are substitution maneuvers?

Fictitious complaints presented for secondary gain can be difficult to distinguish from actual symptoms. To do so, it is necessary to incorporate within the physical examination a number of substitution or distraction maneuvers. These maneuvers take advantage of the clinician's knowledge of wrist anatomy and biomechanics as well as the patient's ignorance. Two of our own substitution maneuvers are presented below. However, even more important than any of these maneuvers is understanding why they are so useful. With that understanding, a myriad of additional substitution maneuvers can be devised.

1. **ANA substitution maneuver.** With the wrist in radial deviation, the ANA junction is obscured by the radial styloid, and no amount of thumb pressure in this region results in pain. With the patient distracted, the wrist is gradually brought into ulnar deviation while the pressure is constantly applied. Only in ulnar deviation, with the ANA junction exposed to thumb pressure, should pain be elicited. Pain described while the wrist is in radial deviation should be noted as a positive substitution maneuver.

2. **Flexor pollicis longus (FPL) substitution maneuver.** A patient attempting to feign hand or wrist weakness will do so without knowledge of muscular innervation patterns. This becomes extremely important during examination for carpal tunnel syndrome, in which the application of a substitution maneuver can be used to assess weakness of the thenar muscles. Such thenar weakness is secondary to compression of the motor branch of the median nerve. The FPL, which is innervated by the anterior interosseous branch of the median nerve, is completely unaffected in the worst case of carpal tunnel syndrome or virtually any wrist disorder. In the cooperative patient it is all but impossible to overcome a fully flexed FPL. Thus, FPL weakness in any patient, other than one with anterior interosseous syndrome, should alert the examiner.

BIBLIOGRAPHY

1. Bottke CA, Louis DS, Braunstein EM: Diagnosis and treatment of obscure ulnar-sided wrist pain. Orthopedics 12:1075–1079, 1989.
2. Brown DE, Lichtman DM: The evaluation of chronic wrist pain. Orthop Clin North Am 15:183–192, 1984.
3. Cuono CB, Watson HK, Masquelet AC: The carpal boss: Surgical treatment and etiological considerations. Plast Reconstr Surg 63:88–93, 1979.
4. Kleinman W: The ballottement test. ASSH Correspondence Newsletter, no. 51, 1985.
5. Pin PG, Young VL, Gilula LA, Weeks PM: Wrist pain: A systemic approach to diagnosis. Plast Reconstr Surg 85:42–46, 1990.
6. Reagan DS, Linscheid RL, Dobyns JH: Lunotriquetral sprains. J Hand Surg 9A:502–514, 1984.
7. Stark HH, Jobe FW, Boyes JH, et al: Fracture of the hook of the hamate in athletes. J Bone Joint Surg 59A:575–582, 1977.
8. Tubiana R, Thomine JM, Mackin E: Examination of the Hand and Wrist. St. Louis, Mosby, 1995.
9. Watson HK, Ashmead D, Makhlouf MV: Examination of the scaphoid. J Hand Surg 13A:657–660, 1988.
10. Watson HK, Ottoni L, Pitts EC, et al: Rotary subluxation of the scaphoid: A spectrum of instability. J Hand Surg 18B:62–63, 1993.
11. Watson HK, Weinzweig J: Physical examination of the wrist. Hand Clinics 13:17–34, 1997.
12. Watson HK, Weinzweig J, Zeppieri J: The natural progression of scaphoid instability. Hand Clin 13:39–50, 1997.
13. Watson HK, Weinzweig J: Intercarpal arthrodesis. In Green DP (ed): Operative Hand Surgery, 4th ed. New York, Churchill Livingstone [in press].
14. Weinzweig J, Watson HK: Triquetral impingement ligament tear [TILT] syndrome. J Hand Surg 21B:36, 1996.
15. Weinzweig J, Watson HK: Examination of the wrist. In Watson HK, Weinzweig J (eds): The Wrist. Philadelhia, Lippincott-Raven (in press).

115. RADIOLOGIC EXAMINATION OF THE WRIST

Viktor M. Metz, M.D., and Louis A. Gilula, M.D.

1. How should the standard posteroanterior (PA) radiogram for examination of the wrist be obtained?

The standard PA view should be obtained with the elbow flexed 90° and the shoulder abducted 90°. The hand (not the wrist) is placed palm flat on the cassette (with no flexion, extension, or deviation). The central beam is perpendicular to the cassette and is centered over the capitate head.

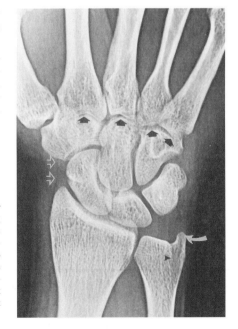

Standard neutral PA view of the wrist showing collinear alignment of the axis of the third metacarpal shaft with the mid axis of the radius. The ulnar styloid process *(curved white arrow)* is projected most ulnar. The extensor carpi ulnaris (ECU) groove *(arrowhead)* is radial to the base of the ulnar styloid. There is parallelism of the articular surfaces of the second through the fifth carpometacarpal joints *(black thick arrows)*, indicating that the palm is flat on the x-ray cassette. The scaphoid fat pad *(open arrows)* is evident on this PA view.

2. What criteria identify an adequate PA view?

1. The third metacarpal shaft has collinear alignment with the mid axis of the radius (indicating the absence of radial or ulnar deviation).

2. The extensor carpi ulnaris groove projects radial to the midpoint of the ulnar styloid (indicating that the elbow is at shoulder height).

3. The second through fifth carpometacarpal joints should be evident by recognizing parallel articular cortices at these joints. Lack of profile of these joints is caused by extension of the wrist or flexion at the MP joints.

3. Why is it important to obtain adequate PA views of the wrist?

Ulnar variance measurements should not be made on a PA view of the wrist that does not meet the above criteria because adducting the elbow toward the patient's side usually makes the ulna more positive (longer in length than the adjacent radius).

4. How should the standard lateral view of the wrist be obtained?

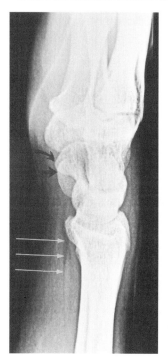

The standard lateral view should be obtained with the elbow flexed 90° and adducted against the trunk. The central beam is perpendicular to the cassette and is centered over the head of the capitate. If the lateral view is performed correctly, the palmar surface of the pisiform bone is located between the ventral cortex of the head of the capitate and the ventral cortex of the distal pole of the scaphoid. This is termed the scaphopisocapitate (SPC) relationship.

Standard lateral radiograph of the wrist. The palmar surface of the pisiform bone *(straight black arrow)* is projected 2 mm dorsal to the distal ventral pole of the scaphoid *(curved black arrow)*. The pronator quadratus fat pad *(long white arrows)* is seen on the lateral view and is straight.

5. What does the scaphoid bone do on a PA view obtained in ulnar deviation?

The scaphoid elongates because it tilts dorsally. In this view the long axis of the scaphoid is seen much better than in the neutral PA view. This view is particularly helpful for detection of scaphoid fractures because the scaphoid waist is more in profile.

6. What are the pronator quadratus and the scaphoid fat pads? What is their importance?

The pronator quadratus fat pad, seen on the lateral radiograph in question 4, lies between the pronator quadratus muscle and the volar flexor tendon sheaths. The scaphoid fat pad (see figure in question 1) lies between the radial collateral ligament and the abductor pollicis longus tendon. These fat pats are disturbed in trauma and may suggest occult fractures. The fat pads are abnormal when they are bowed (convex) away from the adjacent bones.

7. What is a Colles' fracture?

A Colles' fracture is a fracture of the distal radial epiphyseal or metaphyseal area with the distal fracture fragment displaced or angulated in the dorsal direction. The fracture may occur with or without intraarticular involvement. It is the most common fracture of the distal radius and occurs most often in older patients. The mechanism of injury is a fall on the dorsiflexed hand.

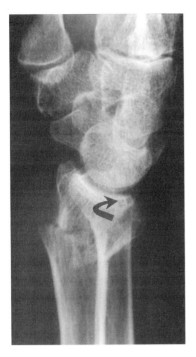

Typical Colles' fracture of the distal radius with the distal fracture fragment angulated in the dorsal direction *(arrow)*.

8. How are Colles' fractures classified?

There are several different classification schemes for distal radius fractures. The classification of Colles' fractures by Frykman has gained wide acceptance in some areas of the world. Frykman divides the fractures into eight types based on the presence of intraarticular involvement of either the radiocarpal or the distal radioulnar joint and the presence or absence of an associated fracture of the ulnar styloid.

9. What is a Smith's fracture?

A Smith's fracture is a fracture of the distal radial epiphyseal or metaphyseal area with the distal fracture fragment displaced or angulated in the volar direction. Like a Colles' fracture, a Smith's fracture may occur with or without intraarticular involvement and with or without an associated fracture of the ulnar styloid. The common mechanism of injury is a fall on the volar flexed wrist.

10. What is the definition of a Barton's fracture?

A Barton's fracture is defined as an intraarticular fracture of the posterior or anterior (reverse Barton's fracture) rim of the distal radius with (in contrast to Smith's and Colles' fractures) accompanying palmar or dorsal displacement of the carpus with the radius fragment, respectively.

11. What is a fracture of the radial styloid process called?

A fracture of the radial styloid process is called a chauffeur's fracture (eponym: Hutchinson's fracture). It is an intraarticular fracture in which the fracture line usually runs through the junction of the scaphoid and lunate fossae of the radius and courses radially in an oblique direction. The mechanism of injury is axial compression of the scaphoid bone against the radial styloid.

12. What is the most frequently fractured carpal bone?

The most frequently fractured carpal bone is the scaphoid. Scaphoid fractures account for 60–70% of all carpal injuries; 70% are located in the waist of the scaphoid, 20% are located in the proximal pole, and 10% involve the distal pole.

13. What are the complications of scaphoid fractures?

Complications of scaphoid fractures include delayed union, nonunion, malunion, and avascular (ischemic) necrosis. The tendency for these complications depends on the fracture site. In general, the prognosis is best in cases of fractures of the distal third and worst in fractures of the proximal third because proximal fractures invariably compromise the blood supply of the proximal fracture fragment. Increased density of the fracture fragment is commonly seen in the healing scaphoid fracture, especially when examined with computed tomography (CT). This finding is due to decreased vascularity of the proximal pole; as a result, the proximal pole does not demineralize as much as the distal pole. Usually with healing, revascularization of the proximal pole occurs and density differences disappear. Less commonly, true necrosis, identified by fragmentation or bone volume loss, may occur.

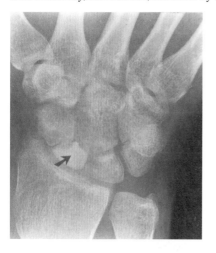

PA radiograph of a patient who suffered a scaphoid fracture, treated with a plaster cast. Clear evidence of increased density of the proximal fracture fragment *(arrow)* indicates decreased vascularity of this proximal pole. Increased density is not synonymous with avascular necrosis. Avascular (ischemic) necrosis with fragmentation and collapse may or may not develop.

14. What is the difference between static and dynamic instabilities of the wrist?

In general, the term *carpal instability* describes abnormalities in the alignment of carpal bones. Static instabilities are constantly present and can be diagnosed on a routine (static) radiographic examination (PA and lateral views). Dynamic instabilities, however, are not always seen on routine static radiographs. Dynamic instabilities need stress or motion to produce the instability and therefore may be diagnosed by obtaining instability series or stress maneuvers recorded with videotape, fluoroscopic spots, or overhead views with applied stress.

15. What is rotary subluxation of the scaphoid (RSS)?

RSS (or scapholunate dissociation) is the most frequent type of wrist instability. The scapholunate joint space is of abnormal width because of rupture of the scapholunate and adjacent ligaments and capsule. In patients with an associated rupture of the volar radiocarpal ligaments, the scaphoid bone tilts volarly. This condition is called RSS. Because of the volar tilting the scaphoid foreshortens and displays a signet-ring shape on the PA neutral view. The signet ring is so called because of the appearance of a stone in the middle of a ring. The shape results from the distal half of the scaphoid overlapping the proximal part of the scaphoid at its waist.

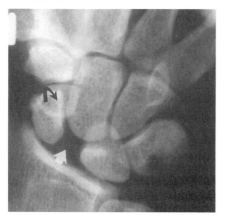

A view of the wrist of a patient with rotary subluxation of the scaphoid. The scapholunate joint space *(arrow)* is abnormally wide because of rupture of the scapholunate ligament. A signet-ring shape of the scaphoid *(curved arrow)* is evident because of its volar tilting due to rupture of adjacent extrinsic ligaments.

16. What are the two major types of carpal dislocations?

Carpal dislocations are divided into two major types: lunate and perilunate dislocations. Under normal conditions on the lateral radiograph, the lunate is centered over the radius fossa, and the capitate is centered over the lunate fossa. In general, whichever bone is centered over the radius (lunate or capitate) is the bone that is considered to be in normal anatomic alignment. In lunate dislocation the lunate is displaced ventrally or dorsally and the head of the capitate is centered over the radius. In perilunate instability the lunate remains in anatomic position, and the capitate is displaced with respect to the radius. If neither the lunate nor the capitate is centered over the radius, the condition is called a midcarpal dislocation because both the lunate and capitate are separated from each other.

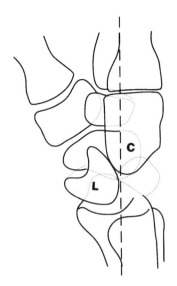

Right, Midcarpal dislocation. The lunate (L) is displaced ventrally, whereas the capitate head (C) is centered over the dorsal portion of the radius. This condition is between a perilunate and a lunate dislocation. Often a perilunate dislocation precedes or is the first stage of a lunate dislocation.

17. What is the role of CT in carpal trauma?

In selected cases, if routine radiograms are inconclusive, CT has become increasingly popular for diagnosing traumatic wrist disorders. CT is useful to evaluate complex carpal trauma, to detect loose intraarticular bodies, to visualize bone graft material, and to determine the degree of fracture healing.

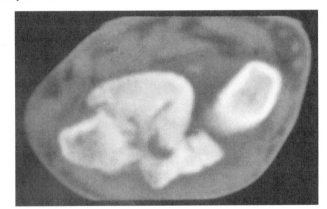

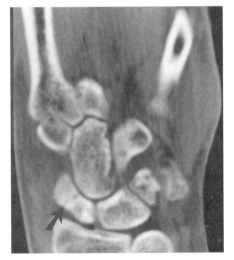

Above, Axial CT of the distal radius and ulna. With CT, intraarticular involvement of a fracture and the degree of fracture fragment displacement are better demonstrated than with conventional radiographs. This example shows an extensively comminuted fracture of the distal radius with involvement of and displacement at the distal radioulnar joint. The top of the image is volar with respect to the bottom.

Left, Coronal CT scan of the wrist demonstrates a scaphoid waist fracture. Sclerotic margins of the fracture fragments and no evidence of bony bridging of the fragments indicate nonunion of the fracture *(arrow).*

18. What are the advantages of MRI for diagnosis of wrist disorders?

MRI is the only imaging technique that allows simultaneous and direct visualization of bony, cartilaginous, and ligamentous structures of the wrist. Because of improvement in examination techniques and development of special wrist surface coils, MRI has become an important imaging technique. It is useful for direct visualization of the intrinsic and extrinsic wrist ligaments and their disorders and extremely sensitive and specific for detection of early stages of avascular necrosis of carpal bones. In addition, MRI has become an important imaging technique for detection of occult wrist fractures.

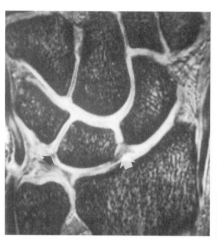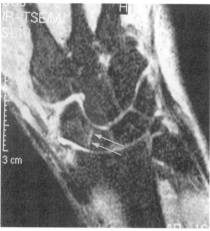

Left, Coronal MRI of the wrist allows precise and direct visualization of the intrinsic interosseous scapholunate and lunotriquetral ligaments *(arrows)* as triangular structures of low signal intensity. *Right,* On the coronal MRI of the wrist in a patient with a clinically suspected scaphoid fracture, a fracture through the proximal third of the scaphoid is evident *(arrows)*. The fracture was not seen on radiographs.

BIBLIOGRAPHY

1. Breitenseher MJ, Metz VM, Gilula LA, et al. Radiographically occult scaphoid fractures: Value of MR imaging in detection. Radiology 203:245-250, 1997.
2. Frykman G: Fracture of the distal radius including sequelae-shoulder-hand-finger syndrome, disturbance in the distal radioulnar joint and impairment of nerve function: A clinical and experimental study. Acta Orthop Scand (Suppl) 108:1–55,1967.
3. Gilula LA (ed): The Traumatized Hand and Wrist. Radiographic and Anatomic Correlation. Philadelphia, W.B. Saunders, 1992.
4. Gilula LA, Yin Y (eds): Imaging of the Hand and Wrist. Philadelphia, W.B. Saunders, 1996.
5. Hardy TH, Totty WG, Reinus WR, Gilula LA: Posteroanterior wrist radiography: Importance of arm positioning. J Hand Surg 12A:504–508, 1987.
6. Heller M, Fink A (eds): Radiology of Trauma. Berlin, Springer, 1997.
7. Stewart NR, Gilula LA: CT of the wrist: A tailored approach. Radiology 183:13-20, 1992.

116. FRACTURES OF THE CARPAL BONES

James Lilley, M.D., Mark Halikis, M.D., and Julio Taleisnik, M.D.

1. What is the relative incidence of carpal fractures?

Scaphoid	79%	Lunate	1%
Triquetrum	14%	Pisiform	1%
Trapezium	2.3 %	Capitate	1%
Hamate	1.5%	Trapezoid	0.2%

2. What is the blood supply to the scaphoid? Why is it important ?

The superficial palmar branch and the dorsal carpal branch of the radial artery feed the distal pole of the scaphoid. Intraosseous vessels flow retrograde to supply the proximal pole. Fractures through the scaphoid's waist can sever the blood supply to the proximal pole, leading to avascular necrosis (AVN) of the proximal fragment in as many as one-third of cases. An even higher incidence of AVN is found in more proximal fractures. AVN is associated with nonunion and persistent symptoms of pain or instability of the wrist.

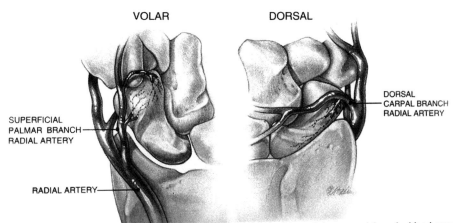

The dorsal blood supply to the scaphoid via the dorsal carpal branch of the radial artery and the volar blood supply via the superficial palmar branch of the radial artery enter the distal pole of the scaphoid. Blood supply to the proximal pole is intraosseous and retrograde. Fractures to the waist of the scaphoid disrupt this intraosseous supply and may lead to avascular necrosis of the proximal pole. (From Amadio PC, Taleisnik J: Fractures of the carpal bones. In Green DP (ed): Operative Hand Surgery, 3rd ed. New York, Churchill Livingstone, 1993, p 801, with permission.)

3. What is the typical presentation of a scaphoid fracture?

The typical patient is a young man who has fallen on an outstretched palm and extended wrist. He presents with pain and swelling of the radial wrist. The presence of tenderness in the anatomic snuffbox should lead to a presumptive diagnosis of fracture until radiographic examination proves conclusively negative.

4. What is the anatomic snuffbox?

It is a small triangular depression just distal and dorsal to the radial styloid. The extensor pollicis brevis (EPB) and abductor pollicis longus (APL) form its volar border as they run together in the first dorsal compartment of the wrist. The extensor pollicis longus (EPL) forms the dorsal border. Extension of the thumb demonstrates the borders best. With ulnar deviation the scaphoid is uncovered by the radial styloid and is palpable at the floor of the snuffbox.

5. What radiographic views should be included in the initial work-up of a scaphoid fracture?

Four views have been found to identify 97% of scaphoid fractures: one posteroanterior (PA), one lateral, and two oblique projections, the supinated and pronated obliques. The clenched fist position or active ulnar deviation in the PA view places the scaphoid more parallel to the film and improves visualization of the fracture. Several authors favor the ulnar deviation PA view in lieu of the supinated oblique. The lateral view helps to visualize fractures in the coronal plane and to assess the degree of scaphoid fracture angulation.

6. What is an occult scaphoid fracture?

A completely nondisplaced fracture or occult fracture may not appear on plain films initially. A period of 10–14 days may be required for resorption to occur at the fracture site before it is visible radiographically. Alternatively, a bone scan may provide this information sooner. A negative scan excludes a fracture; a positive scan may warrant trispiral or computed tomography (CT) studies to confirm the presence of fracture and define its anatomy.

7. What is the navicular fat stripe sign?

It is a small radiolucent line in the soft tissues radial to the carpus as seen on the PA view. A preserved fat stripe or fat pad is evidence that the scaphoid is intact. Fracture leads to radial displacement or (usually) obliteration of the fat stripe.

8. What are the important classification systems of scaphoid fractures?

The middle third or waist of the scaphoid is the most common location of injury. Most treatment recommendations are directed to waist fractures, which Russe subclassifies by the anatomy of the fracture. The plane of the fracture is defined in relation to the long axis of the scaphoid. **Horizontal oblique fractures**, the most frequent of the wrist fractures, are perpendicular to the long axis of the limb but oblique in relation to the longitudinal axis of the scaphoid. These are stable and should heal with 6–8 weeks of immobilization. **Transverse fractures** are less common and less stable, for although perpendicular to the long axis of the scaphoid, they are oblique in relation to the long axis of the limb. Healing occurs in 6–12 weeks. The rare **vertical oblique pattern** is less stable and requires even longer immobilization, because it is more subject to shear forces along the long axis of the limb.

Cooney and others have recognized the importance of fracture displacement and angulation in predicting stability. Nonunion rates climb 10- to 20-fold when displacement of greater than 1 mm is found on any radiographic view. Angulation, which is suggestive of carpal instability, also contributes to nonunion. Examples include scapholunate angles greater than 60° or a radiolunate angle greater than 15°. Herbert published an alphanumeric classification scheme that incorporates fracture anatomy, chronicity, and stability factors. Unstable or type B fractures include distal oblique, complete waist, proximal pole, and transscaphoid perilunate fracture dislocations. Prognostic information is developing from this system as it is adopted by other authors.

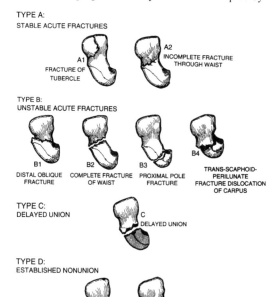

TYPE A:
STABLE ACUTE FRACTURES

A1
FRACTURE OF
TUBERCLE

A2
INCOMPLETE FRACTURE
THROUGH WAIST

TYPE B:
UNSTABLE ACUTE FRACTURES

B1
DISTAL OBLIQUE
FRACTURE

B2
COMPLETE FRACTURE
OF WAIST

B3
PROXIMAL POLE
FRACTURE

B4
TRANS-SCAPHOID-
PERILUNATE
FRACTURE DISLOCATION
OF CARPUS

TYPE C:
DELAYED UNION

C
DELAYED UNION

TYPE D:
ESTABLISHED NONUNION

D1
FIBROUS UNION

D2
PSEUDARTHROSIS

Herbert's alphanumeric classification systems of scaphoid fractures. (From Amadio PC, Taleisnik J: Fractures of the carpal bones. In Green DP (ed): Operative Hand Surgery, 3rd ed. New York, Churchill Livingstone, 1993, p 805, with permission.)

9. How does a scaphoid fracture contribute to wrist instability?

The wrist can be understood as a three-bar linkage with the distal carpal row, the proximal row, and the radius forming links in a chain. Like a chain, this construct is stable in tension but unstable in compression. It requires a stabilizing bar to support compression. The scaphoid provides this stability by its connection distally to the capitate and proximally to the lunate. Disruption of the scaphoid renders the carpus unstable and subject to collapse. The radius, lunate, and capitate are then no longer colinear. Most frequently, the lunate tilts dorsally with the attached proximal pole of the scaphoid. Loading of the distal fragment by the trapezium and trapezoid favors axial compression, causing the distal fragment to flex while the proximal fragment extends and thus creating a volar flexed "humpback" position of the scaphoid. This deformity contributes to delayed healing of the fracture, because it maintains malalignment across the scaphoid waist.

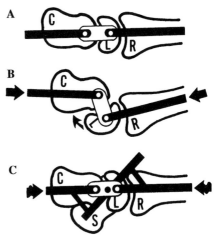

The three-bar linkage model of the wrist predicts stability in tension *(panel A)* and collapse in compression *(panel B)* unless an additional stabilizing link is added to the construct *(panel C)*. S = scaphoid, the stabilizing link; L = the lunate; C = capitate; and R = radius. (From Amadio PC, Taleisnik J: Fractures of the carpal bones. In Green DP (ed): Operative Hand Surgery, 3rd ed. New York, Churchill Livingstone, 1993, p 863, with permission.)

10. What are the essentials of closed treatment of scaphoid fractures?

Unstable scaphoid fractures are treated with open reduction and internal fixation (ORIF) in most cases. Stable or nondisplaced fractures may be treated by closed methods. The use of short- or long-arm casting is controversial. Although reports show a statistically significant decrement in healing time with inclusion of the elbow, short-arm casting of stable scaphoid fractures yields a 95% union rate in an average of 11 weeks. Therefore, stable fractures may be treated in a short-arm thumb spica cast. However, inclusion of the elbow is recommended by several authors for initial immobilization followed by short-arm casting until radiographic union. Electrical stimulators have been used to promote healing of the scaphoid, but prospective double-blind studies that demonstrate efficacy are lacking. This type of therapy is much more costly than casting alone.

11. What are the indications to operate on a fracture of the scaphoid?

Displacement greater than 1 mm or angulation demonstrated by a scapholunate angle greater than 60° or a radiolunate angle greater than 15° are considered significant. Displaced or angulated fractures, fractures that demonstrate no healing at 6–12 weeks, and nonunions that have failed closed treatment after 6 months are best treated surgically. Very proximal fractures, which are at higher risk for nonunion and avascular necrosis, are also good candidates for surgical treatment. Indeed, routine internal fixation is recommended for these proximal fractures.

12. What surgical options are available?

Internal fixation with K-wires is indicated for fracture associated with dislocation or ligamentous instability. Smooth wires are also useful to fix an avascular fragment; a minimum of three wires is needed. The Herbert screw is a proven method for osteosynthesis of the scaphoid. The larger pitch of the leading threads compared with the trailing threads is designed to provide compression across the fracture. The screw is counter-sunk below the articular surface and is generally not removed. The internal fixation provided by the screw allows more rapid mobilization of the wrist. Russe described using iliac crest strips alone for fixation to improve healing potential. Healing rates are comparable to those of the Herbert screw plus bone graft. Recognizing the problems associated with the flexion or "humpback" deformity, Fisk and Fernandez described the use of a volar-placed wedge of bone to reduce the deformity. This corticocancellous graft can be fixed with wires or a screw at the nonunion site. The use of a vascularized bone graft swung on a pedicle has been described for failed grafts. Several techniques are described, including osteotomy of a portion of the pronator quadratus insertion, which is rotated distally with a strip of muscle attached.

13. What differences are seen in pediatric scaphoid fractures?

Most commonly they are in the distal third (59%) and tubercle (33%). Very few are displaced. They can and should be treated by closed technique until skeletal maturity unless grossly displaced.

14. Describe the surgical approaches to the scaphoid.

The key landmarks of the volar or Russe approach are the tuberosity of the scaphoid and the tendon of the flexor carpi radialis (FCR). A curvilinear skin incision that crosses the wrist crease obliquely should allow access to both landmarks. Longitudinal division of the deep fascia radial to the FCR allows radial retraction of the radial artery and ulnar retraction of the FCR and palmar cutaneous branch of the median nerve. The volar radiocarpal joint capsule can be incised to expose the scaphoid. The exposure is extended by division of the thenar origin distally and the pronator quadratus proximally.

The dorsolateral approach to the scaphoid has the disadvantage of crossing the branches of the superficial radial nerve as well as endangering the blood supply to the scaphoid; however, it provides better access to the proximal pole. The nerve is retracted in a dorsal or volar direction as needed. The extensor fascia is divided longitudinally, and the artery is exposed and retracted volarly with care to preserve the dorsal carpal branch. The proximal pole is then well demonstrated by ulnar deviation of the wrist.

15. Can the scaphoid be fixed arthroscopically?

Patients with nondisplaced scaphoid fractures who cannot commit to 8–12 weeks of immobilization are candidates for arthroscopically assisted fixation using the Herbert-Whipple screw, a cannulated modification of the Herbert screw. A guidewire is placed under arthroscopic guidance across the fracture, and a second, parallel wire is used for derotation. The screw is introduced volarly through a small incision and passed over the guidewire.

16. What is Kienböck's disease? How is it related to fractures of the lunate?

Fractures of the lunate are rare when distinguished from Kienböck's disease or AVN of the lunate. The etiology of Kienböck's disease is uncertain. It is possible that in some cases a fracture predisposes the bone to AVN, which leads to later collapse. Alternatively, other factors may impair blood flow to the bone, causing the necrosis, which, in turn, leads to collapse and fracture. (See chapter 117.)

17. What is the typical presentation and work-up of a triquetral fracture?

Isolated triquetral fractures are commonly avulsion or shear fractures from a hyperextension injury with ulnar wrist pain, swelling, and tenderness. Wrist hyperextension may cause the hamate or ulnar styloid to impinge on the triquetrum, causing a dorsal shear fracture. Acute wrist palmar flexion may lead to an avulsion fracture by the dorsal radiotriquetral ligament. Oblique radiographs are the most helpful. Treatment in a splint is adequate. Triquetral fractures are also associated with perilunate fracture dislocation. Simple fractures are treated with splint immobilization.

18. How are pisiform fractures best diagnosed and treated?

Typically resulting from a direct blow, pisiform fractures present with ulnar and volar wrist pain and unmistakable tenderness. Supinated oblique and carpal tunnel radiographic views are most helpful. Cast treatment has not proved to alter the natural history of the injury, but it is recommended by several authors over splinting. Symptomatic nonunions do well with excision of the pisiform.

19. What rare carpal fracture is associated with cyclists?

Trapezial fractures, which are seen best with a Bett's oblique view of the trapezium and may be treated by closed technique in a short-arm thumb spica cast if nondisplaced. Displacement is often intraarticular and requires ORIF. Nonunion is treated with partial or total excision, fusion, or interposition arthroplasty.

20. Which carpal fracture is associated with golf and racquet sports?

Fractures of the hook of the hamate. A dull ache in the ulnar wrist (even dorsally) or hypothenar eminence may be associated with chronic and acute trauma to the area, especially in golf, baseball, or racquet sports. The symptoms are aggravated by lateral movement or flexion of the little finger. Diagnosis requires radiographic evaluation that includes oblique and carpal tunnel views. Standard or computed tomography of the wrist may be needed to clarify the plain film images. Immobilization reduces the risk of nonunion. Excision provides reliable relief for patients who fail conservative therapy for symptomatic nonunion.

21. What is scaphocapitate syndrome?

The scaphocapitate syndrome is caused by fractures through the waist of the capitate and scaphoid waist with rotation of the proximal capitate fragment 90–180°. If recognized early (3–4 weeks), both fractures may be treated with ORIF. Injuries recognized late may be treated expectantly, with arthrodesis reserved for persistent symptoms. Moreover, AVN is a sequel to chronic or acute injury of the capitate because the blood supply to the proximal pole is tenuous.

22. How do scaphoid fractures contribute to wrist arthritis?

Patients with a symptomatic nonunion of the scaphoid have been shown to undergo a predictable pattern of wrist arthritis. Because the distal fragment is unrestrained after fracture, it tends to rotate. This rotation makes the distal articulations incongruous and promotes degenerative change. The proximal articulations are spared because they are spherical and because the proximal fragment remains stabilized by the radioscaphoid and scapholunate ligaments. The pattern of degeneration is similar to that seen in cases of rotatory subluxation of the scaphoid, also known as scapholunate advanced collapse (SLAC) wrist. It refers to a pattern of progressive joint space and cartilage loss that begins at the radial styloid and then progresses down the radioscaphoid articulation. The capitolunate and scaphocapitate articulations are later involved. Still further progression leads to hamatolunate degeneration and scapholunate dissociation as the capitate migrates proximally. The radiolunate articulation is always spared. (See chapter 120.)

BIBLIOGRAPHY

1. Amadio PC, Taleisnik J: Fractures of the carpal bones. In Green DP (ed): Operative Hand Surgery, 3rd ed. New York, Churchill Livingstone, 1993, pp 799–842.
2. Failla JM, Amadio PC: Recognition and treatment of uncommon carpal fractures. Hand Clin 4: 469–476, 1988.
3. Herbert TJ: The Fractured Scaphoid. St Louis, Quality Medical Publishing, 1990.
4. Hoppenfeld S, deBoer P: Surgical Exposures in Orthopaedics: The Anatomic Approach, 2nd ed. Philadelphia, J.B. Lippincott, 1994.
5. Jupiter J: Scaphoid fractures. In Manske PR (ed): 1994 Hand Surgery Update. Englewood, IL, American Society for Surgery of the Hand, 1994, pp 81–85.
6. Ruby L: Fractures and dislocations of the carpus. In Browner B, et al (eds): Skeletal Trauma. Philadelphia, W. B. Saunders, 1992, pp 1025–1027.
7. Szabo RM, Manske D: Displaced fractures of the scaphoid. CORR. 230:30–38, 1988.
8. Taleisnik J: The Wrist. New York, Churchill Livingstone, 1985.
9. Watson HK, Ryu J: Evolution of wrist arthritis. CORR. 202:61, 1986.
10. Whipple TL: Arthroscopic Surgery—The Wrist. Philadelphia, J.B. Lippincott, 1992.

117. KIENBÖCK'S DISEASE

David C. Kim, M.D., and David M. Lichtman, M.D.

1. What is Kienböck's disease?

Avascular necrosis (AVN) of the lunate. To varying degrees, collapse of the lunate is associated with avascular changes. This pathologic process may progress to carpal collapse and ultimately result in pancarpal arthritis.

2. What age group and sex are most commonly affected?

The male-to-female ratio is 2:1. The most common age group affected is 20–40 year olds.

3. What is the cause?

The theories about the cause of Kienböck's disease are numerous and varied. In 1843, before the advent of radiographs, Peste described lunate collapse in anatomic specimens. He attributed this finding to an acute, traumatic event. In 1910, Robert Kienböck noted collapse and sclerosis of the lunate on radiographs and attributed them to progressive vascular compromise resulting from repetitive wrist sprains and contusions. Based on the radiographic association of identifiable fracture lines and lunate collapse, some authors believe that the characteristic lesions result from failure of lunate fractures to unite. Intrinsic factors such as ulnar variance, lunate vascularity, and intraosseous pressure gradients also have been implicated as etiologic agents of Kienböck's disease.

4. What is ulnar variance?

Ulnar variance is the relationship between the distal articular surfaces of the radius and ulna. **Zero variance** refers to level articular surfaces. **Ulnar-minus variance** is a relatively short ulna with respect to the radius or an ulna with a more proximal articular surface. **Ulnar-plus variance** refers to a long ulna relative to the distal radius.

5. What is the significance of ulnar variance to Kienböck's disease?

Data indicate a higher incidence of ulnar-minus variance in patients with Kienböck's disease compared with the general population. Laboratory studies confirm that shortening the ulna results in increased shear stress across the lunate. These forces are translated across the lunate particularly in dorsiflexion and ulnar deviation. However, not all authors agree that ulnar variance is a clinical factor. In certain Asian populations, for example, there is less correlation between variance and Kienböck's disease.

6. Does lunate vascular anatomy influence AVN?

The extraosseous blood supply to the majority of lunates consists of contributions from the radial, ulnar, anterior intraosseous, and deep palmar arch arteries. These arteries coalesce to form a rich vascular plexus on the dorsal and palmar lunate surfaces. Furthermore, most lunates have a complex intraosseous network of anastomoses between the dorsal and palmar vessels. However, some lunates have only a single palmar vessel with minimal internal branching—especially to the proximal surface. These are the lunates that may develop AVN after traumatic arterial disruption. Recent data demonstrate that in Kienböck's disease, intraosseous pressure in the lunate is higher than measurements obtained from the radial styloid, capitate, and normal lunates. This finding may imply that venous congestion rather than primary arterial insufficiency is the precipitating event.

7. What are the symptoms of Kienböck's disease?

The sine qua non of Kienböck's disease is wrist pain. Although the patient may relate a precipitating traumatic event, the symptoms are usually insidious in onset. In the early stages, pain is localized to the area of the lunate and associated with symptoms of inflammation such as swelling and pain with motion. As the disease progresses, patients report stiffness, clicking or grinding, and a concomitant crescendo in pain. Late-stage symptoms are consistent clinically with carpal degenerative arthritis.

8. What are the physical findings?

Varying degrees of swelling may be found along the dorsum of the wrist, particularly in comparison with the contralateral side. Palpation demonstrates tenderness dorsally about the lunate. Depending on the severity of the disease, grip strength may be decreased and range of motion may be painful. Later in the disease the range of motion decreases, and there may be grinding and crepitus with motion.

9. What are the radiographic findings?

Although initially the radiographs may be normal, later they typically demonstrate increased density of the lunate accompanied by fracture lines, fragmentation, and progressive collapse. Advanced collapse is associated with proximal migration of the capitate, increased intercarpal widening of the proximal row, and permanent flexion of the scaphoid. The latter exhibits the characteristic ring sign on an anteroposterior view.

10. What features are found on magnetic resonance imaging (MRI)?

AVN typically involves the lunate in a diffuse pattern. The hallmark finding of AVN is a uniformly decreased signal intensity on both T1- and T2-weighted images.

11. What role does MRI serve in managing Kienböck's disease?

The sensitivity and specificity of MRI for carpal AVN are well suited for the diagnosis of Kienböck's disease. MRI is particularly useful in early stages when clinical findings are suggestive but radiographs are negative. Diagnosis in the early stage provides the basis for instituting the appropriate treatment. Early increased signals on T2 images imply revascularization and a good prognosis.

12. What is the differential diagnosis?

The differential diagnosis most typically includes rheumatoid arthritis, posttraumatic arthritis, synovial-based inflammatory diseases, fractures, carpal instability, and ulnar abutment syndromes.

13. List and describe the stages of Kienböck's disease.

The Lichtman classification is used to evaluate Kienböck's disease and to decide the most appropriate treatment:

Stage I. Radiographs are normal. Technetium bone scans are characteristically "hot," and MRI demonstrates diffuse decreased signals on T1- and T2-weighted images. Physical findings are indistinguishable from a wrist sprain.

Stage II. Density changes isolated to the lunate as indicated by sclerosis. The lunate also may demonstrate fracture lines or minimal collapse on its radial border. However, its overall size, shape, and relationship to the carpal bones are not significantly altered. Clinically stage II is represented by recurrent pain, swelling, and wrist tenderness.

Stage III. Collapse of the lunate. Anteroposterior views exhibit a shortened lunate and elongation in the sagittal plane, accompanied by proximal migration of the capitate. **Stage IIIA** is characterized by no fixed carpal derangements or instability, whereas **stage IIIB** involves fixed rotation of the scaphoid, decreased carpal height, and ulnar migration of the triquetrum. Clinically stage III is characterized by progressive weakness, stiffness, and pain. Clicking and clunking are also noted.

Stage IV. In addition to the radiographic findings of stage IIIB, stage IV is associated with generalized degenerative changes in the carpus. Clinically this stage is indistinguishable from degenerative arthritis of the wrist.

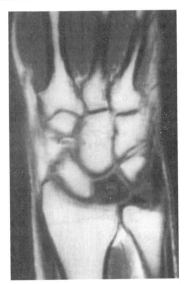

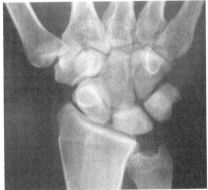

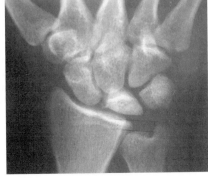

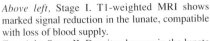

Above left, Stage I. T1-weighted MRI shows marked signal reduction in the lunate, compatible with loss of blood supply.
Top right, Stage II. Density changes in the lunate as indicated by sclerosis. Note the ulnar-minus variance.
Bottom right, Stage IIIA. Collapse of the lunate. There are no fixed carpal derangements.

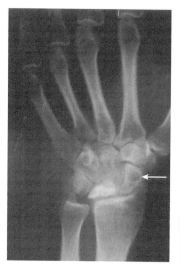 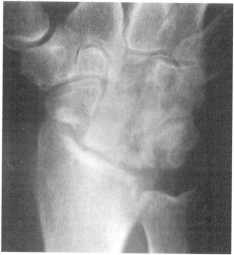

Left, Stage IIIB. Decreased carpal height and proximal migration of the capitate. Note the scaphoid cortical ring sign *(arrow). Right,* Stage IV. Generalized degenerative changes in the carpus.

14. How are the various stages of Kienböck's disease treated?
See algorithm on facing page.

15. Does immobilization have a role in the treatment of Kienböck's disease?
In stage I, immobilization in a well-fitted short cast for up to 3 months is recommended. Although immobilization may not eliminate all axial loads encountered during routine activities of daily living, it may provide an opportunity for the lunate to heal (revascularize).

16. How about simply excising the lunate?
Excising the lunate alone does not prevent proximal migration of the capitate and carpal instability secondary to disruption of perilunate ligaments.

17. What about lunate excision arthroplasty?
Historically both autogenous and synthetic "spacers" have been used for lunate excision arthroplasty. Spacers are rarely used today because placement of an anchovy tendon graft, such as a coiled palmaris longus tendon, precludes direct or indirect lunate revascularization procedures used for early stages of Kienböck's disease. Furthermore, in advanced stages, spacers alone may not provide enough support to inhibit carpal collapse. Artificial spacers such as silicone implants are no longer recommended because of the incidence of complications such as particulate synovitis and cyst formation in adjacent bones.

18. Does altering ulnar variance affect revascularization?
Both clinical and biomechanical studies support the benefit of joint-leveling procedures—either radial shortening or ulnar lengthening. Such operations significantly decompress the lunate by redistributing the axial load from the lunate to the radioscaphoid and ulnocarpal joints. The lunate then presumably will revascularize spontaneously (indirect revascularization). We recommend radial shortening for stage II or IIIA disease before significant lunate collapse occurs. This procedure is indicated only for the typical ulnar-minus case.

19. Can a lunate be revascularized by direct vessel reimplantation?
In the early stages of Kienböck's disease, various direct revascularization techniques have been successful in reversing the progress of lunate collapse. Operations such as vascular bundle transfer of the second dorsal intermetacarpal artery and vein, pronator quadratus pedicled bone grafts, and pedunculated pisiform transfers have demonstrated restoration of lunate viability. The success of

Treatment Algorithm for Kienböck's Disease

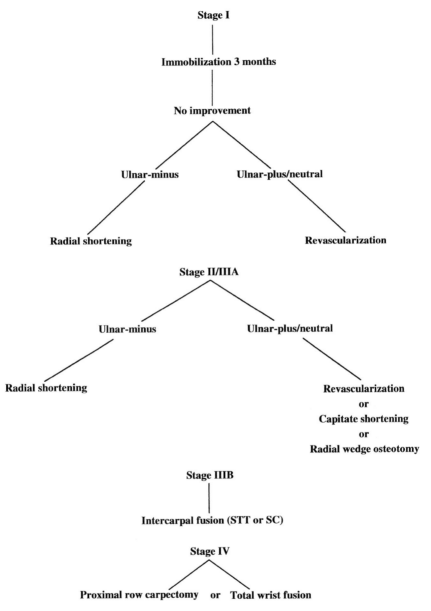

Stage I
|
Immobilization 3 months
|
No improvement

Ulnar-minus   Ulnar-plus/neutral

Radial shortening   Revascularization

Stage II/IIIA

Ulnar-minus   Ulnar-plus/neutral

Radial shortening   Revascularization
or
Capitate shortening
or
Radial wedge osteotomy

Stage IIIB
|
Intercarpal fusion (STT or SC)

Stage IV

Proximal row carpectomy   or   Total wrist fusion

direct revascularization, however, is predicated on performing the procedures before significant collapse occurs. We use them in stage II–IIIA for ulnar-plus cases (in which additional radius shortening is contraindicated).

20. When should intercarpal arthrodesis be considered?

Intercarpal arthrodesis for stage IIIB Kienböck's disease (carpal instability) provides a number of advantages. Although arthrodesis biomechanically unloads the lunate and encourages indirect revascularization, the premise of these procedures in stage IIIB is to address the carpal instability, i.e., proximal migration of the capitate and scaphoid flexion. Furthermore, limited fusions are durable and maintain functional wrist mobility. A necrotic or fragmented lunate should be excised.

21. Which intercarpal arthrodesis is most appropriate?

A triscaphe (STT) or scaphocapitate (SC) fusion is recommended in stage IIIB. Both procedures place the scaphoid in its anatomic position in reference to the scaphoid fossa and provide stability to the midcarpal joint. Other intercarpal fusions have been investigated but do not unload the lunate biomechanically (e.g., triquetrohamate fusion).

22. What salvage procedures are performed for advanced disease?

In the presence of pancarpal arthrosis (stage IV Kienböck's disease) either a proximal row carpectomy (PRC) or total wrist fusion is recommended. Factors such as the patient's physical demands, occupation, preexisting conditions, and the articular integrity of the proximal capitate and lunate fossa of the radius are considered in choosing between the two procedures.

CONTROVERSIES

23. Are radial wedge osteotomies (closing or opening) effective procedures for Kienböck's disease?

Laboratory studies yield conflicting data about the effect of radial wedge osteotomy procedures. Increasing radial angle inclination by an opening wedge osteotomy and decreasing angle inclination by closing wedge osteotomy result in lunate decompression biomechanically. Although it is difficult to understand how both of these procedures can achieve the same biomechanical result, clinical studies to date report good results with closing radial wedge osteotomies.

24. How about vascularized radial bone grafts?

There are several reports of success with reverse-flow vascularized metaphyseal bone grafts for scaphoid nonunions. Described by Zaidemberg, the technique uses a dorsal radius graft based on an ascending branch of the radial artery—the 1,2 intercompartmental supraretinacular artery. Preliminary data about similar techniques for stage IIIA Kienböck's disease appears promising as an adjunct to prevent lunate collapse, relieve wrist pain, and improve grip strength. More data and long-term follow-up are needed before the technique is accepted in the armamentarium for lunate AVN.

25. What procedure is best suited for patients with ulnar-positive variance?

For obvious reasons, radial shortening or ulnar lengthening is contraindicated. We currently recommend direct lunate revascularization for early stages (I–IIIA). Alternatively, a radial wedge osteotomy or capitate shortening may be considered. STT or capitohamate fusion is best reserved for stage IIIB, regardless of variance.

BIBLIOGRAPHY

1. Alexander CE, Alexander AH, Lichtman DM: Kienböck's disease. In Lichtman DM, Alexander H (eds): Disorders of the Wrist. Philadelphia, W.B. Saunders, 1997.
2. Beckenbaugh R, Shives T, Dobyns J, et al: Kienböck's disease: The natural history of Kienböck's disease and consideration of lunate fractures. Clin Orthop 149:98–106, 1980.
3. Gelberman RH, Bauman TD, Menon J, et al: The vascularity of the lunate bone and Kienböck's disease. J Hand Surg 5:272–278, 1980.
4. Jensen CH: Intraosseous pressures in Kienböck's disease. J Hand Surg 18A:355–359, 1993.
5. Miura H, Uchida Y, Sugioka Y: Radial closing wedge for Kienböck's disease. J Hand Surg 21A:1029–1034, 1996.
6. Naksmura R, Horii E, Imaeda T, et al: Current concepts of radial osteotomy for Kienböck's disease. In Vastumaki M (ed): Current Trends in Hand Surgery. Amsterdam, Elsevier Science, 1995, pp 109–112.
7. Schiltenwolf M, Martini A, Mau H, et al: Further investigations of the intraosseous pressure characteristics in necrotic lunates (Kienböck's disease). J Hand Surg 21A:754–758, 1996.
8. Zaidemberg C, Siebert JW, Agrigiani C: A new vascularized bone graft for scaphoid nonunion. J Hand Surg 16A:474–478, 1991.

118. CARPAL DISLOCATIONS AND INSTABILITY

Michael P. Staebler, M.D., Michael Belanger, M.D., and Edward Akelman, M.D.

1. How do carpal dislocations typically occur?
Most carpal dislocations result from extreme hyperextension injuries with intercarpal supination. This mechanism is usually due to violent trauma as in a fall from a height or a motor vehicle accident.

2. What is the difference between a perilunate dislocation and a lunate dislocation?
In a perilunate dislocation the lunate remains aligned with the radius while the rest of the carpus is displaced, usually dorsally. In a lunate dislocation the capitate remains aligned with the radius while the lunate is volarly extruded from the carpus.

3. How do patients with carpal dislocations typically present?
Patients usually describe a high-energy mechanism. However, physical exam findings may not be particularly dramatic initially. Patients usually have diffuse mild-to-moderate swelling when seen early, but swelling is likely to increase significantly with time. Tenderness is diffuse, and range of motion is decreased significantly because of pain. Be aware of possible median nerve injury from direct contusion at the moment of impact, compression of the nerve by the lunate, or swelling within the carpal tunnel.

4. What is progressive perilunar instability? What are the stages?
Progressive perilunar instability (PLI) is a term coined by Mayfield to describe the spectrum of ligamentous injuries involving the wrist. It is based on studies in which cadaveric wrists were subjected to loads in extension, ulnar deviation, and intercarpal supination. Four stages of ligamentous injuries with resulting carpal malalignment that eventually led to lunate dislocations were noted:

Stage I: Scapholunate instability. Tearing of the scapholunate interosseous and volar radioscaphoid ligaments results in scaphoid dissociation.

Stage II: The midcarpal capsule is also disrupted at the capitolunate joint, allowing the capitate to dislocate dorsally.

Stage III: An avulsion fracture of the triquetrum or lunotriquetral ligament disruption results in a perilunate dislocation.

Stage IV: Lunate dislocation. Disruption of the dorsal radiocarpal ligaments allows the lunate to displace volarly, whereas the rest of the carpus remains aligned with the radius.

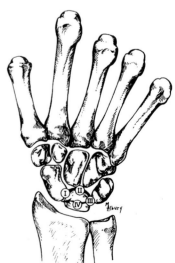

Progressive perilunar instability (PLI). The four stages of PLI, according to Mayfield's sequence of ligamentous injury patterns, result in carpal instability and, eventually, carpal dislocation. (From Green DP: Carpal dislocations and instabilities. In Green DP (ed): Operative Hand Surgery, vol 2, 3rd ed. New York, Churchill Livingstone, 1993, p 869, with permission.)

5. What is the "spilled teacup" sign? What does it signify?

Seen on a lateral wrist radiograph, the spilled teacup represents the lunate and signifies a lunate dislocation. Normally the lunate, shaped like a kidney bean on a lateral radiograph, lies with its convex surface against the distal radial articular surface and its concave surface holding the head of the capitate. In a lunate dislocation, the lunate has flipped volarly on its volar radiolunate ligament hinge so that the concavity (opening of the cup) faces into the carpal tunnel.

6. Describe briefly the various theories of wrist carpal biomechanics.

1. **Proximal and distal rows.** The seven major carpal bones (excluding the pisiform, which is a sesamoid) are arranged in two transverse rows, a proximal and a distal row. The scaphoid acts as the bridge between the two rows. The proximal row includes the triquetrum, lunate, and proximal pole of the scaphoid; the distal row consists of the hamate, capitate, trapezium, trapezoid, and distal pole of the scaphoid. Motion occurs both between rows (intercarpal) and within rows (intracarpal).

2. **Columnar carpus.** Originally described by Navarro and modified by Taleisnik, this theory states that the carpus is composed of three columns: (1) central column (lunate, capitate, hamate, trapezoid, and trapezium); (2) lateral column (scaphoid); and (3) medial column (triquetrum). The central column is the main flexion/extension link along the axis of the radius, lunate, and capitate. The scaphoid acts as the stabilizing or connecting link for the midcarpal joint. The triquetrum is the pivot point around which carpal and hand rotation takes place.

3. **Oval ring concept.** Lichtman considers the carpus as a ring with two mobile links "permitting reciprocal motion between the proximal and distal rows during radial and ulnar deviation." The links include the scaphotrapezial and triquetrohamate joints.

7. What is meant by lesser and greater arc injuries of the carpus?

The lesser arch is an imaginary line or arc around the lunate that includes only soft tissue structures (scapholunate ligament, capitolunate ligament, and lunotriquetral ligament). The greater arc consists of the bony structures around the lunate. Perilunate dislocations may be purely ligamentous or also involve fractures. They are described by the carpal bones involved. For example, a perilunate dislocation with an associated scaphoid and capitate fracture is described as a transscaphoid, trans-capitate perilunate fracture/dislocation.

8. What is the significance of a chauffeur's or radial styloid fracture?

A fracture through the radial styloid may be a harbinger of a more serious ligamentous injury to the carpus. The energy that produced the radial styloid fracture may propagate through the lesser arc, producing a scapholunate disruption or more significant PLI.

9. How can a dorsal perilunate dislocation be reduced?

The technique described by Tavernier is useful. Complete muscle relaxation is essential for atraumatic reduction. This technique entails an initial period of 5–10 minutes of continuous longitudinal traction in fingertraps with 10–15 lb of weight to allow relaxation of muscle forces. After longitudinal traction, manual traction is maintained by the surgeon. The thumb of one hand applies gentle pressure to the volar aspect of the wrist to stabilize the lunate. With the other hand, the patient's wrist is extended while longitudinal traction is maintained. Gradually, the wrist is flexed, allowing the capitate to snap back into the concavity of the lunate.

10. What is the best method of treatment for an acute perilunate/lunate dislocation or fracture/dislocation?

In general, with the significant amount of ligamentous disruption and possible fractures associated with these injuries, nonoperative management with closed reduction and casting is rarely satisfactory. A critical determinant of successful reduction is the position of the scaphoid. A scapholunate angle greater than 80° with a scapholunate gap greater than 3 mm indicates significant residual scaphoid rotatory subluxation and often a poor long-term outcome. Some authors favor closed reduction followed by percutaneous pinning of the scaphoid to the capitate and lunate, but only if anatomic reduction of the scaphoid, lunate, and capitate can be achieved. In many instances, especially with an associated fracture of one or more carpal bones, anatomic reduction cannot be achieved. Most authors now advocate open reduction, ligament repair, and internal fixation of these high-energy injuries.

Many authors favor the combined dorsal and volar approach of Dobyns and Swanson to allow assessment and repair of ligamentous and bony structures on both sides of the wrist.

11. What is Watson's test?

Watson's test, or the "scaphoid shift," as Dr. Watson prefers, is a provocative maneuver used to evaluate scaphoid stability and periscaphoid synovitis. The thumb of one hand is placed on the scaphoid tuberosity (distal pole on volar surface) while the four fingers of the same hand are placed behind the radius. With the patient's wrist initially in ulnar deviation and slight extension, the examiner's opposite hand is used to deviate radially and to flex slightly the patient's wrist. Pressure on the tuberosity prevents the scaphoid from palmarflexing with scaphoid instability or rotary subluxation. The scaphoid thus is "pushed" dorsally out of the radial fossa, producing pain and/or a palpable clunk. A comparison test on the opposite wrist should always be performed. (See chapter 114.)

12. What is a DISI deformity? A VISI deformity?

DISI, which stands for dorsal intercalated segmental instability, occurs when scapholunate ligament disruption results in volar flexion of the scaphoid and dorsal angulation of the lunate. VISI, which stands for volar intercalated segmental instability, signifies a lunotriquetral ligament disruption with volar angulation of the lunate compared with a normally aligned scaphoid.

13. List other radiographic signs of scapholunate dissociation.

1. Foreshortened scaphoid—when the scaphoid is volar flexed, as in scapholunate dissociation, it appears shorter on the anteroposterior (AP) view.
2. Signet ring sign—seen on the AP view; represents an axial view of a significantly volar flexed scaphoid.
3. Lack of parallelism between the articular surfaces of the scaphoid and lunate.
4. Increased capitolunate angle (normally 0° with a normal range of 0–15°).

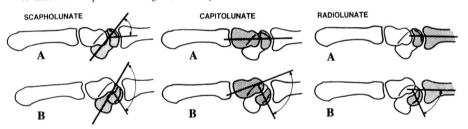

Carpal bone angles. In each case the normal angle is shown *(A)* in comparison with the abnormal angle seen with a DISI deformity *(B)*. The average scapholunate angle is 47°; an angle greater than 80° is indicative of scapholunate dissociation or rotary subluxation of the scaphoid. The capitolunate angle should be 0° with the wrist in neutral; the normal range is 0–15°. The radiolunate angle is abnormal if it is greater than 15°. (From Green DP: Carpal dislocations and instabilities. In Green DP (ed): Operative Hand Surgery, vol 2, 3rd ed. New York, Churchill Livingstone, 1993, p 874, with permission.)

14. Who was Terry Thomas? What is the significance of his name?

Terry Thomas was a famous English film comedian with a wide gap in his front teeth. The "Terry Thomas" sign, seen on an AP of the wrist, indicates a widened scapholunate gap and signifies a scapholunate dissociation. A scapholunate gap > 3mm is considered diagnostic of a scapholunate dissociation.

15. What is the difference between static and dynamic scapholunate dissociation?

Static scapholunate dissociation is associated with a fixed deformity between the scaphoid and lunate as seen on AP and lateral views. In dynamic dissociation there is no radiographic evidence of abnormality with plain views. Any abnormal scapholunate relationship is identified only by stress radiographs, such as a clenched fist AP view.

16. Which radiographs help to make the diagnosis of scapholunate dissociation?

A typical scaphoid series includes the following:
1. True lateral view with the wrist in neutral—useful for evaluation of overall alignment and measurement of carpal angles.

2. Posteroanterior (palm down) view in maximal ulnar deviation—profile view of the scaphoid; helpful for seeing scaphoid fractures.

3. AP view with clenched fist—accentuates a dynamic scapholunate dissociation.

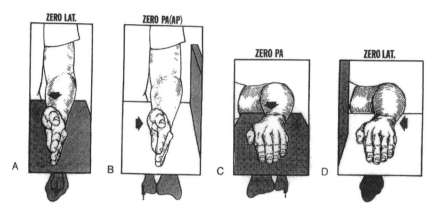

Methods of taking standardized PA and lateral radiographs of the wrist, according to Taleisnik. The arrows indicate the direction of the x-ray beam, which is centered directly over the radiocarpal joint. (From Green DP: Carpal dislocations and instabilities. In Green DP (ed): Operative Hand Surgery, vol 2, 3rd ed. New York, Churchill Livingstone, 1993, p 875, with permission.)

17. What is a normal scapholunate angle? When is a scapholunate angle considered pathologic?

On a lateral view, with the wrist in neutral, a line is drawn through the long axis of the lunate. A second line is drawn through the long axis of the scaphoid. The angle formed by the intersection of the two lines is the scapholunate angle. Normal values range from 30–60° with an average of 47°, as described by Linscheid. An angle greater than 80° should be considered a definite indication of scapholunate dissociation or rotary subluxation of the scaphoid.

18. Other than lunotriquetral tears, what major diagnostic categories must be considered in working up ulnar-sided wrist pain?

Ulnar impaction syndrome, due to the relatively increased length of the ulna with increased load-bearing through the carpus onto the ulnar side of the wrist, may cause painful symptoms similar to lunotriquetral injury. **Triangular fibrocartilage complex** tears can mimic lunotriquetral injuries with similar symptoms of pain and crepitance. Localization of the source of pain via palpation and provocative testing helps to distinguish between possible sources of ulnar-sided pain.

19. How large is the normal angle between the long axis of the triquetrum and the axis of the lunate?

Although it can be difficult to visualize the triquetrum and lunate adequately because of overlap of adjacent carpal bones, the average difference in angulation is 14°. After a lunotriquetral ligament tear, the angle may be decreased significantly and in fact reverse orientation to as much as negative 16°. In chronic cases lunotriquetral joint space narrowing with associated subchondral sclerosis and cysts may be seen.

20. Describe the typical history and examination of a patient with a lunotriquetral ligament tear.

The history is variable, but many patients recall a specific dorsiflexion injury event. Patients may describe a painful palpable or audible click or clunk on the ulnar aspect of the wrist, particularly with ulnar deviation. Complaints also may include weakness and decreased range of motion. Physical findings may demonstrate synovitis or arthritis with periarticular inflammation and swelling. Palpation over the lunotriquetral joint may produce local tenderness. Provocative testing that loads the ulnar carpus may demonstrate increased or pathologic motion compared with the other side. Radiographic examination ranges from completely normal to VISI deformity. The degree of radiographic abnormality most likely depends on the extent of the associated injury to adjacent intercarpal ligaments.

21. Describe a shear or ballottement test of the lunotriquetral joint.

The shear test attempts to demonstrate increased lunotriquetral motion. The examiner places one thumb on the dorsum of the lunate to push volarly and the other thumb on the volar palm at the pisiform, pushing dorsally. Pain, with or without crepitance, is a positive test. Comparison should be made with the unaffected side.

22. How can lunotriquetral instabilities be graded?

Viegas has described three stages of increasing severity:

Stage I: partial or complete disruption of the lunotriquetral interosseous ligament (LTIL) with no clinical or radiographic evidence of dynamic or static VISI.

Stage II: complete disruption of the LTIL and palmar LT ligaments with clinical and/or radiographic evidence of dynamic VISI.

Stage III: compete disruption of the LTIL and palmar LT ligaments, including disruption of the scaphoid and lunate portion of the dorsal radiocarpal ligament, with clinical or radiographic evidence of static VISI.

BIBLIOGRAPHY

1. Dobyns JH, Swanson GE: A 19-year-old with multiple fractures. Minn Med 56:143–149, 1973.
2. Green DP: Carpal dislocations and instabilities. In Green DP (ed): Operative Hand Surgery, vol 2, 3rd ed. New York, Churchill Livingstone, 1993, pp 861–928.
3. Johnson RP: The acutely injured wrist and its residuals. Clin Orthop 149:33–44, 1980.
4. Lichtman DM, Schneider JR, Swafford AR, Mack GR: Ulnar midcarpal instability: Clinical and laboratory analysis. J Hand Surg 6:515–523, 1981.
5. Linscheid RL, Dobyns JH, Beabout JW, Bryan RS: Traumatic instability of the wrist: Diagnosis, classification, and pathomechanics. J Bone Joint Surg 54A:1612–1632, 1972.
6. Mayfield JK, Johnson RP, Kilcoyne RK: Carpal dislocations: Pathomechanics and progressive perilunar instability. J Hand Surgery 3:226–241, 1980.
7. Ruby L: Fractures and dislocations of the carpus. In Browner BD, et al (eds): Skeletal Trauma, vol 2. Philadelphia, W.B. Saunders, 1992, pp 1025–1062.
8. Taleisnik J: Wrist: Anatomy, function, and injury. AAOS Instruct Course Lect 27:61–87, 1978.
9. Watson HK, Ashmead D IV, Makhlouf MV: Examination of the scaphoid. J Hand Surg 13A: 657–660, 1988.
10. Watson HK, Weinzweig J, Zeppieri J: The natural progression of scaphoid instability. Hand Clin 13:39–50, 1997.
11. Watson-Jones R: Fractures and Joint Injuries. 3rd ed. Edinburgh, E & S Livingstone, 1943, pp 568–577.
12. Viegas S, Patterson R, Peterson P, et al: Ulnar-sided perilunate instability: An anatomic and biomechanic study. J Hand Surg 15A:268–278, 1990.

119. ULNAR WRIST PAIN

Arnold-Peter C. Weiss, M.D.

1. What five carpal bones make up the ulnar side of the wrist?

The ulnar carpus encompasses the lunate, triquetrum, pisiform, hamate, and capitate.

2. What structure on the ulnar side of the wrist is frequently injured yet not seen on radiographs?

The triangular fibrocartilage complex (TFCC), which is made up of the ulnar carpal ligaments, ulnar wrist capsule, and triangular fibrocartilage meniscus.

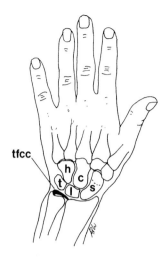

Main structures of the wrist. s = scaphoid, c = capitate, l = lunate, h = hamate, t = triquetrum, tfcc = triangular fibrocartilage complex.

3. What intercarpal ligament is frequently injured along with the TFCC?

The lunotriquetrial ligament is commonly injured along with the TFCC. These two structures are the most likely soft tissue elements of the ulnar wrist to cause pain.

4. Ulnar wrist pain in the hypothenar eminence in golfers is commonly caused by what type of fracture?

A fracture of the hook of the hamate. These fractures are frequently not seen on anteroposterior (AP) and lateral radiographs of the hand or a carpal tunnel view. They are commonly missed but can be documented by computed tomography (CT) of the wrist. Treatment involves cast immobilization, excision of the nonunion fragment if healing does not occur, or open reduction and internal fixation of the hook.

5. What structure on the ulnar side of the wrist is prone to age-related changes?

The TFCC is prone to degenerative tears that are directly proportional to age of the patient.

6. What is ulnar variance?

Ulnar variance refers to the length of the distal ulna compared with the lunate fossa of the distal radius. Patients are described as ulnar-plus, ulnar-neutral, or ulnar-minus. An ulnar-minus variance is associated with the development of Kienböck's disease (avascular necrosis of the lunate), which causes wrist pain. An ulnar-plus variance is associated with ulnar carpal abutment syndrome, in which the ulna is longer than the radius and pushes into the underside of the TFCC, causing degenerative changes and ulnar-sided wrist pain.

7. What diagnostic tests help in differentiating causes of ulnar-sided wrist pain?

Wrist arthrography and magnetic resonance imaging (MRI). Wrist arthrography involves injection of dye into the wrist to visualize the TFCC and intercarpal ligaments. Abnormal leaks of the dye between areas where the structures are supposed to be intact indicate disruption. MRI can also define tears of the TFCC and, to a lesser degree, the intercarpal ligaments.

8. What technique has the best sensitivity, specificity, and accuracy for defining ulnar-sided wrist pain due to soft tissue injuries?

Wrist arthroscopy is more sensitive, specific, and accurate than other diagnostic techniques for defining soft tissue disruption of both the intercarpal ligaments and TFCC.

9. During arthroscopy, loss of what finding may indicate tearing of the peripheral TFCC?

During arthroscopy a probe is used to ballot the TFCC cartilage disc. Normally the cartilage disc is taut and demonstrates a trampoline effect. If the cartilage disc does not rebound to forces provided by the probe, a tear of the peripheral TFCC should be suspected.

10. What is the vascular anatomy of the TFCC?

The TFCC has a rich vascular supply to the peripheral portion, whereas the central portion and attachment to the distal radius are relatively avascular. Tears located in the peripheral TFCC, therefore, have a high propensity to heal if treated by debridement and/or repair, whereas tears of the central component are unlikely to heal with repair alone.

11. What is the main form of treatment for central TFCC tears?

Because this portion of the TFCC is relatively avascular, the redundant portions (i.e., any flaps that may be present) of the meniscal disc itself are debrided. Debridement decompresses the tear itself and does not alter the structural anatomy of the ulnar wrist.

12. In patients who have undergone TFCC debridement but still have ulnar-sided wrist pain, what procedure may be used as an initial salvage procedure for relief of pain?

In patients who have TFCC pain and ulnar-positive variance, an ulnar shortening osteotomy that takes pressure off the underside of the TFCC may be useful after failed TFCC debridements. This procedure is also effective in some patients who have concomitant lunotriquetral ligament and TFCC tears.

13. What vascular anatomy is commonly associated with ulnar-sided wrist pain?

Hypothenar hammer syndrome. Patients who often use their hypothenar eminence as a hammer (e.g., jackhammer operators) may develop a clot in the ulnar artery. Thrombosis causes localized pain, and occasionally a mass is felt in the hyothenar region. The diagnosis can be made by performing an Allen's test, in which loss of refill of the ulnar digits may be noted.

14. What physical tests are used to examine for lunotriquetral ligament tears?

The lunotriquetral shear test (Kleinman or Reagan) and lunotriquetral compression test (Linscheid) are useful for evaluating the lunotriquetral ligament. During either test, pain or a click centered at the lunotriquetral joint may indicate disruption of this ligament.

15. What is the most common diagnostic and therapeutic procedure for lunotriquetral ligament tears?

Wrist arthroscopy (using the 4/5 or 6-R portals) is the best way to identify lunotriquetral ligament tears. Partial tears can often be treated by debridement alone; complete tears also occasionally may be made asymptomatic by debridement of the ligament edges. For patients who have persistent pain, lunotriquetral fusion and four-corner fusion (fusion of the capitate, hamate, lunate, and triquetrum) have been advocated.

16. Why do some authors advocate a four-corner fusion rather than a lunotriquetral fusion for documented lunotriquetral ligament tearing?

The fusion rate obtained with a four-corner fusion is substantially higher than that obtained with a lunotriquetral fusion. Approximately 50% of lunotriquetral fusions result in nonunion.

17. If pain is elicited by the lunotriquetral shear test, what other condition must be ruled out?

Pisotriquetral arthritis. Because the lunotriquetral shear test is performed by putting the thumb over the pisiform and pushing dorsally to provide shear between the lunate and triquetrum, pisotriquetral arthritis rather than any problem at the lunotriquetral ligament may cause pain by compression of this joint. For this reason, testing for pain isolated to the pisotriquetral joint by "shucking" the pisiform against the triquetrum alone should be done.

18. What are the two types of TFCC meniscal tears?

Traumatic and degenerative. Traumatic tears are usually linear and occur at the edges of the TFCC at either the soft tissue attachments or attachment to the distal radius. Degenerative tears generally occur in ulnar impaction syndrome (with an ulnar-plus variance), in older people, and in the midportion of the fibrocartilage meniscus.

BIBLIOGRAPHY

1. Boulas HJ, Milek MA: Ulnar shortening for tears of the triangular fibrocartilage complex. J Hand Surg 15A:415–420, 1990.
2. Buterbaugh GA: Triangular fibrocartilage complex injury and ulnar wrist pain. In American Society for Surgery of the Hand: Hand Surgery Update. Rosemont, IL, American Academy of Orthopaedic Surgeons, 1996, pp 105–115.
3. Osterman AL: Arthroscopic debridement of triangular fibrocartilage complex tears. Arthroscopy 6:1220–1224, 1990.
4. Paley D, McMurty RY, Cruickshank B: Pathologic conditions of the pisiform and pisotriquetral joint. J Hand Surg 12A:110–119, 1987.
5. Palmer AK, Glisson RR, Werner FW: Ulnar variance determination. J Hand Surg 7A:376–379, 1982.
6. Palmer AK, Werner FW: The triangular fibrocartilage complex of the wrist anatomy and function. J Hand Surg 6A:153–162, 1981.
7. Pin PG, Young VL, Gilula LA, Weeks PM: Management of chronic lunotriquetral ligament tears. J Hand Surg 14A:77–83, 1989.
8. Weiss APC, Akelman E, Lambiase R: Comparison of the findings of triple-injection cinearthrography of the wrist with those of arthroscopy. J Bone Joint Surg 78A:348–356, 1996.
9. Weiss APC, Akelman E: Diagnostic imaging and arthroscopy for chronic wrist pain. Orthop Clin North Am 26:759–767, 1995.

120. INTERCARPAL ARTHRODESIS

Jeffrey Weinzweig, M.D., and H. Kirk Watson, M.D.

1. What is an intercarpal arthrodesis?

Intercarpal arthrodesis, also referred to as limited wrist arthrodesis, is the selective fusion of adjacent carpal bones within the wrist. It is a proven method for treating specific carpal pathology that maximizes postoperative wrist motion, function, and strength while eliminating pain and instability.

2. Which wrist joints are responsible for flexion and extension?

Both the radiocarpal and midcarpal joints contribute to all phases of flexion and extension motion of the wrist. Two-thirds of flexion occurs at the radiocarpal joint, whereas one-third occurs at the midcarpal joint. Slightly more extension occurs at the radiocarpal joint than at the midcarpal joint.

3. What is the functional range of wrist motion?

The functional range of wrist motion is 5° flexion, 30° extension, 10° radial deviation, and 15° ulnar deviation. Almost all activities of daily living are completed within these ranges of motion, all of which are usually surpassed with limited wrist arthrodeses. Radioulnar deviation after radiocarpal fusions is the only exception.

4. Is wrist motion lost after intercarpal arthrodesis? If so, how does the loss compare with motion lost after a total wrist arthrodesis?

In the normal wrist adjacent carpal bones demonstrate motion limitations specific to a given intercarpal joint. Fusion of intercarpal joints results in some degree of motion loss; the extent depends on the joint(s) involved in the limited wrist arthrodesis. Fusions crossing the radiocarpal joint (e.g., radiolunate arthrodesis) result in the greatest loss of motion; fusions crossing the proximal and distal rows of the carpus or midcarpal joint (e.g., capitate-lunate-hamate-triquetral arthrodesis or scapholunate advanced collapse [SLAC] reconstruction; see question 18) result in an intermediate loss of motion; and fusions within a single carpal row (e.g., lunotriquetral arthrodesis) result in the least loss of motion (see question 26). When multiple carpal bones undergo fusion, a compensatory increase in motion occurs at the unfused joints, thereby maximizing total wrist motion. This adaptation of the carpus is not usually fully achieved until 9–12 months after intercarpal arthrodesis. Total wrist arthrodesis, however, results in complete loss of all wrist motion.

5. What are the indications for an intercarpal arthrodesis?

Intercarpal arthrodesis addresses a diverse group of wrist disorders, including degenerative disease, rotary subluxation of the scaphoid, midcarpal instability, scaphoid nonunion, Kienböck's disease, carpal osteonecrosis, and congenital synchondrosis or partial fusion of various intercarpal joints.

6. Why is it critical that unaffected intercarpal joints be left unfused? Are there any exceptions?

Unaffected intercarpal joints must be left unfused if motion is to be maintained postoperatively; hence the conceptual basis for selective limited wrist fusion. An exception to this principle is the inclusion of the hamate and triquetrum in SLAC wrist reconstruction to maximize the surface area for bone graft consolidation (see question 18).

7. Why must the normal external dimensions of the carpal bones included in a limited arthrodesis be preserved? Are there any exceptions?

Preservation is essential to maintain normal articulations with adjacent bones. Preservation of the external dimension of the triscaphe (scaphotrapeziotrapezoid [STT]) joint during arthrodesis is accomplished with a temporary spacer that is removed after pin placement. In lunotriquetral arthrodesis, the distal rim of cartilage on the adjacent surface of each bone is left intact. This cartilage is an important guide in maintaining reduction and alignment of the bones before fixation. SLAC wrist reconstruction (see question 18), with fusion of the capitate, lunate, hamate, and triquetrum, presents an exception to this principle. Whereas reduction of the lunate and correction of any dorsal intercalated segmental instability (DISI) is essential, maintenance of the original external dimensions of the four carpal bones is not. No other intercarpal joints remain to be affected. Some collapse of the capitate and hamate on the lunate and triquetrum is tolerated because all loads pass directly through the single fused unit and subsequently through the preserved radiolunate joint.

8. Why must pin fixation include only bones involved in the arthrodesis?

This technique permits any encountered stresses or loads to be dissipated by motion in the adjacent local joints. Inadvertent inclusion of adjoining bones during fixation inhibits the motion of adjacent joints, thus increasing the amount of load transferred through the healing arthrodesis and potentially disrupting the fusion site.

9. Why is the scaphoid susceptible to degenerative arthritic change?

The susceptibility of the scaphoid to degenerative arthritic change is attributable to its anatomy and position within the wrist. The articular surface of the distal radius is composed of two articular fossae, a radial fossa for the scaphoid, and an ulnar fossa for the lunate. The fossa for the scaphoid is ovoid or elliptical, whereas the fossa for the lunate is spherical. Part of the sphere is composed of the most radial portion of the triangular fibrocartilage. The proximal articular surface of the scaphoid resembles a simple teaspoon with its handle immediately dorsal and radial to the position of the relaxed thumb. Flexion and extension occur with full articular contact of the spoon (scaphoid) in the elliptical fossa of the radius. If the spoon handle is brought in front of the little finger and flexed so that the handle is perpendicular to the long axis of the forearm, the contact surface of the spoon in the elliptical fossa is disrupted. When this occurs, the proximal spoon surface (scaphoid) lies on the radial edges of the elliptical fossa, and fairly rapid destruction between the scaphoid and radius occurs in these regions.

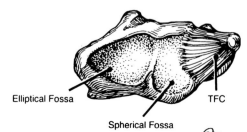

Distal radius and ulna anatomy. An end-on view of the distal radius and ulna demonstrates the elliptical scaphoid fossa and the spherical lunate fossa. The radial portion of the triangular fibrocartilage (TFC) contributes to the support mechanism for the lunate.

Elliptical Fossa

TFC

Spherical Fossa

10. What is a triscaphe arthrodesis?

Triscaphe arthrodesis is a fusion of the scaphoid, trapezium, and trapezoid bones and is often referred to as an STT fusion. A single bony unit is created with external dimensions identical to those of the three carpal bones before fusion. Preservation of the external bony dimensions is necessary to prevent carpal collapse and excessive loading of the capitate, which ultimately result in degenerative change and instability of the lunocapitate column followed by SLAC wrist (see question 15).

Indications for triscaphe arthrodesis include symptomatic rotary subluxation of the scaphoid (see question 11), degenerative disease of the triscaphe joint, nonunion of the scaphoid, Kienböck's disease, scapholunate (SL) dissociation, traumatic dislocations, midcarpal instability, and congenital synchondrosis of the triscaphe joint. Triscaphe arthrodesis provides a stable radial column for load transfer across the wrist to the radius and permits the unloading of carpal units no longer capable of bearing load, such as the lunate in Kienböck's disease. In addition, it provides stability and strength to a wrist affected by the pathomechanics of rotary subluxation of the scaphoid or midcarpal instability.

11. What is rotary subluxation of the scaphoid? How is it treated?

Rotary subluxation of the scaphoid (RSS) is a well-recognized entity in which the scapholunate articulation is disrupted and the wrist develops a pattern of instability with loading. It is classically described as a diastasis between the scaphoid and lunate with dorsal displacement and rotation of the proximal pole of the scaphoid. Disruption of the ligamentous support of the proximal pole permits it to rotate dorsally while the distal pole rotates volarly, producing an increased SL angle on lateral radiographic examination with the scaphoid lying more perpendicular to the long axis of the forearm. This deformity produces a scaphoid with abnormal motion that may subject the radioscaphoid joint to abnormal loading stresses, eventually resulting in destruction of the joint.

Patients with RSS present with various combinations of five consistent complaints: (1) activity pain, (2) postactivity pain, (3) activity modification, (4) carpal tunnel syndrome symptoms, and (5) wrist ganglions. All patients present with at least three of these historical findings; many present with all five. Radiographic findings on the neutral posteroanterior (PA) view may include foreshortening of the scaphoid, a positive ring sign, and an increased scapholunate gap. Radiographic findings on the neutral lateral view may include a scapholunate angle greater than 70° and a DISI deformity of the lunate. RSS is best treated with a triscaphe arthrodesis to stabilize the scaphoid and radial column of the carpus.

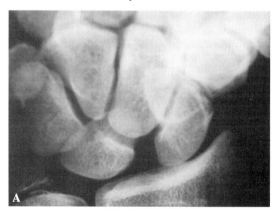
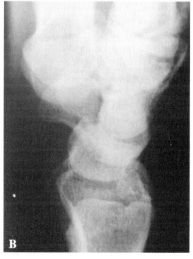

Rotary subluxation of the scaphoid. *A,* The neutral PA view shows foreshortening of the scaphoid, a positive ring sign, and an increased scapholunate gap. *B,* The neutral lateral view shows a scapholunate angle of 90° and a DISI deformity of the lunate.

12. How is a triscaphe arthrodesis performed?

The triscaphe joint is approached through a transverse dorsal wrist incision just distal to the radial styloid. The radial styloid is exposed, and the distal 5 mm of the styloid are resected. The triscaphe joint is approached through a transverse capsular incision between the extensor carpi radialis longus and brevis tendons. The articular surfaces and the subchondral hard cancellous bone of the scaphoid, trapezium, and trapezoid are removed with a rongeur. The cortex dorsal to the articular cartilage on the trapezium and trapezoid is also removed to broaden the surface area for grafting.

Two 0.045-inch Kirschner wires are then passed percutaneously and preset through the trapezoid up to the fusion site to be driven into the scaphoid. The scaphoid is reduced (see below), and a 5-mm spacer, usually the handle of a small hook, is placed into the scaphotrapezoid space to maintain the original external dimensions of the triscaphe joint. The preset pins are then driven from the trapezoid into the scaphoid, avoiding placement into the radioscaphoid joint or radius, and the spacer is removed.

Cancellous bone graft, harvested from the distal radius, is then densely packed into the spaces between the scaphoid, trapezium, and trapezoid. The pins are cut beneath the skin level, and the skin incisions are closed with a single-layer subcuticular monofilament suture. The wrist capsule and extensor retinaculum are simply realigned without suturing. The postoperative dressing consists of a bulky noncompressive wrap incorporating a long-arm plaster splint. The hand is placed in a protected position with the wrist in slight extension and radial deviation, the forearm neutral, and the elbow at 90°.

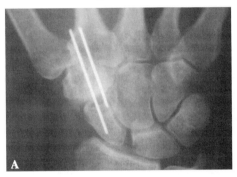 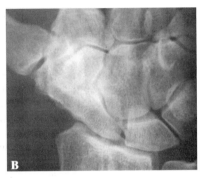

Triscaphe (STT) arthrodesis. *A*, Radiographic examination 6 weeks after triscaphe arthrodesis demonstrates typical pin placement and adequate bony consolidation. *B*, Three months after triscaphe fusion, the arthrodesis is radiographically solid.

13. What is the key to performing a successful triscaphe arthrodesis?

The most important step in triscaphe arthrodesis is reduction of the scaphoid. The normal scapholunate angle is approximately 47° to the long axis of the forearm. Scaphoid reduction is accomplished by placing the wrist in full radial deviation and 45° of dorsiflexion; the scaphoid tuberosity is reduced by the surgeon's thumb to prevent scaphoid overcorrection. Pinning is performed as described, after which the scaphoid should lie at approximately 55° to 60° of palmar flexion relative to the long axis of the radius when seen from the lateral view. This position ensures optimal radioscaphoid congruity and maximizes postoperative range of motion. It is not necessary to correct abnormal rotation of the lunate.

14. Are there any absolute contraindications to a triscaphe arthrodesis?

Triscaphe arthrodesis is contraindicated if significant degenerative change is found at the radioscaphoid joint.

15. What is SLAC wrist?

SLAC wrist is the most common pattern of degenerative disease of the wrist, accounting for 57% of all periscaphoid arthritis. The scaphoid is the weak link in the wrist in regard to degenerative disease, and the specialized radioscaphoid joint is particularly susceptible. Rotation, fracture nonunion, or necrosis of the scaphoid may produce a collapse pattern on the radial side of the wrist, ultimately leading to degenerative disease or SLAC destruction, which occurs first between the radial styloid and the scaphoid (stage IA). With progressive degenerative disease, complete destruction of the radioscaphoid joint occurs with collapse of the articular space (stage IB). Once this collapse has occurred, whether it is secondary to scaphoid instability or scaphoradial in nature, the capitate-lunate joint is unable to bear loads normally. The capitate drives off the radial or dorsal radial portion of the distal lunate articular surface, causing cartilage shear stress with eventual destruction of the capitate-lunate joint and resultant midcarpal SLAC (stage II).

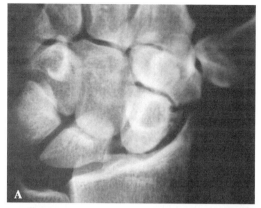

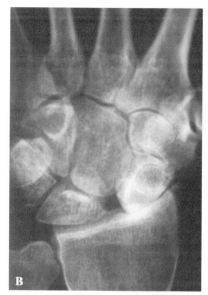

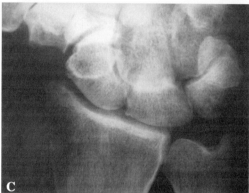

Stages of scapholunate advanced collapse (SLAC) wrist. *A,* SLAC changes are seen earliest at the radial aspect of the radioscaphoid joint beginning at the radial styloid (stage IA). *B,* Subsequently, the remainder of the radioscaphoid joint is involved (stage IB). *C,* Finally, destruction of the capitate-lunate joint occurs (stage II). Isolated involvement of the capitate-lunate joint also may be seen and is referred to as midcarpal SLAC.

16. Which conditions predispose to the development of SLAC wrist?

The most common cause of SLAC wrist is rotary subluxation of the scaphoid followed by scaphoid nonunion. Other conditions that produce SLAC degeneration include Preiser's disease, midcarpal instability, intraarticular fractures involving the radioscaphoid or capitate-lunate joints, and Kienböck's disease (tertiary to the secondary RSS).

17. Which joint in the wrist is virtually never involved in degenerative disease? Why not?

The key to reconstruction of the SLAC wrist lies in the radiolunate joint, which is highly resistant to degenerative change and is preserved at all stages of the SLAC sequence. The articulation of the lunate with the radius is spherical; thus, the lunate can be moved volarly or dorsally, radially or ulnarly, and the proximal articular surface of the lunate will still be perpendicularly loaded (see question 9). Even with significant displacement of the lunate into VISI or DISI, the radiolunate joint usually is preserved.

18. How is SLAC wrist reconstruction performed?

SLAC wrist reconstruction involves excision of the scaphoid and arthrodesis of the capitate, lunate, hamate, and triquetrum. This procedure, also referred to as a four-corner fusion, is performed with two parallel dorsal incisions: one over the radiocarpal joint and one proximally over the distal radial aspect of the radius for bone graft harvest (same incisions as for the triscaphe arthrodesis). After incising the extensor retinaculum along the third compartment, a transverse incision is made through the wrist capsule at the level of the capitate-lunate joint. The scaphoid is approached in the interval between the extensor carpi radialis longus and brevis and removed in piecemeal fashion with a rongeur.

Longitudinal traction on the fingers permits exposure of the radiolunate joint and confirmation that it is well-preserved. Next articular cartilage and subchondral bone are removed from the adjacent surfaces of the capitate, lunate, hamate, and triquetrum. Cancellous bone is then harvested from the distal radius. Three 0.045-inch Kirschner wires are passed percutaneously and preset through the capitate, hamate, and triquetrum up to the fusion site to be driven into the lunate. A fourth wire is preset into the triquetrum to be driven into the capitate. Part of the cancellous graft is then packed in the deep interval between the capitate and lunate. After correction of any DISI deformity of the lunate (see question 19), the preset pins are driven into the lunate from the capitate, hamate, and triquetrum and from the triquetrum into the capitate. Bone grafting, closure, and postoperative dressings are the same as for the triscaphe arthrodesis (see question 12).

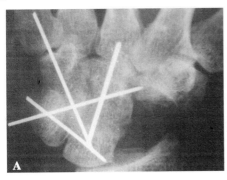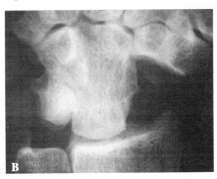

SLAC wrist reconstruction. *A,* Radiographic examination 6 weeks after SLAC reconstruction with limited wrist arthrodesis and scaphoid excision demonstrates typical pin placement and adequate bony consolidation. *B,* Six months after SLAC reconstruction, the arthrodesis is radiographically solid and the radiolunate joint well preserved. Note the ulnar displacement of the capitate on the lunate, which tightens the radioscaphocapitate ligament and prevents ulnar translation.

19. What is the key to performing a successful SLAC wrist reconstruction?

The most important step in SLAC wrist reconstruction is correction of the commonly associated DISI deformity of the lunate. The capitate must be volarly and ulnarly displaced on the lunate to prevent the DISI position and to align the hand over the radius-lunate joint. A buttress pin running dorsally into the lunate abutting the dorsal edge of the radius may be used to maintain the lunate in a slight VISI position. A joker (similar to a Freer) placed across the distal lunate surface and used as a lever will suffice for position control. It is important to bring the capitate ulnarly and to align it centered on the lunate. Inadequate reduction of the DISI deformity of the lunate at the time of arthrodesis not only leads to loss of carpal height but also limits the available arc of radiolunate motion.

20. Are there any absolute contraindications to SLAC wrist reconstruction?

Patients who present with SLAC wrist in conjunction with lunate or radiolunate pathology are *not* candidates for this type of reconstruction. Significant ulnar translation, which disrupts the concentric congruity of the radiolunate articulation and predictably leads to joint destruction, osteonecrosis of the lunate (as in Kienböck's disease), and preexisting radiolunate degenerative change, are absolute contraindications to SLAC wrist reconstruction. The salvage procedures under these conditions include proximal row carpectomy and wrist arthrodesis.

21. What are the most common patterns of degenerative disease of the wrist?

In its normal anatomic position, the scaphoid articulates with the radius at the radiocarpal joint and with the trapezium and trapezoid at the triscaphe joint. It is, therefore, not surprising that approximately 95% of all degenerative disease of the wrist is periscaphoid in origin. Review of more than 4000 radiographs of the wrist yielded 210 films demonstrating degenerative arthritic change. The SLAC pattern of degenerative change was seen in 57%, triscaphe joint arthritis in 27%, and a combination of both in 15%.

22. What is a congenital carpal synchondrosis? Which intercarpal joint is most commonly involved?

Cavitation of a common cartilaginous precursor during the fourth to eighth weeks of intrauterine life results in the formation of individual carpal bones. Incomplete cavitation results in congenital carpal synchondrosis or incomplete separation of the carpal bones, which becomes radiographically apparent as the carpus ossifies. This occurs most commonly at the lunotriquetral joint, where the joint has the pathognomonic appearance of a fluted champagne glass. The distal portion of the joint usually has normal cartilage development, whereas proximally normal joint development has been arrested, predisposing it to degenerative joint disease. The capitate-hamate joint is the next most commonly involved. Such anomalies occur rarely, are generally believed to be asymptomatic, and are usually discovered as incidental findings during radiographic evaluations for minor trauma.

23. Why might a congenitally fused intercarpal joint require subsequent arthrodesis?

Congenital synchondrosis of a joint can be recognized radiographically by the presence of bone where articular cartilage should be found. This unique radiographic finding is diagnostic of this interesting anomaly. In degenerative arthritis, on the other hand, the articular cartilage has developed and subsequently been worn away; as a result, the normal bony surfaces approach one another. The spectrum of synchondrosis ranges from partial to complete fusion, depending on the degree of formation of the articular cartilaginous elements. Degenerative disease may result from motion within a partially fused intercarpal joint that possesses inadequate cartilage to tolerate loading, necessitating a limited wrist arthrodesis.

24. What are the indications for limited wrist arthrodesis of the lunotriquetral joint?

Pathology arising from the lunotriquetral (LT) joint is a known cause of ulnar wrist pain. Indications for limited wrist arthrodesis of this articulation include LT joint instability, degenerative arthritis, and symptomatic congenital synchondrosis or incomplete separation of the lunate and triquetrum. Patients with LT pathology usually experience pain by palpation directly over the LT joint or by shear loading of the joint while performing an LT ballottement test.

25. How is an LT arthrodesis performed?

The LT joint is exposed through a transverse dorsal ulnar incision centered over the joint, and the adjacent articular surfaces are removed with a dental rongeur. The distal margins of cartilage are left intact to preserve the relationship of the two bones and to help maintain alignment during fixation. During removal of the articular surfaces, a biconcave space is created to centralize any loads and to aid in preventing displacement of grafted bone. Two 0.045-inch Kirschner wires are preset into the triquetrum in parallel fashion. The joint is reduced using the preserved margins as guides, maintaining the normal external dimensions of the bones, and the K-wires are driven into the lunate. The biconcave space is then densely packed with cancellous bone graft. A long-arm dressing incorporating a dorsal splint is applied.

26. Which intercarpal arthrodesis results in the greatest loss of wrist motion? Which results in the least loss of motion?

Of the intercarpal arthrodeses, the four-bone SLAC wrist reconstruction results in the greatest loss of wrist motion. This fusion crosses the midcarpal joint and involves four intercarpal joints (lunate-capitate, triquetrum-hamate, lunate-triquetrum, and capitate-hamate joints). The average range of motion after SLAC reconstruction is approximately 60% of the contralateral normal wrist. The average range of motion after triscaphe arthrodesis is approximately 80% of the contralateral normal wrist. Arthrodesis of the LT joint, typically regarded as the tightest joint in the wrist, results in the least loss of carpal motion.

27. What is the optimal bone graft donor site for intercarpal arthrodesis?

The distal radius provides an ample supply of cancellous bone in the same operative field and with minimal morbidity.

28. How is bone graft harvested from the distal radius? The identification of which structure is helpful during graft harvest?

A 3-cm transverse incision is made approximately 3 cm proximal to the radial styloid, extending from the site of Lister's tubercle dorsally to a point just volar to the first dorsal compartment. A flat periosteal surface is exposed between the first and second extensor compartments; this surface is identified by a constant periosteal artery that runs longitudinally in the region. The periosteum is incised longitudinally along this small, dispensable artery and elevated to permit removal of a teardrop-shaped cortical window approximately 2 cm long × 1.5 cm wide with a narrow, straight osteotome. Harvest of the cortical window begins distally on the radial tuberosity. Adequate cancellous bone graft is harvested with an 8-mm curette, and the cortical window is replaced. The cortical window is held securely in place simply by repositioning the overlying periosteum and extensor tendons.

29. Can scapholunate (SL) dissociation be treated with a SL limited wrist arthrodesis?

Absolutely not. SL limited wrist arthrodesis may seem an ideal approach to the management of SL dissociation, but there are several important reasons why this is not so. Perhaps the most obvious is the difficulty of achieving union by fusion of the relatively small articular surfaces of the two bones. Cancellous contact areas are inadequate; therefore, nonunion rates are predictably high. However, there are two other compelling reasons to avoid this procedure. The first reason is that any limited wrist arthrodesis requires sufficient bone to carry the load of the carpus. The banana-shaped SL combination provides inadequate bony volume to carry the loads that this fusion would be required to bear and would result in carpal symptoms. The second reason is based on the fact that the scaphoid and lunate reside in two different fossae on the same bone. A ridge is typically found between the fossae on the radius and is occasionally substantial. Fusing the scaphoid to the lunate would remove the small but necessary degree of motion between the bones and result in decreased range of motion compared with the SLAC reconstruction and degenerative change of the radiocarpal joint.

30. Both scaphoid-capitate arthrodesis and triscaphe arthrodesis are used to treat scaphoid instability. How do the procedures differ biomechanically?

Scaphoid-capitate arthrodesis and triscaphe arthrodesis are two distinct operations. The scaphoid-capitate fusion transmits load directly across the fusion site from the capitate to the scaphoid and then to the radius. With triscaphe arthrodesis, the loads are not transmitted primarily through the fusion site. In fact, most of the load passes from the capitate across normal cartilage to the scaphoid and again across normal cartilage to the radius. Arthrodesis of the triscaphe joint prevents the proximal pole of the scaphoid from displacing beneath the capitate under load, but the fusion does not carry the load. The normally small amount of motion between the capitate and scaphoid gradually increases and provides a significant difference in wrist motion between the two types of limited wrist arthrodesis.

31. What are the indications for a radiolunate arthrodesis in nonrheumatoid patients?

Destruction of the radiolunate joint and ulnar carpal translation are the only indications for radiolunate arthrodesis in nonrheumatoid patients. Destruction usually results from dye-punch fractures involving the spherical lunate fossa on the distal radius. This type of limited wrist arthrodesis also may be indicated for wrist stabilization in the management of ulnar translation. The procedure requires sufficient distal radius bone graft to elevate the lunate and thereby prevent loss of carpal height. Overcorrection of the position of the lunate on the radius by slightly excessive elevation is well-tolerated by the wrist and, in fact, preferred; undercorrection of the lunate position with loss of carpal height results in decreased wrist motion and wrist instability.

32. What is an absolute contraindication to radiolunate arthrodesis?

Destruction of the capitate-lunate joint is an absolute contraindication to this procedure because wrist motion depends on this midcarpal joint after radiolunate arthrodesis.

33. How is the wrist managed after intercarpal arthrodesis?

Our postoperative management is similar for most intercarpal arthrodeses, including triscaphe fusions and SLAC reconstructions. Maximal initial immobilization is mandatory for these small bone fusions. Three to five days after surgery, the bulky intraoperative dressing is removed, and a long-arm thumb spica cast is applied (a short-arm cast is used after LT arthrodesis). The proximal carpal row is easily immobilized by casting the forearm and arm, but it is difficult to maintain adequately the position of the distal carpal row. Therefore, the metaphalangeal joints of the index and middle fingers are flexed to 80–90° and included in the long-arm cast, whereas the interphalangeal joints are left free. The index and middle metacarpals are mortised into the carpals as the "fixed unit" of the hand. Thus, their immobilization tends to maintain the position of the distal carpal row. Because there is relatively free motion at the base of the ring and little metacarpals, they are not included in the cast. As with any thumb spica cast, the thumb is immobilized to the tip. We refer to this type of immobilization as a "Groucho Marx" cast because it is reminiscent of the comedian's classic pose holding a cigar.

Four weeks after limited wrist arthrodesis, the long-arm cast and intracuticular sutures are removed. A short-arm, thumb spica cast is applied for an additional 2–3 weeks. Only the thumb is included in the cast. Six weeks postoperatively, the short-arm cast is removed, and radiographs are obtained. If radiographic evidence of union is seen, the pins are removed and the wrist is mobilized.

34. What is the incidence of complications after intercarpal arthrodesis?
Triscaphe arthrodesis has been an extremely reliable procedure, and complications are relatively few (approximately 1000 procedures have been performed). Nonunion has been extremely uncommon with a rate of 1–3%, depending on the indication for limited wrist arthrodesis. Infection, hematoma, and transient neurapraxias have been rare in our experience. Degenerative change at the radioscaphoid joint, consistent with SLAC wrist, occurred in 1.5% of cases, necessitating subsequent SLAC reconstruction. However, radiolunate degenerative change was not observed in any case.

Complications after almost 300 SLAC wrist reconstructions include nonunion in 1% of cases, wound infection in 1%, and reflex sympathetic dystrophy in 1.5%. Dorsal impingement between the capitate and radius after SLAC reconstruction required revision arthroplasty in 13% of patients. Inadequate reduction of the DISI deformity of the lunate at the time of arthrodesis not only leads to loss of carpal height but also limits the available arc of radiolunate motion. During wrist extension the capitate approaches the dorsal lip of the radius, where impingement may occur with associated pain. Coaxial alignment of the lunate with the capitate is essential for optimal outcome.

Complications after performing 26 LT limited wrist arthrodeses using the cancellous biconcave technique include reflex sympathetic dystrophy in 1 patient and pin migration, necessitating early removal of the Kirschner wires, in 1 patient. There were no nonunions in this series.

BIBLIOGRAPHY

1. Ashmead D, Watson HK, Damon C, et al: Scapholunate advanced collapse wrist salvage. J Hand Surg 19A:741–750, 1994.
2. Ashmead D, Watson HK: SLAC wrist reconstruction. In Gelberman R (ed): The Wrist. New York, Raven Press, 1994, pp 319–330.
3. Ashmead D, Watson HK, Weinzweig J, Zeppieri J: One thousand intercarpal arthrodeses. J Hand Surg 21B:10, 1996.
4. Garcia-Elias M, Cooney WP, An KN, et al: Wrist kinematics after limited intercarpal arthrodesis. J Hand Surg 14A:791–799, 1989.
5. Kirschenbaum D, Schneider LH, Kirkpatrick WH, et al: Scaphoid excision and capitolunate arthrodesis for radioscaphoid arthritis. J Hand Surg 18A:780–785, 1993.
6. McGrath MH, Watson HK. Late results with local bone graft donor sites in hand surgery. J Hand Surg 6:234–237, 1981.
7. Palmer AK, Werner FW, Murphy D, Glisson R: Functional wrist motion: A biomechanical study. J Hand Surg 10A:39–46, 1985.
8. Trumble T, Bour C, Smith R, Edwards G: Intercarpal arthrodesis for static and dynamic volar intercalated segment instability. J Hand Surg 13A:396–402, 1988.
9. Viegas SF, Patterson RM, Peterson PD, et al: Evaluation of the biomechanical efficacy of limited intercarpal fusions for the treatment of scapholunate dissociation. J Hand Surg 15A:120–128, 1990.
10. Watson HK, Ballet FL: The SLAC wrist: Scapholunate advanced collapse pattern of degenerative arthritis. J Hand Surg 9A:358–365, 1984.
11. Watson HK, Fink JA, Monacelli DM: Use of triscaphe fusion in the treatment of Kienböck's disease. Hand Clin 9:493–499, 1993.
12. Watson HK, Goodman ML, Johnson TR: Limited wrist arthrodesis. Part II: Intercarpal and radiocarpal combinations. J Hand Surg 6:223–232, 1981.
13. Watson HK, Hempton RE: Limited wrist arthrodesis. Part I: The triscaphoid joint. J Hand Surg 5:320–327, 1980.
14. Watson HK, Ryu J, Akelman E: Limited triscaphoid intercarpal arthrodesis for rotary subluxation of the scaphoid. J Bone Joint Surg 68A:345–349, 1986.
15. Watson HK, Ryu J, DiBella A: An approach to Kienböck's disease: Triscaphe arthrodesis. J Hand Surg 10A:179–187, 1985.
16. Watson HK, Weinzweig J: Physical Examination of the Wrist. Hand Clin 13:17–34, 1997.
17. Watson HK, Weinzweig J: Intercarpal Arthrodesis. In Green DP (ed): Operative Hand Surgery, 4th ed. New York, Churchill Livingstone (in press).
18. Watson HK, Weinzweig J: Intercarpal arthrodesis. In Watson HK, Weinzweig J (eds): The Wrist. Philadelphia, Lippincott-Raven (in press).
19. Watson HK, Weinzweig J: Treatment of Kienböck's Disease with triscaphe arthrodesis. In Vastamaki M, Vilkki S, Goransson H, et al (eds): Proceedings of the Sixth Congress of the International Federation of Societies for Surgery of the Hand. Bologna, Monduzzi Editore, 1995, pp 347–349.
20. Watson HK, Weinzweig J, Zeppieri J: The natural progression of scaphoid instability. Hand Clin 13:39–50, 1997.
21. Weinzweig J, Watson HK: Wrist sprain to SLAC wrist: A spectrum of carpal instability. In Vastamaki M (ed): Current Trends in Hand Surgery. Amsterdam, Elsevier Science, 1995, pp 47–55.
22. Weinzweig J, Watson HK, Herbert TJ, Shaer J: Congenital synchondrosis of the scaphotrapezio-trapezoid joint. J Hand Surg 22A:74–77, 1997.

INDEX

Page numbers in **boldface type** indicate complete chapters.